Routledge Handbook of Sexuality, Health and Rights

The last two decades have witnessed an explosion of research on sexuality as the social sciences have worked to find new ways of understanding a rapidly changing world. Growing concern for issues such as population, women's and men's reproductive health, and the HIV and AIDS pandemic, has since provided new legitimacy for work on sexuality, health and rights.

A detailed and up-to-date reference work, the *Routledge Handbook of Sexuality, Health and Rights* provides an authoritative overview of the main issues in the field today. Leading academics and practitioners are brought together to reflect on past, present and future approaches to understanding and promoting sexual health and rights. Divided into eight parts, it covers:

* pioneering beginnings;
* language, discourse and sexual categories;
* the reproductive imperative and sexual health;
* how to have sex in an epidemic;
* the choreography of sex;
* the darker side of sex;
* the move from sexual health to sexual rights;
* struggles for erotic justice.

This handbook surveys the state of the discipline and offers an examination and discussion of emerging, controversial and cutting-edge areas. It is an essential reference for academics and researchers in the fields of sexuality studies, sexual health and human rights, and offers key reading for more advanced students.

Peter Aggleton is Professor in Education, Health and Social Care, and Head of the School of Education and Social Work, at the University of Sussex, UK. He is a Visiting Professor in the National Centre in HIV Social Research at the University of New South Wales, Australia, and in the Section for International Community Health at the University of Oslo, Norway. The editor of the journal *Culture, Health and Sexuality*, he has worked internationally on issues of sexuality, sexual health and rights.

Richard Parker is Professor of Sociomedical Sciences at Columbia University, USA. The editor of the journal *Global Public Health*, and the co-convenor of Sexuality Policy Watch (SPW) (www.sxpolitics.org), he has worked extensively on issues of sexuality, health and rights for many years.

Routledge Handbook of Sexuality, Health and Rights

Edited by Peter Aggleton and Richard Parker

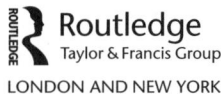

Routledge
Taylor & Francis Group

LONDON AND NEW YORK

First published 2010
by Routledge
2 Park Square, Milton Park, Abingdon, Oxon OX14 4RN

Simultaneously published in the USA and Canada
by Routledge
270 Madison Ave, New York, NY 10016

Routledge is an imprint of the Taylor & Francis Group, an informa business

Typeset in Baskerville by Wearset, Boldon, Tyne and Wear
Printed and bound in Great Britain by CPI Antony Rowe, Chippenham,
Wiltshire

British Library Cataloguing in Publication Data
A catalogue record for this book is available from the British Library

Library of Congress Cataloging in Publication Data
Routledge handbook of sexuality, health and rights / edited by Peter Aggleton
and Richard Parker.
p. ; cm.
Includes bibliographical references.
1. Sex–Handbooks, manuals, etc. 2. Hygiene, Sexual–Handbooks, manuals, etc.
3. Human rights–Handbooks, manuals, etc. 4. Reproductive rights–Handbooks,
manuals, etc. I. Aggleton, Peter. II. Parker, Richard. III. Title: Handbook of
sexuality, health and rights.
[DNLM: 1. Sexual Behavior. 2. Human Rights. HQ 21 R869 2010]
HQ21.R875 2010
306.709–dc22

2009030103

ISBN10: 0-415-46864-7 (hbk)
ISBN10: 0-203-86022-5 (ebk)

ISBN13: 978-0-415-46864-0 (hbk)
ISBN13: 978-0-203-86022-9 (ebk)

For Preecha and Vavá

Contents

Contributors

Peter Aggleton is Professor in Education, Health and Social Care, and Head of the School of Education and Social Work at the University of Sussex, and holds Visiting Professorships at the University of Oslo and the University of New South Wales. He has worked in the fields of sexuality, health and rights for over 20 years and is the editor (with Richard Parker) of *Culture, Society and Sexuality – A Reader* (2006, Routledge) and editor (with Sonia Corrêa, Gary W. Dowsett, Shirley Lindenbaum and Richard Parker) of the Sexuality, Culture and Health (Routledge) series. He is the editor of the journal *Culture, Health and Sexuality*.

Jafari Sinclaire Allen is Assistant Professor in the Departments of Anthropology and African American Studies at Yale University, where he teaches courses on the cultural politics of race, sexuality and gender in black diasporas, black feminist and queer theory, and Cuba and the Caribbean. His current research traces the cultural and political circuits of transnational black queer artistry, activism and intellectual life.

Dennis Altman is Professor of Politics and director of the Institute for Human Security, at La Trobe University in Melbourne. He is the author of 12 books, including *Homosexual: Oppression & Liberation* (1971, Outerbridge & Dienstfrey), *AIDS and the New Puritanism* (1986, Pluto Press) and *Global Sex* (2002, University of Chicago Press). He has been President of the AIDS Society of Asia and the Pacific, and is currently on the Governing Council of the International AIDS Society. In 2007, he was made a member of the Order of Australia.

Ana Amuchástegui is Professor at the Universidad Autónoma Metropolitana-Xochimilco in Mexico City. She has done extensive research on sexuality, subjectivity and rights in Mexico, and has published in journals such as *Sexualities, Reproductive Health Matters* and *Culture, Health and Sexuality*. She has recently edited (with Ivonne Szasz) *'Sucede que me canso de ser hombre' ... Relatos y experiencias de hombres y masculinidades en México* (2007, El Colegio de México), and is conducting research on the subjective processes different groups experience when advancing rights related to sexuality.

José Ricardo Ayres is Professor in Primary Health and Preventive Medicine at the University of São Paulo, Brazil. His interests lie within the field of young people's health, reproductive health and rights and HIV/AIDS.

Iván C. Balán is a clinical psychologist and researcher at the HIV Center for Clinical and Behavioral Studies at the New York State Psychiatric Institute/Columbia

University in New York. His current research interests include understanding the relationship between mental health and HIV risk behaviour, particularly among minority men who have sex with men.

Carmen Barroso became the Regional Director of IPPF/WHR in March 2003. A widely acknowledged leader in the field of sexual and reproductive health, she served for 12 years as Director of Population and Reproductive Health of the John D. and Catherine T. MacArthur Foundation. She was a founding member of DAWN, a network of Third World women, and of the Funder's Network on Population, Reproductive Health and Rights.

José Bauermeister is Assistant Research Professor in the Department of Health Behavior and Health Education at the University of Michigan School of Public Health. His research focuses on interpersonal prevention and health promotion strategies for high-risk adolescents and young adults, particularly young men who have sex with men.

Evelyn Blackwood is Associate Professor in the Department of Anthropology at Purdue University. She is the co-editor of two award-winning anthologies on women's same-sex sexualities and female masculinities, *Female Desires: Same-sex Relations and Transgender Practices across Cultures* (1999, Columbia University Press) and *Women's Sexualities and Masculinities in a Globalizing Asia* (1997, Palgrave Macmillan). She was awarded the 2008 Martin Duberman Fellowship by the Center for Lesbian and Gay Studies, City University of New York.

Cristiane S. Cabral is a doctoral student in public health at Social Medicine Institute, Rio de Janeiro State University (IMS/UERJ) and a Researcher of Latin American Center on Sexuality and Human Rights (CLAM/IMS/UERJ), in Brazil. She is interested in the studies of youth sexuality, gender relations and reproductive health and contraception.

Carlos F. Cáceres is Professor in the School of Public Health at Cayetano Heredia University, Lima, and Director of the Unit on Health, Sexuality and Human Development at that same university. He has worked in the fields of sexuality, HIV/AIDS and sexual health for the past two decades. He is an associate editor of the journal *Sexualidad, Salud y Sociedad* and chairs the Board of the International Association for the Study of Sexuality, Culture and Society.

Alex Carballo-Diéguez is Professor of Clinical Psychology in the Department of Psychiatry at Columbia University and Associate Director and Senior Research Scientist at the HIV Center for Clinical and Behavioral Studies at New York State Psychiatric Institute. His research focuses on the determinants of sexual risk behaviour among men who have sex with men and the application of information technology tools to social and behavioural research.

Héctor Carrillo is Associate Professor of Sociology and Gender Studies at Northwestern University. He is the author of the award-winning book *The Night Is Young: Sexuality in Mexico in the Time of AIDS* (2002, University of Chicago Press). He currently conducts research on sexuality and HIV with Mexican immigrant populations in the USA. He was principal investigator of the Trayectos Study, a large ethnographic study of Mexican gay and bisexual immigrant men in California.

Radhika Chandiramani, a clinical psychologist working on issues of sexuality and rights, is the Executive Director of TARSHI and the South and Southeast Asia Resource Centre on Sexuality. She is a recipient of the MacArthur Fellowship for Leadership Development and the Soros Reproductive Health and Rights Fellowship. She has co-edited *Sexuality, Gender and Rights: Exploring Theory and Practice in South and Southeast Asia* (2005, Sage).

Ellen Chesler is Distinguished Lecturer and Director of the Eleanor Roosevelt Initiative at the Roosevelt House Public Policy Institute at Hunter College of the City University of New York. She is a biographer of Margaret Sanger and author of numerous articles and reviews in the fields of reproductive health and women's rights. She spent most of her career in government and in philanthropy, most recently with the Open Society Institute.

Eli Coleman is the Director of the Program in Human Sexuality at the University of Minnesota in Minneapolis, Minnesota. He is the author of articles and books on compulsive sexual behaviour, sexual offenders, sexual orientation, gender dysphoria, chemical dependency and family intimacy. He is the editor of the *International Journal of Sexual Health* and past president of the World Association for Sexual Health.

Sonia Corrêa is co-chair of Sexuality Policy Watch (SPW) and is based at the Brazilian Interdisciplinary AIDS Association (ABIA) in Rio de Janeiro. She is the author of *Population and Reproductive Rights: Feminist Voices from the South* (1994, Zed) and co-author (with Richard Parker and Rosalind Petchesky) of *Sexuality, Health and Human Rights* (2008, Routledge).

Sarah H. Costa is Director of Special Projects and New York Representative at the Global Fund for Women. Before that, she has worked for the Ford Foundation, managing programmes on sexuality and reproductive health, HIV/AIDS and women's rights. With an academic background in demography and social medicine, she has published numerous papers and articles on women's health and reproductive rights.

Jane Cottingham was until recently Team Coordinator for Gender, Reproductive Rights, Sexual Health and Adolescence in the Department of Reproductive Health and Research at the World Health Organisation in Geneva. She co-founded ISIS, the Women's International Information and Communication Service, and served as the organisation's director for 13 years. She is a member of the Editorial Advisory Board of the journal *Reproductive Health Matters*.

Rafael M. Díaz is by training a social worker and a developmental psychologist. He is director of César Chávez Institute in San Francisco, which conducts research pertaining to the impact of social oppression on the health, education and well-being of disenfranchised communities in the USA. Prior to his present post, he conducted research on Latino gay men and HIV at the Center for AIDS Prevention Studies at the University of California, San Francisco.

Curtis Dolezal is a research scientist at the HIV Center for Clinical and Behavioral Studies at New York State Psychiatric Institute and Columbia University. He has researched sensation seeking, drug and alcohol use, couple relationship quality, childhood sexual experiences, psychoendocrinology and sexual risk behaviour as well as methodological issues such as self-reported honesty in sex interviews, and the use of web-based instruments to assess sexual behaviour.

Gary W. Dowsett is Professor and Deputy Director at the Australian Research Centre in Sex, Health and Society at La Trobe University, Melbourne. A sociologist by background, he has long been interested in sexuality research, particularly in relation to the rise of modern gay communities and the HIV epidemic. In 2003, he was elected to the International Academy of Sex Research, and in 2008, he was admitted as a Fellow of the Academy of the Social Sciences in Australia.

R. Danielle Egan is Associate Professor of Gender and Sexuality Studies at St. Lawrence University in New York. Her current research on childhood sexuality is featured in her book (with Gail Hawkes) entitled *Theorizing the Sexual Child* (2010, Palgrave Macmillan) and in several articles. Her ethnography on exotic dance is entitled *Dancing for Dollars and Paying for Love* (2006, Palgrave Macmillan).

Katherine Frank is a faculty associate at College of the Atlantic in Bar Harbor and a scholar-in-residence in the Department of Sociology at American University. Her current research explores understandings of and approaches to monogamy. Past publications have examined strip clubs and the sex industry, the motivations and experiences of male customers of strip clubs, swinging and polyamory, third wave feminism, popular culture, cosmetic surgery and research methods.

Claudia Garcia-Moreno is Senior Adviser on gender, violence and HIV/AIDS with the World Health Organization. She is coordinator of the WHO Multi-country Study on Women's Health and Domestic Violence and has been active for the past 20 years in women's health, sexual and reproductive health. She has published on all these topics and, more specifically, on violence against women.

Sasha Gear is a researcher at the Centre for the Study of Violence and Reconciliation in South Africa. She coordinates the Sexual Violence in Prison Project, conducting research to gain understanding on the nature and circumstances of sexual violence and coercion happening in men's prisons. She has published on violence in prisons and the gendered dimensions of male rape. Her primary interest is in masculinities and how different understandings of manhood feed into and shape experiences of violence.

Gloria González-López is Associate Professor of Sociology at the University of Texas at Austin. She is author of *Erotic Journeys: Mexican Immigrants and Their Sex Lives* (2005, University of California Press). Her research interests include sociology of gender, sexuality and diversity; migration studies; sexual violence; masculinities; religion; and sociology of family life. She is currently conducting sociological research on incest in four of the largest urban areas in Mexico.

Sofia Gruskin is Associate Professor of Health and Human Rights and Director of the Program on International Health and Human Rights at the Harvard School of Public Health, where her work emphasises the conceptual, methodological, policy and practice implications of linking health to human rights, with particular attention to HIV/AIDS, women, children, gender issues and vulnerable populations.

Abigail Harrison is Assistant Research Professor at Brown University's Population Studies and Training Center, and the Warren Alpert School of Medicine. She is a social scientist whose work focuses on the interdisciplinary application of medical anthropology, demography and epidemiology in public health. Her current research addresses the social determinants of HIV infection in young people in South Africa.

Gail L. Hawkes is Senior Lecturer in Sociology at the University of New England in Armidale, Australia. She is the author of the books *A Sociology of Sex and Sexuality* (1996, Open University Press) and *Sex and Pleasure in Western Culture* (2004, Polity). Her research since 2005 on the history of ideas about the sexual child has been undertaken with Danielle Egan.

Maria Luiza Heilborn is a social anthropologist and Assistant Professor in the Instituto de Medicina Social at the Universidade do Estado do Rio de Janeiro in Brazil and joint coordinator of Centro Latino-Americano em Sexualidade e Direitos Humanos. She is active in the International Association for the Study of Sexuality, Culture and Society and the author and editor of many articles and books within the field of sexuality.

Julia R. Heiman is the Director of the Kinsey Institute for Research in Sex, Gender, and Reproduction and a professor of psychology and clinical psychiatry at Indiana University. Her career has focused on understanding patterns of sexuality from an integrated psychosocial-biomedical perspective. She has served as President of the International Academy of Sex Research, President of the American Board of Family Psychology, and Editor-in-Chief of the *Annual Review of Sex Research*.

Gilbert Herdt is a cultural Anthropologist, founding Professor of Sexuality Studies and Anthropology, and the Director of the National Sexuality Resource Center (NSRC). Previously he has taught at Stanford University and the University of Chicago. His books on the Sambia of Papua New Guinea, gay and lesbian youth, sexual development and sexual culture are well known. His latest work is *Sex Panics/Moral Panics* (2009, New York University Press).

Jenny A. Higgins is a feminist researcher and sexual health advocate and Assistant Professor of Population and Family Health at Columbia University in New York. She has written about pleasure, sexuality, unintended pregnancy and HIV/AIDS.

Jennifer S. Hirsch is Associate Professor of Sociomedical Sciences at Columbia University. Her research focuses on gender, sexuality and reproductive health, USA to Mexico migration and migrant health, the applications of anthropological theory and methods to public health research and programmes, and faith-based approaches to public health. Her major publications include *A Courtship After Marriage: Sexuality and Love in Mexican Transnational Families* (2003, University of California Press) and a co-authored volume, *The Secret: Love, Marriage and HIV* (2009, Vanderbilt University Press).

Peter A. Jackson is Senior Fellow in Thai History in the Australian National University's College of Asia and the Pacific. He is Editor-in-Chief of *The Asian Studies Review* and a general editor of Hong Kong University Press' 'Queer Asia' monograph series. He has published extensively on same-sex and transgender cultures in Thailand and is currently editing a forthcoming collection of essays entitled *Queer Bangkok: 21st Century Markets, Media and Rights.*

Susan Kippax is Professorial Research Fellow at the National Centre in HIV Social Research in the Faculty of Arts & Social Sciences at the University of New South Wales, and a Fellow of the Academy of the Social Sciences of Australia. Her contribution to HIV/AIDS social research is internationally regarded and she has published extensively. She is a member of the Global HIV Prevention Working Group and the UNAIDS Prevention Reference Group.

Robert Lorway is a medical anthropologist and Assistant Professor in the Department of Community Health Sciences at the University of Manitoba. He has published essays on the lives of 'queer' Namibians in journals such as *Culture, Health and Sexuality, American Ethnologist* and *Medical Anthropology.* Currently, he completing a new book on Namibian sexualities. He is also engaged in action research among male sex workers in Karnataka, South India.

Paula Sandrine Machado is Assistant Professor in the Graduate Program in Public Health at the Universidade do Vale do Rio dos Sinos, Brazil, and an associate researcher in the Núcleo de Pesquisa em Antropologia do Corpo e da Saúde at the Universidade Federal do Rio Grande do Sul, Brazil. Her work centres on intersexuality, medical decision making and the anthropology of the body and health. Together with Mauro Cabral, she coordinates the Latin American Consortium on Intersex Issues.

Pardis Mahdavi is Assistant Professor of Anthropology at Pomona College in Los Angeles, California. A medical anthropologist, she works on sexuality, sexual politics and sexual and reproductive rights and health in the Middle East.

Lenore Manderson is Research Professor in the School of Psychology, Psychiatry and Psychological Medicine, Faculty of Medicine, Nursing and Health Sciences, and School of Political and Social Inquiry, Faculty of Arts, at Monash University, Melbourne, Australia. The author and editor of over 35 books and guest edited issues of journals, she is a founding member of the International Association for the Study of Sexuality, Culture and Society, and was its President between 2001 and 2003.

Diane di Mauro is a faculty member of the New York State Psychiatric Institute and the Sociomedical Sciences Department of the Mailman School of Public Health at Columbia University. She is the Program Director of the MAC AIDS Fund Leadership Initiative run jointly by Columbia University, UCLA, and the Human Sciences Research Council of South Africa. She has worked for over 20 years in the field of reproductive rights and human sexuality.

Andrea J. Melnikas is Program Coordinator for the Poverty, Gender and Youth Program at the Population Council, New York. Her research interests include young people's sexual health and youth empowerment programmes.

Miguel Muñoz-Laboy is Associate Professor and Director of the Doctor in Public Health programme in the Department of Sociomedical Sciences at the Mailman School of Public Health at Columbia University. He has conducted ethnographically informed research with youth and young adults on issues related to masculinity, bisexuality, HIV and sexually transmitted infections, unintended pregnancy and alcohol, tobacco and other drugs.

Cheikh Ibrahima Niang is a researcher and Lecturer at Cheikh Anta Diop University in Dakar, Senegal. He has conducted several studies of male same-sex relations in Senegal, The Gambia and Burkina Faso. He has served as the Director of the Gender Institute of the Council for the Development of the Research on Social Sciences in Africa (CODESRIA) and serves as the West Africa Regional Coordinator of the SAHARA (Social Aspects of HIV/AIDS Research Alliance) Network.

Mark B. Padilla is Assistant Professor in the Department of Health Behavior and Health Education and an adjunct assistant professor in the Department of Anthropology at the University of Michigan. He is a medical anthropologist with training in public health, and has worked for 10 years on HIV/AIDS in Latin America and the Caribbean. His books include *Caribbean Pleasure Industry: Tourism, Sexuality and AIDS in the Dominican Republic* (2007, University of Chicago Press).

Vera Paiva is Professor in the Department of Social Psychology at the University of São Paulo, Brazil and co-coordinator of the Interdisciplinary AIDS Prevention Studies Unit (NEPAIDS-USP). She has published extensively on sexuality, HIV prevention and care technologies within a human rights and vulnerability framework.

Richard Parker is Professor of Sociomedical Sciences at Columbia University in New York City and Director and President of the Brazilian Interdisciplinary AIDS Association (ABIA) in Rio de Janeiro, as well as the co-chair of Sexuality Policy Watch (SPW). His most recent books include *Sexuality, Health and Human Rights* (2008, Routledge, co-authored with Sonia Corrêa and Rosalind Petchesky) and *Bodies, Pleasures and Passions: Sexual Culture in Contemporary Brazil* (2nd edn, 2009, Vanderbilt University Press). He is Editor-in-Chief of the journal *Global Public Health*.

Rodrigo Parrini is a researcher with the Programa Universitario de Estudios de Género of the Universidad Nacional Autónoma de México. His research interests include sexuality and masculinity. His publications include the book *Panópticos y Laberintos: subjetivación, deseo y corporalidad en una cárcel de hombres* (2007, El Colegio de México). He is currently a researcher with the Centro Nacional de Control y Prevención del VIH/SIDA in México.

Mario Pecheny is Professor of Political Science at the University of Buenos Aires. He completed doctoral studies in political science at the University of Paris III and works on human rights, health and sexuality issues in Argentina and other Latin American countries. He has published and edited several books, including *Todo sexo es político* (2008, Del Zorzal).

Rosalind Petchesky is Distinguished Professor of Political Science at Hunter College and the Graduate Center at the City University of New York. She is also a member of the Steering Committee of Sexuality Policy Watch (SPW). Her recent books include *Global Prescriptions: Gendering Health and Human Rights* (2003, Zed) and *Sexuality, Health and Human Rights* (2008, Routledge, co-authored with Sonia Corrêa and Richard Parker).

Ken Plummer is Emeritus Professor of Sociology at the University of Essex, editor of the journal *Sexualities* and co-editor with John Macionis of *Sociology: A Global Introduction* (4th edn, 2008, Pearson Prentice-Hall). He has written many books and over 100 articles on sexualities, critical humanism and symbolic interactionism. His most recent book is *Intimate Citizenship: Private Decisions and Public Dialogues* (2003, University of Washington).

Kane Race is Senior Lecturer in the Department of Gender and Cultural Studies at the University of Sydney. His research has focused primarily on the impact of antiretroviral therapy on gay cultures and HIV discourse. His book, *Pleasure Consuming Medicine: The Queer Politics of Drugs* (2009, Duke University Press) investigates the political signification of drug regimes in neoliberal contexts, and corresponding practices of 'counterpublic health'.

Gayatri Reddy is Associate Professor in the Gender and Women's Studies Program and Department of Anthropology at the University of Illinois at Chicago. Her research focuses on the intersections of sexuality, gender, health and the politics of subject and community formation in India, and more recently, within the diasporic South Asian queer community in the USA. She is the author of *With Respect to Sex: Negotiating Hijra Identity in South India* (2005, University of Chicago Press).

Vasu Reddy is Acting Research Director in the Human Sciences Research Council (South Africa). He is also an honorary associate professor and research fellow in gender studies at the University of KwaZulu-Natal. He is the co-founder of the Durban Lesbian and Gay Community Centre and Chairperson of the Board of OUT LGBT Well-being (South Africa) and the editor of *From Social Silence to Social Science: Same-Sex Sexuality, HIV/AIDS and Gender in South Africa* (2009, HSRC Press).

Robert H. Remien is Professor of Clinical Psychology in the Department of Psychiatry at Columbia University and director of the Global Community Core and senior research scientist at the HIV Center for Clinical and Behavioral Studies at the New York State Psychiatric Institute. His research interests include sexual risk behaviour and adherence interventions for HIV-infected adult men and women and the development of behavioural interventions for people with acute HIV infection.

Matthew S. Rowe is a doctoral student in sociology at the University of California at Berkeley. His previous work has addressed sexuality, culture and the institutional and cultural responses to HIV and AIDS.

John S. Santelli is the Harriet and Robert H. Heilbrunn Professor and Chair of the Heilbrunn Department of Population and Family Health at Columbia University's Mailman School of Public Health. His research focuses on improving research in family planning and reproductive health in the USA and globally, with a focus on young people's sexual health. He is co-editor of *Adolescent Health: Understanding and Preventing Risk Behaviors* (2009, Jossey-Bass).

Rebecca Schleifer is with Human Rights Watch's Health and Human Rights Division. She has conducted research on a variety of human rights issues, including government restrictions on access to HIV/AIDS information for young people and injection drug users, access to HIV prevention and other post-rape services by survivors of sexual violence and other abuses against people living with and at high risk for HIV/AIDS in Bangladesh, Jamaica, South Africa, Thailand, Ukraine and the USA.

Fernando Seffner is Associate Professor of Education at the Federal University of Rio Grande do Sul in Porto Alegre, Brazil. He is trained in history as well as education, and his research focuses on the study of pedagogical methods, the construction of masculinity, homosexuality and bisexuality and social vulnerability in relation to HIV.

Sylvia Tamale is a feminist activist and academic based in Kampala, Uganda. She is Associate Professor and immediate outgoing Dean of Law at Makerere University. She founded and serves as coordinator of the Gender, Law & Sexuality Research Project within the Law Faculty, and has won several awards for defending the human rights of marginalised social groups.

Veriano Terto Junior is Executive Director of the Brazilian Interdisciplinary AIDS Association. He is trained in psychology, anthropology and public health, and his work has focused on the social construction of homosexuality, the social dimensions of HIV and AIDS and HIV treatment access.

Deborah L. Tolman is Professor of Social Welfare at Hunter College School of Social Work and The Graduate Center, City University of New York. She was previously director of the Center for Research on Gender and Sexuality at San Francisco State University. She is a developmental psychologist whose research has focused on young people's sexuality, gender development and gender equity. She has published widely on these topics and is a frequent speaker at professional associations and schools.

Ana Ventuneac is a social psychologist and a research project manager at the HIV Center for Clinical and Behavioral Studies at the New York State Psychiatric Institute and Columbia University. Her research focuses on sexual risk behaviour and HIV prevention among gay and bisexual men.

Jeffrey Weeks is Professor Emeritus of Sociology at London South Bank University, and a Visiting Professor at Cardiff University and at the Institute of Education, University of London. He has been a pioneer in developing historical approaches to the understanding of sexuality and intimate life, and has published over 100 articles and over 20 books, chiefly on these topics. Recent books include *Same Sex Intimacies* (2001, Routledge), *Sexualities and Society: A Reader* (2003, Polity) and *The World We Have Won* (2007, Routledge).

Bianca D. M. Wilson is a community psychologist and Assistant Professor of Psychology at California State University, Long Beach. Prior to this, she was a postdoctoral fellow at the University of California, San Francisco Institute for Health Policy Studies and the Lesbian Health and Research Center. Her research focuses on the relationships between culture, oppression and sexual health among African American same-gender loving people.

Acknowledgements and permissions

We would particularly like to thank Rakhi Kabawala at the Thomas Coram Research Unit, Institute of Education, University of London, who liaised with contributors and prepared the manuscript for publication.

Special thanks as well to the authors and publishers who gave permission to reprint material included in this volume:

Simon & Schuster, Inc., for permission to reprint parts of *Woman of Valor: Margaret Sanger and the Birth Control Movement in America* (1992) by Chesler, E. Copyright © 1992 by Ellen Chelser. Afterword Copyright © 2007 Ellen Chesler.

Duke University Press, for permission to reprint parts of 'Transnational Discourses and Circuits of Queer Knowledge in Indonesia' (2008) by Blackwood. E., *GLQ: Journal of Lesbian and Gay Studies*, 14, 481–507.

Taylor & Francis, for permission to reprint, in abbreviated form, 'Hidden Love: Sexual Ideologies and Relationship Ideals in the Context of HIV/AIDS in South Africa' (2008) by Harrison, A., *Culture, Health and Sexuality*, 10, 2, 175–89.

Taylor & Francis, for permission to reprint parts of 'Geographies of Contagion: Hijras, Kothis, and the Politics of Sexual Marginality in India' (2005) by Reddy, G., *Anthropology and Medicine*, 12, 3, 255–70.

Taylor & Francis, for permission to reprint parts of 'Intersexuality and Sexual Rights in Southern Brazil' (2009) by Machado, P., *Culture, Health and Sexuality*, 11, 3, 237–50.

ABC-CLIO, for permission to reprint material from *Sexual Health*, Volume 1: Psychological Foundations (2007) by Tepper, M. & Owens, A. F. (eds) (pp. 7–35: 'Sexual Health: Definitions and Construct Development'. Copyright © Eli Coleman). Westport, CT: Praeger Publishers.

Taylor & Francis, for permission to reprint, in abbreviated form, 'Is "Bareback" a Useful Construct in Primary HIV-prevention? Definitions, Identity and Research' (2009) by Carballo-Diéguez, A., Ventuneac, A., Bauermeister, J., Dowsett, G. W., Dolezal, C., Remien, R. H., Balán, I. and Rowe, M., *Culture, Health and Sexuality*, 11, 1, 51–65.

Taylor & Francis, for permission to reprint parts of 'The Hip-hop Club Scene: Gender, Grinding and Sex' (2007) by Muñoz-Laboy, M., Weinstein, H. and Parker, R., *Culture, Health and Sexuality*, 9, 6, 615–28.

Taylor & Francis, for permission to reprint, in abbreviated form, 'Passionate Uprisings: Young People, Sexuality and Politics in Post-revolutionary Iran' (2007) by Mahdavi, P., *Culture, Health and Sexuality*, 9, 5, 445–57.

Taylor & Francis, for permission to reprint parts of 'Black Lesbian Gender and Sexual Culture: Celebration and Resistance' (2009) by Wilson, B., *Culture, Health and Sexuality*, 11. 3, 297–313.

Taylor & Francis, for permission to reprint pages 212–24 of *Sexuality, Health and Human Rights* (2008) by Corrêa, S., Petchesky, R. and Parker, R.

HURIPEC, Makerere University, for permission to reprint in a revised form elements of 'Paradoxes of Sex Work and Sexuality in Modern-day Uganda' (2009) by Tamale, S., *East African Journal of Peace and Human Rights*, 5, 1.

1 Introduction

Peter Aggleton and Richard Parker

Over the course of the past three decades, there has been a veritable explosion of work in the field of sexuality, both conceptually and methodologically. From a relatively limited field, dominated primarily by biomedical and sexological inquiry, the study of sexuality has expanded across a wide range of social sciences. The signs of a field 'coming of age' are everywhere: new scholarly and scientific journals have been launched; new interdisciplinary research centres have been formed; innovative academic degree programmes have been created; established foundations and research funding agencies have made sexuality a programmatic priority; and the volume of publications reporting sexuality research findings has rapidly increased. While much of this development has taken place in leading intellectual centres of resource-rich countries, the trend is clearly global, with important new developments taking place as much in the south as in the north.

Many factors have influenced the changes that have taken place. First, social science disciplines such as history, anthropology, sociology and psychology sought to find new ways of understanding a rapidly changing world in which sex and sexuality are highly visible. Second, growing attention towards sexuality – both academically and in policy terms – has been triggered by a set of increasingly visible social movements. These include the feminist, gay and lesbian and men's movements that emerged from the 1960s but whose influence reached ascendancy in the 1970s and the 1980s. Finally, growing concern for issues such as population and development, women's and men's reproductive health, HIV and AIDS and young people's rights has provided new legitimacy for work of relevance to sex, sexuality and health.

As a result of these different sources of impetus, there has been growing concern to investigate and understand aspects of life that can be defined as broadly 'sexual'. These include the social, economic, historical and cultural factors shaping sexuality in different settings, as well as the complex and often contradictory meanings associated with sexual experience both for individuals and social groups. Of special concern, at least within the fields of population science and public health, have been efforts to delineate the individual determinants of sexual behaviour and behaviour change, most usually defined in terms of demographic correlates or the variable present within psychological models of behaviour change. The focus of much of this work has been on the promotion of reproductive health – defined most usually in terms of the absence of sexually transmitted infections (including HIV) and unwanted pregnancy.

In recent years, the focus has shifted yet again to engage more explicitly with other forms of explanation and a rather different set of social goals. The notion of sexual health as 'absence of disease' has itself been questioned, with some research-ers and policymakers calling for more affirmative understandings of the concept. The intimate relations between sexuality, sexual expression and power have been unpicked by feminist scholarship examining women's roles and gender violence as well as by research within the fields of lesbian and gay studies and masculinity studies. Even more recently, postmodern research and queer theory have encour-aged an understanding of sexuality and sexual expression as performance, linked to 'positionality' and location within the social structure.

Increasingly, too, there have been calls for a clearer specification of the links between sexuality, sexual health and rights – including the human rights already recognised in national laws and international human rights documents and other consensus statements, but extending beyond these to include specifically *sexual* rights – including the right to the highest attainable standard of sexual health; the right to seek, receive and impart information related to sexuality; the right to respect for bodily integrity; the right to decide to be sexually active or not; the right to consensual sexual relations; the right to decide whether or not, and when, to have children; and the right to pursue a satisfying, safe and pleasurable sexual life.

Together, these multiple sources of impetus have extended, and to some extent fractured, the terrain of what counts as sexuality – calling into question hitherto unproblematised notions of sex and sexual relations, what it might be to be sexually healthy, and what it might mean to exercise one's sexual rights. It is against this backcloth that this *Handbook* has been developed, to offer in one location an author-itative introduction to key writers, key material and key debates. By far the majority of chapters take the form of original contributions, although a small number of papers have been reprinted in abridged form from elsewhere. Our goal is to offer readers an authoritative overview of current understanding within the interrelated fields of sexuality, sexual health and sexual rights. We trace the origins of big debates, describe the current state of play in particular fields and hint at where the future might be taking us.

Our aim has been to offer a comprehensive yet accessible account of these and related concerns. The book is organised into eight main sections, each of which concerns both a particular historical moment and a specific set of issues. We begin with pioneering beginnings, or what might be loosely called the genealogy of the present. Here, we learn from the work of Margaret Sanger, an early pioneer for women's reproductive rights, who was imprisoned in 1917 for distributing dia-phragms to immigrant women in Brooklyn, New York. We learn, too, of the work of Alfred Kinsey whose background in biology and whose work on sexual behaviour in women and men laid the foundations for generations of research to come. Anthro-pology's contribution to the developing field of sexuality has been immense through the work of scholars as diverse as E. E. Evans-Pritchard, Bronislaw Malinowksi, Claude Lévi-Strauss, Ruth Benedict and Margaret Mead, to name but a few. Finally, the contribution of historical and sociological explanation – and the seminal contri-bution of scholars such as Michel Foucault, John Gagnon and William Simon – needs to be acknowledged, both for its capacity to illuminate the diverse aspects of sexuality, and for the value of particular frameworks of understanding in advancing understanding of the field.

The second part of the handbook moves the reader forward in time but picks up on the theme of symbolism and meaning in the work of anthropologists and symbolic interactionist sociologists. Its focus is on language, discourse and sexual categories, examining the different ways in which sexuality has been constructed linguistically and discursively. All the chapters here highlight the ways in which sexual acts take their meaning from particular cultures, norms and beliefs about the self and the world. Sexual practices are socially produced, having little meaning outside the context in which they take place or are enacted. The same is true for self-understandings in general and sexual self-understandings in particular, with language being central to the construction of sexual identities. Chapters examine the ways in which *tombois* and their girlfriends understand and construct their sexuality in Indonesia, the growth and proliferation of minority sexual identities in Thailand, and the social identities of same-sex attracted men in Senegal. Because all constructions of sexuality have a past that must be appreciated in order to understand the present, history and context are given centre stage. By analyzing the experiences of *goor-jigeen* (man–woman) in Senegal, *hijra* (an indigenous transgender category) in India and modern day 'gay men' in Thailand, contributors reveal how political power, religious and spiritual influence, colonialism and globalisation, all have a role to play in shaping individual lives and sexual communities. The impact of biopower and the biomedical gaze is also explored in relation to intersexuality and gender determination, as well as in public health practice.

A rather different set of issues is explored in Part III, which focuses on the emergence of, first, reproductive and, later, sexual health. Paralleling interest in language, discourse and meaning were efforts by researchers, policymakers, activists and practitioners to intervene in sex. Many early interventions – particularly within the field of sexology but also in relation to childhood sexuality – aimed to normalise the 'abnormal', eradicate the 'unacceptable' and improve sexual function. Autoeroticism and childhood masturbation were a focus for much early intervention, as were efforts to 'cure' homosexuality and same-sex activity. But also of importance were efforts to prevent unplanned pregnancies through family planning and population control. In their earliest incarnations, these different concerns (albeit in different ways) sought to constrain the expression of sexuality to reproduction. Masturbation and same-sex activity were wrong because they misdirected sexual energies away from their 'natural' ends. Intervention was necessary to correct these deviations. Increasingly, biomedicine was thought to provide the answers, giving rise both to sexology and to demography as 'scientific' disciplines, firmly encompassing sexuality within the field of health. Both sought both to normalise and to control – with sexology focusing on the individual and demography the population as a whole. With the passage of time, however, and under the influence of diverse forces of feminism, technological development, libertarianism and lesbian and gay activism, a growing concern with pleasure and rights emerged. This caused both an expansion of what hitherto had been understood as the 'sexual' (radically decoupling its links with reproduction), and a growing concern with responsibilities and rights. Sex broke free from narrow confines the reproductive, giving rise to a diversity of expression. Pleasure seeking and sexual enjoyment were placed centre stage, being viewed as central to any understanding of how sexual life is lived and organised. In their different ways, chapters within Part III engage with these themes, highlighting concern with childhood sexuality, the growth of sexology, concern for reproductive health and the emergence of sexual health. They highlight, too, the importance of social factors in influencing understandings of sexuality both negatively or more positively – in moral panic over teenage pregnancy or in struggles for the rights of all people to sexual autonomy, sexual integrity and sexual freedom.

The fourth part of the *Handbook* looks at the profound impact that HIV has had on sexuality research and practice. Social science research attention to issues of sexuality had begun to gradually increase during the 1970s, and international research was almost completely dominated by demography and population studies, when AIDS was first recognised in the early 1980s. Not surprisingly, the initial research response to the epidemic, in North America, western Europe and the countries of the global south, was shaped by the concerns of behavioural medicine and population sciences, and tended to focus on surveys of sexual behaviour with the goal of both better understanding the behavioural dynamics of sexual transmission and providing information on cognitive and behavioural interventions to reduce the risk of infection. From the very beginning of the epidemic, however, serious questions were raised – often by the members of affected communities – about the kinds of knowledge that would be necessary to respond positively to HIV and AIDS. Indeed, this section of the *Handbook* takes its title from a well-known book, *How to Have Sex in an Epidemic: One Approach,* co-authored by AIDS activists, Michael Callen and David Berkowitz, together with Joseph Sonnabend, which outlined the tenets of safe sex from a gay community-based perspective long before public health officials or institutions had begun to come to terms with the need for explicit and detailed approaches to the epidemic. Over the course of the 1980s and the 1990s, in work carried out by social researchers such as Dennis Altman, Herbert Daniel, Cindy Patton, Paula Treichler and Simon Watney, with strong links to community activism around HIV and AIDS, a critical alternative approach to HIV and AIDS research began to emerge that has shaped much of the most important work being carried out on these issues over the course of the 1990s and up to the present day. This work has raised important and ongoing questions that are explored in this part of the *Handbook* about the epistemological assumptions that have guided HIV and AIDS research, as well as about the political dynamics that have shaped the ways in which narrow approaches developed in resource rich settings have often been exported to and uncritically imposed in often strikingly different social and cultural environments. As these selections suggest, the complex interplay between sexual risk and other health-related and recreational practices has become an important focus for research, as have been the forms of sexual practice engaged in by people living with HIV as well as those living in affected communities.

One of the important consequences of increased research attention given to sexuality and sexual practices in the wake of HIV and AIDS was new attention to the social organisation of sexual performances. This emphasis had important precursors or antecedents in some of the earliest work on the sociology of sexuality, particularly in the work of John Gagnon and William Simon on sexual scripts. While the metaphor of sexual scripts has had major impact, in seeking to document and interpret the structure of sexual practices much recent work has shifted attention from the dramaturgical language of scripts and performances to more multidimensional and sensual metaphors of dance, as exemplified in the fifth part in this *Handbook*. Work along these lines has sought to characterise the unfolding of sexual meanings and interactions in their materiality and corporality not merely as a script but as a kind of enactment, a kind of complex dance in which both predetermined steps and unexpected improvisations can take place. As the chapters in this part suggest, the notion of choreography can be taken quite literally, as in chapters focusing on the social universe of exotic or erotic dancers or on the interactions of urban minority youth in hip-hop clubs and related venues. But it can also be far more metaphorical, as a way of thinking about the symbolic 'mating' and 'partnering' dances that play themselves out in the social and sexual interactions of young people, male sex workers and their partners, gay and bisexual men and others who cannot be neatly characterised by any of these labels – and in settings as different as the cities of contemporary Iran, the beaches and resort towns of tropical Dominican Republic, the gay communities of current day Australia and the erotic urban landscapes of urban Brazil.

It should be clear from what has been said that both sex and sexuality hold both empowering and destructive possibilities, and it is to the darker side of sex that Part VI turns. In both rich and poor world contexts, so much of sex ties not to autonomy, reciprocity and mutuality but to the expression of power and control. We can see this in extreme forms in the case of gender violence, sexual abuse and rape. But other more subtle forms of expression take place in everyday relationships – in name calling, harassment and verbal abuse; in stereotyping and discrimination; and in general unwillingness to accept the rights of sexual minorities such as lesbian, gay, bisexual and trans individuals. Many of these negative actions have their origins in deeper structures of gender, age, class and race but give rise to damaging forms of misogyny, sexism and homophobia. Part VI of the *Handbook* engages with a broad range of relevant concerns focusing first on sexual and intimate partner violence with a particular focus on women's experience globally. In explaining well-documented patterns of abuse, it is important to look at structural factors influencing women's and men's roles, expectations and behaviours, including the importance of social reputation and opportunity structure determining sexual misbehaviour, unfaithfulness and abuse. The mass media have an important role to play in promoting negative stereotypes and practices as well as positive ones, establishing a taken for granted sense of normalcy that influences both women's and men's actions. Yet the 'normal' carries with it a darker side. Some of the least talked about forms of sexual abuse take place in family settings – in the form of incest, sexual exploitation and gender violence. Difficulty talking about these makes them appear unusual, abnormal and strange, yet they may constitute the normative experience of many young women and men all over the world. In all-male environments such as the military and prisons, sex may be used both as a weapon and as a commodity, turning some men into 'women' and reasserting in the male perpetrators of sexual violence and rape a misplaced sense of their own masculinity. Finally, in contexts where legal, political and religious systems provide legitimacy for sexual violence and abuse, practices such as the 'corrective rape' of lesbians may prevail, being sanctioned both by the local community and society at large. These are but a few of the issues examined here. Each on its own is major cause for concern. Collectively, they demonstrate the necessity for wider struggles for justice and sexual rights.

It is precisely because of such concerns that among the most significant developments in work focusing on sexuality during recent decades has been the growing attention that has focused on issues of sexual rights. As we emphasise throughout this *Handbook*, it is important to understand that this recent work has deep roots and important historical antecedents – many of the very earliest figures in sexology and sexological medicine viewed themselves as social reformers and progressive advocates for sexual freedoms. These longstanding historical precursors were also reinforced in important ways by many of the leading figures in the social science of sexuality that took shape in the 1970s and the 1980s – many of the first historians, anthropologists and sociologists who began to carry out research on sexual topics during this period were participants in progressive political movements, and frequently had to work outside the structures of traditional academic life as independent scholar/activists. As work on sexual health began to take on growing importance over the course of the 1980s and the 1990s, both in relation to the fields of population and reproductive health and in relation to HIV and AIDS, growing concern began to focus on the ways in which gender and sexuality are frequently implicated in, and impacted by, the most horrific forms of abuse and violence – not only through the kinds of action and circumstance discussed in chapters included in Part VI, but also through the very structures and practices of medicine, science and other contemporary social institutions. In both the field of reproductive health and of HIV and AIDS, by the early 1990s leading thinkers and activists had become convinced of the need to move from a focus on health, in and of itself, to a new emphasis on rights – and on the relationship between health and rights. In the field of reproductive health and rights, this new turn became especially evident in the build-up to the global conferences of the mid-1990s, the United Nations Conference on Population and Development held in Cairo in 1994 and the Fourth World Conference on Women held in Beijing in 1995, as the global women's movement mobilised around efforts to move reproductive and sexual rights from the periphery to the centre of meaningful debate. In very similar fashion, in work focusing on HIV and AIDS, what initially began as a defence in the face of widespread stigma and discrimination was increasingly transformed into proactive efforts first on the part of activists and civil society advocates, but increasingly also on the part of official agencies and governmental institutions to make health and human rights the overarching conceptual architecture for approaching sexuality.

As articulated in Part VII of the *Handbook*, this framework has increasingly been expanded over the course of the past decade and a half, through efforts to defend the rights of young people (among others) to information and education about sexuality, the rights of those who fall outside the strictures of normative patterns in relation to gender and sexuality, and of all those who suffer abuse and violence for any reason linked to gender or sexuality. But these chapters also explore the political limits of 'victimisation' as a strategy for social protection and the complex nuances of assuming (or not) specific sexual identities in relation to both health and sexuality. They tell a compelling story of the long struggle, at a global level, to move beyond reproductive rights to a more all-encompassing conception of sexual rights. And they tell a perhaps somewhat surprising (at least for some) story of how much some supposedly well-to-do and advanced societies can learn in this regard from work on sexual rights that is being carried out at the local level by frontline, community-based organisations even in some of the most resource-poor or resource-constrained settings.

Finally, in Part VIII, the chapters that have been included to round out this collection focus on a range of the most cutting edge struggles for erotic justice that are currently underway in diverse communities around the world in defence of sexual rights and sexual citizenship on the part of people at the grassroots seeking to build better sexual lives for themselves and their communities. While these battles are often waged at a very local level, far from the transnational networks and the formal spaces of rights discourses, they offer clear evidence of the broad relevance and that deep power that values such as equity and justice can have in the most diverse settings. In the lives of Ugandan sex workers, young people living with HIV in Brazil, queer South Africans, sexual immigrants from Latin America seeking asylum in the USA, Cuban queers in the black diaspora and black lesbians struggling with normative social and cultural structure of both mainstream society and alternative lesbian and gay communities, we find examples of struggles for sexual freedoms that vividly characterise life in the early twenty-first century.

In bringing together the contributions that make up this *Handbook*, we have worked hard to develop a text that offers a scholarly yet accessible overview of the diverse and rapidly developing field of sexuality studies today. In doing so, we have sought not to privilege any one particular perspective but rather to offer an up-to-date overview of the field of sexuality, health and rights. By describing past origins, present trends and future possibilities, we want to offer readers insight into an area of work that has captured our own imaginations for many years now. We hope you find this book helpful and a useful source of reference for many years to come.

Part I

Pioneering beginnings

The genealogy of the present

2 Margaret Sanger

Her legacy reconsidered[1]

Ellen Chesler

Margaret Sanger went to jail in 1917 for distributing diaphragms to immigrant women from a makeshift clinic in a tenement storefront in the Brownsville section of Brooklyn, New York. When she died nearly 50 years later, the cause for which she defiantly broke the law had achieved international stature. Although still a magnet for controversy, she was widely eulogised as one of the great emancipators of her time.

A visionary if sometimes quixotic thinker, a relentless agitator and gifted organiser, Sanger lived just long enough to savour the historic US Supreme Court decision in *Griswold* v. *Connecticut*, which established privacy protections as a framework for legalising basic reproductive rights. Elderly and frail, she watched Lyndon Johnson finally incorporate family planning into US social welfare and foreign policy programmes, although he refused her a much coveted Presidential Medal of Freedom, for fear of provoking controversy with Catholic voters. She saw the birth control pill developed and marketed by a team of doctors and scientists she had long encouraged and found the money to support. She watched a global family planning movement descend from her own international efforts.

The years since have not been as good to Sanger, even as they have witnessed measurable progress for women in achieving reproductive freedom. Today, outside of a small minority of countries in sub-Saharan Africa and in parts of the Middle East, which are now high-profile exceptions to the global norm, a typical woman bears no more than two children over the course of several years and spends another 30 to 40 years avoiding pregnancy. More than 60 million women around the world use oral contraception daily, a dramatic increase since organised interventions began. The right of women to plan their families remains at least for the time being enshrined in the US Constitution and in international human rights law, where it is widely recognised as a necessary condition to improve women's status, and in turn to sustain democratic institutions, promote social and economic progress and help sustain fragile environments.

Still, universal standards for women's human rights offer no sure cure for violations that persist with uncanny fortitude and often unimaginable cruelty in so many places around the world. Harsh fundamentalisms are resurgent in many countries, where women's bodies remain an arena of intense political conflict, as a perhaps predictable response to the social dislocations resulting from changing gender roles and to the larger assaults on traditional cultures from the many real and perceived injustices of modernisation and globalisation. Counted among these are the abuses of technologically driven and demographically targeted population programmes, which have spawned understandable outrage and, despite many well-realised efforts at reform in recent years, continue to spark controversy, especially around Sanger to whom they are linked, however indirectly.

Even in the USA, decades of substantial progress by women have fuelled a fierce backlash. With an intensity that few would have predicted in 1992 when Bill Clinton was elected as America's first pro-choice president, a powerful conservative minority has eroded abortion rights along with funding for family planning at home and abroad, while dollars have surged instead for abstinence programmes known to be ineffective and often harmful. We have tolerated the impunity of daily campaigns of intimidation and outright violence against courageous providers of contraception and abortion. And Sanger herself has become a collateral victim of this frenzy, her reputation savaged by rightwing zealots who deliberately misrepresent what has been a heated but usually respectful academic discourse about the history of birth control to circulate scurrilous, false accusations about her on the internet.[2]

Reproductive and sexual rights are attacked, on the one hand, for fostering a corrosive individualism that threatens the presumed cohesion of traditional families and communities. At the same time, if somewhat contradictorily, they are criticised for demanding a fearsome conformity that homogenises cultures and denies rights of self-determination to minority groups, a point on which critics across a political spectrum from right to left often concur (Roberts 1997).

Conceptions of the past are never stable. We are, in fact, prisoners of our own experience. We bring to history the preoccupations of our own age. In the context of a reproductive and sexual rights discourse that is at once vibrant and expansive but also fiercely contested, we are obliged to re-examine Margaret Sanger one more time and interrogate her unquestioning confidence in the power of medicine and science to shape human conduct and alleviate suffering, a confidence that fuelled her interest in trying to make birth control serve as a tool of both individual liberation and social betterment.

Sanger's contribution and legacy

Margaret Sanger's fundamental heresy was in claiming women's right to experience their sexuality free of consequence, just as men have always done. Following in the footsteps of a first generation of educated US women who had proudly forgone marriage in order to seek fulfilment outside the home, she offered birth control as a necessary condition to the resolution of a broader range of personal and professional satisfactions. The hardest challenge in writing about her for modern audiences, for whom this claim has become routine, is to explain how absolutely destabilising it seemed in her own time.

Even with so much lingering animus toward changes in women's lives around the world, it is difficult to inhabit an era in our own history when sexuality was considered more an obligation of women than a pleasure. It is hard to remember that well into Sanger's own time motherhood was accepted as a woman's principal purpose and primary role. It is even harder to fathom that US women, a mere century ago, were still largely denied identities or rights of their own, independent of those they enjoyed by virtue of their relationships with men, and that this principle was central to the enduring opposition they encountered in seeking access to full rights of inheritance and property, to suffrage and, most especially, to birth control. This unyielding principle of male covertures defined women's legal identities even with respect to physical abuse in the family, which the US Supreme Court condoned in 1910, denying damages to a wife injured by violent beatings on that the grounds that to do so would undermine the peace of the household.

Re-examining this history in the context of the recent expansion of human rights to incorporate women's autonomy underscores Sanger's originality as a feminist theorist who first demanded civil protection of women's claims to reproductive liberty and bodily integrity, in and outside marriage. Recent scholarly works have made all the more clear that as a result of private arrangements and a healthy trade in condoms, douches and various contraptions sold largely under the subterfuge of feminine hygiene, the country's birth rate began to decline long before she came on the scene (Brodie 1994; Tone 2001). But it was she who invented 'birth control' as a comfortable, popular term of speech, and, in so doing, gave the practice essential public and political currency. It was she who first recognised the far reaching consequences of bringing sexuality and contraception out in the open and claiming them as fundamental women's rights. And by winning medical validation for specific contraceptive practices, she also helped lift the religious shroud that had long encased reproduction in myth and mystery and secured houses of worship as primary arbiters of sexual behaviours and values.

When Sanger opened her clinic and deliberately staged an arrest in 1916, she challenged anachronistic obscenity laws that remained on the books as the legacy of the notorious anti-vice crusader, Anthony Comstock, whose evangelical fervour had captured Victorian politics and led to the adoption by the states and Federal government of broad criminal sanctions on sexual speech and commerce, including all materials related to contraception and abortion. Her critique, however, was not just of legal constraints on obscenity, but of legal constraints on women's place. In this respect, I would argue, she helped inaugurate the modern human rights movement that moves beyond traditional civil and political claims of liberty on behalf of women to embrace social and cultural ones. She understood that to advance women's rights it is necessary to address – and the state has an obligation to protect – personal as well as public spheres of conduct. It must establish broad safeguards for women and intervene to eliminate everyday forms of discrimination and abuse.

Sanger was fortunate to witness the fulfilment of at least part of this vision when the Supreme Court finally protected the private use of contraception in its landmark 1965 decision in *Griswold* v. *Connecticut.* The extension of that privacy doctrine to abortion eight years later in *Roe* v. *Wade,* and the court's reinterpretation of the law in *Planned Parenthood* v. *Casey* in 1992, moved it further in the direction of achieving her intent by explicitly ruling that women are not obliged to seek spousal consent in decisions about whether or not to bear a child. But as feminist legal theorists from Justice Ruth Bader Ginsburg to Catherine McKinnon have since pointed out, privacy is not a secure judicial philosophy for women, since it only protects couples from unwarranted state interference and does not mandate positive state obligation for their equal protection under the law.[3]

Those intentions, they both would argue and I would agree, are more fully realised today in international human rights constructs than in US constitutional law – in an intellectual architecture that builds on the Universal Declaration of Human Rights of 1948, the first formal document to claim that discrimination against women is an appropriate matter for international concern, not a category privileged and protected by local sovereignty or by traditional cultural or religious practices governing women's civil status or their marriage and family relations. The Universal Declaration of Human Rights quite deliberately guarantees rights to all 'human beings' not just to men, establishes broad protections for women as citizens and workers and specifically accords them the right to free consent in marriage and divorce and to the necessary provisions to care for their children when abandoned or widowed.

Drafted by Eleanor Roosevelt, who was, incidentally, long a friend and follower of Sanger's, the Universal Declaration paved the way for vigorous participation in the UN Commission on the Status of Women (CSW) by women from India, Latin America, the Caribbean and later from African and other newly independent states, a fact that disputes common accusations that this ambitious women's rights agenda has largely been a product of western feminism. Years of incremental but significant gains by the CSW occurred over the next 30 years and were then finally codified with adoption in 1979 of CEDAW, the Convention to Eliminate All Forms of Discrimination against Women, one of the UN's five pillars of human rights implementation, along with its agreements on civil and political rights, torture, social and economic rights and racial discrimination.

CEDAW acknowledges the importance of women's traditional obligations with the family but also establishes new norms for their participation in all dimensions of life. It provides binding protection to a broad range of rights in marriage and family relations, including property, inheritance and access to healthcare, with an explicit mention of family planning. It demands equality for women as citizens with full access to suffrage, political representation and other legal obligations and benefits. It declares their right to education, including professional and vocational training and the elimination of gender stereotypes and segregation, and establishes their rights as workers deserving equal remuneration, social security benefits and protection from sexual harassment and workplace discrimination on the grounds of marriage or maternity.

In 1992 CEDAW was expanded so that gender-based violence is also formally identified as a form of discrimination in violation of fundamental human rights and recognised as a problem of epidemic proportions worldwide, veiled by traditions of privacy, guilt and shame. International human rights law thus moves beyond traditional constructs guaranteeing sex-neutral norms measured by male standards to obligate state response to what is now finally understood as pervasive and systematic discrimination against women.

In 1994 the UN International Conference on Population and Development in Cairo, reacting to heavy-handed practices in population programmes, created a framework for state responsibility to ensure programmes allowing women to make free and informed decisions about their bodies, while also guaranteeing them access to quality healthcare services, including family planning. A year later, in Beijing, the international community overcoming considerable conservative resistance, committed to a wide range of practical interventions to advance women's rights, and while paying required deference to the plurality of religious values around the world, reaffirmed the universality of human rights over local custom and culture. With strong leadership from a US delegation assembled by the Clinton administration, the Beijing Platform of Action, while stopping short of creating a new category of explicit sexual rights that in the eyes of some would have licensed same-sex partnerships and abortion, is quite direct in claiming that: 'The human rights of women include their right to have control over and decide freely and responsibly on matters related to their sexuality, including sexual and reproductive health, free of coercion, discrimination and violence'.

The Beijing Platform received unanimous endorsement, although 29 countries, including many Islamic states, filed reservations about the sexual and reproductive health and rights language and, in the years since, of course, the USA under George W. Bush substantially eroded prior commitments to sexual and reproductive health and rights, even as it waged two wars in Afghanistan and Iraq, ostensibly in pursuit of securing human freedoms. Meanwhile, CEDAW has now been endorsed by 185 countries, with the notable exception of the USA itself, which signed the document in 1980 when Jimmy Carter was president but has never since been able to achieve the two-thirds majority vote in the Senate required for ratification – a worthy goal now back on the agenda of the Obama administration.

From the past to the present

Observing the contorted politics of sexuality in recent years has only reinforced my sympathy for Margaret Sanger's predicament as a wildly polarising figure and clarified the logic of her decision after the First World War to abandon radicalism and mainstream her movement by identifying reproductive autonomy as a necessary foundation for broader improvements in public health and social welfare. Moreover, her decision to adopt the socially resonant content of 'family planning over birth control', when the Great Depression encouraged attention to collective needs over individual ones and when the New Deal created a blueprint for bold public endeavours, continues to seem inventive, not cynical. Neither, as some of her harshest critics then and since have charged, did she ever define family planning as right of the privileged, but as a duty or obligation of the poor, any more than we do so today when we call for increased public expenditure on it as a matter of simple justice. To the contrary, I would argue that Sanger showed considerable foresight in lobbying for voluntary family planning programmes to be included among the benefits of any sound public investment in social security. Had the New Deal included public health and access to contraception in its social welfare package, as most European countries were then doing, protracted conflicts over welfare and healthcare policy in the years since in the USA might well have been avoided. Where she went wrong was in failing to anticipate the force of the opposition her proposal would generate from a coalition of urban Catholics and rural fundamentalist Protestants to whom Roosevelt Democrats became captive, much as Republicans have become in recent years.

What is harder to deconstruct and understand is Sanger's engagement with eugenics during these years, the widely respectable and popular movement of her era that addressed the manner in which biology and heredity affect human intelligence and ability. Like many well-intentioned secularists and social reformers of her day, Sanger took away from Darwin the essentially optimistic lesson that men and women's common descent in the animal kingdom makes us all capable of improvement, if only we apply the right tools. Eugenics held the promise that merit would replace birthright and social status as the standard for mobility in a democratic society.

Eugenics most enduring if still controversial legacy is standard IQ testing, its most damning and unfathomable, a series of state laws upheld by a progressive majority of the US Supreme Court in 1927, including Justices Oliver Wendell Holmes and Louis Brandeis, who in *Buck* v. *Bell* authorised the compulsory sterilisation of a poor young white woman with an illegitimate child, on grounds of feeble mindedness that were never clearly established, a decision, incidentally, also accepted by civil libertarians such as Roger Baldwin and civil rights advocates, including W. E. B. DuBois of the National Association for the Advancement of Colored People, both of whom Sanger counted among her supporters and friends.

Orthodox eugenics opposed birth control on the grounds that the fit should procreate. Sanger countered by disdaining what she called a 'cradle competition' of class, race or ethnicity. She opposed immigration restrictions and racial and ethnic stereotypes. She framed poverty as a matter of differential access to resources, including birth control, not as the immutable consequence of low inherent ability or poor character, a view many eugenicists embraced. She argued for broad government safety nets for social welfare and public health. And she proudly marshalled clinical data to demonstrate that most women, even among the poorest and least educated populations, did use birth control successfully when it was provided them.

At the same time, however, she was capable of shrill rhetoric about the growing burden of large families among individuals of low intelligence and defective heredity, which may well have provoked exactly the intolerance she claimed to oppose. In endorsing compulsory sterilisation, and also on several occasions the payment of pensions or bonuses to women of low intelligence who would with this inducement agree to the procedure, she seems to have considered neither the fundamental rights questions raised by such practices nor the validity of the aptitude assessments on which determinations of low intelligence were based. Living in an era indifferent to the firm obligation to respect and protect the rights of individuals whose behaviour does not always conform to prevailing mores, she did not always fulfil it.

The challenge for historians has been to reconcile these apparent contradictions in Sanger's views. She was actually an advanced thinker on race for her day, one who condemned discrimination and encouraged racial reconciliation. She opened an integrated clinic in Harlem in the early 1930s and then facilitated birth control and maternal health programmes for rural black women in the south, when local white health officials denied them access to the New Deal's first federally funded programmes. She worked on this project with behind-the-scenes support from Eleanor Roosevelt, whose advanced views on race were well known but whose support for birth control was silenced by her husband's Catholic political handlers, at least until he was safely ensconced in the White House for a third term. Historically specific circumstances of this complexity, however, are hard to untangle and convey, and Sanger's legacy has been compromised accordingly.

Michel Foucault, perhaps better than any other thinker about sexuality, must be summoned in conclusion to help explain the complicated politics of reproduction, which has so long ensnarled Margaret Sanger and all others who have tried to discipline it. As so many scholars writing under Foucault's broad influence have observed, reproduction is by its very nature experienced individually and socially at the same time.[4] In claiming women's fundamental right to control their own bodies, Margaret Sanger, was also mindful of the dense fabric of cultural, political and economic relationships in which those rights are exercised (Wolin 2006; Clarke 1998;

Murphy 2004; Petchesky 2003). And almost if obviously not always, she tried to encourage a balance in the behaviours she prescribed between the contentment that derives from the right of individual self-expression and the contrary obligation to participate in a shared human experience, governed by common mores, rules and laws.

This same tension, I would argue, exists at the heart of the movement today that is formulating principles by which to incorporate sexuality within a framework of universal human rights at once protective and empowering. That Sanger in a long and mostly honourable career failed to get the balance quite right should not discourage us from continuing to try and do so. Like the deities of ancient lore, perhaps, she can inspire us with awe and fear at the same time.

Notes

1 This chapter is a new contribution but draws on E. Chesler (1992, 2007) *Woman of Valor: Margaret Sanger and the Birth Control Movement in America*, New York: Simon & Schuster; and E. Chesler (2005) 'Introduction', in Chavkin, W. and Chesler, E. (eds) (2005) *Where Human Rights Begin: Health, Sexuality, and Women in the New Millennium*, New Brunswick, NJ: Rutgers Press.
2 Some of this material can be found in *Margaret Sanger Papers Project Newsletter*, 42 (Spring 2006), 'Searching for Sanger in the Land of Google', 1–4, available at www.nyu.edu/ projects/sanger.
3 For more on the limitations of the privacy doctrine and of the 'undue burden' standard established in *Casey*, see US Senate Committee on the Judiciary, Nomination of Ruth Bader Ginsburg to be Associate Justice of the Supreme Court of the United States, July 20–23 1993, at www.gpoaccess.gov/congress/senate/judiciarysh 103–482 (MacKinnon 2005; Wharton *et al.* 2006).
4 Wolin, R. 'Foucault the Neohumanist?', *The Chronicle of Higher Education*, 1 September 2006, 12–14, contains a provocative discussion of the tensions in Foucault's writings between his early celebration of non-conformity and difference, for which he has been canonised, and a later reconsideration of humanist values and liberal political traditions guaranteeing individual rights and expanding civic freedom that he had once rejected as inherently suppressive. For contrasting analyses of the politics of disciplining reproduction, also see Clarke 1998; Murphy 2004; and Petchesky 2003.

References

Brodie, J. F. (1994) *Contraception and Abortion in 19th Century America*, Ithaca and London: Cornell University Press.

Chesler, E. (1992, 2007) *Woman of Valor: Margaret Sanger and the Birth Control Movement in America*, New York: Simon & Schuster.

Chesler, E. (2005) 'Introduction', Chavkin, W. and Chesler, E. (eds) *Where Human Rights Begin: Health, Sexuality, and Women in the New Millennium*, New Brunswick, NJ: Rutgers Press.

Clarke, A. M. (1998) *Disciplining Reproduction: Modernity, American Life Sciences, and the Problems of Sex*, Berkeley: University of California Press.

MacKinnon, C. (2005) *Women's Lives: Men's Laws*, Cambridge, MA: Harvard University Press.

Margaret Sanger Papers Project Newsletter (2006) 'Searching for Sanger in the Land of Google', Spring, 42: 1–4. Available at www.nyu.edu/projects/sanger/ (accessed 27 April 2009).

Murphy, M. (2004) 'Liberation through Control in the Body Politics of U.S. Radical Feminism', in Daston, L. and Vidal, F. (eds) *The Moral Authority of Nature*, Chicago: University of Chicago Press.

Petchesky, R. (2003) 'Introduction', in Petchesky, R. and Judd, K. (eds) *Global Prescriptions: Gendering Reproductive Health and Rights*, London: Zed Books.

Roberts, D. (1997) *Killing the Black Body: Race, Reproduction, and the Meaning of Liberty*, New York: Pantheon Books.

Tone, A. (2001) *Devices and Desires: A History of Contraceptives in America*, New York: Hill & Wang.

Wharton, L. J., Frietsche, S. and Kolbert, K. (2006) 'Preserving the Core of *Roe:* Reflections on Planned Parenthood v. Casey', *Yale Journal of Law and Feminism*, 18 (2): 319–87.

Wolin, R. (2006) 'Foucault the Neohumanist?', *The Chronicle of Higher Education*, 1 September: 12–14.

3 Anthropological foundations of sexuality, health and rights

Gilbert Herdt

To examine the nexus between sexuality, health and rights in the foundations of anthropology requires a historical review of the emergence of the 'culture' concept and cultural relativism in studies of sexuality, allowing a perspective on how ethnographic work, over the period from approximately 1920 to 2000, created a new way of thinking about sexual meanings and practices. During this time, older theoretical approaches evolved and died out, new voices emerged and the colonial history of anthropology ended, leading to a call for a different and more interdisciplinary vision of sexual, gender and reproductive rights and health in research, policy and advocacy.

In the social sciences in the USA, anthropology and sociology played pivotal roles in the twentieth-century reaction to evolutionary and social Darwinist approaches (Harris 2001; D'Emilio and Freedman 1988) in medicine and sexology. By the beginning of modern anthropology around the time of the First World War, these discourses on sexuality were so heavily influenced by the language of pathology that the label 'medicalised' in respect to such work seems apt (Irvine 2000). Creation of a unified concept of 'culture' (defined here as a system of meanings and social practices) during this period, and the rise of the epistemology of 'cultural relativism' (the world view that all cultures have equally good knowledge sets) was foundational to this reaction and subsequent social learning and environmental or ecological perspectives on sexuality, sexual meanings, roles and scripts (Bell *et al.* 2001; Gagnon 2004; Herdt 1997; Laumann *et al.* 1994; Rubin 2002).

Anthropology's critical role in the invention of functionalism, too, and then structural-functionalism in theory and methodology, allied with sexuality study early on, was paradoxical, however, in that the work of the early pioneers was all but forgotten until decades later, an hiatus that led anthropology to 'rediscover' sexuality after the advent of Foucault, explained below (Vance 1999; Herdt 2004; Herdt and Stoller 1990). Activism in anthropology has always been complicated and with regard to sexuality, this long silence on sex created a formidable barrier, even in the fight against AIDS and HIV.

Early anthropological pioneers in sexuality

The colonial origins of anthropology are foundational to understanding the invention of the culture concept and contextual sexual ethnography. I take my cue in reflecting on this history from the most influential American anthropologist of the late twentieth century, Clifford Geertz (1988). Although not interested in sexuality per se, Geertz's prime examples come from anthropologists who were (Malinowski, Benedict, Mead, Evans-Pritchard, Lévi-Strauss, K. E. Read).[1] Reacting to the hegemonic evolutionary thinking of the nineteenth century, by extending the culture concept through the participant–observation method of ethnography, anthropology found a means of grounding social study in the lived experience of learning another language and culture.

Yet Geertz (1988: 82) argues that this pioneering work contained two distinct and perhaps oppositional images of authority: the anthropologist as *Pilgrim* and the anthropologist as *Cartographer*. The Pilgrim was on a romantic journey, told as a 'quest story' (p. 42), describing the anthropologist in highly contextual and emotional but persuasive terms as a 'seeker' (p. 45), whose compassion could provide deep insight and understanding. Conversely, in reaction to this image, another school of thought viewed the role of classical anthropology as objective; mapping out a culture by 'being there' in exotic places, 'seeking through to the foundations of strange looking lives, not through 'personal immersion' (p. 48) as is so commonly believed, but by analyzing the cultural productions of each society – its myths and rituals, art and history. Thus, it is helpful to think about how anthropology's romantic rebellion against the Enlightenment (Shweder 1990) gave impetus to the theme of the Pilgrim in sexual study, which years later infused a variety of rights movements.

Malinowski's (1929) magisterial classic, *The Sexual Life of Savages*, was thus not only the premier attempt of an anthropologist to establish how a Pilgrim from another world would chart an exotic sexual culture. His work showed the 'objective' and 'scientific' manner in which sex 'functions' to maintain that society, even when the folk culture lacks a category of 'sex'. Sexual customs thus 'maintained' marriage and kinship in tandem with other major institutions such as religion, to use the functionalist theory and language of the founder of social anthropology and 'participant–observation'.

> The reader will find that the natives treat sex in the long run not only as a source of pleasure, but, indeed, as a thing serious and even sacred. Nor do their customs and ideas eliminate from sex its power to transform crude material fact into wonderful spiritual experience, to throw the romantic glamour of love over the technicalities of love making … it is in this richness and multiplicity of love that lies its philosophic mystery, its charm for the poet and its interest for the anthropologist.
>
> (Malinowski 1929: xxiv)

This passionate, exoticising and romantic voice captured, in Geertz's terms, the conjoining of sex in both the Pilgrim and Cartographer roles, ensuring fascination by the public and scientific acceptance by academics: what John Gagnon (1997: 24) later aptly called the 'dense assemblage of collective myth and individual fantasy' belonging to the era.

Prior to the 1980s, while sexuality clearly remained peripheral to the mainstream of theory and fieldwork, sexual (and reproductive) rights as such were treated as wholly contextual; they were densely connected, if at all – to reproduction (Paige and Paige 1981); to kinship and family and childbearing, and sometimes to religious roles. However, cultural relativism was background to all sexual customs.

Malinowski's (1929) famous description, for example, of Trobriand Islanders biting their lover's eye-lashes at the peak of sexual excitement is thus of no less or more *meaning* than any other element of culture (Herdt 1999), although it was connected to the sense in which Trobriand sexual culture was egalitarian and complementary to the rights of women. Yet because these accounts of local sexual culture were pockets of colonial time and space (Newton 1993), often omitted from the study or erased in the ethnography (Appadurai 1996), the sexual ethnographies became suspect and were mostly ignored in later decades: they ignored critical historical change, encapsulation by western authorities and the sense in which local customs were in decline (Lévi-Strauss 1955).

The anthropologist in this ideology should look, but not touch; the taboo suggested that anthropologists again were Innocents, even Celibates, having what the British anthropologist E. E. Evans-Pritchard (1957: 81–2) dared to call 'a certain kind of character and temperament'. Suffice it to say that the sexual engagement with the natives, whether in fantasy or reality, was removed from the ethnography. The Cartographer account was antiseptic and clean, without an erotic slant. In fact, of course, since the time of Malinowski's (1967) posthumously published diary, this image has been unsustainable (Herdt and Stoller 1990). The majestic biography of Malinowski (Young 2004: 405) reveals just how deeply flawed the idea is, in view of Malinowski's sexual fantasies of local girls and his racist revulsion and fear of caste pollution regarding them, all part of the Catholic conscience within his own thoughts.

Sexuality was handled, if it were handled at all, as an individual need or biological function in this approach (Vance 1999), and same-sex relationships were treated as a form of deviance, pathology or mental illness (Rubin 1984), rather than as a social issue or matter of social difference (Herdt 2004). This same colonial legacy discursively linked the sexual ethnography to the medical discourse in sexology (Foucault 1980). No doubt a significant reason for this approach was Freudian developmentalism (Herdt 1991; Robinson 1967). The Freudian influence on early anthropology, as in virtually all of the social and behavioural sciences (Harris 2001: 422–48), was nearly hegemonic, countered by the Marxism, which, of course, typically ignored sexuality; for the materialist, sex is marginal to the production of goods and services, not a prime mover but a decoration on the cake of political economy (Harris 2001).

Freudian universalism opposed the cultural relativism of the times, particularly when it came to the interpretation of sexual 'abnormality' and 'perversion' (Herdt 1991), was nonetheless the cultural mode of describing sexuality in its day. The unfortunate effect of Freudian developmentalism in combination with sexology was to treat sexuality as an individual psychological problem that relied on Freudian diagnostic language, pathologising much of native cultures. For example, the sexual ethnography of the Mohave Indians typifies this trend, in such areas as masturbation, sexual play in childhood, homosexuality and Two-spirit (Berdache) roles (to name but a few of the significant psycho-cultural patterns), described by Georges Devereux (1937), the French-American anthropologist turned psychoanalyst. By adherence to an Oedipal framework, as in the case of Mead's work (1935, 1949) or by reaction to it, as in the case of Malinowski's *Sex and Repression in Savage Society* (1927; see Spiro 1982), the possibility of contextual rights was undermined. Not until the decisive counter-hegemonic influence of Foucault's *History of Sexuality* filtered in the 1980s (Knauft 1994) did Freudianism decline, and rights begin to have a clearer modern profile. Even Mead's (1935) allusion to 'sexual exceptionalism' in *Sex and Temperament* could not escape this pathologising tendency (reviewed in Herdt 1991).

The same schism between Pilgrim and Cartographer, local and universal, is apparent in the neo-Freudian accounts of Ruth Benedict and Margaret Mead, teacher and student, two of the great American anthropologists. They were intent on bringing sexuality more clearly into the ethnographic approach and they succeeded to a considerable extent (Herdt 1997: 11ff). Benedict clearly believed that homosexuality was normal, and Mead was of the conviction that bisexuality was the best sexual identity, although neither of them could say so publicly (Banner 2003: 119, 150, 348–51). Curiously, however, to note a convergence of gender and sexual ideas in this early work, Mead disliked the Freudian active/passive dichotomy; disliked the concept of homosexuality because it merged identity and behaviour, linked gendered masculinity/femininity to sexual expression; and disliked passivity in homosexuals (Banner op cit.: 357–8).

Transition to the later twentieth century

The upsurge of social science interest in deviance as a problem of social development and sexual behaviour formed a cornerstone of anthropology's latter transformation. A significant conference in Hanover, New Hampshire, in 1934, showed the differences in attitudes about sexual normality among key anthropologists of the times, ranging from the negative and homophobic (Edward Sapir) to the enlightened feminist critiques of Mead (Banner 2003: 351). Benedict's (1938) subsequent essay on discontinuities in cultural conditioning actually used 'ritual homosexuality' as an example of how cultures may intervene into development in positive and negative ways, implicitly connecting sexuality, culture and rights, as these ideas would be understood 50 years later (Herdt 1997).

Virtually in tandem with this anthropological work was the hugely influential Chicago school of sociological community studies. Gayle Rubin's (2002) masterful review of this work and the reformulation of 'deviance' as normal or presentational demonstrates how 'subculture' and 'deviance theory' typified American symbolic interactionist approaches following George H. Mead, defined by functional-structural theory or grounded theory (Kurt Lewin and, later, Erving Goffman). British sociology Cohen (1972) also followed with the construct of 'moral panics' in relation to youth culture, sexuality and subcultural deviance (reviewed in Herdt 2009). Symbolic interactionism grew from this paradigm, through the work of Goffman (1959), which was highly influential in the creation of symbolic anthropology in the 1960s and 1970s – paving the way for feminist anthropology, gender studies and subsequent forms of sexual ethnography (Weston 1991).

Goffman's landmark study, *Stigma* (1963), a brilliant functionalist analysis of 'the natural cycle' of passing as a homosexual, was perspicacious for its time, anticipating the impact of cultural stigma on health and rights. But this approach also led to the influential work of John Gagnon and William Simon (1973), collaborating at the Kinsey Institute in the late 1960s, which laid the foundations for later social constructionist accounts of sexuality, same-sex relations and HIV studies. Gagnon's (2004) major pieces about culture and sexual scripts are also foundational here.

Major work being conducted nowadays on minority stress, following the research of Meyer and Northridge (2007)) provides new and still to be studied insights into issues of sexual health and minority status.

The post-Second World War influence of famed zoologist Alfred Kinsey largely passed by anthropology, in part because of the tendency of Kinsey to treat 'culture' as the enemy of sexual freedom (Herdt 2009). However, it paved the way for the emergence of second-wave feminism, gay and lesbian social movements and anthropological studies of gender and later sexuality (Herdt and Stoller 1990; Ginsburg and Rapp 1995). Oriented toward issues of women's gender roles, reproduction and the subsequent break between the sexual and reproductive, this work responded (at least in part) to the invention of the contraceptive pill in the early 1960s, the advent of what Laumann *et al.* (1994) have referred to as the paradigm of 'sex as recreation'. Rosado and Lamphere's (1974) classic anthology illustrates new and older ideas, such as the neo-Freudian approach of sociologist Nancy Chodorow (2008), whose work was highly influential in anthropological and sociological construction especially during the 1980s.

As Rubin (1984) critiqued this work, the feminist approach toward sexuality was sometimes hostile, and the politics created complications both for rights and health. Feminism during this period was, of course, also labouring under the difficulties of various identity splits between heterosexual and lesbian identities (Lewin 1996) and white middle class versus women of colour voices (D'Emilio and Freedman 1988), which were anticipated by events that unfolded in the women's health movement in the 1970s (Schneider 1997). A critical overview of these social movements reveals a trend toward a new thinking about health, gender and rights (Epstein 1999), which is especially productive of asking questions about social policy. The role that women began to take vis-à-vis the HIV epidemic paved the way for a different approach to sexuality. There is no question but that the obstacles to sexual and reproductive health coming out of very detailed case studies, for example, in South America (Shepard 2006) reveal themes of continuity with this past, and new moves away from it, as for example, toward a different conception of sexual citizenship (Weeks 1985), recently taken up in US LGBT marriage rights debates (Herdt and Kertzner 2006).

Beginning in the 1970s, same-sex behaviour began to be an explicit object of study in anthropology, indirectly through the cultural performance study of Newton's (1972) *Mother Camp*, well reviewed in Rubin (2002). Explicit new ethnographies of same-sex behaviour then got underway, such as my own studies of age-structured boy-inseminating practices among the Sambia of Papua New Guinea (Herdt 1981). As I have reviewed this paradigm of work in Melanesia (Herdt 1984), it was not there were no prior ethnographic mentions or vignettes, they just were not investigated in depth; certainly they were not theorised. In fact, heterosexual male ethnographers who worked in Melanesia for decades (and the vast majority of ethnographers *were* men) found the expression of same-sex practices repellent or embarrassing; theoretically, they were completely unequipped to deal with these remarkable symbolic and material practices (Herdt 2003). In other words, there was no anthropology of the body (Burton 2008), a lack of a critical medical anthropology that was concerned with sexuality, and the absence of a theory of agency that might connect sexual subjectivities to desires (Hostetler and Herdt 1998), compounding the difficulty of how to handle the ethics of sexual study in the perspective of cultural relativism.

With the emergence of the HIV and the AIDS social movements and their focus on the health and health provider impact of HIV on individuals and communities (Herdt and Lindenbaum 1992), a whole new range of sexual ethnography emerged (Parker 1991). As has been so well conceptualised, HIV resulted in a huge transformation in anthropology and social science study in general, leading not only to new conceptions of sexuality (Parker and Gagnon 1995), but also to a more explicit theory of the body, of the role of qualitative ethnography in these endeavours and the place of sexual health in culture theory. The subsequent emergence of queer theory as a distinctive voice in the early 1990s, and the ways in which high theory was to be somewhat detrimental to the expansion of thinking about rights, are not easily reviewed but definitely played a decisive force during this period. Certainly, the work of medical anthropologists and those who have followed in the tradition of the early anthropology of sexuality has gone in other directions (Teunis and Herdt 2006), for example, in understanding how transgender rights are grounded in a variety of indigenous cultural practices (Herdt 1993; Valentine 2007). Here again we see the tension between playing out the historical roles of Pilgrim and Cartographer in the field of sexuality studies.

Conclusion

Anthropology's rediscovery of sex in the past three decades has introduced new and vital work into work on rights and health. Our enduring contribution is, of course, cultural relativism and the respect for each culture in its own context in relation to sexual and reproductive rights and health. Anthropological forms of cultural constructionism of sexuality remained largely peripheral to the development of rights and health (Cowan *et al.* 2001; Corrêa *et al.* 2008). Even in the extraordinary work of the medical anthropologist Paul Farmer (1999), who is rightly cited in both articulating and in making popular the structural violence framework, sexuality played a very small role in its foundations, in spite of the HIV discourse (Teunis and Herdt 2006). There is an epistemological reason for this hiatus: the source of this work, including liberationist theology, applied medical anthropology and the radical pedagogy of Paolo Freire, largely omitted sexuality from its view of human nature. On the practice side, however, Parker (2007) has written well concerning another problem for the field: the emergent rights discourses came from the grassroots, with academics largely lagging behind.

The lag between the trenches and the Academy has occurred in many policy areas, such as the emergence of HIV and AIDS research and interventions, which began among activists in response to huge impact of the loss of friends and lovers, while academics were slow to catch up – psychology preceding other disciplines, such as anthropology (Herdt and Lindenbaum 1992). In this work, we see the continuing struggle between local context and universalism; between the respects for each culture as unique, which is suggested by cultural relativism; and the commitment to find support for each unique human being's struggle for rights.

The struggle between the Pilgrim and Cartographer in anthropology remains in place, and, in some ways, this tension is productive of new forms of thinking, including research and activism on rights. It is true that anthropology has been remiss in its lack of support for empirically based advocacy, as some have argued, and that its contributions on culture and relativism have made few inroads into American society. In the USA, for example, sexual rights are often placed together with reproductive rights in rightwing discourse (DiMauro and Joffe 2009), and moral panics continue to surround the basic right to full sexual citizenship. Not so curiously, the USA as a society remains gripped by a fundamental preconception that sex is 'natural', a huge barrier to advocacy for human rights; we shall have to see if greater sexual literacy emerges. In these ways, the emergent field of rights and health is helping to change opinion and lead toward a different future. Where once this was a drag on theory and a barrier to policy formation, the situation now suggests a necessary and healthy tension between local experience and universal claims to rights in all times and places.

Note

1 These classics include but are not limited to: Malinowski *Sexual Life of Savages* (1929), Ruth Benedict's *Patterns of Culture* (1934), Margaret Mead's *Sex and Temperament in Three Primitive Societies* (1935), Lévi-Strauss' (1955) *Triste Tropiques*, and K. E. Read's *The High Valley* (1965).

References

Appadurai, A. (1996) *Modernity at Large*, Minneapolis: University of Minnesota Press.

Banner, L. W. (2003) *Intertwined Lives: Margaret Mead, Ruth Benedict, and Their Circle*, New York: Vintage Books.

Bell, L. S., Nathan, A. J. and Peleg, I. (eds) (2001) *Negotiating Culture and Human Rights*, New York: Columbia University Press.

Benedict, R. (1934) *Patterns of Culture*, New York: Houghton-Mifflin.

Benedict, R. (1938) 'Continuities and Discontinuities in Cultural Conditioning', *Psychiatry*, 1: 161–7.

Burton, J. (2008) *Culture and the Human Body: An Anthropological Perspective*, New York: Waveland Press.

Chodorow, N. (2008) *The Reproduction of Motherhood*, 6th edn, New York: Columbia University Press.

Cohen, S. (1972) *Folk Devils and Moral Panics*, New York: St. Martin's Press.

Corrêa, S., Petchesky, R. and Parker, R. (2008) *Sexuality, Health and Human Rights*, New York: Routledge.

Cowan, J. K., Dembour, M. and Wilson, R. A. (2001) *Culture and Rights: Anthropological Perspectives*, New York: Cambridge University Press.

D'Emilio, J. and Freedman, E. (1988) *Intimate Matters*, New York: Harper & Row.

Devereux, G. (1937) 'Institutionalized Homosexuality among the Mohave Indians', *Human Biology*, 9: 498–527.

DiMauro, D. and Joffe, C. (2009) 'The Religious Right and the Reshaping of Sexual Policy: Reproductive Rights and Sexuality Education during the Bush Years', in Herdt, G. (ed.) *Moral Panics/Sex Panics*, New York: New York University Press.

Epstein, S. (1999) 'Gay and Lesbian Movements in the United States: Dilemmas of Identity, Diversity and Political Strategy', in Adam, B. D., Duyvendak, J. W. and Krouwel, A. (eds) *The Global Emergence of Gay and Lesbian Politics*, Philadelphia, PA: Temple University Press.

Evans-Pritchard, E. E. (1957) *Essays in Social Anthropology*, London: Clarendon.

Farmer, P. (1999) *Infections and Inequalities: The Modern Plagues*, Berkeley: University of California Press.

Foucault, M. (1980) *The History of Sexuality* (trans. R. Hurley), New York: Viking.

Gagnon, J. (1997) 'Others have Sex with Others: Captain Cook and the Penetration of the Pacific', in Herdt, G., *Sexual Cultures and Migration in the Era of AIDS*, Oxford: Clarendon.

Gagnon, J. (2004) *An Interpretation of Desire*, Chicago: University of Chicago Press.

Gagnon, J. and Simon, W. (1973) *Sexual Conduct: The Social Sources of Human Sexuality*, Chicago: Aldine.

Geertz, C. (1988) *Works and Lives: The Anthropologist as Author*, Stanford, CA: Stanford University Press.

Ginsburg, F. and Rapp, R. (1995) *Conceiving the New World Order*, Berkeley: University of California Press.

Goffman, E. (1959) *Presentation of Self in Everyday Life*, New York: Doubleday.

Goffman, E. (1963) *Stigma*, Englewood Cliffs, NJ: Prentice-Hall.

Harris, M. (2001) *The Rise of Anthropological Theory*, 2nd edn, Walnut Creek, CA: Altamira Press.

Herdt, G. (1981) *Guardians of the Flutes: Idioms Of Masculinity*, New York: McGraw-Hill.

Herdt, G. (1984) 'Ritualized Homosexuality in the Male Cults of Melanesia, 1862–1982: An Introduction', in *Ritualized Homosexuality in Melanesia*, Berkeley: University of California Press.

Herdt, G. (1991) 'Representations of Homosexuality in Traditional Societies: An Essay on Cultural Ontology and Historical Comparison', *Journal of the History of Sexuality*, 2 (2): 603–32.

Herdt, G. (1993) *Third Sex, Third Gender: Beyond Sexual Dimorphism in Culture and History*, New York: Zone Books.

Herdt, G. (1997) *Same Sex, Different Cultures*, Colorado Springs, CO: Westview Press.

Herdt, G. (1999) *Sambia Sexual Culture*, Chicago: University of Chicago Press.

Herdt, G. (2003) *Secrecy and Cultural Reality*, Ann Arbor: University of Michigan Press.

Herdt, G. (2004) 'Sexual Development, Social Oppression, and Local Culture', *Sexuality Research and Social Policy*, 1: 1–24.

Herdt, G. (2008) 'Kinsey', in *International Encyclopedia of the Social Sciences*, 2nd edn, Detroit: Macmillan.

Herdt, G. (2009) *Moral Panics/Sex Panics*, New York: New York University Press.

Herdt, G. and Kertzner, R. (2006) 'I Do, but I Can't: The Impact of Marriage Denial on the Mental Health and Sexual Citizenship of Lesbians and Gay Men in the United States', *Sexuality Research and Social Policy: Journal of the NSRC*, 3 (1): 33–49.

Herdt, G. and Lindenbaum, S. (eds) (1992) *The Time of AIDS*, Thousand Oaks, CA: Sage.

Herdt, G. and Stoller, R. J. (1990) *Intimate Communications: Erotics and the Study of Culture*, New York: Columbia University Press.

Hostetler, A. and Herdt, G. (1998) 'Culture, Sexual Lifeways, and Developmental Subjectivities: Rethinking Sexual Taxonomies', *Social Research*, 65 (2): 249–90.

Hunt, L. (2007) *Inventing Human Rights: A History*, New York: Norton.

Irvine, J. (2000) *Disorders of Desire*, Philadelphia, PA: Temple University Press.

Knauft, B. (1994) 'Foucault meets South New Guinea', *Ethos*, 22: 391–438.

Laumann, E. O., Gagnon, J. H., Michael, R. T. and Michaels, S. (1994) *The Social Organization of Sexuality*, Chicago: University of Chicago Press.

Lewin, E. (ed.) (1996) *Inventing Lesbian Cultures in America*, Boston, MA: Beacon Press.

Lévi-Strauss, C. (1955) *Triste Tropiques*, Paris: Librairie Plon.

Malinowski, B. (1927) *Sex and Repression in Savage Society*, New York: Harcourt, Brace, & Company.

Malinowski, B. (1929) *The Sexual Life of Savages*, London: Routledge.

Malinowski, B. (1967) *A Diary in the Strict Sense of the Term*, London: Routledge & Kegan Paul.

Mead, M. (1935) *Sex and Temperament in Three Primitives Societies*, New York: Norton.

Mead, M. (1949) *Male and Female*, New York: Norton.

Meyer, I. and Northridge, M. E. (eds) (2007) *The Health of Sexual Minorities: Public Health Perspectives on Lesbian, Gay, Bisexual and Transgender Populations*, New York: Springer.

Newton, E. (1972) *Mother Camp*, Chicago: University of Chicago Press.

Newton, E. (1993) *Cherry Grove, Fire Island*, Boston, MA: Beacon Press.

Paige, K. E. and Paige, J. M. (1981) *The Politics of Reproductive Ritual*, Berkeley: University of California Press.

Parker, R. (1991) *Bodies, Pleasures and Passions*, Boston, MA: Beacon Press.

Parker, R. (2007) 'Sexuality, Health and Human Rights', *American Journal of Public Health*, 96: 972–3.

Parker, R. and Gagnon, J. (1995) *Conceiving Sexuality*, New York: Routledge.

Read, K. E. (1965) *The High Valley*, New York: Charles Scribners Sons.

Rosado, M. and Lamphere, L. (1974) *Woman, Culture and Society*, Stanford, CA: Stanford University Press.

Robinson, P. (1967) *The Modernization of Sex*, New York: Harper & Row.

Rubin, G. (1984) 'Thinking Sex: Notes for a Radical Theory of the Politics of Sexuality', in Vance, C. S. (ed.) *Pleasure and Danger: Exploring Female Sexuality*, New York: Routledge & Kegan Paul.

Rubin, G. (1997) 'Elegy for the Valley of the Kings: AIDS and the Leather Community in San Francisco, 1981–1996', in Levine, M. P., Nardi, P. M. and Gagnon, J. H. (eds) *In Changing Times: Gay Men and Lesbians Encounter HIV/AIDS*, Chicago: University of Chicago Press.

Rubin, G. (2002) 'Studying Sexual Subcultures: Excavating the Ethnography of Gay Communities in Urban North America', in Lewin, E. and Leap, E. (eds) *Out in Theory*, Urbana: University of Illinois Press.

Schneider, B. (1997) 'Owning an Epidemic: The Impact of AIDS on Small City Lesbian and Gay Communities', in Levine, M. P., Nardi, P. M. and Gagnon, J. H. (eds) *In Changing Times*, Chicago: University of Chicago Press.

Shweder, R. (1990) 'Cultural Psychology, What is It?', in Stigler, J. W., Shweder, R. A. and Herdt, G. H., *Cultural Psychology*, New York: Cambridge University Press.

Shepard, B. (2006) *Running the Obstacle Course to Sexual and Reproductive Health*, New York: Praeger.

Spiro, M. E. (1982) *Oedipus in the Trobriands*, Chicago: University of Chicago Press.

Teunis, N. and Herdt, G. (2006) 'Sexual Inequalities: Introduction', in *Sexuality Inequalities and Social Justice*, Berkeley: University of California Press.

Valentine, D. (2007) *Imagining Transgender: Ethnography of a Category*, Durham, NC: Duke University Press.

Vance, C. (1999) 'Anthropology Rediscovers Sexuality: A Theoretical Comment', in Parker, R. and Aggleton, P. (eds) *Culture, Society and Sexuality*, London: University College London Press.

Weeks, J. (1985) *Sexuality and Its Discontents*, London: Routledge & Kegan Paul.

Weston, K. (1991). *Families We Choose: Lesbians, Gays, and Kinship*, New York: Columbia University Press.

Young, M. W. (2004) *Malinowski: Odyssey of an Anthropologist*, New Haven, CT: Yale University Press.

4 The importance of being historical

Understanding the making of sexualities

Jeffrey Weeks

We are living in the midst of a long, unfinished but profound revolution that is transforming sexual and intimate life. Across the globe, but especially in the late modern (and capitalist) societies of the old 'west', there have been dramatic changes in family, marital and erotic behaviour, sexual identities, parenting patterns, relationships between men and women, men and men, women and women, adults and young people, and in laws, norms and values. Many of these changes have been, or are still, bitterly contested, but others have been rapidly assimilated. As a result, the true nature of the transformation is easily forgotten, and the complex histories that produced them can all too easily be obliterated. Without a sense of history, and an understanding of the ways we lived in the past, we have no benchmarks by which to measure the magnitude of change, no way of really understanding the present or preparing ourselves for the future (see Weeks 2007). That is why sexual history as it has developed since the 1970s is so important.

The American historian, Vern Bullough (1976: 1–17), famously complained at the beginning of the 1970s that sex in history was a 'virgin field'. Ken Plummer (1975) similarly noted that sociology had sorely neglected sexuality. The study of sexuality was marginal to the key academic disciplines, and threatened to marginalise those who ventured onto the landscape. It made you, in Plummer's phrase, 'morally suspect' (Plummer 1975: 4).

Much has changed. We now know a great deal about such topics as marriage and the family, prostitution and homosexuality, forms of legal and medical regulation, moral codes and religious traditions, masculinities and femininities, women's bodies and health, illegitimacy and birth control, rape and sexual violence, the evolution of sexual identities and sexual practices, transgenderisms and heteronormativities, social networks and oppositional sexualities, and the impact of colonial and postcolonial regimes of power, domination and resistance (Phillips and Reay 2002; Weeks 2000). Historians have deployed sophisticated methods of family reconstitution and demographic history, have intensively searched for new, or interrogated old, documentary sources and made full use of oral and life history interviews to reconstruct the subjective or the tabooed experience. Encouraged by a vigorous grassroots' history, fed by modern feminism and gay and lesbian politics and made urgent by the impact of the HIV crisis, there is now an impressive library of articles, pamphlets, books, films, videos and a mass of cyber-dialogue about all aspects of sexual history, as well as a well-honed critique in the form of queer theory (Weeks 2009).

But having said this, we are still left with a dilemma: What is the magic element that defines some things as sexual and others not? The rejection of essentialist theories gave the sexual a fluidity that challenges as it stimulates intellectual curiosity. The history of sexuality is, as Robert Padgug (1979) suggested, a history of a subject in constant flux. But that, as it has turned out, has become the strength of sexual history. Its originality lies in a willingness by its practitioners to question the naturalness and inevitability of the sexual categories and assumptions we have inherited – including the category of the sexual itself. Gagnon and Simon talked in their pioneering study of *Sexual Conduct* in the early 1970s of the need that may have existed at some unspecified time in the past to *invent* an importance for sexuality (Gagnon and Simon 1973). Michel Foucault, clearly aware of such theorising, was more specific:

> Sexuality must not be thought of as a kind of natural given which power tries to hold in check, or as an obscure domain which knowledge tries gradually to uncover. It is the name that can be given to a historical construct.
>
> (Foucault 1978: 105)

This thesis has been enormously influential. But it has always been wrong to see Foucault in isolation. His work made a vital contribution to the history of sexuality precisely because it grew out of work that was already creatively developing in challenging naturalistic assumptions about the sexual. From social anthropology, sociology and post-Kinsey sex research came a growing awareness of the vast range of sexual practices that exist in other cultures and within our own culture, offering a mirror to our own transitoriness. The 'new social history', with its emphasis on the history of populations and of 'mentalities', the experiences and beliefs of the downtrodden and oppressed as much as the powerful, has posed new questions about what we mean by 'the present' as well as about the 'history of the past' (Weeks 2000). It has also shown the importance of language and discourse in not simply reflecting but constituting the 'real'.

Finally, and most powerfully of all, the emergence of new social movements concerned with sex have challenged many traditional certainties, producing new insights into the power and domination that shapes our sexual lives. The politics of homosexuality have placed on the historical agenda questions about the social explanations of sexual preference, the making of identities, the arbitrariness of sexual categorisations, the significance of entrenched homophobia and the nature of heteronormativity. The women's movement has forced a recognition of the multiple forms of female sexual subordination, from male violence and misogyny to sexual harassment and a pervasive language of sexual denigration and abuse. It has dramatised the institutionalised nature of 'compulsory heterosexuality' (Rich 1984). It has demanded recognition of women's rights over their own bodies by reposing questions about consent and reproductive rights, desire and pleasure.

What the new sexual history, born out of these diverse influences, has done is to open the whole field of the erotic to critical analysis and assessment. What became known as the 'social constructionist' approach to sexuality has been centrally concerned precisely with the diverse ways in which our emotions, desires, erotic practices and intimate relationships are shaped by the societies in which we live (Stein 1992). It is fundamentally concerned with the ways in which sexualities have been shaped in a complex history, and in tracing how sexual patterns have changed over time.

Understanding the present

Despite the hegemony of constructionist approaches, however, sexual history remains a battleground for differing interpretations of the past and present (Weeks 2008a). A naive progressivism, a sort of Whig interpretation of sexual history, which sees the present as an inevitable result of liberalising forces, has long lost any resonance as history has failed to walk in a straight line. But it is in danger of being replaced by a declinist vision that laments the passing of a lost world of social order and family harmony before the 'Great Disruption' (Fukuyama 1999); or by a strange melange of arguments – from neo-Marxists, feminists, queer theorists – that seem to suggest that nothing has really changed at all.

The late modern individual, the argument goes, is forced to live the illusion of freedom while actually being wrapped in the gilded cords of late capitalism (Hennessy 2000; Binnie 2004; Elliott and Lemert 2006). Critics of neoliberalism argue that ideas of individual autonomy and self-responsibilisation are not so much illusory or deceptive as the very forms of regulation that can be most effectively articulated with the current form of capitalist organisation (see Weeks 2007: Chapter 6). As applied to sexuality and intimacy, critiques of neoliberalism often deploy a particular reading of the work of Foucault (for example, Rose 1999; cf. Weeks 2005), which stresses the discursive construction of subjectivities within specific regimes of power. Under neoliberal imperatives, individuals become 'entrepreneurs of themselves, shaping their own lives through the choices they make among the forms of life available to them' (Rose 1999: 230). This elaborate and sophisticated form of subjectivity/subjectification identifies self-governance as the principal form of social regulation.

Recent liberalising sex reforms have been read in this light. Critics of same-sex marriage, for example, have seen it as a move toward creating the respectable gay as opposed to the transgressive, disruptive and challenging queer. 'Respectability' involves a voluntary regulation of the sexual self in the interests of full acceptance and citizenship (Richardson 2004). Some have seen this process working its way through the management of HIV in the 'post-crisis' world (in the west, at least). A surveillance medicine, based on a risk rationality, replaces hospital medicine, with the aim of creating self-reflexive, self-managing subjects. People with HIV learn to calculate and manage risk, using their knowledge of their HIV status, their T-cell count and viral load and the likelihood of infection to negotiate sexual partnerships (Adkins 2002; Davis 2005). An emphasis on individual freedom and rights, and the importance of self-surveillance and regulation for the individual who has internalised the norms and goals of liberal forms of governance, is central to the new society (Richardson 2004).

There are two major problems to my mind in such arguments. First, they tend to deny the reality of many if not most of the changes that have taken place, certainly in the west, and the real gains in terms of human freedom and social justice. The long revolution has been overwhelmingly beneficial to the vast majority of people who have experienced it, despite the problems, inequalities, prejudices and discriminations that remain. Second, they ignore the agency of people, in their millions, who have actually made the changes. Collective struggles – of feminism and lesbian and gay movements especially – have contributed to, complemented, but also often obscured the reality of myriad individual struggles by women and men over many years to gain control over the conditions of their lives – in controlling fertility, entering into freely chosen or escaping oppressive relations, challenging sexual ignorance, battling against sexual violence, affirming sexual identities, having sexual pleasure, avoiding sexual pain. These have been, in Giddens' (1992: 4–17) phrase, 'everyday experiments' in which people have created the conditions for post-traditional ways of life. Unless we understand the impact of these two elements it is impossible to make sense of the history that is making us, and that we make.

The great transition

Between the 1960s and the 2000s, most parts of the western world underwent a historic transformation in sexual beliefs and intimate behaviour – what I call the 'Great Transition'. There was no single cause, no regular pattern across regions and countries, no common agenda for its main actors, chiefly members of the baby-boom generation. The process was messy, contradictory and haphazard. But in the end it drew in and involved millions of people, reimagining and remaking their lives in many different ways.

Among the most important effects are: the separation of sex and reproduction; the separation of sex and marriage; the separation of marriage and parenting; the separation of heterosexuality and parenting; and the separation of heterosexuality and marriage. Together they signal the effective demise of the traditional model of sexual restraint and opened the way to a new moral economy – one that was less hierarchical and more democratic, more hedonistic, more individualistic, more selfish, perhaps, but also one that was vastly more tolerant, experimental and open to diversity and choice in a way that had been inconceivable just a generation earlier. These changes can be traced across a range of historic actors (see Weeks 2008b, on which the following is based).

The position of women remains the most sensitive marker of deep-structured change. On most of the key issues – of education, employment opportunities, family roles, reproductive and sexual choice – there have been major shifts. The category of gender itself has been fundamentally challenged by the emergence of movements of transgendered people (Ekins and King 2006). The gender order (Connell 1987, 1995, 2002) has been shaken, even destabilised.

Many factors underlie the transformations, but a key one has been the dramatic changes in the social relations of reproduction. There was birth control before the pill, and dramatic falls in the birth rate before the 1970s. But the pill, as a woman-controlled and relatively reliable contraceptive, both helped to realise and symbolised a massive shift, a world historic shift indeed: the separation of sex and reproduction (McLaren 1999; Cook 2005).

The issue of reproductive rights has wider resonances: the right to have children as well as not, the right to terminate pregnancies in defined situations as well as to go ahead with them, the right to control fertility and to enhance it. There are also complex issues about non-traditional means of conception and the rights of non-heterosexual parents. Above all, there are fundamental questions of access to resources, of power and opportunity, on a global scale (Petchesky 2003).

The impact of these changes has been uneven. Even the most self-confident women still hear the 'male in the head' (Holland *et al.* 1998) calling them back to sexual subordination. Even the most enlightened men find it difficult to cast off their privileges. Reproductive rights remain a battleground on a global scale. We remain locked in relationships of superiority and subordination at various levels. Violence and abuse still police the boundaries. What has genuinely shifted, however, are the fundamental terms of the debate. The story is not so much that men and women are now equal or treated equally. The real achievement is that inequality has lost all its moral justification.

As the heterosexual nexus linking the gender order, family and sexual reproduction has changed, so homosexuality has come out of the shadows. The sharp binary schism between heterosexuality and homosexuality that defined and distorted the western sexual regime for the past couple of centuries, and perhaps reached a peak in the determined reassertion of the domestic ideology of the 1950s, has been fundamentally undermined as millions of gays and lesbians, bisexuals and transgendered people have not so much subverted the established order as lived as if their sexual difference did not matter (Adam *et al.* 1999; Altman 2001). Perhaps the most significant evidence of this is the growing toleration of same-sex relationships in most western countries: no longer a sin or a sickness, barely a transgression, with same- sex marriage apparently the key issue in many jurisdictions, LGBT lives are in danger of seeming ordinary (Weeks 2007).

That is not, of course, the end of the story. Homosexuality may have come out into the open, it may have made institutionalised heterosexuality porous, but even in the advanced cultures of the west is still subjected to the minoritising forces that excluded it in the first place. In other parts of the world social obloquy, imprisonment, even death (by stoning or beheading) remains the fate of many homosexuals (Bamforth 2005). For far too many, that face of Otherness remains shrouded in mystery and fear, and the result is a terror that makes homosexuality as a way of life impossible. But in large parts of the world the question of same-sex personhood is no longer at issue. The challenge remains to work out the full implications of this in terms of policy and practice, and of equity and social justice.

The gender revolution and the challenge to heteronormativity are underpinned, and accelerated, by a profound change in the ways in which men and women, men and men and women and women relate to one other, by a transformation of intimate life. The transformation, Giddens (1992) argues, is towards egalitarian, open and disclosive relationships, marked by the 'pure relationship'. Same-sex relationships have been seen as especially important to this transformation, as leading the way to more egalitarian forms of relationships and creative life experiments (Weeks *et al.* 2001). There are many critics of this position (see Jamieson 1998, 1999), but behind the controversies there is a longer term trend at work, towards an informalisation and democratisation of intimate life, which has yet unrealised and unsettling implications for the relationship between private passions and public life (Wouters 2004, 2007; Weeks 2007).

Gayle Rubin (1984) famously spoke of the advance of the perverse sexualities out of the pages of Krafft-Ebing onto the stage of history. Today the very category of the perverse has all but disappeared from the diagnostic standards. People proudly proclaim not only their gayness, bisexuality, sado-masochisms, trans-identities, fetishisms and fantasies in all their infinite variety, they can satisfy them through the infinite possibilities of e-media and the internet. We dwell in a world of polymorphous non-perversities (Giddens 1992). But this is only a part of the radical diversity that characterises contemporary life. There are different ways of life, shaped by 'race' and ethnicity, class and geography, age, (dis)ability and so on. There are also, as Gilroy (2004: xi) has argued, new forms of 'conviviality', which defy such simple categorisations and can be said to represent the fraying of difference if not yet the disappearance of divisions.

As this suggests, we can now tell our sexual stories in a huge variety of different ways. Michel Foucault (1978) wrote of the discursive explosion since the eighteenth century which produced sexual modernity. But that was defined by rules on who could speak, in what circumstances and on whose authority. Now we can hear everyone who wants and is able to speak – in talk shows and home movies, in parliaments and in the media, on the streets and in personal blogs. Through stories – of desire and love, of hope and mundane reality, of excitement and disappointment – told to willing listeners in communities of meaning, people imagine and reimagine who and what they are, what they want to become (Plummer 1995, 2003). Now there are many would-be authorities competing cacophonously, especially in the anarchic democracy of cyberspace. By no means all of these voices are progressive by any definition of the word – there are evangelical Christian or radical Islamicist voices as loud as any liberal or libertarian voices. There are threats as well as opportunities in the hypermarket of speech. But we can no longer doubt the power of narratives and the ways in which we can make and remake ourselves through them in the new age of globalisation (Altman 2001; Plummer 2003).

If we can see the globalisation of sexuality as a reordering of risk, then at the heart of the risks facing the world today is the inexorable presence and spread of HIV (see the chapters by Altman, Dowsett and Kippax elsewhere in this volume). Twenty years ago it was possible to write about it largely as a threat to the gay populations of North America, Europe and Australasia. Today the wealthy countries have found ways of managing the progression of the virus. But globally, the statistics, and behind them the realities of everyday life, remain sobering. Here sexuality has become entwined in the nexus of poverty, ignorance, fear and prejudice on a massive scale. The pandemic reveals as nothing else the impossibility of separating the sexual and the intimate from other social forces, and the inevitable flows, in an increasingly globalised world, of sexual experiences and tragedies from nation to nation, continent to continent. AIDS has become the symbol, if not the only example, of the risks of rapid sexual change in a world uncertain of its values and responses.

Uncertainty breeds conflict, the danger of culture wars and the rise of fundamentalisms, both secular and religious. Fundamentalisms especially can be seen as a response to uncertainty, confronting the ambiguities and ambivalences of the world with an absolute certainty about truth, history and tradition (Ruthven 2004). The various forms of fundamentalism, whether Islamic, Christian, Hindu or Jewish, are very much products of late modernity, utilising its technologies and global linkages brilliantly (Bhatt 1997). At their heart is the wish to restore fraying demarcations between men and women, reaffirm heterosexual relationships and extirpate perversity. In their most extreme manifestations, they enforce their will through the bullet, the knife and the hangman's noose. But though the tone and the tenor might be different, the religious and socially conservative movements of the USA and elsewhere, in their affirmation of traditional values and opposition to abortion, homosexuality, same-sex marriage, sex education, evolutionism and the like, share some common assumptions with them: a belief that there is an essential truth to sexuality that they alone know the key to. 'Culture wars' are the inevitable result.

It is in this context that new discourses about sexual or intimate citizenship have emerged (Plummer 1995). Citizenship is about belonging, about being recognised, about reciprocal entitlements and responsibilities. Historically, it has been restricted – racially, xenophobically, by gender and by sexuality (Brandzel 2005). We forget how recent has been the achievement of full citizenship rights for women, to what extent our prized welfare states have been built on assumptions about the right way to live, and on the exclusion of minorities and deviants from the rights and obligations of full citizenship. Sexual or intimate citizenship is about the recognition of these exclusions and about moves to inclusion (Weeks 1998; Bell and Binnie 2000; Richardson 2000a, 2000b; Plummer 2003). The steps in the process have been erratic, and in many jurisdictions, including the most wealthy and most powerful, not yet fully realised. Yet without the idea of full citizenship, we cannot measure how far we have come; and without the ideal of equal citizenship, we have no measure of how far we have yet to go.

This becomes especially challenging in the context of globalisation and 'global sex' (Altman 2001; Corrêa *et al.* 2008). Sexuality has a 'central significance within global regimes of power' (Hemmings *et al.* 2006: 1), and this is manifest in persistent inequities between cultures and in continuing sexual injustices, especially against women, children and lesbian, gay or transgendered identified peoples. At the same time, we see the emergence of global standards of what constitutes justice. We can learn to accept difference and human variety, various ways of being sexual, and this has become a new imperative as we get to know more and more about other cultures. We can understand the power differentials that underpin difference. But, increasingly, in a world not just of different but of conflicting values, many people are also seeking common standards by which to measure behaviours. We have become aware of sufferings across the world where 'before they might have gone unnoticed' (Baird 2004: 8). We can no longer easily fail to notice when the survivors of injustices can tell us of their sufferings across the globalised media, from the internet to television, and when waves of people begin to appear at our own doorsteps, seeking refuge from persecution. Globalisation has made us aware of sexual wrongs across the world, and has awakened us to the significance of sexual rights.

A conclusion

It has become a cliché that sexuality has a history, indeed many histories. But it is easy to forget as we live our own sexual history, that alongside us people are living theirs', and their experience might be quite different from ours. What a historical approach to sexuality can do is make us aware of our commonalities and differences. It should alert us to the ways in which the erotic is shaped in complex relations of power. But it should also make us aware of our contingency.

No one in the 1950s and 1960s, within the lifetime of the postwar baby-boomers who have helped define the era we live in, could have foreseen the world we now inhabit and have helped to remake. We live in a different world. But if we forget our history we are in danger of having to relive it. Perhaps one of the greatest achievements of the long revolution is that it has made us reflexive, sensitive to our own historicity and to the profoundly challenging notion that if we have made our own history we can remake it. There lies the true importance of being historical.

References

Adam, B. D., Duyvendak, J. W. and Krouwel, A. (eds) (1999) *The Global Emergence of Gay and Lesbian Politics: National Imprints of a Worldwide Movement*, Philadelphia, PA: Temple University Press.

Adkins, L. (2002) *Revisions: Gender and Sexuality in Late Modernity*, Buckingham: Open University Press.

Altman, D. (2001) *Global Sex*, Chicago: University of Chicago Press.

Baird, V. (2004) *Sex, Love and Homophobia: Lesbian, Gay, Bisexual and Transgender Lives*, London: Amnesty International.

Bamforth, N. (2005) *Sex Rights*, Oxford Amnesty Lectures, Oxford and New York: Oxford University Press.

Bell, D. and Binnie, J. (2000) *The Sexual Citizen: Queer Politics and Beyond*, Cambridge: Polity Press.

Bhatt, C. (1997) *Liberation and Purity: Race, New Religious Movements and the Ethics of Postmodernity*, London: University College London Press.

Binnie, J. (2004) *The Globalization of Sexuality*, London, Thousand Oaks and New Delhi: Sage.

Brandzel, A. L. (2005) 'Queering Citizenship? Same-sex Marriage and the State', *GLQ: A Journal of Lesbian and Gay Studies*, 11 (2): 171–204.

Bullough, V. L. (1976) 'Sex in History: A Virgin Field', in Bullough, V. L., *Sex, Society and History*, New York: Science History Publications.

Connell, R. W. (1987) *Gender and Power*, Cambridge: Polity Press.

Connell, R. W. (1995) *Masculinities*, Cambridge: Polity Press.

Connell, R. W. (2002) *Gender*, Cambridge: Polity Press.

Cook, H. (2005) *The Long Sexual Revolution: English Women, Sex, and Contraception 1800–1975*, Oxford: Oxford University Press.

Corrêa, S., Petchesky, R. and Parker, R. (2008) *Sexuality, Health and Human Rights*, New York and London: Routledge.

Davis, M. D. M. (2005) 'Treating and Preventing HIV in the Post-crisis Situation: Perspectives from the Personal Experience Accounts of Gay Men with HIV', unpublished PhD thesis, Institute of Education, University of London.

Ekins, R. and King, D. (2006) *The Transgender Phenomenon*, London, Thousand Oaks and New Delhi: Sage.

Elliott, A. and Lemert, C. (2006) *The New Individualism: The Emotional Costs of Globalization*, London and New York: Routledge.

Foucault, M. (1978) *The History of Sexuality: Volume 1: An Introduction*, Harmondsworth: Penguin.

Fukuyama, F. (1999) *The Great Disruption: Human Nature and the Reconstitution of Social Order*, London: Profile Books.

Gagnon, J. H. and Simon, W. (1973) *Sexual Conduct: The Social Sources of Human Sexuality*, London: Hutchinson.

Giddens, A. (1992) *The Transformation of Intimacy: Sexuality, Love and Eroticism in Modern Societies*, Cambridge: Polity Press.

Gilroy, P. (2004) *After Empire: Melancholia or Convivial Culture*, Abingdon: Routledge.

Hemmings, C., Gedalof, I. and Bland, L. (2006) 'Sexual Moralities', *Feminist Review*, 83, 1–3.

Hennessy, R. (2000) *Profit and Pleasure: Sexual Identities in Late Capitalism*, New York and London: Routledge.

Holland, J., Ramazanoglu, C., Sharpe, S. and Thomson, R. (1998) *The Male in the Head*, London: Tufnell Press.

Jamieson, L. (1998) *Intimacy: Personal Relationships in Modern Societies*, Cambridge: Polity Press.

Jamieson, L. (1999) 'Intimacy Transformed: A Critical Look at the "Pure Relationship"', *Sociology*, 33 (3): 447–94.

McLaren, A. (1999) *Twentieth-Century Sexuality: A History*, Oxford: Blackwell.

Padgug, R. A. (1979) 'Sexual Matters: On Conceptualizing Sexuality in History', *Radical History Review*, 20: Spring/Summer.

Petchesky, R. (2003) 'Negotiating Reproductive Rights', in Weeks, J., Holland, J. and Waites, M. (eds) *Sexualities and Society: A Reader*, Cambridge: Polity Press.

Phillips, K. M. and Reay, B. (eds) (2002) *Sexualities in History: A Reader*, New York and London: Routledge.

Plummer, K. (1995) *Telling Sexual Stories: Power, Change and Social Worlds*, London: Routledge.

Plummer, K. (1975) *Sexual Stigma: An Interactionist Account*, London: Routledge & Kegan Paul.

Plummer, K. (2003) *Intimate Citizenship: Private Decisions and Public Dialogues*, Seattle: University of Washington Press.

Rich, A. (1984) 'Compulsory Heterosexuality and Lesbian Existence', in Snitow, A., Stansell, C. and Thompson, S. (eds) *Desire: The Politics of Homosexuality*, London: Virago.

Richardson, D. (2000a) *Rethinking Sexuality*, London and Thousand Oaks: Sage.

Richardson, D. (2000b) 'Claiming Citizenship? Sexuality, Citizenship and Lesbian/ Feminist Theory', *Sexualities*, 3 (2): 255–72.

Richardson, D. (2004) 'Locating Sexualities: From Here to Normality', *Sexualities*, 7 (4): 391–411.

Rose, N. (1999) *Governing the Soul: The Shaping of the Private Self*, 2nd edn, London and New York: Free Associations Books.

Rubin, G. (1984) 'Thinking Sex: Notes for a Radical Theory of the Politics of Sexuality', in Vance, C. S. (ed.) *Pleasure and Danger. Exploring Female Sexuality*, London and Boston: Routledge & Kegan Paul.

Ruthven, M. (2004) *Fundamentalism: The Search for Meaning*, Oxford: Oxford University Press.

Stein, E. (ed.) (1992) *Forms of Desire: Sexual Orientation and the Social Construction Controversy*, New York and London: Routledge.

Weeks, J. (1998) 'The Sexual Citizen', *Theory, Culture and Society*, 15 (3–4): 35–52.

Weeks, J. (2000) *Making Sexual History*, Cambridge: Polity Press.

Weeks, J. (2005) 'Remembering Foucault', *Journal of the History of Sexuality*, 14 (1/2): 186–201.

Weeks, J. (2007) *The World We Have Won: The Remaking of Erotic and Intimate Life*, Abingdon: Routledge.

Weeks, J. (2008a) 'Traps We Set Ourselves', *Sexualities*, 11 (1/2): 27–32.

Weeks, J. (2008b) 'Rewriting Sexuality and History', in Edwards, R. (ed.), *Researching Families and Communities: Social and Generational Change*, Abingdon and New York: Routledge.

Weeks, J. (2009) *Sexuality*, 3rd edn, Abingdon, New York: Routledge.

Weeks, J., Heaphy, B. and Donovan, C. (2001) *Same Sex Intimacies: Families of Choice and other Life Experiments*, London: Routledge.

Wouters, C. (2004) *Sex and Manners: Female Emancipation in the West, 1890–2000*, London, Thousand Oaks and New Delhi: Sage.

Wouters, C. (2007) *Informalization: Manners and Emotions since 1890*, Los Angeles, London, New Delhi and Singapore: Sage.

5 Research innovation
Alfred C. Kinsey's legacy and the Kinsey Institute for Research in Sex, Gender, and Reproduction

Julia R. Heiman

A core belief of those engaged in sex research is that broad and deep knowledge about sexuality and reproduction is a necessary perquisite for a healthy society and respectful human rights. Simply put, knowledge can and does save lives. Research is one pathway to knowledge and is valuable because its methods are 'public' and available for critique, replication, confirmation or revision. In this chapter, I aim to connect together the initial and current trajectory of the Kinsey Institute's efforts to research sex, gender and reproduction with the larger attempt to understand and improve the human condition with regard to sexuality. While there might be many approaches to this topic, I have selected the theme of innovation with which to organise these comments. Innovation emphasises two key aspects of research: to truly innovate, one must be aware of the past, and, since innovation is trying to exert a change in an uncertain or unwilling environment, there is a greater risk of failure.

Historical elements

There are few research efforts in any field including sex research that have convincingly made an impact on the field and the broader society. Alfred C. Kinsey's work with his colleagues is one of those efforts. This research emerged in response to something missing – the lack of data on sexual behaviour as Kinsey prepared to teach a course to college students in large university (Indiana University) in a small town (Bloomington, Indiana) in the middle of the USA. Kinsey, importantly, was a biologist interested in evolution via the taxonomy of gall wasps, used to travelling significant distances with his graduate students to find his specimens, and convinced that large samples, especially in several selected locations, contributed to knowledge (e.g. Kinsey 1944). Kinsey's uniquely driving intellect, as evidenced from his collection of over seven million gall wasps at the Museum of Natural History (New York City), then turned to the topic of human sexual behaviour. It is no wonder that he thought collecting sexual history data on 100,000 individual humans in the USA could be accomplished and why the over 18,000 he did collect was (for him) not sufficient. But the man and the research team are only part of the answer to what made their work impactful. The postwar country was almost ready to listen to the report on males, in 1948, the date of the first book on male sexual behaviour (Kinsey *et al.* 1948). It was at least bearable, although still shocking, that men were sexual (albeit hard to acknowledge they also were so frequently masturbating, having extramarital affairs and reporting same-sex experiences). Kinsey's work was upsetting but, more or less tolerably so until the second book on females in 1953 (Kinsey *et al.* 1953). Statistical sampling issues were part of the criticism that the research faced. But it was primarily public reactions to the mirror held up to female sexuality, perhaps combined with Kinsey's being outspoken about his opinions about the data, which were particularly perceived as outrageous. Funding problems followed. The data and what they revealed, in how different they were from public assumptions about sexuality, were the primary fuels in the reactions.

What might be instructive for us, including most of us who are 'post-Kinseyian', in the sense that our work methods and assumptions are not based on his directly? We know that he opened a door for inquiry into sexuality in an important data-based way. Behind that critical step was an essential confluence of factors that allowed his innovative work to have impact:

1 the identification of missing information and the lack of understanding or problem of importance;
2 an accomplished scientist leading the team who was willing to charge ahead into a different field and methodology, from gall wasp taxonomy to human behaviour;
3 a strong and determined personal will and committed team to get the project done in spite of obstacles;
4 a culture that was energised, having emerged from a consuming depression and world war into rapid economic expansion, to react on many levels (legal, medical, media), which increased the impact of the data.

But there was another important issue, namely the Institute for Sex Research (its name changed in 1981 to the Kinsey Institute for Research in Sex, Gender, and Reproduction) was established in 1947 at Indiana University as a non-profit corporation, to help protect its work and collections from the pressures that Indiana University faced as a publicly funded institution in a conservative state. The university president at the time, Herman Wells, was responsible for helping to set up this structure, and was himself directly and forcefully involved in defending academic freedom and the right to study all types of topic, including sexuality (Christenson 1971).

Do all innovative studies of sex research need this kind of formula to succeed? Not necessarily, but they clearly need more than bright minds, hard work and well-meaning individuals. A broader social structure to support the forging of new directions is valuable, although rare. Instead, allies in key places (funding, political, community) can be essential to protect the conduct of socially sensitive work.

It is clear that innovation is not a safe and predicable path. Innovation can take an unexpectedly long time to show results, and it may fail to produce anything of value or produce something that current society does not want to accept. Innovative efforts are often not welcomed but instead challenged, especially if they are too different from current perspectives. William Masters and Virginia Johnson's (1966, 1970) research observing and measuring human sexual response in a laboratory setting and then suggesting the non-medical treatment of sexual dysfunctions were shocking at the time, even for some professional groups. Masters was ostracised from mainstream gynaecological practice even though he had been known to be an excellent surgeon. They were also severely critiqued by those currently treating sexual disorders, who distrusted the new 'sex therapy' techniques for treatment that focused on couples doing sexual assignments in private. Kinsey encouraged Masters, whose photo, taken when Masters was visiting the Institute, is still displayed on the Institute's entry walls.

It is fair to say that the Kinsey Institute has been supportive of pursing rare or new ideas since its inception. Among the specific groundbreaking ideas of the time, emerging from his data on human histories, was that sexual orientation, taking experience and 'psychic reactions' into account, was best represented as a continuum between exclusive heterosexuality and exclusive homosexuality, resulting in his seven-point rating scale (Kinsey *et al.* 1948). It seemed, beginning with Kinsey himself, that the Institute created a safe territory to take intellectual chances and as a result attracted researchers with a bent toward forging new (sometimes unsafe) paths. Examples of people who spent significant periods of time based at the Institute, for example, include John Gagnon, William Simon, Martin Weinberg, Collin Williams, and directors such as Paul Gebhard, June Reinisch and John Bancroft. Others were visiting scholars over time, including Anke Ehrhardt, Gunther Schmidt and many others. In addition, the work of an array of researchers or clinicians, including William Masters, Harry Benjamin and John Money, were to varying degrees impacted by the Institute. Traditionally, the Institute works to attract researchers whose work has been innovative and help new young researchers for ideas that show promise. Thus, an effort to encourage innovation has been one theme of the Kinsey Institute research tradition that continues today. For discussion here, I will single out two areas where innovation remains in high demand for the field: methodology and theory/model development.

Methods and innovation

Regarding methodology, one could arguably say that sampling and measurement are the most central issues. Sampling remains a significant and often under-considered problem in psychological and medical research (less so in sociological) and does ultimately determine the extent to which the findings can be generalised. In fact, Kinsey's sampling method was rather innovative but it ultimately lost to the rising and now dominant valuing of random probability sampling (Laumann *et al.* 1994). The Institute has not itself championed sampling strategy innovations or the related issues of statistical solutions, opting instead to work with the expertise of colleagues.

Measurement, by way of contrast, is a significant focus and concern of the Institute. Measurement in sexuality research is underdeveloped, and funding limitations in the field have contributed to this problem. Measurement is the basis of constructing any database, whether the database is made up of the narratives study participants give us or the physical responses and fluids we collect. The Kinsey Institute has fostered, in its own work and that of others:

• the construction of and testing of new measures;
• and openness to combining physiological and self-report measurement.

Examples of the former are researchers hired or collaborated with who had worked, prior to joining the Institute, on new measurement approaches to genital sexual arousal, such as the vaginal photoplethysmograph developed at Stony Brook University (Sintchak and Geer 1975; Heiman 1977) and the use of pelvic MRI imaging, first explored at the University of Washington School of Medicine, to study clitoral sexual arousal patterns (Maravilla *et al.* 2003, 2005). A labial photopletymograph was also developed at the Institute (Prause *et al.* 2005). Work currently underway (2009) has been funded to help test a promising new measure of female sexual response developed by a team in Massachusetts (Sachtler 2008).

In terms of self-report measures, the principles and content of sexual history interviewing, not technically a self-report measure but an interview format, was established by the Kinsey team and is written about in the original work (Kinsey *et al.* 1948, 1953). Since then, scale development examples include the Sexual Inhibition and Sexual Excitation Scales (SIS/SES) by Janssen and colleagues (2002a, 2002b) to begin to tap into the dual process theory they were developing. Other Kinsey Institute researchers worked on a different, focus group-based version for women (Graham *et al.* 2006). A Mood and Sexuality Questionnaire (Bancroft *et al.* 2003a, 2003b) was developed to test the effect of acute mood on sexual response and risk taking. As with physiological instruments, some researchers came to the Institute with a history of working on measurement development as a collaborative enterprise. This includes sexual function measurement in cancer survivors (Syrjala *et al.* 2000), sexual functioning in women (Rosen *et al.* 2000; Quirk *et al.* 2002) and sexual distress in women (Derogatis *et al.* 2002). Collaborating with those interested in behavioural genetics similarly has underscored the relative value of other measurement approaches (Harris *et al.* 2008).

New measures allow for questions to be researched that otherwise could not be pursued. Coincidentally, given that every measure has limitations, the weaknesses of any given measure may become more 'accepted' or defended and slow efforts to improve on it. For sexuality, the issue of genital measurement is instructive. The use of genital measurement has been somewhat of a battle both in the research community and politically. A reasonably good, albeit of limited application, genital measure for women's sexual arousal was designed in the 1970s (Sintchak and Geer 1975), and pelvic imaging has been used more recently to document anatomical structures during sexual response (Suh *et al.* 2004). Only when the PDE-5 medications (sildenafil citrate, Viagra™ being the first) proved so successful for men were women's genitals again of research interest, at least of commercial interest, freeing up some funding to document genital changes during sexual response studies. From the research side, there has been a tendency among some researchers to view genital measurement as irrelevant and reductionist. In addition, the HIV epidemic research captured much sex research attention between 1980 and today, pursuing a focus on other non-genital measures related to risk of HIV transmission.

In addition to measurement development, the past 20 years of the Institute's work has fostered a combination of physiological and subjective measures where appropriate to a given research question. Often this has been in laboratory contexts with exposure to various stimuli and measurement of physiological signs of sexuality, stress, negative or positive affect and, more recently, sexual interest and reward dependency. This combined measure approach is especially useful when studying clinical conditions or samples at risk (Rowland and Heiman 1991; Kuffel and Heiman 2006; Janssen *et al.* 2009). The use of functional magnetic resonance imaging (fMRI) methods in order to incorporate menstrual cycle phases and sexual decision making, is helping to more directly test theories of mate choice and risk taking (Rupp *et al.* 2009a, 2009b).

Researchers at the Institute and the University of Amsterdam are currently collaborating on a project combining two physiological measures, two implicit measures, subjective measures and standardised and new self-report scales to study women's sexual desire. Not every study could and should be this extensive but for the questions we are posing, the willingness to combine measurements can help reveal both the stability and flexibility of sexual response and its relationship to sexual desire. We are still quite a long way from understanding exactly how response patterns vary at different ages and under different psychological (stress, depression, anxiety) or physical (alcohol, hormonal conditions, medication) conditions (see Janssen 2007).

Theory and theoretical model development

Theory, especially a general encompassing theory of human sexuality, remains incompletely articulated. Kinsey's own work started from an evolutionary stance but he never fully applied evolutionary theory to explain the wide variation in sexual patterns. The term 'evolution' is not indexed in the male volume and it occurs in the female volume primarily when phylogenic origins of patterns are discussed. Kinsey was most likely predisposed to value variability as he looked for that in his gall wasp work and it is the basis from which evolution can selectively proceed. Today, evolutionary theory is often invoked to explain sex differences, mate choice and even sexual risk taking but, unlike evolutionary biology, evolutionary psychology has a limited and contentious level of acceptance and testable applicability.

While the Institute does not have a steady history in theory construction, two lines of theoretical development deserve mention. One is Gagnon and Simon's theoretical work (1973) on sociosexual scripting. Gagnon was at the Institute from 1959 to 1968 and Simon from 1965 to 1968. Their published work during that period was more focused on sexual deviance addressing social deviance and the violation of cultural norms more broadly. Their remarkable collaboration later resulted in one of the more enduring theoretical perspectives to date that can in fact be tested or used heuristically. Social scripting theory deeply connects the individual's development with the accompanying social pressures in a way that permits fluidity and change on a human timescale. Biological events are secondary to the power of the narrative and accompanying role provided by that narrative. Scripting theory has expanded its relevance as the HIV epidemic, sexual dysfunction treatment and sexual and gender identity issues became more part of the social fabric especially in the USA (see, for example, Gagnon 1990).

A less developed but potentially very integrative model arising from collaboration at the Institute is the dual control model of Bancroft and Janssen (2000) originally articulated for erectile dysfunction in men but more recently broadened to women (Bancroft *et al.* 2009). The model posits that sexual responses involve an interaction between sexual excitatory and sexual inhibitory processes that vary across individuals and contribute to the wide variability seen in human sexuality. While the theoretical model is relatively untested, it has the potential for being able to inform research from the molecular to the social level. The authors have also developed self-report scales to tap parts of the constructs (see earlier) and propose a relevance to gender differences and similarities, sexual development across the lifespan and sexual desire. Further research will determine the value and the applicability of the model.

Future directions

The most likely major influences on the conduct of sex research are economics worldwide and social forces impacting human health and migration. Changes in these areas will require innovation to address them. In the near future – the next 5–10 years – I expect that greater use of the internet to gather and disseminate research-based information worldwide will be crucial, especially for younger generations. The growth of online communities and virtual worlds may also have significant impact on sexual patterns and mate choice. The recognition of genetic and epigenetics research and its reproductive implications will be important to track and, for the social sciences, to work with, as it is clear that genetics will not fully explain who we are sexually or what we do with our sexuality in different cultural contexts. The task of sex research will be to be at least as innovative as the changes coming our way.

References

Bancroft, J. and Janssen, E. (2000) 'The Dual Control Model of Male Sexual Response: A Theoretical Approach to Centrally Mediated Erectile Dysfunction', *Neuroscience and Biobehavioral Reviews*, 24: 571–9.

Bancroft, J., Graham, C. A., Janssen, E. and Sanders, S. (2009) 'The Dual Control Model: Current Status and Future Directions', *Journal of Sex Research*, 46: 121–42.

Bancroft, J., Janssen, E., Strong, D., Carnes, L., Vukadinovic, Z. and Long, J. S. (2003a) 'The Relation between Mood and Sexuality in Heterosexual Men', *Archives of Sexual Behavior*, 32: 217–30.

Bancroft, J., Janssen, E., Strong, D. and Vukadinovic, Z. (2003b) 'The Relation between Mood and Sexuality in Gay Men', *Archives of Sexual Behavior*, 32: 231–42.

Christenson, C. V. (1971) *Kinsey: A Biography*, Bloomington: Indiana University Press.

Derogatis, L. R., Rosen, R. C., Leiblum S., Burnett, A. and Heiman, J. R. (2002) 'The Female Sexual Distress Scale (FSDS): Initial Validation of a Standardized Scale for Assessment of Sexually Related Personal Distress in Women', *Journal of Sex and Marital Therapy*, 28: 317–30.

Gagnon, J. H. and Simon, W. (1973) *Sexual Conduct: The Social Sources of Human Sexuality*, Chicago: Aldine.

Gagnon, J. H. (1990) 'The Explicit and Implicit Use of the Scripting Perspective in Sex Research', *Annual Review of Sex Research*, 1: 1–43.

Graham, C. A., Sanders, S. A. and Milhausen, R. R. (2006) 'The Sexual Excitation/Sexual Inhibition Inventory for Women: Pyschometric Properties', *Archives of Sexual Behavior*, 35: 1–13.

Harris, J. M, Cherkas, L. F., Kato, B. S., Heiman, J. R. and Spector, T. D. (2008) 'Normal Variations in Personality are Associated with Coital Orgasmic Infrequency in Heterosexual Women: A Population-based Study', *Journal of Sexual Medicine*, 5: 1177–83.

Heiman, J. (1977) 'A Psychophysiological Exploration of Sexual Arousal Patterns in Females and Males', *Psychophysiology*, 14: 266–74.

Janssen, E. (2007) *The Psychophysiology of Sex*, Bloomington: Indiana University Press.

Janssen, E., Goodrich, D., Petrocelli, J. and Bancroft, J. (2009) 'Psychophysiological Response Patterns and Risky Sexual Behavior in Heterosexual and Homosexual Men', *Archives of Sexual Behavior*, 38: 528–50.

Janssen, E., Vorst, H., Finn, P. and Bancroft, J. (2002a) 'The Sexual Inhibition (SIS) and Sexual Excitation (SES) Scales: I. Measuring Sexual Inhibition and Excitation Proneness in Men', *Journal of Sex Research*, 39: 114–26.

Janssen, E., Vorst, H., Finn, P. and Bancroft, J. (2002b) 'The Sexual Inhibition (SIS) and Sexual Excitation (SES) Scales: II. Predicting Psychophysiological Response Patterns', *Journal of Sex Research*, 39: 127–32.

Kinsey, A. C. (1944) 'Isolating Mechanisms in Gall Wasps', *Biological Symposia*, 6: 251–69.

Kinsey, A. C., Pomeroy, W. B. and Martin, C. E. (1948) *Sexual Behavior in the Human Male*, Bloomington: W. B. Saunders Company.

Kinsey, A. C., Pomeroy, W. B., Martin, C. E. and Gebhard, P. H. (1953) *Sexual Behavior in the Human Female*, Bloomington: W. B. Saunders Company.

Kuffel, S. W. and Heiman, J. R. (2006) 'Effects of Depressive Symptoms and Experimentally Adopted Schemas on Sexual Arousal and Affect in Sexually Healthy Women', *Archives of Sexual Behavior*, 35: 163–78.

Laumann, E. O., Gagnon, J. H., Michael, R. T. and Michaels, S. (1994) *The Social Organization of Sexuality. Sexual practices in the United States*, Chicago: University of Chicago Press.

Maravilla, K. R., Cao, Y., Heiman, J. R., Garland, P. A., Peterson, B. T., Carter, W. O. *et al.* (2003) 'Serial MR Imaging with MS-325 for Evaluating Female Sexual Arousal Response: Determination of Intrasubject Reproducibility', *Journal of Magnetic Resonance Imaging*, 18: 216–24.

Maravilla, K. R., Cao, Y., Heiman, J. R., Yang, C., Garland, P. A., Peterson, B. T. *et al.* (2005) 'Noncontrast Dynamic Magnetic Resonance Imaging for Quantitative Assessment of Female Sexual Arousal', *Journal of Urology*, 172: 162–6.

Masters, W. H. and Johnson, V. E. (1966) *Human Sexual Response*, Boston, MA: Little Brown.

Masters, W. H. and Johnson, V. E. (1970) *Human Sexual Inadequacy*, Boston, MA: Little Brown.

Prause, N., Cerny, J. and Janssen, E. (2005) 'The Labial Photoplethysmograph: A New Instrument for Assessing Genital Hemodynamic Changes in Women', *Journal of Sexual Medicine*, 2: 58–65.

Quirk, F. H., Heiman, J. R., Rosen, R., Laan, E., Smith, M. D. and Boolell, M. (2002) 'Development of a Sexual Function Questionnaire (SFQ) for Clinical Trials of Female Sexual Dysfunction (FSD)', *Journal of Women's Health and Gender-based Medicine*, 11: 277–89.

Rosen, R., Brown, C., Heiman, J., Leiblum, S., Meston, C., Shabsigh, R. *et al.* (2000) 'The Female Sexual Function Index (FSFI): A Multidimensional Self-report Instrument for the Assessment of Female Sexual Function', *Journal of Sex and Marital Therapy*, 26: 191–208.

Rowland, D. and Heiman, J. (1991) 'Self-reported and Genital Changes in Sexually Functional Men following a Sex Therapy Program', *Journal of Psychosomatic Research*, 35: 609–19.

Rupp, H. A., James, T. W., Ketterson, E. D., Sengelaub, D. R., Janssen, E. and Heiman, J. R. (2009a) 'The Role of the Anterior Cingulate in Women's Sexual Decision Making', *Neuroscience Letters*, 449: 42–7.

Rupp, H. A., James, T. W., Ketterson, E. D., Sengelaub, D. R., Janssen, E. and Heiman, J. R. (2009b) 'Women's Neural Activation in Response to Masculinized versus Feminized Male Faces; Mediation by Hormones and Psychosexual Factors', *Evolution and Human Behavior*, 30: 1–10.

Sachtler, W. L. (2008) 'Female Sexual Dysfunction Diagnostic Tool Development. 2R44DK066877-02A1', National Institutes of Health: National Institute of Diabetes and Digestive and Kidney Diseases.

Sintchak, G. and Geer, J. H. (1975) 'A Vaginal Plethysmograph System', *Psychophysiology*, 12: 113–15.

Suh, D. D., Yang, C. C., Cao, Y., Heiman, J. R., Garland, P. A. and Maravilla, K. R. (2004) 'MRI of Female Genital and Pelvic Organs during Sexual Arousal: Initial Experience', *Journal of Psychosomatic Obstetrics and Gynaecology*, 25: 1531–62.

Syrjala, K. L., Schroeder, T. C., Abrams, J. R., Atkins, T. Z., Brown, W. S., Sanders, J. E. *et al.* (2000) 'Sexual Function Measurement and Outcomes in Cancer Survivors and Matched Controls', *Journal of Sex Research*, 37: 213–25.

6 The social reality of sexual rights

Ken Plummer

When people define situations as real they become real in their consequences.

(Thomas 1932: 572)

A person has as many selves as there are situations.

(James 1985: 93)

A separate individual is an abstraction unknown to experience, and so likewise is society when regarded as something apart from individuals. The real thing is human life.

(Cooley 1956: 36–7)

This chapter suggests a way of looking at issues of human sexual rights. It focuses on how human beings are symbol manipulating creatures living their lives embodied and embedded in different kinds of historical and social situation. Human life unfolds precariously in a heaving universe of contingency and change.

At its heart there is an ontology of the human being as a bundle of potentials and capabilities that need appropriate social conditions in order to flourish. Without the right social conditions, human life becomes flawed and damaged and prone to too much suffering: lives become 'wasted.' In the important work of Amartya Sen (1999) and Martha Nussbaum (1999), there is a listing of what these human capabilities could be for all human beings. They include: life; health; bodily integrity; senses, imagination and thought; emotions; practical reason; affiliation and recognition; the ability to play; some control over one's environment; and, finally, an ability to live with other species expressed in a concern for and in relation to animals, plants and the world of nature. Such a list offers a good starting point for thinking about what a human life needs to develop if it is to flourish.

My critical focus in this humanist task is through one focused route into this position: namely, the century-old stance of symbolic interaction.

Symbolic interactionism, critical humanism and sexual conduct

The traditions of symbolic interactionism are long, and not without schisms and controversies. Interactionist thought have their origins in the Stoical philosophical traditions of the ancients. In recent times, they were born again in the philosophies and pragmatism of William James, John Dewey, Charles S. Peirce, George Herbert Mead; in the poetics of Emerson, Thoreau and Whitman; in the more formal theorising of Georg Simmel and others; and in the down-to-earth fieldwork of sociologists and reformers like Robert Park, W. I. Thomas and Jane Adams. The term symbolic interactionism was coined in 1937 by Herbert Blumer and its ideas informed the work of Everett Hughes, Howard S. Becker and Anselm Strauss. It has undergone a philosophical renewal in the work of Richard Rorty and Sidney Hook. And there are many affinities with cultural anthropology, cultural historians, humanistic social psychologies and (some) postmodern and cultural theorists.

At its heart, symbolic interaction offers a grounded, practical and everyday approach to social life and social understanding. It sees human beings as bundles of potentials living everyday lives in local contexts through doing things together, and struggling to make meaning in their daily lives. The symbolic nature of human life is central to understanding; these meanings are never transcendental, essential or fixed but are ambiguous and contested. Social life is emergent. At its heart lies the process of language and communication and the ability to recognise, interpret and understand 'others.' But it is deeply and always precarious and unfolding.

All human beings dwell in what we might call 'Otherness.' To live, like it or not, we have to become attuned to others – to develop role-taking ability, to acquire sympathy and to empathise with fellow humans, and sometimes other animals. If we fail this, social life as we know it simply could not continue. Life is embroiled in metaphor – it can be seen as a journey and a struggle in the acquisition of meaning as we tell the stories of our lives and our times. And so we come to define ourselves, our bodies and others; our pasts, our presents and our futures. It matters hugely how we make these definitions and how we construct our symbols: we must be cautious, for, when people define situations as real they may well become real in their consequences.

Symbolic interactionism is one of a range of accounts of the world that, taken together, may be called *critical humanism*. The core of their ontology is a fragile sense of what it is to be a human being. We are indeed specks of dust in a boundless universe, being, as Ernest Becker once argued, profoundly, the 'little Gods who shit' (Becker 1973: 58). We are little animals striving to make sense of our lives through elaborate symbols in a universe so vast it defies comprehension. And yet, at the same time, we need to grasp our human vulnerability and place it at the heart of our thinking. The grand abstraction and the search for universals is bound to falter and we are usually better working with a theory of the human being that is grounded, practical and charged with doing things, usually together with others.[1]

Understanding sexualities

Flowing from this view of social life is a distinctive view of sexualities: one that is largely at odds both with popular naturalistic and biological accounts ('sex is natural') and with more sophisticated Freudian theories (who tend to 'read' sex and desire into everything). My approach is a much more practical and down-to-earth approach to sexuality that focuses on the ways in which sexual symbols and meanings are generated and transformed constantly in everyday life, across lives and across history. Culture, power and ethics play crucial roles in the organisation of such negotiated meanings, which connect closely with emotions, bodies and selves.

This way of thinking has a long lineage but started to gain popularity in the 1960s through the work of John Gagnon and William Simon, two sociologists who were working at the Kinsey Institute for Sex Research. They drew from their Chicago-based training in fieldwork, were influenced by the work of the literary theorist Kenneth Burke for whom 'symbolicity' was so central; and borrowed ideas from their influential peer – Erving Goffman, and his idea of dramaturgy and social stage-craft. The peak point of their writing was the syntheses of papers they created in *Sexual Conduct: The Social Sources of Human Sexuality*, first published in 1973 and reprinted, in slightly revised form in 2005. The book, as Simon said years later, 'was actually a series of essays rather than a coherent linear text' (Simon 1999: 130). But it has been hugely influential.

Their most influential idea was the metaphor of sexual scripting. Rather than seeing sexuality as a biological drive or gender as a fixed essence, sexuality should be seen as meanings organised loosely into scripts that suggest *who* people are sexually and what *others* they can desire sexually, *what* they can do sexually, *where* and *when* they can do it and also explain to them *why* they do it. Such scripts change from society to society, group to group, person to person and even within the same person. Scripts are not fixed but are wide open to improvisation. They can be examined at a wide *social* level (historical, cultural), at an *interpersonal* level (what people do with each other) and psychically (how people come to inhabit their own emotional and symbolic sexual worlds and sexual scripts).

This is account of sexualities shaped a great deal of further thinking and research. It encourages us to look for symbols of sexualities: look for the meanings and the histories of self, of conduct, the stories we tell about it and the wider cultural sense of it. It makes us think about how we give meaning to our bodies and our feelings, our fantasies and our relationships, our lives and our histories. It encourages attention to be focused on the ways in which sexualities are moulded through interactional webs and networks. Finally, it sees sexuality as emergent: not as a fixed essence or thing but always on the move, flowing, developing and changing. The question here is to find ways of capturing – albeit momentarily – this flux and flow: the doings, feelings and tellings of our meaning-making sexualities assembled with others, in a world of profound divisions and inequalities (cf. Plummer 2005).

Some theses on human rights

With these background issues in mind, I want now to turn to human rights. Although 'human rights' have a long history, I take them to be a thoroughly contested field. Across the world, the issues the idea raises have been widely challenged and debated. Those who suggest that rights are straightforward, inalienable, uncontested – and many do – work from a shallow and culturally limited ideas of rights. One day being active in any of the multitudinous social movements working for human rights, or reading the massive and polarised literatures on human rights – in law, in politics, in sociology – would surely reveal just how contested notions of human rights are. Symbolic interactionism and critical humanism provide one major tool into thinking about all this.

Pragmatism and everyday life

Human social life is a grounded, practical affair. This is also true of human rights. Human rights are everyday matters of great practical importance to the everyday lives of practical people as they go about their daily rounds of sufferings and joys. Hence, while there are indeed some great philosophical writings and some hugely important abstract documents of rights – notably the Declaration of Independence, 1776; the Declaration of the Rights of Man and Citizen, 1789; and the Universal Declaration of Human Rights, 1948 – these have all been born of blood and human suffering: the French Revolution, the War of Independence, the two world wars, the Holocaust, the Stalinist/Maoist purges. Millions have been slaughtered both in the name of rights and in order that such grand statements could be produced. Such grand abstract documents conceal a multitude of battles (cf. Grayling 2007; Hunt 2007).

Although rights can be analysed abstractly (and usually are), the task for social researchers is to become intimately familiar with the crusaders, their claims and the social processes through which rights emerge and are made public. There is an important need to see 'rights' as part of the day-to-day world of lived meaning, and not simply belonging to the theoretical and philosophical or even legal heavens. Thus, when we hear the term human rights we always need to ask: Whose rights? What rights? Why are rights being claimed here? And where and when? The very idea means many things to many people and it has throughout different cultures and different historical periods.

Claims for sexual rights are recent (see Coleman and Cottingham elsewhere in this volume) – they are not to be found in the classical statements as such, but have to be read into them. All rights work takes place in morally grounded activities and political practices; and with issues of sexual rights traditional moralities clash furiously with those advocating progressive changes (Hunter 1990). There is a major conflict over defining what it means to live a good life and to be human. Abstractions may be used in the arguments; but the actual battles are very down to earth and we need to understand how they take place (Plummer 2003).

Meanings, signs and symbols

Human social life can only be understood with due attention to its symbolic nature and the full range of ever ambiguous human meaning. This is also true of human rights. Human rights are powerful symbols, but their meanings constantly shift across times, spaces, groups. The term has variously meant 'security' (Hobbes), 'life, liberty and property' (Locke), 'freedom' (Kant), 'life, liberty, and the pursuit of happiness' (Paine) and so on. These days notions of rights are often linked to ideas of citizenship (see Corrêa and Petchesky elsewhere in this volume), and there are many versions of this too: economic, legal, welfare, intimate, cultural, feminist, global and so on (Isin and Turner 2002).

The idea of human rights is always an emergent and contested symbol. Symbolic interactionism places the symbol at the centre of its thinking – and stresses the triadic nature of meaning for humans. Thus meaning appears as we approach an object such as human rights, it is then handled and manipulated as we try to put it into action and then is itself further modified as it emerges through its outcomes. Human rights are not – by their very symbolic character – ever capable of standing still. They are always ambiguous and emergent. We may declare human rights in various declarations – but behind these declarations exist huge human struggles for meanings. We know too that when we read seemingly much approved and agreed on documents such as the United Nations Universal Declaration of Human Rights (1948), many people have spent thousands of hours debating and analyzing in order to make sense of their arguments and applications. Finally, the outcomes of any rights framework is never clear – they emerge as new sets of understandings that then themselves become open to further interpretation. It is important to grasp the flow of meanings, the contestations, the ambiguities of the symbolic (Blumer 1969).

Cultures as emergent complexities

Human cultures are mosaics of multilayered, negotiable and ever emergent symbolic interactions. Human rights are part of these cultures. Cultures are never tight, fixed or agreed on but are multilayered 'mosaics of social worlds'. As Seyla Benhabib (2002: 9) says: 'The interpretation of cultures as hermetic, sealed, internally self consistent wholes is untenable and reflects the reductionist sociology of knowledge.' There are innumerable social worlds that are constantly contradictory and tensionful. Cultures are 'the scraps, patches and rags of daily life' (Benhabib 2002: 36); they are the layered, daily lived, toolboxes of ideas and materials that are constantly in flow and flux to help us resolve daily problems of living. Ideas of human rights have become part of this toolbox. But there is nothing clear, unified or established about this. Thus, when we are looking *across* cultures, we should never be at all surprised to find enormous differences: the trouble is that we are sometimes too surprised when we look *inside* specific cultures that we also find these differences.

Cultures do not speak to consensus and uniformity: by their nature, they cannot. Thus to speak of sexual cultures as harmonious, well-ordered consensual wholes is nonsense. To talk of 'Muslim culture', 'women's culture', 'British culture' or even 'gay culture' is, in truth, to immediately step into social worlds of massive ambiguities, contradictions, tensions – never worlds of agreed on consensus. Social life as lived times grows out of these tensions. It is important to grasp this – because some views of cultures flatten them and turn them into monologic, monolithic and monomoral overly stable forms. Human rights debates over sexualities can become lost if they work with this naive, dead and overly simple view of culture.

Thus, while it is useful to sense the pervasiveness of multiculturalism, this can also bring the danger of seeing a different culture as if it were fixed, different and lacking dynamics of change. It is more useful to recognise their ceaseless dynamism, overlaps, continuities and contestations. Cultures, and human rights, are always lived actions: in *bricolage*, in mobilities and complexities; and they are always negotiated and deeply contested. This is what breathes persistent life into culture, what animates it. Without it, culture dies. Multicultures are not separate essences apart from one other, but are always overlapping and emergent as well as internally contested.

Interaction and others

Human social life is always made, acted, constructed through the interactions of living people in a society. People do things together and build social life. This is how societies work. Human rights too are constructions of people doing things together. Rights are not given in nature merely waiting to be found. Rights are inventions created by human agents through symbolic interactions. They involve the collective conduct and social meaning of many, and come into being through the interpretive work of social movements and a diverse range of moral crusaders and entrepreneurs: from kings, prophets and philosophers to governments, social movements, writers and non-governmental organisations. We need to study collective behaviour and social movements as part of this web of ceaseless negotiated interactions.

Self, others and dialogue

Symbolic interaction always depends on an idea of imagining others – of dialoguing with, at least linking to, and maybe even empathising or sympathising, with others. Human social life could not exist without awareness of others in the social world. The social human is always contingent on other people. There is no way that individuals can function in this world on their own. And in large part this is because human beings have selves predicated on communication and dialogues with others. In a very profound sense, 'we live in the minds of others without knowing it' (Cooley 1998: Chapter 13; Scheff 2006: 33). Language, communication and the self are bound together and to be social requires that we acquire and develop an idea of self. And doing this always hovers on the edge of a moral imagination that invites all people to consider how these others – who are inescapably present and bound up with our lives – should actually be handled within our lives.

In this, we are never monologic in the sense that we have unitary and single voices: rather we always dialogic – in discussion with others – even as we forget this. How are these others to be connected to ourselves? In my view, we cannot understand humanity – or sexuality or human rights – without taking a dialogical and reflective stance. Our rights must be linked to the idea of otherness – we depend on others for the rights we can have. Rights imply mutuality – and usually obligations as well as rights; so rights can only exist in dialogue with others. We have no social claims to *our* rights if we have no sense of the *others* who can give us these rights, and if we have this, then we need to be aware of *their* rights too. We are all bound together.

These dialogues are dependent on what the symbolic interactionists – through James, Mead and Goffman – called 'role taking': but there are many closely connected words that suggest this: empathy, sympathy, recognition, being attuned to another, being aware of someone's needs. Thus, being attuned to the other requires a communication network – even patches of communal cultures – that enables us to take seriously the presence of others. Some of these others will be near to us and close, our significant others; but others will be much more distant and far away (from generalised others to abstract others). We feel less for them and we are shaped less by them. And part of the self-process is not just awareness of others but also a feeling of self-regard concerning how we come to see ourselves and place ourselves in the social world.

People nowadays may claim human rights for themselves; but for such rights – including sexual rights – to make sense we need to know something about the wider contexts in which such claims are made. And one of these most surely derives from an imaginative understanding of what is meant by both the self and the other: the self who has rights and the other who may or may not have rights. Sexual rights demand a close attention to the sexual worlds of others as well as of ourself. They connect to what might be called a moral imagination – the capacity to empathise with others and to see the possibilities for ethical actions (McCollough 1991: 63).

Storytelling and narratives

Social life is shaped by the definitions of situations we make, and the stories and narratives we tell. Cultures construct narratives with diverse moral meanings for the self that can be connected to human rights. Part of the search for self and other, along with the conception of just what rights a human might have, will arise from the significant and generalised others with whom one is linked: real people in real life. These are the key players in shaping our social worlds and our senses of rights. But there are also wider, broader features of a culture which foster our sense of empathy, role taking and comprehension of other worlds.

One argument developed in the past few decades highlights the significance of storytelling and narrative for the construction of the self (Holstein and Gubrium 2000). Lynn Hunt (2007) in her recent history of human rights, for example, places great store on the rise of the eighteenth-century novel as a key factor in shaping a wider sensitivity to other. Accounts of violence and torture, for example, helped people imagine the pain of others. Novels gave people new ideas about how the self worked, and 'imagined empathy' in a range of areas sensitised more and more people to ideas of the rights of others. Before her, the philosophers Martha Nussbaum (1999) and Richard Rorty (1989) placed great store on the role of reading novels and art more generally as a keystone for comprehending moral and political life.

There is always the possibility, then, that when people define situations as real they become real in their consequences. This is also true of human rights. The stories we construct that tell of sufferings and joys help direct us to a world we wish to become and a world where human rights are recognised. 'Good stories' can be the harbingers of human rights. They have often arisen from telling us about the truly dehumanising things that people do to each other in the form of genocides, war, torture, slavery and oppression as well as in the everyday simple nastiness of some people. But they also can tell about the importance of equality, the value of lives, of what it is to be fully functioning human being.

Kay Schafer and Sidonie Smith (2004) talk of *Human Rights and Narrated Lives* in their examination of the traumatic past in apartheid South Africa, the underground literature that circulated during this time and the subsequent Truth and Reconciliation Commission. They look also at Aboriginal experiences in Australia and the struggle for indigenous rights; at the stories of abduction and forced sexual slavery during the Second World War by poor Korean women in Japanese 'comfort stations'; at prison narratives and political prisoners – especially in the USA. The stories they tell sensitise readers to terrible things that have happened and pathways ahead through human rights dialogues. As they say:

> This book is a testimony to the efficacy of stories: stories silenced by and emerging from fear, shame, trauma and repression; stories enlivened by hope,

connection, commitment and affiliation; stories fed by calls for justice, fuelled by empathy and an ethics of equality and human dignity; stories framed by faith in international covenants calling for dignity, justice and freedom. These stories, taken together, mount a powerful argument for the efficacy of storytelling in advancing the ongoing and constantly transforming pursuit of social justice, emanating from, but not limited to, the human rights project inaugurated by the United Declaration of Human Rights.

(Schafer and Smith 2004: 233–4)

The same has been happening in the field of sexual rights. Narratives of sexual difference, sexual suffering and sexual survival are required to progress the development of sexual rights: for in them lies a wider understanding of the selves and worlds of others that are so closely linked to our sexualities and our humanities.

Political cultures and social movements

Human social life is embedded in power and moral relations and always has to be negotiated – societies are contested negotiated orders animated by schisms and fracturings. Rights work involves a continuous round of negotiated collective actions to interpret, rationalise and define both social identities and related rights. It is a core feature of the work of social movements, and entails 'claims and counterclaims', often animated by quasi-arguments and storytelling. It is endemically schismatic and political.

Social movements can be seen as arising out of subterranean worlds where people are resisting dominant powerful forces. Under conditions of stress and crisis, people engage in collective activity that produces claims and help frame arguments about the nature of their lives and their problems. From this, they work to mobilise resources and get organised. By the nineteenth century, social movements had become international, playing a key role in participation linked to the 'expansion and contraction of democratic possibilities' (Tilly 2004: 3). Three factors mark out the development of social movements after 1750: the prominence of sustained campaigns beyond any single event; the use of a wide range of tools (from pamphleteering to demonstrations); and organisations' ultimate sense of their own worthiness, unity, size and commitment (Tilly 2004).

Sexual rights have become an important part of this work – in the women's movement, the homophile/queer movement and the transgender movement. The gay movement may have culminated in Stonewall in 1969 and the formation of the London Gay Liberation front in 1970. But, like all social movements, such a movement did not arise overnight; and without such movements no rights claims could be made. Now, the actions of such movements and claims for sexual rights are firmly on the international agenda.

The significance of emergence and history

Human social life is processual, emergent and flowing: there is always a history to it. This is also true of human rights. Rights work moves through certain phases, histories and stages. At one point, it is invisible and hardly articulated; at another it finds a voice; and at a later stage it can become habitualised and institutionalised. But it is never fixed and is always on the move. Claims for human rights have long histories.

In her study of the history of human rights, Micheline Ishay (2004) suggests five major waves: early times, the Enlightenment, socialism and the industrial age, the world wars and international rights and the global age. For most of recorded history, religions have been the seedbeds of rights – they have provides rules, codes, commandments, 'ways of living' for societies to observe, and although these are not rights per se, they often hint at rights to come. Yet in most of these codes, same-sex relations are strongly condemned. 'Humanitarian' as they often are in providing a seedbed of values for how to live a good life, they are also harbingers of hate in marking out the despised sexual other and advocating the hatred of such groups.

In recent times, there has been growing concern for rights within the field of sexuality. As Rosalind Petchesky comments, they are 'the newest kid on the block' (2000: 81–103). There were odd hints of such rights in nineteenth-century feminism; hints that grow in a few countries during the twentieth century. Historians have documented a substantial tradition of gay life during the early part of the twentieth century (Houlbrook 2005; Doan 2001). Likewise, in Germany and to a lesser extent in the USA, there were significant pushes towards homosexual emancipation (Weeks 1977, 2007). In the UK, the scandals of Oscar Wilde forced homosexuality deeply underground, extensive though it was. In the twentieth century, the cases of Wildeblood and Montagu[2] led to the Wolfenden Report, which, in turn, created organizations that lobbied for homosexual law reform and, ultimately, legal changes in 1967 in the UK. But such concerns do not become part of global sexual citizenship debates until the 1990s.

The global and the cosmopolitan

Human social life is global

While it is grounded in the self, it is also intrinsically linked to an awareness of the others in the wider world. George Herbert Mead classically located the ways in which the self moved out from the significance of others in the immediate world to the existence of a 'generalised other', initially the community but later to the international global community. In the twenty-first century, social commentators now presume the significance of the global – they see global markets, global media, global governance and global cultures. They stress that social processes of globalisation proceeding alongside those of globalisation, and have reinvoked the ancient idea of cosmopolitanism to flag the significance of being citizens in the wider cosmos or world (Toulmin 1990).

George Herbert Mead was a dedicated internationalist (Aboulafia 2001: 18). Speaking in the 1920s, he suggests that:

> The organised 'other' … is a community of narrow diameter. We are struggling now to get a certain amount of international-mindedness. We are realising ourselves as members of a larger community. The vivid nationalism of the present should, in the end, call out for an international attitude of the large community … If we assert our rights, we are calling for a definite response just because they are rights that are universal – a response which everyone should, and perhaps will, give.
>
> (Mead 1934: 167, 260)

Struggles over such rights now take place not only in local arenas but also in global ones. They are part of universalising attitudes, emergent global flows and what has now become the search for global standards of human rights and a global citizenry. We see it embodied in the work of many non-governmental organisations and in the work of the United Nations. Kant's famous principle – the peoples of the earth have entered into a universal community – has now developed to the point where a violation of rights in one part of the world is starting to be felt everywhere.

The hopeful news now is to be found in writers who have detected the rise of a new cosmopolitan attitude within the world and the arrival of a cosmopolitan self (and with it, perhaps, a cosmopolitan sexuality?). Cosmopolitanism, above all else, sees us all as universally part of the same world but as incorrigibly different. People everywhere are different and there is much to be learned from these differences. But at the same time, 'humankind' is one (Appiah 2006; Beck 2006; Fine 2007).

Conclusion

In this chapter, I have tried to continue my journey as a critical humanist. Despite our differences, dreams and desires, we are all part of the same small species in a vast universe. We are busy practical beings with our different enterprises, sufferings and joys and are here but for a very short time on our planet. By seeing our social lives as symbolic, emergent and interactive, we may deepen our understanding of our sexualities, our rights and, ultimately, our human capabilities.

Notes

1 I have outlined much of this in Plummer 2000. See also Denzin 1992.
2 In the 1950s, there was a series of sensational trials of homosexuals – of which that of Peter Wildeblood was most famous. For a brief account, see Houlbrook (2005: 254–63).

References

Aboulafia, M. (2001) *The Cosmopolitan Self: George Herbert Mead and Continental Philosophy*, Urbana: University of Illinois Press.

Appiah, K. A. (2006) *Cosmopolitanism: Ethics in a World of Strangers*, London: Allen Lane.

Beck, U. (2006) *Cosmopolitan Vision*, Cambridge: Polity Press.

Becker, E. (1973) *The Denial of Death*, New York: Macmillan/Free Press.

Benhabib, S. (2002) *The Claims of Culture: Equality and Diversity in the Global Era*, Princeton: Princeton University Press.

Blumer, H. (1969) *Symbolic Interactionism*, Englewood Cliffs, NJ: Prentice-Hall.

Clark, C. (1997) *Misery and Company: Sympathy in Everyday Life*, Chicago: University of Chicago Press.

Cooley, C. H. (1956) *Human Nature and the Social Order*, Glencoe, IL: Free Press.

Cooley, C. H. (1998) 'On Self and Social Organisation', in Schubert, H.-J. (ed.) *On Self and Social Organisation*, Chicago: University of Chicago Press.

Denzin, N. (1992) *Symbolic Interactionism and Cultural Studies*, Oxford: Blackwell.

Doan, L. (2001) *Fashioning Sapphism: The Origins of a Modern English Lesbian Culture*, New York: Columbia University Press.

Fesmire, S. (2003) *John Dewey and the Moral Imagination: Pragmatism in Ethics*, Bloomington: Indiana University Press.

Fine, B. (2007) *Cosmopolitanism*, London: Routledge.

Gagnon, J. and Simon, W. (2005) *Sexual Conduct: The Social Sources of Sexuality*, 2nd edn, Chicago: Aldine.

Grayling, A. C. (2007) *Towards the Light: The Story of the Struggles for Liberty and Rights that Made the Modern West*, London: Bloomsbury.

Holstein, J. and Gubrium, J. F. (2000) *The Self We Live By: Narrative Identity in a Postmodern World*, Oxford: Oxford University Press.

Houlbrook, M. (2005) *Queer London: Perils and Pleasures in the Sexual Metropolis 1918–1957*, Chicago: University of Chicago Press.

Hunt, L. (2007) *Inventing Human Rights: A History*, New York: Norton.

Hunter, A. (1990) *Culture Wars*, New York: Basic Books.

Ishay, M. R. (2004) *The History of Human Rights: From Ancient Times to the Globalization Era*, Berkeley: University of California Press.

Isin, E. F. and Turner, B. S. (eds) (2002) *Handbook of Citizenship Studies*, London: Sage.

James, W. (1985) *Psychology: The Briefer Course*, Boston, MA: Harvard University Press.

Mead, G. H. (1934) *Mind, Self and Society*, Chicago: University of Chicago Press.

McCollough, T. (1991) *The Moral Imagination and Public Life: Raising the Ethical Question*, Chatham, NJ: Chatham House.

Nussbaum, M. (1999) *Sex and Social Justice*, Oxford: Oxford University Press.

Oberleitner, G. (2007) *Global Human Rights: Between Remedy and Ritual*, Cambridge: Polity Press.

O'Byrne, D. J. (2003) *Human Rights: An Introduction*, London: Pearson.

Petchesky, R. (2000) 'Sexual Rights: Inventing a Concept, Mapping an International Practice', in Parker, R., Barbosa, R. M. and Aggleton, P. (eds) *Framing the Sexual Subject: The Politics of Gender, Sexuality and Power*, Berkeley: University of California Press.

Plummer, K. (1982) 'Symbolic Interactionism and Sexual Conduct: An Emergent Perspective', in Brake, M. (ed.) *Human Sexual Relations*, New York: Pantheon Books.

Plummer, K. (1995) *Telling Sexual Stories: Power, Change and Social Worlds*, London: Routledge.

Plummer, K. (2000) 'Symbolic Interactionism in the Twentieth Century', in Turner, B. (ed.) *Blackwell Handbook of Social Theory*, Oxford: Blackwell.

Plummer, K. (2003) *Intimate Citizenship: Private Troubles and Public Discourses*, Washington, DC: University of Washington Press.

Plummer, K. (2005) 'Intimate Citizenship in an Unjust World', in Romero, M. and Margolis, E. (eds) *The Blackwell Companion to Social Inequalities*, Oxford: Blackwell.

Rorty, R. (1989) *Irony, Contingency and Solidarity*, Cambridge: Cambridge University Press.

Schafer, K. and Smith, S. (2004) *Human Rights and Narrated Lives: The Ethics of Recognition*, Basingstoke: Palgrave.

Scheff, T. J. (2006) *Goffman Unbound! A New Paradigm for Social Science*, Boulder, CO: Paradigm.

Sen, A. (1999) *Development as Freedom*, Oxford: Oxford University Press.

Simon, W. (1999) 'Sexual Conduct in Retrospective', *Sexualities*, 2: 126–33.

Taylor, C. (1994) 'The Politics of Recognition', in Appiah, K. A. (ed.) *Multiculturalism*, Princeton: Princeton University Press.

Thomas, W. I. (1932) *The Child in America*, New York: Knopf.

Tilly, C. (2004) *Social Movements 1768–2004*, Boulder, CO: Paradigm.

Toulmin, S. (1990) *Cosmopolis: The Hidden Agenda of Modernity*, Chicago: University of Chicago Press.

United Nations (1948) *Universal Declaration of Human Rights*, United Nations, available at www.un.org/Overview/rights.html (accessed 17 April 2009).

Weeks, J. (1977) *Coming Out: Homosexual Politics in Britain from the Nineteenth Century to the Present*, London: Quartet.

Weeks, J. (2007) *The World We Have Won: The Remaking of Erotic and Intimate Life*, London: Routledge.

7 Recent developments in US sexuality research

Diane di Mauro

The history, evolution and current status of sexuality research in the USA is a continuing story of fits and starts at progressive moments and snags and hindrances in regressive eras.[1] Modern research in sexuality in the USA began over 50 years ago with the work of Alfred Kinsey to whom the professional title 'sex researcher' was first given. Since then, sexuality research has been conducted in numerous fields and disciplines and its history is entwined with a variety of political, social and educational forces. Yet, while the contributions of many sexuality researchers have provided legitimacy to the scientific study of sexuality in the past half century, it did not establish a tradition of systematic and cumulative research in the USA – primarily due to longstanding political controversies surrounding such work, beginning with Kinsey's own research (see Chapter 5) and continuing more recently, a situation that has constituted a persistent impediment over time.

The origins and evolution of this field of sexuality research has been traced by many scholars who have highlighted its early foundation in the US public health surveys of the early 1900s to large-scale demographic survey research in the 1950s, to research focusing on reproduction and fertility in the 1960s and 1970s, to research on sexual behaviours and risk prevention among specific populations following the emergence of HIV and AIDS globally in 1980s and 1990s (di Mauro 1995; Ericksen 1999; Hunt 1999; Irvine 2004; Parker 2008). As the first decade of the new millennium comes to a close, the recent epoch might best be described as one that has witnessed an unprecedented expansion of research on a variety of sexual topics and issues, from sexual arousal and response, to the shifting terrain of sexual identity, to what can be regarded as sexual transgression across cultures – all of which constitutes research that questions 'scientific certainty about the nature of sexual life' (Parker 2008: 84).

This chapter aims to outline some of this development, highlighting the field's progressive and regressive movement over the past 15 years. In noting both the achievements and continuing needs/obstacles, it makes a number of suggestions for further legitimising the field and advancing research and training endeavours that, with sufficient support, may lay the foundation for the continued cultivation of a future generation of scholars capable of addressing the contextual nature of human sexuality and exploring links across disciplines, methods and issues.

So where do we begin?

Almost 15 years ago, an assessment of sexuality research in the social and behavioural sciences was commissioned by a group of private foundations to identify research trends and gaps, priority topics and critical issues (di Mauro 1995). The report noted that:

> Comprehensive data on contemporary sexual behaviors, attitudes and practices are not available, nor is it understood how they are shaped by different societal, cultural and familial contexts ... there is no consistent support to conduct behavioral and social science research focusing on human sexuality ... the lack of which has created a substantial dearth of knowledge which in turn has sustained many of the social crises evident in the U.S. today.
>
> (di Mauro 1995: 2)

Findings highlighted a driving force behind research was one that dictated a preventive health agenda in which research – typically as part of a larger disease prevention or public health initiative – best served the need to identify high-risk sexual behaviours and/or motivate behavioural change. In its recommendations for much needed change, the report called for sufficient and consistent support for sexuality research to expand the scope of existing inquiry, support new research and improve research dissemination; provide more formalised opportunities for training in sexuality research in the form of fellowships and specialised curricula in higher education and postgraduate venues; and build a constituency to advance sexuality research by establishing a coordinating support network of researchers, providers and policymakers working in the field and in related areas.

Recent developments

An expanded research agenda and many more researchers

One notable outcome of the report was the launching in September 1995 of the Sexuality Research Fellowship Program (SRFP) hosted by the Social Science Research Council based in New York, which provided fellowships to the first cohort of dissertation and postdoctoral scholars for social and behavioural research on a range of sexuality issues. Between 1996 and 2005 the SRFP selected over 150 fellows and their mentors, providing them with research support to address the complexity and contextual nature of human sexuality; to promote methodological diversity and innovation; and through their research, to link the study of human sexuality to the intellectual trajectory of their own disciplines. Given its scope and longevity, the programme significantly strengthened the sexuality research field in the USA in terms of 'seeding' the next generation of sexuality researchers in the social sciences and humanities.[2]

Alongside this development and prompted by it to a significant extent, a diversification and contextualisation of the sexuality research agenda is evident, one that promotes a continuing legitimisation of such work. While the preventive health agenda continues to drive much funded work (especially that supported by large Federal government grants), there is an assumed understanding across disciplines, perhaps in the form of bemoaning what inevitably gets funded, that the field is in need of significant support to complement its current disease prevention research focus by focusing on the more positive aspects of sexual health and wellbeing. A proliferation of relevant research on a wide range of issues and topics across disciplines and research arenas is evident, and there is also an increasing number of scholars identifying as sexuality researchers, although only a minority of them have successfully obtained consistent and sufficient support for their work and more often than not, researchers are compelled to 'hide' the nature of their research and/or to incorporate sexuality components to existing, funded health-based research. Typically based in universities and small research centres, scholars and researchers representing a wide swathe of disciplines are conducting research in the biomedical/physical sciences, public health, the social sciences and humanities, as well as in disparate fields such as demography, economics, education, ethics, cultural and women's studies, political science, nursing and law.

This continuing legitimisation of the field over the past 15 years has promoted a profound change in awareness and attitude, such that it is increasingly understood that it is both legitimate and feasible to pursue a professional career in sexuality research within a wide variety of academic disciplines that are not directly linked to public health. Beyond this, it has spawned a new generation of scholars who are willing to take risks in terms of what they choose to investigate about sexuality and whom they engage in the process, within limits, of course (Epstein 2006).

Diversified research foci

Since 1995, this proliferation of research on sexuality across disciplines can be characterised as representing a more nuanced view of the subject area, one that seeks to decipher its historical significance and construction, approaching it primarily as a mutable entity, in its social, physiological and/or evolutionary expression. Eschewing the neat dichotomy of nature *versus* nurture, the research gaze over the past 15 years has become increasingly wide reaching as it seeks to decipher the diversity and distribution of sexual values, beliefs and behaviours across various populations and their experiential and subjective meanings for individuals as they are situated within culture and society.

More specifically, sexuality research focusing on the individual has included a wide range of topics and issues, such as the factors and processes that shape sexuality at different developmental junctures across the lifecourse; the sexual physiology of sexual arousal, response and functioning within the context of experience and perception; the diversity of sexual practices (within and across cultures) and the concomitant fluidity of sexual response (especially for women); reproductive health, including how reproductive behaviours, decisions, technology and status influence sexuality; the conceptualisation, enactment and meaning given to gender identity; the impact of physical and mental disability on sexual functioning and behavioural response; and the effect(s) of drug, alcohol and pharmaceutical use on sexual arousal and response.

In terms of the individual in the context of institutional arenas, research has focused on religious institutions, schools and the role of the family/parents in establishing, maintaining and shaping sexual norms, values, attitudes and behaviours. Included here also is research on the media, information technology/ internet systems and experiences as emerging, prevalent venues of sexual intimacy and sexual education and primary sources of sexual information and networking. Moreover, with regard to sexual and social networks among and between men and women, the research highlights the behavioural and motivational dynamics of sexual 'coupling', intimacy and relationships within the context of sexual orientation and lifestyle.

Last, as a result of social and political change/movement(s) triggered by globalisation across geographical regions and within cultural arenas, the research gaze is increasingly directed to the diverse processes of sexual socialisation (both as an expression and impact of immigration and migration) and to the intersection of gender, power, violence and sexuality, including analyses of pornography, forced migration and sexual slavery. Included here as well is research on STIs, HIV/AIDS, sexual politics and sexual rights, such as analyses of stigma and discrimination and historical and contemporary analyses of sexual science and social movements and sexual citizenship across time and space.

As well, moving away from the larger representative samples of population surveys, researchers are increasingly using smaller, focused samples representing situational or 'experiential' status instead of demographic characteristics such as (reproductive) age, gender etc. Such work includes studies as diverse as those researching: gay, lesbian and transgender individuals who are also homeless (e.g. Cochran *et al.* 2002; Meyer 2003 and Whitbeck *et al.* 2004); gay and lesbian couples who parent (e.g. Kurdek 2004; Tasker and Bigner 2007); people working in the pornography industry (e.g. Bernstein 2007; Frank 2002; Stoller and Levine 1996; Weitzer 2000); the experience of love and intimacy for transmigratory populations (e.g. Cantu 2009; Carrillo 2001; Gonzáles Lopez 2006; Padilla 2007); teachers and administrators as players in the sexuality education debate (e.g. Fields 2008); subjective measures of arousal among women (e.g. Chivers *et al.* in press; Diamond 2009; Peterson *et al.* in press; Suschinsky *et al.* 2009); sexual intimacy among men with cerebral palsy (e.g. Shuttleworth 2000, in press); semen and egg donors motivated to assist infertile couples (e.g. Becker 2000; Fielding *et al.* 1998; Yee 2009); couples taking Viagra and sexual (dis)satisfaction and negotiation (e.g. Meika 2001; Potts 2003; Simons and Carey 2004); and women observing Jewish purity laws and *mikvehs*, who embrace sexual passion (e.g. Kaufman 1991; Wasserfall 1999).

In diversifying and contextualising the research agenda, sexuality researchers over the past 15 years have critically expanded the knowledge base on human sexuality and in the process have promoted a more nuanced understanding of a wider range of sexual inquiry, theory and practice.

Current challenges and needs

The backdrop: continuing controversy

Beneath the surface of these more positive developments in sexuality research, continuing needs and obstacles are very much evident. These include an inconsistent and modest financial support for this work, on the part of both public and private sectors, an adamant hesitancy to publicly promote its value and relevancy for public health and lingering issues of legitimacy and professional identity for researchers across disciplines. Moreover, although human sexuality has been inquired into since the early twentieth century (Ericksen 1999) the field continues to lack a coordinating structure that could provide financial, logistical or political support to its professionals. Especially in the USA, conservative pressure to eliminate funding for research on sexuality from the early 1990s and through the G. W. Bush years, has severely curtailed the production and dissemination of knowledge about sexuality (Epstein 2006). As a result, while sexuality research is conducted across a wide range of fields within the social sciences, public health and humanities disciplines of academia, it is rarely used as a primary source for evidence-based policy development and implementation.

As well, sexuality researchers have little participation in the US political arena, which, until recently, has been dominated by conservative organisations, ideological views often substantiated by faith rather than by research, to bear on legislators and policymakers (Epstein 2006; Herdt in press; Hunt 1999; Irvine 2002). At the same time, a range of well-funded and highly effective conservative organisations that do not view human sexuality as a legitimate area of inquiry have proved their continuing skill at lobbying and interfacing with the media and government agencies to effectively shape public opinion and forcefully hinder support for this work (Herdt in press; Klein 2008; Lane 2006). In sum, there remains considerable misperception of the work of sexuality researchers with scarce understanding of its potential for health and wellbeing. Substantial support is needed to promote sexuality research, ensure its potential, and sustain those who conduct it, both within and outside academic arenas.

The need for training

A key priority in building capacity for sexuality research is training. While there exists some formalised training opportunities in sexuality research, these primarily take the form of short summer institutes or periodic, short training courses or workshops that typically precede or follow the annual meetings of professional sexuality organisations such as the American Association of Sex Educators, Counselors, and Therapists; the International Academy of Sex Research; the International Association for the Study of Sexuality, Culture, and Society; the International Society for the Study of Women's Sexual Health; the Society for the Scientific Study of Sexuality; and the Society for Sex Therapy and Research; and the World Association for Sexual Health.[3] However, such training efforts remain small in number, are insufficiently and inconsistently supported, and are in need of a consistent source of qualified mentors with comprehensive knowledge of methodology and theoretical frameworks, or who have a keen understanding of the complexity and contextual nature of human sexuality.

Specifically, a critical need remains for comprehensive training in both innovative and traditional methodologies that can advance theory and/or test new methodology and promote *practical* applications for public wellbeing and policy formation. Formalised training in sexuality research is needed at all levels in order to provide a rigorous foundation in theory and methodology and to ensure a sufficient mix of qualified researchers to the field. While those conducting research in academic venues may be trained as part of the curriculum requirements of a degree programme, little attention has been given to the content and quality of training or the creation of a coordinating entity to determine whether such training is rigorous, consistent and relevant across institutions.

Training is also needed to adequately prepare scholars in the art of multi- and interdisciplinary research. This requires familiarity with diverse methods, terminology, analyses and interpretations, and could be provided by fellowship programmes with training components, short-term training specialised institutes, senior scholar resident programs linked to mentoring and other 'customised' efforts. Concurrent with this, research training programmes that target health practitioners are sorely needed – especially physicians, public health practitioners, medical students and residents whose work requires close interaction with the public and whose lack of training in and understanding of human sexuality is a serious limitation.

The need for policy-relevant research

A long-term inadequacy of sexuality research is the dire need for the utilisation of research findings in policy development and implementation. While lip service is given to the need for such work and there is some evidence of a more applied, potentially policy-relevant research approach in the field, what remains rare are initiatives attuned to integrative research methodologies, and dedicated to more useful research dissemination, both of which would be inherently useful to policy-relevant research. A well-conceptualised approach and guiding framework with which to effectively forge links between sexuality research and policy arenas is vital, both within and outside academia. Such an approach would help ensure the effective application of sexuality research to local, state and national policy issues, would promote the inclusion of sexuality issues in current policy work, and would encourage researchers to engage in policy-related issues as an integral part of their professional and academic careers.

Research funding

Wherever sexuality research is conducted, the primary sources of support are either the public or private sector – as in government grants, philanthropic or corporate support. In the USA, public sector support is typically provided in the form of Federal government grants for large HIV/AIDS or population/reproduction prevention research initiatives in which a small 'add-on' (and often hidden) component of the initiative focuses on sexuality. Private sector support is provided to a large extent by pharmaceutical companies funding research that focuses primarily on the physiology of the body, as in, for example, the deciphering of universal 'laws' of sexual response for men and women as binary categories of sexual reality, or in the pursuit of new chemical aphrodisiacs to resolve sexual 'dysfunctions' in arousal and response.

To a lesser extent, private sector support is provided by private foundations that have a history of funding such work, especially in the area of reproductive health and population management and control. The earliest record of such funding took place in 1921, when the concern over increasing immorality led the National Research Council to form the Committee for Research in Problems in Sex with funding by the American Social Hygiene Association by the Rockefeller Foundation (di Mauro 1995). Following the publication of the Kinsey reports on male and female sexuality and the ensuing controversy, the foundation diverted its support from sexuality research to reproductive health and population.

With regard to public sector support, the challenge for the field lies in disentangling research inquiry about sexuality from the preventive, behavioural straitjacket of HIV/AIDS and population/demographic research. Regarding pharmaceutical support, the challenge is to counteract the 'propensity to reduce the question of sex to an underlying … biological or psychological imperative that determines the meaning of even the most disparate beliefs and practices, sex as natural force that exists in opposition to civilisation, culture, or society' (Parker 2008: 107). With respect to private foundations, the challenge is to encourage a more consistent and substantial level of support for sexuality research, including collaborative research initiatives with training components. As well, foundations are uniquely positioned to leverage their support for sexuality research with large-scale public sector initiatives, providing crucial support for specific research and training components that dovetail with their specific funding priorities or mission.

Future directions

Briefly, future directions for sexuality research are likely to include the following foci.

Lifecourse/quality of life

As life expectancy rises and the concomitant 'greying' of the population takes place, a lifecourse approach is likely to become particularly significant for sexuality research. Here, the research gaze should be on sexual health as it is experienced over the lifespan, on the quality and urgencies of life and health; the reality of aging and increasing reliance on pharmaceutical products and medical interventions and on the impact on sexuality in terms of deficits/compromises in physical and mental health with aging.

Institutional analysis relevant for policy development

Research here may usefully focus on the significance and impact of key institutions on sexuality, as they function as socially constructed structures and mechanisms of social order – especially the institutions of the government, family, education and religion. The resulting policy-relevant research will increasingly inform those working in various arenas, such as youth development, criminal justice and reproductive health. As well, the media and internet arenas will be of research significance as an increasing source for sexual information, networking, communication and policy development.

Processes/experiences/language

Cognitive research will increasingly focus on the various informational processes involved in knowledge acquisition and sexual response and arousal, with emphasis on individual experience, perception, motivation and behaviour. Such research will inform clinical work on sexual functioning and dysfunctioning and as well, the development of biopsychosocial theoretical frameworks of gender- and age-specific sexual response and behaviour.

Sexuality in time, space and the body

While the disciplines of history, psychology and anthropology will probably continue to represent the majority of sexuality research in the social sciences, they will need to pay increasing attention – perhaps in collaboration with biomedical research – to the interaction of biology and behaviour within social, cultural, historical, political and economic contexts. A wide-ranging research agenda would tackle such disparate areas as psychosocial adjustment, self-esteem, body image and sexual functioning as well as hormonal influence on sexuality across over women's and men's lifecycles.

Movements

Closely related to policy research, research initiatives might usefully focus on the significance of social movements, struggles and processes over time, and increasingly, human/sexual rights within the context of industrialisation, population growth, sexwork, gender discrimination and economic globalisation. There will continue to be a significant expansion of research on social and political movements and sexual politics focusing on issues of power, coercion and discrimination, and their relevance for identity politics (e.g. sexual and/or gender identity) within the arena of sexual and human rights, activism and advocacy.

Conclusion

If either the public or private sector were to provide sufficient support for sexuality research with the intent of having a significant impact, it could potentially, over time, motivate increased support from both sides and thereby generate a formalised public/private sector partnership that could assess and adequately address the needs of the field. In addition to funding at the individual level (e.g. research fellowships and training at various levels), funding could be available at the institutional level, creating a variety of programmatic initiatives based in research centres nationwide. Such support could have significant impact were it to be provided for initiatives such as the creation of a single coordinating entity to serve as a clearinghouse for research initiatives that could synchronise research initiatives across institutions and research venues, and publicly promote and support sexuality research and training as a cohesive field of inquiry, investigation and mentoring.

Beyond this, however, there is a need for a major collaborative effort in the form of linked, parallel research initiatives in tandem, initiatives that cross over theoretical and methodological divides. This effort could be designed to unify research methodological approaches, involving teams of researchers with expertise in qualitative and quantitative methodology and representing diverse fields such as history, economics, biomedicine and medical anthropology. In this process, researchers would collaborate on an initiative with singular research foci but utilise a variety of distinct yet complementary theoretical approaches to the initiative.

That said, nothing short of long-term substantial support will spur further development of this field on the scale and scope of what is needed as described here. Building human capacity and promoting its development by strengthening a research field is a long-term process, and the level of support for sexuality research has been woefully inadequate to date. Despite the disappointment from inadequate support to date and the frustration of continuing controversy prompted by conservative ideology, there exist strong expectations from within the field that significant support should be forthcoming both from the public sector and from the private sector, especially by the charitable foundations that have historically been of support. However, given that the economic downturn towards the end of the first decade of the twenty-first century sets limits on what might be hoped for and achieved, it is instead perhaps more reasonable to imagine that the field will continue to develop for the foreseeable future in much the same way that it has – making do with limited, inconsistent support, with little coordination of funded initiatives across institutions and venues.

As the earlier assessment of the field intimated:

> If there is any optimal moment for expanding support … the time is now, [for] the ingredients are all in place … a plethora of opportunities for interdisciplinary work and a pronounced need for relevant and applied research in this area.
>
> (di Mauro 1995: 61–2)

This chapter began with the observation that the history of sexuality research is a continuing story of fits and starts at progressive moments and snags and hindrances at its regressive eras. For now, we will have to continue to wait for the next 'fit and start' cycle, at which time support for sexuality research may, in addition to all the potential gains already noted, 'promote a much needed view of sexuality not as a source of problems and risks, but as a domain of well-being and human potential' (di Mauro 1995: 62), and as well, as a domain which seek to promote our inalienable right to sexual health.

Notes

1 While there are many similarities and parallel developments between the USA and other parts of the world, the historical evolution and current status of the sexuality field as described in this chapter focuses on US experience, which is unique in comparison both to the developing world as well as other parts of the developed world (e.g. the history/status of sexology and more recently sexuality studies in western Europe).
2 This initiative was made possible with support from the Ford Foundation. A report can be downloaded at http://programs.ssrc.org/sexuality/publications/Sexuality-Research-in-the-US/ (accessed 15 June 2009).
3 For listing of professional associations and contact information, see resource link from Kinsey Institute website: www.kinseyinstitute.org/resources/professional.html (accessed 15 June 2009).

References

Becker, G. (2000) *The Elusive Embryo: How Men and Women Approach New Reproductive Technologies*, Berkeley: University of California Press.
Bernstein, E. (2007) *Temporarily Yours: Intimacy, Authenticity and the Commerce of Sex*, Chicago: University of Chicago Press.
Cantu, L., Naples, N. and Vidal-Ortiz, S. (2009) *The Sexuality of Migration: Border Crossings and Mexican Immigrant Men*, New York: New York University Press.
Carrillo, H. (2001) *The Night is Young: Sexuality in Mexico in the Time of AIDS*, Chicago: University of Chicago.
Chivers, M. L., Seto, M. C., Laan, E., Lalumière, M. L. and Grimbos, T. (in press) 'Agreement of Genital and Subjective Measures of Sexual Arousal: A Meta-analysis', *Archives of Sexual Behavior*.

Cochran, B., Stewart, A., Ginzler, J. and Cauce, A. (2002) 'Challenges Faced by Homeless Sexual Minorities: Comparison of Gay, Lesbian, Bisexual and Transgender Homeless Adolescents with their Heterosexual Counterparts', *American Journal of Public Health*, 921: 773–7.

Corrêa, S., Petchesky, R. and Parker, R. (2008) (eds) *Sexual Health and Human Rights*, London and New York: Routledge.

Diamond, L. (2009) *Sexual Fluidity: Understanding Women's Love and Desire*, Cambridge, MA: Harvard University Press.

di Mauro, D. (1995) *Sexuality Research in the United States: An Assessment of the Social and Behavioral Sciences*, New York: Social Science Research Council.

Epstein, S. (2006) 'The New Attack on Sexuality Research: Morality and the Politics of Knowledge Production', *Sexuality Research and Social Policy Journal*, 3: 1–12.

Ericksen, J. (1999) *Kiss and Tell: Surveying Sex in the Twentieth Century*, Cambridge, MA: Harvard University Press.

Fielding, D., Handley, S., Duqueno, L. Weaver, S. and Lui, S. (1998) 'Motivation, Attitudes and Experience of Donation: A Follow-up of Women Donating Eggs in Assisted Conception Treatment', *Journal of Community & Applied Social Psychology*, 8: 273–87.

Fields, J. (2008) *Risky Lessons: Sex Education and Social Inequality*, New Brunswick, NJ: Rutgers University Press.

Frank, K. (2002) *G-Strings and Sympathy: Strip Club Regulars and Male Desire*, Durham, NC: Duke University Press.

González Lopez, G. (2006) 'Confesiones de Mujer: The Catholic Church and Sacred Morality in the Sex Lives of Mexican American Women', in Teunis, N., Herdt, G. and Parker, R. (eds) *Sexual Inequalities and Social Justice*, Berkeley: University of California Press.

Herdt, G. (ed.) (in press) *Moral Panics, Sex Panics: The Fear and the Fight over Sexual Rights*, New York: New York University Press.

Hunt, M. (1999) *The New No-Nothings: The Political Foes of the Scientific Study of Human Nature*, New Brunswick, NJ: Transaction Press.

Irvine, J. (2004) *Talk About Sex: The Battles over Sex Education in the United States*, Berkeley: University of California Press.

Kaufman, D. (1991) *Rachel's Daughters: Newly Orthodox Jewish Women*, New Brunswick: NJ: Rutgers University Press.

Klein, M. (2008) *America's War on Sex: The Attack on Law, Lust and Liberty*, Westport, CT: Greenwood Publishing.

Kurdek, L. (2004) 'Are Gay and Lesbian Cohabiting Couples "Really" Different From Heterosexual Married Couples?', *Journal of Marriage and Family*, 4: 880–90.

Lane, F. (2006) *The Decency Wars: The Campaign to Cleanse American Culture*, Amherst, NY: Prometheus Books.

Meika, L. (2001) 'Fixing Broken Masculinity: Viagra as a Technology for the Production of Gender and Sexuality', *Sexuality and Culture*, 5: 97–125.

Meyer, I. (2003) 'Prejudice, Social Stress and Mental Health in Lesbian, Gay and Bisexual Populations: Conceptual Issues and Research Evidence', *Psychological Bulletin*, 129: 674–97.

Padilla, M. (2007) *Caribbean Pleasure Industry: Tourism, Sexuality and AIDS in the Dominican Republic*, Chicago: University of Chicago Press.

Peterson, Z., Janssen, E. and Laan, E. (in press) 'Straight and Lesbian Women's Sexual Responses to Straight and Lesbian Erotica: The Role of Stimulus Intensity, Affective Reaction, and Sexual history', *Archives of Sexual Behavior*.

Potts, A., Gavey, N., Grace, V. and Vares, T. (2003) 'The Downside of Viagra: Women's Experiences and Concerns', *Sociology of Health and Illness*, 25: 697–719.

Shuttleworth, R. P. (2000) 'The Search for Sexual Intimacy for Men with Cerebral Palsy', *Sexuality and Disability*, 18: 263–82.

Shuttleworth, R. P. (in press) 'Disabled Men: Expanding the Masculine Repertoire', in

Hutchinson, B. and Smith, B. (eds) *Gendering Disability*, New Brunswick, NJ: Rutgers University Press.

Simons, J. and Carey, M. (2004) 'Prevalence of Sexual Dysfunctions: Results from a Decade of Research', *Archives of Sexual Behavior*, 30: 177–218.

Stoller, R. and Levine, I. S. (1996) *Coming Attractions: The Making of an X-Rated Video*, New Haven, CT: Yale University Press.

Suschinsky, K., Lalumière, M. L. and Chivers, M. L. (2009) 'Sex Differences in Patterns of Genital Arousal: Measurement Artifact or True Phenomenon?', *Archives of Sexual Behavior*, 38: 559–73.

Tasker, F. and Bigner, J. (2007) *Gay and Lesbian Parenting: New Directions*, New York: Haworth Press.

Tiefer, L. (2008) *Sex is Not a Natural Act and Other Essays*, 2nd edn, Boulder, CO: Westview Press.

Wasserfall, R. (1999) *Women and Water: Menstruation in Jewish Life and Law*, Waltham, MA: Brandeis University Press.

Weitzer, R. J. (2000) *Prostitution, Pornography and the Sex Industry*, New York: Routledge.

Whitbeck, L., Chen, X., Hoy, D., Tyler, K. and Johnson, K. (2004) 'Mental Disorder, Subsistence Strategies and Victimization among Gay, Lesbian and Bisexual Homeless and Runaway Adolescents', *Journal of Sex Research*, 41: 329–42.

Yee, S. (2009) '"Gift without a Price Tag": Altruism in Anonymous Semen Donation', *Human Reproduction*, 24: 3–13.

Part II

Language, discourse and sexual categories

8 'Lesbians', modernity and global translation

Female sexualities in Indonesia

Evelyn Blackwood

From a western viewpoint, sexuality constitutes an essential or core attribute of identity; individuals are said to have fixed sexual identities or orientations. Sexuality as it is understood in the USA and western Europe, however, often bears little resemblance to sexual relationships and practices across cultures. Theorists such as Michel Foucault (1978) and Judith Butler (1990) argue that sexuality itself is a social product. According to this view, sexual acts, or what *appear* to be sexual acts, take their meaning from particular cultures, norms and beliefs about the self and the world. Social processes do not act as constraints on a 'natural' sexuality, but actually produce sexualities through discourses of desire, religion, gender and so on. In this chapter, I draw on feminist and queer theories, particularly those that constellate around social construction theory, in order to understand the meanings of sexualities among females in Indonesia.

Many academics now attend to the ways in which sexual acts are culturally produced, but since the early 1990s growing attention has been focused on the intersection of global and local processes. Plummer (1992) pointed out that same-sex experiences are increasingly fashioned through the interconnectedness of the world. He argued that lesbian and gay studies should pay close attention to the 'international connectedness yet local uniqueness' of diverse practices (1992: 18), thereby giving both global and local processes and practices a distinct role. In contrast, Altman (2001) initially spoke confidently about the 'apparent globalisation of postmodern, gay identities', arguing that new 'globalised' queer identities would replace older indigenous identities, resulting in a homogeneous global gay identity. Feminist theorists Grewal and Kaplan (2001) move beyond the limited and simplistic dichotomy of local–global by using the term 'transnational sexualities', which refers to the way in which genders and sexualities are produced through and intersect with a large number of processes implicated in globalisation. The term 'transnational' points to the lines that crosscut binaries of local/global; it suggests that the global and local thoroughly infiltrate one another (Grewal and Kaplan 2001).

At the same time that global interconnections among emerging gay and lesbian communities and networks create new visions of and spaces for women's and men's same-sex relations, some significant oversights persist. Global gay discourse tends toward an effacement of sexualities that do not have the appearance of same-sex identities emblematic of the lesbian and gay liberation movements of western Europe and North America (Bacchetta 2002). Activist lesbian discourse, in particular, holds the expectation that modern lesbian subjects will express a consciousness or self-awareness of sexual identity as 'lesbians' and as 'women'. The traditional/

modern dichotomy of western thought is perpetuated in this discourse; those individuals who do not reflect modern identities are marginalised because they appear to lack the grammar of fully liberated modern queers (Grewal and Kaplan 2001). Queer discourses rely on this dichotomy to create a developmental teleology that situates other sexualities as premodern, that is, not yet lesbian or gay, while placing western sexualities at the pinnacle of modern, autonomous sexuality (see also Cruz-Malavé and Manalansan 2002; Gopinath 2002). In this universalising turn, transnational queer discourses bypass the historicity and specificity of queer subjects outside the west, relegating their stories to the margins of queer movements. The effacement of postcolonial, non-western queer subjects is particularly disabling for lesbians, who are less visible in global gay (male) movements and narrowly defined in global lesbian feminist organising (Bacchetta 2002; King 2002).

The fixity of identities promoted by such terms as lesbian, gay, bisexual and transgender needs to be reconsidered in light of the tombois, lesbian men and other masculine females whose lives blur the boundaries of lesbian and transgender (see also Blackwood and Wieringa 1999; Morgan and Wieringa 2005). Evident throughout Asia in both cities and rural areas are masculine females whose own identities are firmly located in localised gender regimes as well as in global signifiers apparent in the proliferating forms of the English term 'tomboy' that they use to identify themselves (see Wieringa *et al.* 2007). These individuals, like their activist peers in major urban centres in southeast Asia, are influenced by global feminist and queer organising as well as by localised processes, which they negotiate to construct the particular forms of sexuality and gender evident in Asia today. Although seemingly divergent, these gendered and sexual subjectivities are part of and responsive to global queer discourse.

In Padang, West Sumatra, tombois and their girlfriends, who identify themselves as masculine and feminine respectively, access global circuits of queer knowledge and see themselves as part of a global community, but maintain subject positions that are distinct from the identities promoted and encouraged by activist lesbian organisations in Indonesia. In this chapter, I offer insights into the asymmetries of queer knowledge and the consequent multiplicity of desires and subjectivities as a way to challenge fixed identity categories and incorporate the diversity of queer subjectivities within a global gay ecumene.

In the particular case discussed here, I use the terms that individuals in Padang use to make sense of their lives, mainly *lesbi* and *tomboi*. Despite being cognates of English terms (lesbi/lesbian, tomboi/tomboy), these two Indonesian terms do not share the same meanings and resonances as their English counterparts. Also, by using terms such as 'queer knowledge' and 'queer discourses' in relation to Indonesia, I mean to suggest that these discourses are inflected by and participate in the globalised discourses of sexualities.

Tombois and their girlfriends

The subject positions that tombois and their girlfriends take up are informed by a wide array of global discourses at the same time that these subject positions respond to localised discourses.[1] The city of Padang, which sits on the coast of West Sumatra in Indonesia, is a sprawling metropolis of over 700,000 people. It has been a major trading port in southeast Asia for hundreds of years. Located near the equator, this sultry city is currently the provincial capital of West Sumatra and a province of the state of Indonesia. A regional metropolis, Padang is cosmopolitan and globally connected.

Being lesbi in Padang is generally understood as an expression of gender rather than a form of sexuality engaged in by two women (see also Blackwood 2005, 2010). By this I mean that a lesbi couple comprises two individuals who express distinctly different genders. Tombois do not see themselves as women; they consider themselves masculine or like men. I asked Tommy, a tomboi in h/er mid-twenties, how men treat h/er.[2] S/he said: 'They consider me a guy and treat me like one, not like a female. That's also because I consider myself a guy'. In regard to h/er family, Tommy said: 'My family understands that I'm more like a guy, even to the extent of sleeping [overnight] anywhere I want. It's not a problem. They know I can protect myself'. When asked how s/he sees h/erself, Robi, another tomboi, answered: 'I feel like a guy because my behaviour is more like a guy's. Really, there is no difference between me and men. We're the same'. Tombois are marked by their short hair, their rowdy, boisterous behaviour and their habit of smoking in public.

Tombois' performances of masculinity include the ability to move in spaces dominated by men, to work in men's jobs and to participate in behaviours that are allowed only for men, such as smoking, drinking and staying over at friends' houses. The ability to access some of men's privileges and to move in men's world assures tombois of their status as men. The men's world in Padang is found in the public spaces predominantly occupied by men, such as cafés, pool halls, bars, street corners, and for the more religious, the prayer house where religious studies and devotions are held. For young unmarried men in Padang this pattern means that they are generally free from familial supervision and control. Tommi's statement earlier that s/he can sleep overnight anywhere s/he wants substantiates h/er ability to move in the men's world. The everyday activities that tombois emphasise as part of their masculine life include: sleeping anywhere (especially not at home), doing anything they want, associating with whomever they want, going out, travelling alone, staying out late, doing men's work, smoking and drinking and hanging out with men. Being able to participate in the men's world substantiates their sense of self as masculine.

In contrast to tombois, girlfriends, who dress in the same style as other young women in West Sumatra, are generally polite, restrained and considerate in public. In fact, girlfriends see themselves as indistinguishable from other women. Jeni, who was in her early twenties at the time, explained to me: 'I am the same as other women. I wear feminine clothes, sometimes even skirts, and put on makeup'. She defines women as 'neat, polite, and warm hearted'. Being 'the same as other women' refers not only to the attributes they possess but the occupations they take up. Nila and Jeni manage a food stall, for which they do all the cooking themselves. Another is a maid, a fourth a seamstress. In addition to their occupations, they prioritise domestic interests. Epi said: 'I like to cook a lot – things like cake and cookies (*kuê*)'. Jeni said she likes to take walks, cook and read popular magazines when she is not busy. Girlfriends define themselves as normative women who are attracted to men; they happen to be lesbi at this point because their boyfriends are female bodied.

Tombois' and girlfriends' views of each other join together in supporting their differences. Jeni said: 'Girlfriends like a lot of attention just like other women. They like to be loved and spoiled'. In contrast, 'Tombois are just like guys', she said. 'They can be very crude and egotistical'. Noni stated that tombois are not afraid of anything, but for her: 'I'm very afraid to go out at night alone. I'm a woman. Someone might try to rape me!' Girlfriends speak of their relationships in hetero-normative terms, finding the masculine traits of their partners desirable. Jeni said: 'With Andri [her tomboi partner], I feel safe and protected'. Their traits and desires accord well with the gendered expectations for men and women. By demonstrating that they are not what women are, tombois feel confident in their knowledge of themselves as men. At the same time, girlfriends do not need to question their own desires because their self-presentation of femininity properly contrasts with that of the tombois.

All these comments underscore the reality of binary gender for these individuals and the importance of maintaining gender difference. Lesbi in Padang envision themselves as either masculine or feminine, men or women. In conversations among themselves, they use slang terms such as 'cowok' and 'cewek', meaning guy and girl, for masculine and feminine partners, respectively. These terms describe tombois and their partners in specifically gendered ways, bringing into being and reinforcing for each a gendered sense of self that contrasts with one's partner.

Falling into the lesbi world

Although tombois and their girlfriends place themselves at opposite ends of a gender spectrum, they see themselves at the same time as part of a lesbi world (*dunia lesbi*) that intersects in varying ways and to varying degrees with national and transnational queer discourses and movements. The means by which these discourses circulate globally are quite varied, including newspapers, magazines and films. Although in mainstream media such information is typically couched in negative terms, it still offers the possibility of imagining difference. Since the early 1980s, Indonesian media attention to an increasingly international gay and lesbian movement brought into common use the terms *lesbi* and *gay*, derived from the English terms lesbian and gay (Boellstorff 2005; Gayatri 1996). Stories about abusive or suicidal lesbian couples, the love interests of internationally famous lesbian and gay figures and reports of same-sex marriage and sex-reassignment surgeries offered an understanding of non-normative sexualities not available in everyday discourse. These stories provide a major source of information about lesbian, gay and trans-gender identities and lifestyles to Indonesian youth.

Other sites of knowledge transmission are the small urban communities of lesbi, gay and *waria*, each with their own particular knowledges and their different connections to global queer discourses. Waria is one of the Indonesian terms for male-bodied individuals who act like women and take men as lovers. Urban activist groups model themselves after and gain resources from international lesbian and gay organisations. While waria have been acknowledged and visible in Indonesia for many decades, the early 1980s saw the appearance (and disappearance) of several small organisations, primarily on the island of Java, formed by individuals who identified as gay or lesbi (see Boellstorff 2005; Howard 1996; Oetomo 2001; Wieringa 1999). One of the longest lasting groups, GAYa Nusantara, which is primarily a gay group but has included a few lesbi and waria, was organised in the mid-1980s. The first lesbian group was organised and disbanded in the early 1980s (Wieringa 1999).

Since 1998 two activist lesbian organisations, Swara Srikandi, the internet-based lesbian group in Jakarta, and Sector 15 of the Indonesian Women's Coalition (Koalisi Perempuan Indonesia, KPI), have developed a significant presence in Indonesia. These organisations, usually headed by well-educated, well-travelled, English-speaking activists from the upper echelons of Indonesian society, have looked to the lesbian and gay movements and literatures of western Europe and the USA for models and resources but have also created their own Indonesian understanding of gender and sexual identities.

Queer knowledge circulates unevenly in Indonesia, less dependent on institutional spaces or publications than on the everyday interactions and travels of lesbi, gay and waria individuals. For those in Padang not linked directly to international lesbian and gay organisations, and not actively participating in or seeking information from national activist groups, queer discourses travel primarily by word of mouth as tombois visit or live for brief periods of time in Jakarta and elsewhere in Indonesia. One of the best ways to illustrate the uneven circulation and reception of queer knowledge is to track the movement of particular linguistic terms and phrases. The terms lesbi, lesbian and gay were taken up by lesbi and gay groups in Jakarta as their identifiers in the early 1980s despite media-influenced associations with deviance, crime and illness (see Gayatri 1993). These terms circulated not only in the media but on the streets and among the social networks of those in same-sex relationships (Murray 1999; Wieringa 1999). In appropriating western labels, these groups lay claim to certain meanings attached to those labels but they were not simply imitating western identities. Rather, activists tended to rely on those terms and definitions as a way to validate their own existence and connect with a global movement.

Tombois who travelled to Jakarta, like Tommi, heard the word lesbi used by others like themselves in places where lesbi and gay congregated. But the activist definition of lesbi as 'women who are attracted to women' was not the meaning s/he attached to the word. The prevalence of 'butch' lesbians in working class contexts helped bolster tombois' view of themselves as lesbi who are like men (see Murray 1999). When asked why s/he sees h/erself as lesbi, Tommi replied: '[B]ecause I fell in love with a woman', creating a connection between lesbi and tombois' desires for women. Girlfriends are also included under the label lesbi because they are with someone who is a tomboi. Tommi's girlfriend Lina said: 'A woman with a tomboi is definitely a lesbi'. For girlfriends this attraction is consonant with their attraction to men in general, and yet their desire for tombois brings them under the label lesbi.

At the same time that they stand under the label lesbi, tombois and girlfriends shift its meaning. Because partners are differently gendered, a lesbi in their understanding of the term is not a *woman* attracted to other *women*, but a *female* who is attracted to the other gender. Lesbi, in this sense, serves as an umbrella term that incorporates their different subjectivities. For tombois and girlfriends, the label lesbi includes individuals with different histories and different routes into the lesbi world. Lesbi then serves as an identifier, signifying a group that occupies a space distinct from the rest of the world. Consequently, lesbi as a circulating category is not a stable term throughout Indonesia but is appropriated and reconstituted to fit particular meanings.

Other idioms circulate in lesbi, gay and waria circles in Jakarta and travel to West Sumatra to become part of tombois' and girlfriends' speech. Gay men in Jakarta use the phrase 'falling into the gay world' (*terjun ke dunia gay*) to describe becoming involved with another man (Howard 1996). The phrase 'the lesbian world', which appeared in various newsletters in the 1990s and 2000s, employs the same concept of a separate world, in this case for lesbi. This phrase travelled to Padang via tombois such as Tommi, who had spent nearly two years in Jakarta. When talking about a young woman who had become involved with her first tomboi, one tomboi said: '[She] fell into the lesbian world' (*terjun ke dunia lesbi*). This phrasing signifies movement from the everyday world of family and kin into a new world populated by others like themselves. Girlfriends are seen as 'falling into' the lesbi world while their tomboi partners seem always to have been there. *Dunia lesbi* is not the world of tombois, however, but the world of lesbi couples, both tombois and their girlfriends. While Jakarta activists imagine this world to be composed of women attracted to other women, in Padang the same terminology is used for a world comprising individuals with two very different subjectivities: that of normative females/women (the girlfriends) and physical females/men (the tombois).

Thus *dunia lesbi* is not localised but inclusive of a lesbian world populated by global others. In the selective reception of queer knowledge these others are read as sharing the same understanding of lesbi as those in Padang. Famous lesbians such as Martina Navratilova and Melissa Etheridge, whose stories of betrayal by 'femme' lovers are well known in Indonesia, secure a strong connection between lesbi in Padang and a global *dunia lesbi*. Both women are read as tombois and their girlfriends as femmes who, unsurprisingly to tombois in Padang, left their partners for men. Thus, while images of famous lesbians connect tombois and their girlfriends to a global lesbian world, these images are read in a way that supports a gendered construction of sexuality. In the circulation of queer knowledge, lesbi in Padang use their own culturally available models to interpret global queer discourses and arrive at meanings that make sense to them, creating their own particular version of the lesbi world.

Conclusion

Queer discourses are accessed by lesbi in Padang in ways circumscribed by their class location. Because their location limits access to certain circuits of knowledge, their lesbi subjectivities reflect the particularities of place. Despite their lack of access to new technologies and print media published by national lesbian and gay activist organisations, lesbi are not isolated from global networks; these networks are accessed through different, often indirect, means. This queer knowledge is used to construct a sense of community of like-minded individuals that includes lesbi, waria and gay in Indonesia and beyond. Tombois and their girlfriends should not be seen as existing on the backward edge of a social movement whose full weight has yet to be felt. They are already part of and interconnected with the larger global queer community. While their subjectivities reflect their particular location within larger national and transnational queer discourses and movements, their particular differences are part of the global shifts in sexual and gender subjectivities.

Part of the problem of global translation lies in the misrecognition of gender-based sexualities, which happens when females who 'act like men' are said by scholars and activists to lack an awareness of their sexual identity. Lesbi in Padang are not lacking in awareness: they are a product of modern national and transnational processes in the same way as their counterparts in the west. The diversity of gendered and sexual subjectivities in Indonesia demonstrates that there is neither a homogeneous global nor national queer identity, suggesting that strategies to address sexual rights must be sensitive to the differences within and across groups, nations and regions of the world.

Notes

1 During 2001 and 2004, I conducted extensive research on lesbi subjectivities in Padang. I met 28 individuals who were either tombois or girlfriends of tombois. Of those 28, I formally interviewed 16 individuals whose families range from somewhat poor to average income.
2 When referring to tombois, I use the pronominal constructions 's/he' and 'h/er' as a way to disrupt the binary genders of the English language. No English pronouns adequately convey the Indonesian usage, in which the third person pronoun is gender neutral.

References

Altman, D. (2001) *Global Sex*, Chicago: University of Chicago Press.

Bacchetta, P. (2002) 'Rescaling Transnational "Queerdom": Lesbian and "Lesbian" Identitary Positionalities in Delhi in the 1980s', *Antipode: A Radical Journal of Geography*, 34: 947–73.

Blackwood, E. (2005) 'Transnational Sexualities in One Place: Indonesian Readings', *Gender & Society*, 19: 221–42.

Blackwood, E. (2010) *Falling into the Lesbi World: Desire and Difference in Indonesia*, Honolulu: University of Hawaii Press.

Blackwood, E. and Wieringa, S. E. (eds) (1999) *Female Desires: Same-Sex Relations and Transgender Practices across Cultures*, New York: Columbia University Press.

Boellstorff, T. (2005) *The Gay Archipelago: Sexuality and Nation in Indonesia*, Princeton: Princeton University Press.

Butler, J. (1990) *Gender Trouble: Feminism and the Subversion of Identity*, New York: Routledge.

Cruz-Malavé, A. and Manalansan IV, M. F. (2002) 'Introduction: Dissident Sexualities/Alternative Globalisms', in *Queer Globalizations: Citizenship and the Afterlife of Colonialism*, New York: New York University Press.

Foucault, M. (1978) *The History of Sexuality. Vol. 1: An Introduction*, New York: Vintage Books.

Gayatri, B. J. D. (1993) 'Coming Out but Remaining Hidden: A Portrait of Lesbians in Java', paper presented at the International Congress of Anthropological and Ethnological Sciences, Mexico City, Mexico.

Gayatri, B. J. D. (1996) 'Indonesian Lesbians Writing their Own Script: Issues of Feminism and Sexuality', in Reinfelder, M. (ed.) *Amazon to Zami: Towards a Global Lesbian Feminism*, London: Cassell.

Gopinath, G. (2002) 'Local Site/Global Contexts: The Transnational Trajectories of Deepa Mehta's *Fire*', in Cruz-Malavé, A. and Manalansan IV, M. F. (eds) *Queer Globalizations: Citizenship and the Afterlife of Colonialism*, New York: New York University Press.

Grewal, I. and Kaplan, C. (2001) 'Global Identities: Theorizing Transnational Studies of Sexuality', *GLQ: Journal of Lesbian and Gay Studies*, 7: 663–79.

Howard, R. S. (1996) 'Falling into the Gay World: Manhood, Marriage, and Family in Indonesia', unpublished thesis, University of Illinois, Urbana.

King, K. (2002) 'There are no Lesbians here: Lesbians, Feminism and Global Gay Formations', in Cruz-Malavé, A. and Manalansan IV, M. F. (eds) *Queer Globalizations: Citizenship and the Afterlife of Colonialism*, New York: New York University Press.

Morgan, R. and Wieringa, S. (2005) *Tommy Boys, Lesbian Men and Ancestral Wives: Female Same-Sex Practices in Africa*, Johannesburg: Jacana Media.

Murray, A. J. (1999) 'Let Them Take Ecstasy: Class and Jakarta Lesbians', in Blackwood, E. and Wieringa, S. E. (eds) *Female Desires: Same-sex Relations and Transgender Practices across Cultures*, New York: Columbia University Press.

Plummer, K. (1992) 'Speaking its Name: Inventing a Lesbian and Gay Studies', in Plummer, K. (ed.) *Modern Homosexualities: Fragments of Lesbian and Gay Experience*, London: Routledge.

Oetomo, D. (2001) *Memberi Suara pada yang Bisu* [Giving Voice to the Mute], Yogyakarta: Galang Press.

Wieringa, S. E. (1999) 'Desiring Bodies or Defiant Cultures: Butch-femme Lesbians in Jakarta and Lima', in Blackwood, E. and Wieringa, S. E. (eds) *Female Desires: Same-sex Relations and Transgender Practices across Cultures*, New York: Columbia University Press.

Wieringa, S. E., Blackwood, E. and Bhaiya, A. (eds) (2007) *Women's Sexualities and Masculinities in a Globalizing Asia*, New York: Palgrave Macmillan.

9 Hidden love

Sexual ideologies and relationship ideals in rural South Africa

Abigail Harrison

In sub-Saharan Africa, about two-thirds of HIV infections occur among young people aged 15–24 (UNAIDS 2006). An estimated 15.5 per cent of South African women aged 15–24 are HIV infected, compared to 4.8 per cent of men (Pettifor *et al.* 2005) and 15 per cent of the world's HIV-infected population aged 15 to 24 lives in the country (Hallman 2004). Unequal gender and power relations mean that women are particularly vulnerable to HIV (Susser and Stein 2000; Campbell and MacPhail 2002; Jewkes *et al.* 2003). Within heterosexual relationships, women often lack the power to negotiate with whom, how and when to have sex (Bhana *et al.* 2007). These vulnerabilities are further compounded by age, constraining prevention choices (Dowsett and Aggleton 1999; MacPhail and Campbell 2001; Harrison *et al.* 2001). Both sexual coercion, which is common, and the practice of partnering with older men increase young women's HIV risk (Dunkle *et al.* 2004; Gregson *et al.* 2002). In southern Africa, historical inequalities, widespread social dislocation and long-term disruption in family and social organisation reinforce these gender dynamics (Gilbert and Walker 2002).

Entrenched gender beliefs also influence young people's socialisation regarding sexuality, and often mandate deferential behaviour for young women in sexual relationships (Varga 2003). Understanding the social construction of young people's sexuality requires attention to the range of meanings and definitions attached to sexuality and relationships. Studies of African young people's sexualities highlight several common themes. First, a rising age of marriage has created an extended adolescence, making premarital sexual activity more common (Mensch *et al.* 1998). Second, sexuality is contested, highlighting generational differences between youth and their parents, who remain invested in sexual regimes based on marriage and reproduction (Smith 2000; Wight *et al.* 2006). Third, young people often rely on peers for information (Rivers and Aggleton 2000), which may reinforce unsafe behaviours. Fourth, the stigma or shame associated with sexual activity outside marriage may further constrain access to appropriate advice and information (Harrison 2002; Morrell 2003; Haram 2005). Ultimately, young people rely on a range of competing social influences to negotiate and construct their sexuality, often drawing simultaneously on conservative social norms, modern romantic aspirations about relationships and the community discourse through which these changes are contested (Dilger 2003).

In South Africa, there has been intense recent public scrutiny of young women's sexual mores (Harrison *et al.* 2000; LeClerc-Madlala 2001; Scorgie 2002). Yet most scholarship on sexuality has addressed either the historical context (Delius and

Glaser 2002; Reid and Walker 2005), the evolution of cultural practices, such as virginity testing (LeClerc-Madlala 2001) or changes in men's behaviour (Hunter 2004).

In contemporary discourse (Burns 2007), popular notions of sexuality are generally assumed to reflect African 'traditions', often with little examination of historical practice (Delius and Glaser 2002; Burns 2007). This 'neo-traditionalism' is often highly conservative, interpreting cultural practices as static and immutable rather than dynamically contested and adaptive (Spiegel and Boonzaier 1988). However, ethnographic accounts provide historical insight into the management of young people's sexuality in Zulu culture. Puberty rituals (*umhlonyane*) prepared young women for marriage, with an emphasis on premarital morality and decorum, as well as sex and procreation (Krige 1950), after which a young woman became eligible for courtship (Gluckman 1950). Communication about sexual matters was conducted through older girls or elder 'sisters' (*amaqikiza*), who introduced suitors and provided instruction in sexual conduct, including *ukusoma*, non-penetrative 'thigh sex' permissible prior to marriage (Krige 1950). Engagement and marriage proceeded through a series of formal steps, including public acceptance of a lover (*ukuqoma*) and payment of bridewealth (*ilobolo*). A girl's moral status and virginity were central to this negotiation, with higher bridewealth accorded young women deemed chaste and pure (Ngubane 1981).

In the late nineteenth century, Christian missionaries sought to eliminate such 'primitive' or 'backward' practices (Gaitskell 1982; Marks 2002). Over time, Christian beliefs became interwoven with cultural practices, so that 'traditions' owe as much to a Christian as to an Africanist heritage (Burns 2007). The recent rise of 'independent' churches based on both Africanist and Christian beliefs, and Pentecostalism, as in the popular Zionist and Apostolic churches, has reinforced this (Muller 1999).

This chapter uses qualitative data to examine how young men and women engage with these sociocultural influences to construct and enact their sexuality in rural KwaZulu/Natal, South Africa, with discussion of the implications for HIV prevention, an urgent priority given South Africa's severe HIV epidemic.

Research setting

KwaZulu/Natal with a population of 10 million is South Africa's largest province. The rural areas, home to about half the population, are among the country's most economically disadvantaged areas (UNDP 2006). KwaZulu/Natal also has the highest HIV prevalence, with 14.1 per cent of young people and 16.5 per cent of the general population HIV infected (Shisana *et al.* 2005). Labour migration, along with colonial and apartheid era policies, deeply affected the social organisation of rural KwaZulu/Natal, and, given continued rural underdevelopment, migration to urban areas remains common.

Data and methods

Selection of participants

The study was conducted among school-going young people in one subdistrict. Nearly 80 per cent of young South Africans aged 15–19 currently attend school (Statistics South Africa 2004). To select participants, 16 high schools comprising grades 8–12 were separated into three homogeneous groups based on school size and geographic characteristics. One school was then randomly selected from each group. Participants were selected for peer group discussions through responses to a self-administered questionnaire on HIV prevention knowledge and sexual behaviour that was given to all students in selected grades. Eligibility was based on age and grade level, reported sexual experience, availability during non-school hours and willingness to notify parents regarding participation. No refusals from schools, teachers or parents occurred. Data collection occurred between January 2000 and March 2001. Six categories of young people were defined at the outset of the study: younger (14–15 years) and older (16–19 years) teenage women, younger and older teenage men and sexually inexperienced women and men. These categories reflected assumptions about likely differences between those groups (i.e. gender, age, sexual experience), with the research designed to explore those differences. All peer groups were single sex and included 5–10 participants each, meeting weekly over a 3-month period.

Data collection

Two qualitative research methods were used: peer group discussions (PGD) and in-depth interviews (IDI).

Peer group discussions

Peer group discussions are similar to standard focus groups, but comprise repeat sessions with the same group (Balmer *et al.* 1997). Like focus groups, they rely on discussion generated among relatively homogeneous groups, and are useful for identifying and clarifying group norms, values and beliefs (Kitzinger 1995). In this study, group discussions were deemed appropriate due to the sensitive nature of the topic and the paucity of data on normative behaviour and peer influences on sexuality in this setting. Repeat discussions allow for the development of trust and rapport within groups, provide a dynamic understanding of change over time, validate reports and help to evaluate complex or sensitive topics.

Discussions occurred during eight separate peer group sessions. Each focused on one topic and used a structured question guide for each session. Interviewers were trained to facilitate open-ended discussions and to follow participants' own narrative accounts, 'giving voice' to their values, concerns and language.

In-depth interviews

Twelve in-depth interviews with selected peer group participants were conducted to complement the peer group discussions. These were intended to elicit personal narratives and experiences about sexual life histories, yielding personal information that did not emerge in the groups.

Conducting the research

The peer group discussions and in-depth interviews were conducted by two female facilitator–interviewers of roughly the same age as the participants. All group discussions and interviews were conducted in *isiZulu*, taped using a micro-cassette recorder, and then translated and transcribed by the interviewers. Sessions were conducted privately in schools or in a selected venue outside the school.

A four-step analytical process was used for both peer group and interview data. This involved structured reading of the transcripts; identifying core themes and development of a structured coding scheme; identifying major analytical domains; and creating matrices to allow comparison between groups. In addition, the iterative analytical process permitted comparison and validation of data from the peer group discussions and the in-depth interviews.

Findings

Attitudes toward sexuality

Good behaviour

Both young women and men emphasised the importance of 'good behaviour' in their prospective partners. The word for behaviour in isiZulu, *nokuzipatha*, conveys the broader meaning of comportment or decorum. Although *nokuzipatha* was used to express all the desirable characteristics of a person, it was most commonly used to comment on sexual conduct, with 'good behaviour' an essential characteristic for a girlfriend:

MZ: The thing that affects me is to see a young girl misbehaving.
FACILITATOR 1: What do you mean by misbehaving
MZ: I mean changing boys [having many boyfriends] now and then.
FACILITATOR 2: So how does that affect you?
MZ: When I grow up I want to marry someone, so I have some problem in choosing the girl because I will never know which is the right one because they are all doing the same thing.

(PGDs, teenage men)

In this gendered portrayal, a young woman's 'inappropriate' behaviour is cited. This could include having more than one sexual partner or simply not remaining a virgin. Young women also referred to the 'behaviour' of female friends and young men: 'What he said to me was that he was a well-behaved guy, didn't have a girl-friend and also that he wasn't someone who liked women. He spends most of his time alone and not with women'. (IDI, 18 year old woman). For young women, 'good behaviour' also included decency, honesty and coming from a good family, in addition to sexual modesty.

Sex is wrong

Becoming openly sexually active at a young age clearly violated standards of 'good behaviour'. For young men and women, sexual relationships were the province of 'older' people, and the late teens or early twenties viewed as the 'right age and time to have sex'. Younger teenage women in relationships, whether sexually active or not, risked strong family and community disapproval. Reflecting these social mores, most younger teenage women regarded their relationships and sexual activity as 'wrong'. As one young woman said: 'I realised what I was doing was wrong because I was still young'.

These views produced a pronounced ambivalence about sexual activity: 'It [sex] is not important and it's not the way you can show someone that you love him or her'. Younger teenage women viewed abstinence as the 'right' thing to do, and also a preferred HIV prevention strategy. Their own failure to remain abstinent did not hinder these feelings, but influenced self-perceptions of their behaviour as transgressing accepted community norms.

Notions of the ideal relationships

Young women and men had strongly romantic ideas, which coexisted and contrasted with perceptions of relationships as inappropriate. The phrase 'proposing love' (*ukushela*) describes the romantic process of initiating relationships. 'Proposing love' proceeds according to socially approved guidelines that are clearly understood among peers, with young men responsible for initiating interest. When 'proposing love', young men emphasised romance and courtship. Among young women, first relationships were both anticipated and feared, due to negative community attitudes toward young women's sexuality.

Descriptions of ideal partners captured these conflicts: 'I want someone with style and who would respect my parents because some boys don't respect parents. They call you even in front of your parents, I don't like that type of person' (PGD, younger teenage women). Since parents often oppose relationships, teenage men and women sought partners who would be acceptable to their families. However, teenage women also expected boyfriends to conform to expectations of 'modernity':

PD: I want someone who is active, handsome, dresses smartly, loves people ...
NM: Maybe at college or at university level and not a person who is not working.

(PGDs, younger teenage women)

Clandestine relationships

Hiding relationships from adults was another strategy to accommodate social expectations, particularly for teenage women who experienced enormous anxiety about relationships being discovered. Boyfriends from school or other communities were desirable since a girl's family would not recognise them. As one young woman described it:

PR: She [girl's mother] says that I shouldn't have boyfriends.
FACILITATOR 1: Does she say until when?
PR: Until I finish school. And then she says that I can then introduce that person at home once I've finished school if I think he is worth the introduction ...
FACILITATOR 1: Does she know that now you are involved in a relationship?
PR: No she doesn't know ... I normally visit my boyfriend when she is not home.

(IDI, 15-year-old woman)

Although young men did not feel the same pressure to hide their relationships, they were not entirely open. As one said: '[O]ur parents do not even know we are having sex' (PGDs, older teenage men). More often, they protected their girlfriends by hiding the relationship, a situation that sometimes benefitted young men, as they could more easily have additional partners.

Entering a 'serious' relationship

Many of the younger teenage women defined even their short-term relationships as 'serious', and spoke of 'introducing a boyfriend at home', Since families generally viewed serious relationships as acceptable, they could be conducted openly:

> I stopped him when he wanted to go home to show himself to my parents [to initiate the formal engagement process]. I told him that I still want to finish my schooling first. But my mother knows about our relationship. The way I see it, he is serious ...

> (IDI, 16-year-old woman)

Another woman discussed expectations for her boyfriend to 'come home': '[I]t all depends on how you live your lifestyle. The first time I had sex was with my current boyfriend. I always refused to have sex with him until he formally met my parents' (IDI, 17-year-old woman). Another 17-year-old woman described her hopes for the future: 'He always says that maybe by the end of this year he'll be working and ... [then in five years] ... we'll be married'.

Relationship type

The serious relationships described by young women were referred to as *ukuqoma*, or 'committed', and were customarily a formal part of the Zulu marriage process (Krige 1950). In contemporary terms, when relationships become openly known to both families, young women no longer have to hide the relationship or sexual activity. As one woman described:

N: *Ngiqomile* [I am committed].
FACILITATOR 1: If you say you are *qomile*, what do you mean?
N: It's not a hidden relationship ... I would say it's a serious relationship.
FACILITATOR 1: Why do you say that?
N: First of all, I am not *jolaring, ngiqomile* [I am committed]. So whatever we have done is not a secret, we did everything openly and it's clear to everyone.

(IDI, 16-year-old woman)

In contrast, *ukujola* (from the South African word 'jol', meaning 'to have a good time'), refers to a relationship for fun, without an expectation of commitment, which is more acceptable for young men. None of the teenage men reported more serious *ukuqoma* relationships, most likely due to their young age. Pressure from older brothers or friends to pursue *ukujola* relationships was common, with sexual activity seen as integral to male development.

Sexual activity

Young women often sought to characterise their relationships as *ukuqoma* once sexual activity began, so that the relationship would be open and legitimate in the eyes of the community. Although most women did not view sexual intercourse as necessary, it was regarded as a key component of relationships. Young women had little power to prevent or resist sexual activity, and male partners controlled sexual decision making. As one said: 'You realise that you are ready [to have sex] once your boyfriend asks for it' (PGD, older teenage women). These ambiguities were present in most discussions about sexual activity, and there was little discussion of sexual pleasure or even intimacy. With younger women, discussions of sexuality were characterised initially by frequent silences, hesitation and fear. Most women said they were not prepared or ready for their first intercourse.

Proving virginity

The practice of 'proving virginity', whereby a young woman has sexual intercourse to establish her virginity, was prominently discussed by both young women and men. The young men universally felt that virginity was a desirable characteristic and reflected a young woman's good behaviour and high moral standard: 'If you have a virgin, you know that you got a right partner' (IDI, 17-year-old man). Once in a relationship, however, boyfriends often insisted on sexual intercourse to establish that a girlfriend was still a virgin. Young women's reluctance to have sexual intercourse often disappeared in the face of these demands, as they perceived they were 'saving' their virginity for the right partner.

None of the young men mentioned virginity as desirable for themselves neither did any of the participants discuss the clearly paradoxical nature of this practice, whereby a young woman lost her valued virgin status in order to 'prove' virginity. However, some young women recognised the dangers:

ZN: Boys like girls who are virgins. Sometimes even if they don't love you but just because they know that you are a virgin, they try by all means to get you and the next day they go proud telling their friends that they had sex with a virgin.

(PGD, older teenage woman)

As another woman said: 'Maybe someone would have heard that you've never had a boyfriend and they wish to be the first one to sleep with you'. One young woman discussed the importance of losing her virginity to her boyfriend: 'I always ask him not to let me down, like if he's not serious about us he should make it clear from the start. He shouldn't play around with my virginity' (IDI, 16-year-old woman). In reality, 'proving virginity' often acted against young women's best interests, with the idealised notion of saving virginity for the right partner contrasting sharply with reality.

Discussion

Young participants in this research articulated a clear moral framework regarding sexuality and relationships, rooted in a sexual ideology that views sexual activity as 'inappropriate' and 'wrong'. Consequently, relationships are often hidden, and sexual expression is legitimate only in serious relationships (*ukuqoma*) deemed acceptable to the community. These relationships were perceived as favourable and 'safe' because they could be conducted openly and offered the prospect of a long-term commitment. In reality, *ukuqoma* relationships appear no safer than any other relationship, as young women still expressed fear and hesitation regarding sex, and lacked power to resist male partners' demands.

Other research on African youth sexualities has similarly noted the importance of abstinence as an idealised behaviour (Wight *et al.* 2006), although normative values surrounding sexuality rarely inhibit sexual activity (Dowsett and Aggleton 1999). Where sexuality is hidden, young women are placed at risk, both of HIV and of unwanted sexual attention, including coercion (Haram 2005). Other research has noted young women's use of 'serious' relationships to legitimise sexual expression, with disastrous consequences for prevention (Holland *et al.* 1991).

In this study, young people's approach to relationships and prevention was rife with paradoxes and contradictions, perhaps most evident in the sexually active young women whose preferred prevention method was abstinence. Instead of a viable prevention method, abstinence was an ideology that placed them at risk. Yet there was logic in this approach: How can someone in a hidden relationship seek condoms or contraceptives publicly, for example, when her highest priority is to ensure no one knows she is being sexually active? Women's consent to sexual intercourse in order to 'prove virginity' was also paradoxical, although in keeping with gendered constructions of sexuality and femininity (Varga 2003; Pattman 2005; Reddy and Dunne 2007).

The peer group methodology paired with in-depth interviews represents one strength of this research. Structuring the peer groups by age and gender permitted an understanding of variation within the lifecourse, particularly differences between older and younger women. This emphasised the vulnerabilities of the younger women – those aged 14–15, instead of the voices of older, more sexually experienced respondents dominating. Thus, a picture emerged of the development of sexuality and risk in the early sexual lives of teenagers in this setting. Teenage men and older teenage women, aged 16–19, were more comfortable and open in discussions of their sexual life histories. Normative views about sexuality emerged primarily from the peer group discussions, with important consensus between the different age and gender groups.

Importantly, the findings from this study highlight the absence of a constructive and positive discourse surrounding sexuality and prevention. Most young South Africans are well informed about HIV and AIDS, and about condoms as a prevention strategy (Pettifor *et al.* 2005). At the same time, 'cultural' approaches to HIV prevention have achieved prominence, emphasising abstinence and virginity testing among other methods. Rather than educating and preparing young people for sexual life, these restrict sexuality and reinforce gender inequality, and young people have largely been left alone to make sense of these competing discourses. In a context in which young women experience some of the highest HIV levels in the world, this has had severe consequences.

Yet there are 'cultural' forms of sexuality education that could be appropriate for contemporary adaptation, including the use of 'elder sisters' (*amaqikiza*) for sexuality education, or promotion of non-penetrative thigh sex (*ukusoma*) as a safer alternative to intercourse for those entering sexual activity. Recent research calls for interventions to address the social context of sexual risk, focusing on ways to alter social norms that contribute to sexual risk behaviours (Wellings *et al.* 2006). In rural South Africa, broad-based sexuality education could challenge harmful social norms and promote greater openness around sexuality. Sexual activity will never be safe as long as young people are told that sexual expression is bad, dangerous and wrong, or where it remains hidden and stigmatised. In addition, there are enormous gaps in HIV prevention. At minimum, young people need accurate information about sexuality, to ensure better preparation for sexual life and healthy relationships. Opportunities to promote such changes do exist, including revitalisation of the national Life Skills programme, intended to provide sexuality education to school-going youth (Morrell 2003). Ultimately, however, success will lie not in changing one intervention but in altering existing discourse about gender and sexuality, and expanding HIV prevention options for young people.

References

Balmer, D. H., Gikundi, E., Billingsley, M. C., Kihuho, F. G., Kimani, M., Wang'ondu, J. *et al.* (1997) 'Adolescent Knowledge, Values and Coping Strategies: Implications for Health in Sub-Saharan Africa', *Journal of Adolescent Health*, 21: 33–8.

Bhana, D., Morrell, R., Hearn, J. and Moletsane, R. (2007) 'Power and Identity: An Introduction to Sexualities in Southern Africa', *Sexualities*, 10 (2): 131–9.

Burns, C. (2007) 'Book Review: Special Issue of Culture, Health and Sexuality', *Sexualities*, 10 (2): 263–5.

Campbell, C. and MacPhail, C. (2002) 'Peer Education, Gender and the Development of Critical Consciousness: Participatory HIV prevention by South African Youth', *Social Science and Medicine*, 55 (2): 331–45.

Delius, P. and Glaser, C. (2002) 'Sexual Socialisation in South Africa: A Historical Perspective', *African Studies*, 61 (1): 27–54.

Dilger, H. (2003) 'Sexuality, AIDS and the Lures of Modernity: Reflexivity and Morality among Young People in Rural Tanzania', *Medical Anthropology*, 22: 23–52.

Dowsett, G. and Aggleton, P. (1999) 'Young People and Risk-taking in Sexual Relations', in Aggleton, P., Dowsett, G., Rivers, K. and Warwick, I. (eds) *Sex and Youth: Contextual Factors affecting Risk for HIV/AIDS: A Comparative Analysis of Multi-site Studies in Developing Countries, Part I*, Geneva: UNAIDS. Available at www.unaids.org/html/publications/irc-pub01/jc096-sex_youth_en_pdf.pdf (accessed 19 September 2006).

Dunkle, K. L., Jewkes, R. K., Brown, H. C., Gray, G. E., McIntyre, J. A. and Harlow, S. D. (2004) 'Gender-based Violence, Relationship Power, and Risk of HIV Infection in Women attending Antenatal Clinics in South Africa', *Lancet*, 363 (9419): 1415–21.

Gaitskell, D. (1982) 'Wailing for Purity: Mothers, Daughters and Christian Prayer Unions in South Africa', in Marks, S. and Rathbone, R. (eds) *Industrialisation and Social Change in South Africa: African Class Formation, Culture, and Consciousness, 1870–1930*, New York: Longman.

Gilbert, L. and Walker, L. (2002) 'Treading the Path of Least Resistance: HIV/AIDS and Social Inequalities. A South African Case Study', *Social Science and Medicine*, 54 (7): 1093–110.

Gluckman, M. (1950) 'Kinship and Marriage among the Lozi of Northern Rhodesia and the Zulu of Natal', In Radcliffe Brown, A. R. and Forde, D. (eds) *African Systems of Kinship and marriage*, London: University of London Press.

Gregson, S., Nyamukapa, C., Garnett, G., Mason, P. R., Zhuwau, T., Carael, M. *et al.* (2002) 'Sexual Mixing Patterns and Sex-differentials in Teenage Exposure to HIV Infection in Rural Zimbabwe', *Lancet*, 359 (9321): 1896–903.

Hallman, K. (2004) *Socioeconomic Disadvantage and Unsafe Sexual Behaviours among Young Women and Men in South Africa.* Policy Research Division Working Paper No. 190, New York: Population Council.

Haram, L. (2005) '"Eyes have no Curtains": The Moral Economy of Secrecy in Managing Love Affairs among Adolescents in Northern Tanzania in the Time of AIDS', *Africa Today,* 51 (4): 57–75.

Harrison, A. (2002) 'The Social Dynamics of Adolescent Risk for HIV: Using Research Findings to design a School-based Intervention', *Agenda,* 2002 (53): 43–52.

Harrison, A., Montgomery, E., Lurie, M. and Wilkinson, D. (2000) 'Barriers to Implementing South Africa's Termination of Pregnancy Act: Case Study from Rural KwaZulu/Natal Province', *Health Policy and Planning 2000,* 15 (4): 424–31.

Harrison, A., Xaba, N. and Kunene, P. (2001) 'Understanding Safe Sex: Gender Narratives of HIV and Pregnancy Prevention by Rural South African School-going Youth', *Reproductive Health Matters,* 9 (17): 63–71.

Holland, J., Ramazanoglu, C., Scott, S., Sharpe, S. and Thomson, R. (1991) 'Between Embarrassment and Trust: Young Women and the Diversity of Condom Use', in Aggleton, P., Hart, G. and Davies, P. (eds) *AIDS: Responses, Interventions and Care,* London: Falmer Press.

Hunter, M. (2004) 'Masculinities, Multiple Sexual Partners, and AIDS: The Making and Unmaking of *Isoka* in KwaZulu/Natal', *Transformation,* 54: 123–53.

Jewkes, R. K., Levin, J. B. and Penn-Kekana, L. A. (2003) 'Gender Inequalities, Intimate Partner Violence and HIV Preventive Practices: Findings of a South African Cross-sectional Study', *Social Science and Medicine,* 56 (1): 125–34.

Kitzinger, J. (1995) 'Introducing Focus Groups', *British Medical Journal,* 311: 299–302.

Krige, E. J. (1950) *The Social System of the Zulus,* Pietermaritzburg: Shuter & Shooter.

LeClerc-Madlala, S. (2001) 'Virginity Testing: Managing Sexuality in a Maturing HIV/AIDS Epidemic', *Medical Anthropology Quarterly,* 15 (4): 533–52.

MacPhail, C. and Campbell, C. (2001) '"I think Condoms are Good but, aai, I hate those Things": Condom Use among Adolescents and Young People in a Southern African Township', *Social Science and Medicine,* 52: 1613–27.

Marks, S. (2002) 'An Epidemic waiting to Happen? The Spread of HIV/AIDS in South Africa in Social and Historical Perspective', *African Studies,* 61 (1): 13–26.

Mensch, B. S., Bruce, J. and Greene, M. (1998) *The Uncharted Passage: Girls' Adolescence in the Developing World,* New York: Population Council.

Morrell, R. (2003) 'Silence, Sexuality and HIV/AIDS in South African Schools, *Australian Educational Researcher,* 30 (1): 41–62.

Muller, C. A. (1999) *Rituals of Fertility and the Sacrifice of Desire: Nazarite Women's Performance in South Africa,* Chicago: University of Chicago Press.

Ngubane, H. (1981) 'Marriage, Affinity and the Ancestral Realm: Zulu Marriage in Female Perspective', In Krige, E. J. and Comaroff, J. L. (eds) *Essays on African Marriage in Southern Africa,* Cape Town: Juta & Company, Ltd.

Pattman, R. (2005) '"Boys and Girls should Not be too Close": Sexuality, the Identities of African Boys and Girls and HIV/AIDS Education', *Sexualities,* 8 (4): 497–516.

Pettifor, A., Rees, H., Kleinschmidt, I., Steffenson, A., MacPhail, C., Hlongwa-Madikizela, L. *et al.* (2005) 'Young People's Sexual Health in South Africa: HIV Prevalence and Sexual Behaviours from a Nationally Representative Household Survey', *AIDS,* 19 (14): 1525–34.

Reddy, S. and Dunne, M. (2007) 'Risking It: Young Heterosexual Femininities in South African Context of HIV/AIDS', *Sexualities,* 10 (2): 159–72.

Reid, G. and Walker, L. (2005) 'Sex and Secrecy: A Focus on African Sexualities', *Culture, Health and Sexuality,* 7 (3): 185–94.

Rivers, K. and Aggleton, P. (2000) *Adolescent Sexuality, Gender and the HIV Epidemic,* New York: United Nations Development Programme.

Scorgie, F. (2002) 'Virginity Testing and the Politics of Sexual Responsibility: Implications for AIDS Interventions', *African Studies*, 61 (1): 55–75.

Shisana, O., Rehle, T., Simbayi, L. C., Parker, W., Zuma, K., Bhana, A. *et al.* (eds) (2005) *South African National HIV Prevalence, HIV Incidence, Behaviour and Communication Survey*, Cape Town: HSRC Press.

Smith, D. (2000) ' "These Girls Today *na war-o*": Premarital Sexuality and Modern Identity in Southeastern Nigeria', *Africa Today*, 47 (3/4): 98–120.

Spiegel, A. and Boonzaier, E. (1988) 'Promoting Tradition: Images of the South African Past', in Boonzaier, E. and Sharp, J. (eds) *South African Keywords. The Uses and Abuses of Political Concepts*, Cape Town: David Phillip.

Statistics South Africa (2004) *Census 2001: The People of South Africa Population Census. Primary Tables, KwaZulu/Natal*. Pretoria: Statistics South Africa.

Susser, I. and Stein, Z. (2000) 'Culture, Sexuality and Women's Agency in the Prevention of HIV/AIDS in Southern Africa', *American Journal of Public Health*, 90 (7): 1042–8.

UNAIDS (2006) *Report on the Global HIV/AIDS Epidemic*, Geneva: Joint United Nations Programme on HIV/AIDS (UNAIDS).

United Nations Development Programme (UNDP) (2006) *Human Development Report, 2006*, New York: United Nations Development Programme.

Varga, C. A. (2003) 'How Gender Roles influence Sexual and Reproductive Health among South African Adolescents', *Studies in Family Planning*, 34 (3): 160–72.

Wellings, K., Collumbien, M., Slaymaker, E., Singh, S., Hodges, Z., Patel, D. *et al.* (2006) 'Sexual Behaviour in Context: A Global Perspective', *Lancet*, 368: 1706–28.

Wight, D., Plummer, M. L., Mshana, G., Wamoyi J., Shigongo Z. S. and Ross, D. A. (2006) 'Contradictory Sexual Norms and Expectations for Young People in Rural Tanzania', *Social Science and Medicine*, 62: 987–97.

10 Thai (trans)genders and (homo)sexualities in a global context

Peter A. Jackson

Since the early 1990s many authors (e.g. Plummer 1992; Altman 1996a; Drucker 2000; Jackson 2000) have identified the proliferation of new same-sex and transgender identities, such as the Indonesian *waria*, Brazilian *travesti* and Thai *tom-dee* couples, as a significant instance of cultural globalisation. Dennis Altman has labelled this phenomenon 'global queering',[1] (Altman 1996a) and in a 1997 article 'Global Gaze/Global Gays', he observed: 'What strikes me is that *within* a given country, whether Indonesia or the United States, Thailand or Italy, the *range* of constructions of homosexuality is growing' (Altman 1997: 424, emphases in original). While we still lack definitive answers to the question of what has produced a variety of apparently similar transgender and homosexual identities in diverse social, political and cultural settings, recent research on global queering in Asia has clarified the scope and nature of the phenomenon by challenging some earlier accounts of the globalisation of homosexual and transgender identities. In this chapter, I summarise key findings of this research as a basis for interpreting the modern histories of homosexuality and transgenderism in Thailand, providing one case study response to the question of what have been the sources of this global queering.

Globalisation is not homogenising world queer cultures

Comparative research on Asia's diverse queer cultures (e.g. Jackson 1995, 2004; Garcia 1996; McLelland 2000; Sinnott 2004; Martin 2004) has questioned earlier views that '(g)lobalisation has helped create an international gay/lesbian identity' (Altman 2001: 86). Recent studies have revealed a proliferating diversity of sexual and gender identities that in some, but not all, countries have drawn on English identity categories such as 'gay' and 'lesbian'. As Tom Boellstorff (2007) notes, the adoption of labels such as 'gay' in Asian queer cultures more often reflects the emergence of new local patterns of sexual and gender identity than the simple borrowing of western models.

Jeffrey Weeks observes that recent comparative studies of queer globalisation are, 'helping to dissolve the idea of a single universal lesbian or gay identity' (Weeks 2007: 219) and he concludes that, '[T]he Western gay is not seated at the top of an evolutionary tree ... notions of what it is to be sexually different are likely to be radically modified as the "perverse dynamic' at the heart of so many cultures ... confronts the imperatives of global interconnectedness' (Weeks 2007: 218). Research on Asia's queer cultures confirms Arjun Appadurai's account of cultural globalisation as a multifaceted phenomenon: '[G]lobalisation is ... (an) uneven and even *localising* process. Globalisation does not necessarily or even frequently imply homogenisation or Americanisation' (Appadurai 1996: 17, emphasis in original).

Contemporary Asian transgenders are not 'traditional'

Early research, including my own (Jackson 1995), often opposed m-t-f transgenderism, imagined as premodern, pre-capitalist and traditional, to gay male homosexuality, represented as modern, transgressive, commodified and western influenced. This is a view I have since had to revise (Jackson 2003). Recent research reveals Asia's gay, lesbian and m-t-f transgender cultures to all be modern forms that differ from both western queer cultures *and* the premodern gender/sex cultures of their own societies. Regarding transgenderism, Boellstorff observes:

> [M]ale transvestites in Southeast Asia are not legacies of prior 'traditions'. Rather the available evidence suggests that male transvestites emerged as 'commodified transgender' subject positions only in the late nineteenth century or early twentieth.
>
> (Boellstorff 2007: 192)

Recent research on Thai queer genders and sexualities reveals that patterns of *kathoey* transgenderism are just as recent and as different from premodern forms as Thai gay sexualities, with Thailand's *kathoey* cultures taking their contemporary forms as a result of a twentieth-century revolution in Thai gender norms (Jackson 2003). Research on Asian queer cultures confirms Altman's (2001) contention that capitalism has played a central role in global queering. Indeed, new Asian transgender identities have emerged within the same context of market capitalism that Altman argues has supported the globalization of gay-type identities.

Americanisation is not the main source of global queering

As Ara Wilson observes, early discussions of global queering assumed what she calls 'an import–export calculus' that new queer subjectivities beyond the West 'derive from US-inflected Western modes of sexuality or from Western-based systems of modernity, such as capitalism' (Wilson 2006). Empirical research on queer Asia challenges the simplistic view that globalising capitalism has provided an avenue for exporting American sex cultural forms. Boellstorff notes:, 'A frequent Western misunderstanding is that gay tourism or international gay organisations have played a significant role in the translocation of "gay" subjectivities to Southeast Asia, an assertion commonly made without a shred of supporting evidence' (Boellstorff, 2007: 198).

Linguistic evidence played a key role in arguments that the borrowing of western homosexual identities has been the main driver of global queering. The fact that increasing numbers of homosexual men in both western and non-western societies use the label 'gay' was central to arguments about the global gay (Altman 1997). In contrast, Adam *et al.* argue:

> [S]imilarities in activities, styles, symbols, institutions, language, and so on ... do not imply the identities are the same ... [A]pparent commonalities must not

blind us to differences that exist in the meanings of these practices. Country-specific elements remain important.

(1999: 348)

Historical evidence also challenges the view that cultural borrowing from the west provided the prime impetus for the development of modern Asian queer cultures. The 'import–export calculus' (Wilson 2006) of global queering assumes that the west has imposed its form of modernity on the rest of the world, whether by imperialism in the colonial era or neo-imperialism since the Second World War. This view is assumed even in some comparative queer studies research (see various chapters in Cruz-Malavé and Manalansan 2002). However, not all modernisation in Asia has resulted from colonial rule or neo-colonial expansionism. It is often forgotten that not all of Asia was colonised by the west. Japan and Siam[2] both remained independent throughout the colonial era and, significantly, it is in these two countries that Asia's first modern homosexual communities emerged.[3] The import–export model of global queering does not explain why Tokyo and Bangkok were the first to emerge as Asian 'gay capitals' rather than the metropolitan centres of former colonies, such as Jakarta, Bombay and Hanoi, where direct rule by Europeans extended over many decades if not centuries. The import–export model does not explain why modern Asian homosexualities emerged first in those societies that suffered the *least* direct impact from western imperialism. Contact with the west, at least in its imperialist colonising form, delayed rather than assisted the development of modern gay cultures in Asia. Rather than being cultural consequences of Asia's subordination to the west, it is clear that the relative *autonomy* of politically independent Siam and Japan was central to the early emergence of modern gay cultures in both countries.

Global queering began before 'globalisation'

Some discussions of global queering have suggested that new Asian queer identities emerged only in the 1990s as part of the most recent wave of post-Cold War globalising influences. For example, Chris Berry *et al.* state: 'The recent emergence of gay and lesbian communities in Asia and its diaspora is intimately linked to the development of information technology in the region' (Berry *et al.* 2003: 1). However, this historical sequence, which positions non-western queer cultures as emerging after sex-cultural transformations that it is assumed took place first in the USA in the 1960s, is inaccurate. Global queering has a considerably deeper history than is represented in many accounts of the phenomenon, with new forms of sexual subjectivity being apparent in Thailand since at least the early 1960s (see Jackson 1999).

George Chauncey (1994) maintains that 'the sexual regime now hegemonic in American culture, is a stunningly recent creation' (Chauncey 1994: 13), and he identifies the mid-twentieth century as the period when modern US ideas of homosexuality emerged. This chronology of US sex cultural shifts is very close to the periodisation revealed in my research on Thailand (Jackson 1999, 2000), where contemporary understandings of both the transgender *kathoey* and gay male identity emerged in the years after the Second World War. The central question for global queering research is why sexual cultures in parts of Asia and the west *both* underwent major transformations in similar, but also distinctive, ways over the same period of the twentieth century. Given the discrediting of the import–export model of global queering, answers will need to identify common transnational processes that have impacted on both Asian and western sexual cultures. Understanding the emergence of new Asian queer genders and sexualities will need to draw on a more complex model in which both local sex cultural differentiation *and* transnational convergence are seen as equally modern phenomena.

Reading and rereading Thai queer history

In earlier work, I have tried to bring a comparative perspective to studies of global queering by exploring the histories of Thailand's new queer cultures in light of the results of the research summarised already in this chapter. I began by tracing the emergence of new same-sex and transgender identity categories into public discourse in the Thai press and gay and lesbian publications (Jackson 1997, 1999, 2000, 2003). This research revealed that from the early 1960s there was a rapid differentiation of queer identities and an expansion in publicly visible transgender and homosexual cultures. This explosion of Thai queer identities had both similarities with and differences from the west. Sexuality-based gay identities very similar to those in the west emerged. However, for the female homosexual *tom-dee* (butch-femme) and transgender *kathoey* cultures, masculine/feminine gender difference rather than sexuality was the most important determinant of identity. Crucially, the post-Second World War explosion of Thai identities was thus a proliferation of queer genderings as well as queer sexualities. I suggest that hybridising the alternative queer historiographies presented by Michel Foucault (1980), Randoph Trumbach (1987), and John D'Emilio (1993), respectively, may provide a starting point for understanding the complexities of modern Thai queer history.

Foucault: biopower in Thailand?

From the basis of research on Thai language sources, I have tried to consider whether Foucault's (1980) account of the origins of modern European homosexualities might also account for the explosion of Thai queer genders and sexualities. Foucault argued that nineteenth-century modes of biopower (mediated through the law, medicine, education and religion) linked to western Europe's transformation to an industrial society radically restructured patterns of sexual identity. Critically, however, the forms of power that Foucault identified as the sources of modern European homosexualities were mobilised in Thailand *after* the new queer genders and sexualities had emerged. (Jackson 1997) Medical, educational, and other forms of biopower were adapted from western models in the 1970s as part of a state-based regime to control and suppress non-normative genders and sexualities. A biomedical regime over homosexuality and transgenderism arrived late in Thailand, being established in an ultimately unsuccessful attempt to put the genies of the new queer genders and sexualities back into the bottle of Thai tradition. This finding left two key questions. First, where did the new Thai queer identities come from if not via a Foucauldian mechanism and, second, why was gender difference rather than sexuality the dominant domain over which so many of the new identities had emerged? In seeking answers to these questions I could not fall back on the notion that the new identities reflected the persistence of premodern Thai gender culture. The historical record left no doubt that all the gay, *tom, dee* and *kathoey* identities had taken their current forms in recent times.

Trumbach (via Foucault): Thailand's gender revolution

The discursive and representational dominance of queer genderings in modern Thailand led me to Trumbach's (1987) argument that an early eighteenth-century revolution in gender norms in Britain preceded and laid the foundations for modern homosexualities. Trumbach's findings prompted me to revisit the Thai archive for signs of a possible gender transformation, and retracing the historical record I found that the modernising Thai state had enforced a restructuring of normative gender culture that largely ignored homosexuality and transgenderism until the 1970s and 1980s (Jackson 2003). In the late nineteenth and early twentieth centuries, Foucauldian forms of biopower had indeed been instituted in Thailand via reforms of the law, education and other domains. But the aim of these reforms was to refashion heteronormative male and female genderings as 'civilised' and 'modern' rather than to establish normative patterns of sexual behaviour.

In the second half of the nineteenth century, Siam's increasing engagement with the imperialist west led to the society's gender culture – in particular, what Europeans perceived as the 'androgyny' of male and female fashions – becoming an object of elite concern. The British and French viewed the relative lack of difference between Siamese men's and women's fashions, hairstyles and occupations as signs of a 'semi-barbarous' lack of civilisation. Siam's ruling royal elites responded to these criticisms by using state instrumentalities to 'civilise' the populace and ensure that Siamese men and women dressed and looked differently from each other. In responding to western critiques of 'semi-barbarous' androgyny, the Siamese state drew on new forms of power to institute a regime of European-styled masculine–feminine gender differentiation. That is, the forms of biopower that Foucault identified as the source of the homosexual/heterosexual divide in Europe were adapted in Siam to institute a masculine/feminine binary across cultural fields that previously had not been strongly marked by gender difference.

This research, using a gender-focused hybridisation of Trumbach's and Foucault's ideas, explained the predominance of gender over sexuality in modern Thai queer cultures: it has emerged from a self-modernising regime of biopower that focused intensely on the public performance of heteronormative gendering but largely overlooked private sexual practice. However, another major question remained. Gay identities based on notions of homosexuality had also emerged as part of the explosion of Thai queer subjectivities. While Trumbach's ideas helped in developing a gender-focused Foucauldian account to understand the modern proliferation of Thai transgenderism, it did not explain the parallel emergence of sexuality-based gay homosexualities. This gap indicated that yet other historical processes had also been in train. In reflecting on this situation, I realised that while Foucault and Trumbach had led me to consider the place of state power in modern Thai queer history, I still had no clear picture of the role that capitalism may have played in the explosion of Thai identities. In seeking to redress this gap, I turned to D'Emilio's account of the place of capitalist urbanisation in the origins of modern homosexual identities.

D'Emilio: capitalism and queer autonomy beyond the west

D'Emilio (1993) argues that in nineteenth-century USA, the marketisation of labour broke down heteronormative restrictions of family-based subsistence farming communities, while urbanisation provided spaces for the emergence of new sex cultural networks. D'Emilio's account of modern US homosexualities as indigenous forms of sex cultural differentiation produced by market processes within the USA provides a model for understanding other new homosexual cultures as equally local consequences of the rise of other national varieties of capitalism. In contrast to recent accounts of cultural globalisation that emphasise the impact of transnational capitalism, D'Emilio considered capitalism in an earlier, national-level phase. As noted earlier, new queer identities emerged in Thailand before the 1990s intensification of globalising forces. In considering the impact of capitalism on Thai homosexual cultures we need to reflect on relations between the market, sexuality and gender in the pre-globalisation era.

Drawing on D'Emilio, I have explored the extent to which national, not transnational, forms of capitalism have been sources of some of the commonalities that now link gay and transgender cultures across borders (Jackson 2009). I have sought to understand the key finding of first-generation global queering studies – transnational queer similarities are emerging in the context of the expansion of capitalism – in terms of the central conclusion of comparative research that modern queer cultures beyond the west are expressions of local agency. My aim has been to develop a narrative of global queering that decouples the spread of capitalism from cultural westernisation by considering how the growth of market economies may enhance queer autonomy beyond the west.

While more research on capitalism and Thai queer history needs to done, case studies from twentieth-century Thai gay and *kathoey* history confirm that global queering has emerged at least in part from national-level, market-based sex cultural differentiation. For example, the commodified cultural forms of male sex work and gay magazines emerged in Bangkok from local commercial conditions in an urban mass market. Only *after* these market-based sex cultural forms appeared locally did they subsequently come into contact with similar commercial phenomena in the west. Wilson (2004) has studied the place of the market in Thailand's contemporary female same-sex *tom-dee* culture, and she points out that shopping malls are key sites of *tom-dee* socialising and that small trading and franchise businesses provide a basis for some *tom*-identified women to attain a degree of sexual autonomy. This research reveals that while the west's political and economic dominance has impacted on Thailand, the arrival of capitalism does not necessarily lead to an imposition of western forms of cultural modernity that destroy local identities. Capitalism is indeed central to global queering, but in its national as much as its transnational varieties, and it deracinates premodern traditions and produces novel cultural forms time and again in each society in which it takes root.

Conclusions

Better understanding global queering requires further empirical and theoretical work. The empirical task is to incorporate the histories of more queer cultures beyond the west into an expanded narrative. The analytical task is to negotiate tensions between different schools of queer historiography. Reading Foucault in conversation first with Trumbach and subsequently with D'Emilio has proved highly productive, leading me to engage the Thai archive from a number of perspectives and revealing the diverse processes that underpin global queering. However, drawing on these different authors also entails negotiating tensions within the notion of global queering that emerge from a disjuncture between the frameworks that the two elements of this compound expression respectively derive from. On the one hand, accounts of the 'global' are typically understood in terms of the impact of transnational capitalism. On the other hand, 'queer' is usually, although not exclusively, understood in Foucauldian terms, in which shifting relations of power and discourse are emphasised more than the effects of capital. To bring these different streams of queer historiography into closer dialogue will require augmenting Foucauldian accounts of biopower with D'Emilio's political economy of modern homosexual history.

A queer political economy of proliferating gender and sexual difference

Altman argues that 'current debates around changing forms of homosexuality [present] a choice between political economy, which argues for universalising trends, and anthropology, which argues for specificities' (Altman 1996b: 87). I agree with him that '(w)e badly need a political economy of sexuality ... which recognises the interrelationship of political, economic, and cultural structures' (Altman 2001: 157). This political economy of queer sexualities and genders needs to relate the market to *both* the localising and the transnational dimensions of cultural globalisation, and it needs to explain how capitalism produces both modern forms of sex/gender cultural differentiation in some domains alongside homogenisation in others. In contrast to US-centred models, we need a political economy of global queering that represents globalisation as multicentred. If capitalism is the engine of cultural globalisation, and if, as revealed by research on queer Asia, local sex cultural differentiation and transnational homogenisation are equally salient and coexisting trends, then the task is to explain how the market produces new local forms of sexual difference as well as transnational commonalities.

I have tried to begin addressing this analytical gap by bringing the universalist political economy and particularist anthropological approaches to global queering into dialogue. In contrast to Altman (2001: 158–9), I do not believe a political economy approach to global queering entails abandoning queer theory. Research on Thai queer history shows that no current account of queer history, whether following Foucault or D'Emilio, fully explains the emergence of new forms of transgenderism and gender-normative homosexuality in that country. Queer theory is part of, not apart from, the development of a more adequate political economy of global queering. The place to begin building such theory is in a conversation among contributing streams of political economy and queer studies analysis. Such a theoretical conversation may provide a first step to developing a hybridised model of global queering that is better able to account for the hybridising processes that are at work in all contemporary sexual and gender cultures societies, western and non-western.[4] Comparative research exploring processes of sex cultural differentiation and convergence in the context of globalisation will help us assess the extent to which the ideas of Foucault, Trumbach, D'Emilio and indeed other queer theorists capture the processes of change that are at work in all of the world's sexual and gender cultures.

Notes

1 While used widely in English-speaking countries to refer collectively to diverse gay, lesbian, bisexual, transgender and transsexual identities, the term 'queer' is not used in all societies. Nonetheless, the growing influence of queer studies in Asia was reflected in the more than 160 papers presented at the *1st International Conference of Asian Queer Studies* convened in Bangkok in July 2005. See http://bangkok2005.anu.edu.au.
2 The country was called Siam until 1939, when the name was changed to Thailand.
3 For accounts of the modern history of male homosexuality in Japan, see McLelland 2000.
4 In collaboration with Fran Martin, Mark McLelland and Audrey Yue, I have elsewhere considered global queering through the lens of theories of cultural hybridity (see Martin *et al.* 2008).

References

Adam, B. D., Duyvendak, J. W. and Krouwel, A. (1999) 'Gay and Lesbian Movements Beyond Borders? National Imprints of a Worldwide Movement', in *The Global Emergence of Gay and Lesbian Politics: National Imprints of a Worldwide Movement*, Philadelphia: Temple University Press.

Altman, D. (1996a) 'On Global Queering', *Australian Humanities Review,* July 1996; internet edition available at www.lib.latrobe.edu.au/AHR/archive/Issue-July-1996/altman.html#1) (accessed 17 June 2007).

Altman, D. (1996b) 'Rupture or Continuity? The Internationalisation of Gay Identities', *Social Text*, 14 (3): 77–94.

Altman, D. (1997) 'Global Gaze/Global Gays', *GLQ: A Journal of Gay and Lesbian Studies*, 3 (4): 417–36.

Altman, D. (2001) *Global Sex*, Crows Nest, NSW: Allen & Unwin.

Appadurai, A. (1996) *Modernity at Large: Cultural Dimensions of Globalisation*, Minneapolis: University of Minnesota Press.

Berry, C., Martin, F. and Yue, A. (2003) 'Introduction: Beep – Click – Link', in *Mobile Cultures: New Media in Queer Asia*, Durham, NC and London: Duke University Press: 1–18.

Boellstorff, T. (2007) *A Coincidence of Desires: Anthropology, Queer Studies, Indonesia*, Durham, NC: Duke University Press.

Chauncey, G. (1994) *Gay New York: Gender, Urban Culture, and the Makings of the Gay Male World, 1890–1940*, New York: Basic Books.

Cruz-Malavé, A. and Manalansan, M. F. (eds) (2002) *Queer Globalizations: Citizenship and the Afterlife of Colonialism*, New York and London: New York University Press.

D'Emilio, J. (1993) 'Capitalism and Gay Identity', in *The Lesbian and Gay Studies Reader*, New York and London: Routledge.

Drucker, P. (2000) 'Introduction: Remapping Sexualities', in *Different Rainbows*, London: Gay Men's Press.

Foucault, M. (1980) *The History of Sexuality Volume 1: An Introduction* (trans. R. Hurley), New York: Vintage Books.

Garcia, J. N. C. (1996) *Philippine Gay Culture, The Last Thirty Years: Binabai to Bakla, Silahis to MSM*, Diliman, Quezon City: University of the Philippines Press.

Jackson, P. A. (1995) *Dear Uncle Go: Male Homosexuality in Thailand*, Bangkok: Bua Luang Books.

Jackson, P. A. (1997) 'Thai Research on Male Homosexuality and Transgenderism and the Cultural Limits of Foucaultian Analysis', *Journal of the History of Sexuality*, 8 (1): 52–85.

Jackson, P. A. (1999) 'An American Death in Bangkok: The Murder of Darrell Berrigan and the Hybrid Origins of Gay Identity in 1960s' Bangkok', *GLQ: A Journal of Lesbian and Gay Studies*, 5 (3): 361–411.

Jackson, P. A. (2000) 'An Explosion of Thai Identities: Global Queering and Reimagining Queer Theory', *Culture, Health and Sexuality*, 2 (4): 405–24.

Jackson, P. A. (2003) 'Performative Genders, Perverse Desires: A Bio-History of Thailand's Same-sex and Transgender Cultures', *Intersections: Gender, History & Culture in the Asian Context*, 9; internet edition available at http://intersections.anu.edu.au.

Jackson, P. A. (2004) '*Gay* Adaptation, *Tom-Dee* Resistance, and *Kathoey* Indifference: Thailand's Gender/Sex Minorities and the Episodic Allure of Queer English', in *Speaking in Queer Tongues: Globalisation and Gay Desire*, Urbana: University of Illinois Press.

Jackson, P. A. (2009) 'Capitalism and Global Queering: National Markets, Sex Cultural Parallels, and Queer Autonomy Beyond the West', *GLQ, A Journal of Gay and Lesbian Studies*, 15 (3): 357–95.

McLelland, M. (2000), *Male Homosexuality in Modern Japan: Cultural Myths and Social Realities*, Richmond, VA: Curzon.

Martin, F. (2004) *Situating Sexualities: Queer Representation in Taiwanese Fiction, Film and Public Culture*, Hong Kong: Hong Kong University Press.

Martin, F., Jackson, P., McLelland, M. and Yue, A. (2008) *AsiaPacifiQueer: Rethinking Gender and Sexuality in the Asia-Pacific*, Urbana: University of Illinois Press.

Plummer, K. (1992) 'Speaking its Name: Inventing a Gay and Lesbian Studies', in *Modern Homosexualities: Fragments of Lesbian and Gay Experience*, London: Routledge.

Sinnott, M. (2004) *Toms and Dees: Transgender Identity and Female Same-sex Relationships in Thailand*, Honolulu: University of Hawaii Press.

Trumbach, R. (1987) 'Sodomitical Subcultures, Sodomitical Roles, and the Gender Revolution in the Eighteenth Century: The Recent Historiography', in *'Tis Nature's Fault: Unauthorized Sexuality During the Enlightenment*, Cambridge: Cambridge University Press.

Weeks, J. (2007) *The World We Have Won: The Remaking of Erotic and Intimate Life*, London and New York: Routledge.

Wilson, A. (2004) *The Intimate Economies of Bangkok: Tomboys, Tycoons, and Avon Ladies in the Global City*, Berkeley: University of California Press.

Wilson, A. (2006) 'Queering Asia', *Intersections: Gender, History and Culture in the Asian Context*, 14, November; internet edition available at http://intersections.anu.edu.au/issue14/wilson.html (accessed 27 August 2008).

11 *Hijras*, 'AIDS cosmopolitanism' and questions of *izzat* in Hyderabad[1]

Gayatri Reddy

A few years ago, the first organisation offering medical services for 'men who have sex with men (MSM) and kothis' was established in the south Indian city of Hyderabad. On hearing about the organisation, members of the *hijra* community (the so-called third sex or indigenous transgendered category) asked me, the itinerant anthropologist, to find out more about this much needed clinic – 'our *kothi* clinic' – as they referred to it, invoking the category and social formation loosely translated in anthropological and public health literature as an effeminate man who is most often the recipient in male same-sex encounters. 'Last month, one of my "customers" from Saudi [Arabia] told me about it. I believe this clinic is only for us – *kothis* here and in the Garden [a popular same-sex cruising area in the city]', Shanti, a *hijra* sex worker, explained, including in her lexical label both her fellow *hijras* and the *kothis* in the Garden. Later that same week, when speaking to self-identified *kothis* in the Garden, I was reassured that the clinic was indeed going to be established and that it was for 'all MSM and kothis ... but please tell *hijras* to come only on Sundays'. On further inquiry, I was told that this request was on account of the *hijras*' stigma and its potential contagion: 'If *hijras* come during the week, what will people think? Everyone will know this is a "homosex" clinic then, and our *izzat* (respect) will go. You can understand how this will look ... So you tell them', Rakesh told me.

In Rakesh's statement, *hijras* are clearly included as a recognisable MSM subjectivity/community, even as they are simultaneously excluded on the basis of respect (*izzat*) and the shame (*sharm*) of visibility. For *hijras*, this incorporation into the MSM or 'men who have sex with men' rubric, while a welcome avenue through which to access their 'right' to healthcare, is nevertheless an awkward habitation; in most contexts, they see themselves neither as 'men' nor as necessarily 'sexual', invoking instead their 'traditional' perception as divinely blessed *a*sexual figures. Further, even as *hijras* articulate themselves within a *kothi* framework – a category and social formation widely acknowledged to have originally derived from *hijra* discourse/practice (Cohen 2006) – they do not necessarily accept the moral logics dictating their insertion into this social landscape and the economies of care outlined by Rakesh in the earlier vignette.

Drawing on such differential constructions of sexuality, stigma, respect and the need for care, this chapter explores the fraught deployments of the signifiers 'MSM', '*kothi*' and '*hijra*' in Hyderabad, and their increasingly complex and fluid circulations within the semantic fields of AIDS and sexual rights discourses. In the altered landscape of post-AIDS enterprise India – what Lawrence Cohen refers to in

a recent article as 'AIDS Cosmopolitanism', i.e. 'an imagined formation of dislo-
cated agents using the economically fortified enterprise of AIDS prevention to
support its own covert agendas' (2006: 271) – it is these kinds of friction between
and among such frameworks that reveal their complex genealogies and the moral
logics of self and other making in the contemporary sexual terrain of India. Reflecting on these kinds of tension, Cohen ends his article with an interesting question:
'What kind of ethics and what kind of care are possible and likely under contingent
instances of particular global conjunctures?' (2006: 301).

In this chapter, I engage this question/issue – the ethics and politics of care –
addressing how these play out in the lives of *hijras*, deeply implicated and simultaneously marginalised as they are in the terrain of AIDS cosmopolitanism. Specifically,
I refract this question through the plural and particular logics at play between the
cosmopolitanisms of *hijras* and their public health interlocutors in Hyderabad. I
argue that the seeming ineffectiveness of existing health programmes, translated in
hijras' understanding to a lack of care, needs to be understood through several dia-
lectical tensions – between emerging definitions of *hijras* as rights-bearing sexual
minorities and their continued representations as stigmatised social figures, between
local moral economies of *izzat* (respect) and *sharm* (shame), and between representations of self and other in terms of sexual and asexual difference.

Hijras and visible regimes of difference

In much of the early literature, *hijras* have been represented as social pariahs, stigmatised and set apart on the basis of their transgressive gender identification and
their location beyond the domain of procreative sexuality (Vyas and Shingala 1987,
among others). Stemming in part from their bodily disfigurement (an ideal but not
always realised genital excision) and from their ambiguous gender identification,
hijras are often constructed in the popular imaginary as 'dirty', socially marginal
outcasts who 'do not have any *sharm* [shame]' in the words of my next-door neighbours (see also Sharma 1989). *Hijras* in turn contribute to this construction by
explicitly engaging in practices that subvert norms of middle-class morality, such as
threatening to expose their lack of genitalia if their demands are not met. From the
perspective of mainstream, middle-class society, *hijras*, defined as they are by and
through their lack of a normal procreative body and their subsequent lack of potential for shame, are among the most *recognisably* marginalised figures in Indian
society, indelibly located on the margin, as physically, socially and morally stigmatised bodies.

Given this marginalised location, their election, *as hijras*, to political office in
north India a few years ago is arguably a very significant event in their recent history
(Bearak 2001). Apparently, it was precisely their gendered and sexual *difference* as
asexual 'neutralists' that provided their transcendent morality in the political
sphere. Explicitly projecting themselves as individuals without the encumbrances of
family, gender and caste affiliations, and thereby 'freed' from greed and nepotism,
hijras successfully declared themselves as perfect antidotes to the rampant corruption and immorality of Indian politics. As one *hijra* candidate's slogan stated, 'you
don't need genitals for politics; you need brains and integrity'. In fact, it is expressly
the *lack* of genitals and any expression of gendered, sexed and kinship-mediated ties
that apparently makes (or made) *hijras* ideal political leaders.

But what does this emphasis on their *difference*, their location beyond the social categories of gender, procreative sexuality and kinship mean for *hijra* marginality? As I argue elsewhere (Reddy 2003), invocations of marginality on the basis of sexuality and kinship, far from remaking normative institutions, appear to reinscribe their hegemonic importance, thereby undercutting *hijras'* subversive potential. Such mobilisations tie into popular negative constructions of *hijras* and often increase their stigma and suffering, as evinced by recent studies that document the violence directed at this community (PUCL 2003; Narrain 2004).

In recent years, one manifestation of *hijras'* stigma and suffering has been the devastation of the community by AIDS. With little access to healthcare, seroprevalence rates have skyrocketed, crossing 68 per cent in at least one early study (Kumta *et al.* 2002). This study, conducted in a municipal hospital in Mumbai, was the first to collect data specific to *hijras* – or in public health discourse, the transgendered (TG) community, and it is only since 2004 that the National AIDS Control Organisation (NACO) has begun to disaggregate MSM and TG data. Of the various high-risk groups in recent NACO sentinel surveillance data – female sex workers, injecting drug users, migrants, MSM and TG – it is only the last two groups that record an increase in HIV prevalence rates from data pertaining to the same city, Mumbai. And while the increase in these figures between 2006 and 2007 surveillance data is less than 1 per cent in the MSM category/group (from 7.6 per cent to 8.4 per cent), it is over 12 per cent in the TG group, with HIV prevalence rates rising to 42.2 per cent in 2007, from 29.6 per cent in 2006 (NACO 2008; see also Setia *et al.* 2006).

While sentinel surveillance data are more scarce for Hyderabad, my personal experience with *hijras* in the city warrants similar conclusions. Within the last decade, of the approximately 32 sex workers I knew well, 11 have died, most if not all from AIDS-related causes. Four are currently infected with HIV and have left Hyderabad to throw themselves at the mercy of the families they had been forced out of a decade earlier. Three others live together in a small town a few hours' distance from the city. The rest are scattered across the city and state, eking out their existence as best they can with their limited (and rapidly shrinking) resources. Given this scenario and growing rates of seroprevalence, perhaps the most urgent questions we need to ask are *why* there have been few public health efforts directed at this community, and why the few that exist have been so ineffective, despite efforts to attend to so-called 'indigenous' communities at risk through the funding-saturated AIDS enterprise.

One potential answer, I argue, lies in the ways that stigma and 'othered' difference get refracted along the faultlines of sexuality, gender and class, and play themselves out along individualised pathways mediated by behavioural public health models of 'subjects/groups at high risk', with devastating consequences for *hijras*, among others. As the opening vignette of this chapter illustrated, anxieties about *visible* signs of (homo)sexual stigma reveal the social and political geographies of blame – from its initial attachment to western *gay* bodies to the supposedly indigenous transgendered (TG) body of the *hijra*. And it is through negotiations of value within the moral economies of *izzat* and *sharm* that such mappings acquire their ethical force, especially in the imagined terrain of AIDS cosmopolitanism.

'Sexual' targets of risk behaviour: geographies of innocence and blame

Since the first detection of HIV in India in 1984, the numbers of HIV-positive individuals have increased at an alarming rate. In 2007 the official government estimate indicates 2.31 million people living with HIV/AIDS in India, with an estimated adult HIV prevalence of 0.34 per cent, with much higher estimates within high-risk groups, as noted earlier (NACO 2008).

With the help of the World Bank, other multilateral organisations and NGOs, the Indian government has in recent years actively begun to address this challenge. In this endeavour, it has been helped by a partial reconceptualisation of the epidemiological categories through which the public health community addresses the issue. In a bid to be more 'culturally sensitive', that is, partly in response to acknowledging the existing cross-cultural variation in constructions of sexual subjectivity, the CDC adopted the category of MSM or men who have sex with men to replace the earlier category 'homosexual'. Within this new classification, communities such as *hijras* and *kothis* – who do not necessarily identify as homosexual – are now targeted as MSM.

Corresponding to this discursive change, there has been an explosion of sexual health organisations in India. In Hyderabad alone, there are at least six NGOs working on sexual health, at least two of which are working explicitly on issues relating to *male* sexual health, wherein the primary objective is educating the community about its sexual rights in addition to safe sex practices and the transmission of HIV. This is particularly so in the wake of the recent police raids and arrests of HIV-prevention workers under Section 377 (anti-sodomy law) of the Indian Penal Code. Following one such incident in Lucknow, a supportive lawyer posted the World Association for Sexology declaration of sexual rights on one of India's largest lesbian–gay list serves, adding the following: 'Sexual rights are universal human rights. It is really important that all of us know what our sexual rights are so that we can *all* fight for our rights under the constitution'. As he stated in *Pukaar*, an English-language quarterly published by the NGO, Naz Foundation, the lawyer declared: 'I speak for the concerns of *all* sexual minorities in India, be they lesbian, gay, bisexual, transgendered, *kothi*, *hijra* or any other traditional name by which they choose to call themselves ... [and I] call upon the Indian government to ensure that the human rights of all in India are respected, protected and promoted' (Bondopadhyay 2002: 3).

Hijra *and the 'sexual rights' paradigm*

Interestingly, it is perhaps for the first time in *hijra* history that they are now publically perceived as *sexual* (rather than *a*sexual) figures, as metonymic figures of 'sexual difference' in compendia of lesbian, gay, bisexual and transgendered (LGBT) studies, on the one hand, and as an integral part of the MSM or *kothi* sexual culture, on the other. While *hijras* might have thought themselves a part of this wider *kothi* universe and engaged in male same-sex behaviour for some time, it appears to be only recently that their sexual practices have become commodified and that they are now primarily perceived as 'sex workers' or victims of HIV/ADS.[2] In the popular Indian imaginary, rather than sexual subjects, *hijras* have traditionally been viewed as either *asexual*, auspicious, religious figures – blessed by a Hindu goddess through whose power they get their power to confer fertility – or, more often, as objects of ridicule because of their asexuality and lack of any one gendered, religious or caste affiliation. It is largely with the emergence of the HIV/AIDS epidemic that *hijras* have been reconceptualised as 'MSM' and are now actively targeted by public health interventions. Given the public health imperative to identify target communities of those 'at risk', this discursive elaboration of a MSM category – and the inclusion of *hijras* under this rubric – is to a large extent a consequence of mobilising around the HIV/AIDS epidemic, rather than a prior commitment to any sexual identity.

With respect to HIV and AIDS, on the one hand, the *hijra* community is, no doubt, being devastated by this epidemic, partly due to the stigma directed at their visibly flamboyant sexual and gender transgressions. On the other hand, following the onset and rapid spread of the epidemic, an egalitarian ethic of equal rights for *all*, irrespective of sex, gender, caste or religion is being simultaneously posited. The recognition of such sexual rights appears to have become particularly salient for *hijras* in recent years. As a spokesperson declared at the 2004 *Hijra* Festival in Bangalore: '*Hijras* are a part of the wider community of sexual minorities. It is important for us to assert our rights as sexual minorities and get what we want from the government'.

As noted earlier, in their recent election campaigns, *hijras* have begun to position themselves as authentic cultural signifiers beyond the factional and corruptible politics of gender, sexuality and caste. At the same time, they are also asserting this citizen construction as a collective identity and are developing a public political consciousness (Altman 1997). This invocation of a *hijra* community and its group rights culminated a few years ago in a movement to declare a 'World Eunuch Day', and in the proposal by the recently elected *hijras* to launch a national political party for *hijras*. More recently, *hijras* moved the Chennai High Court to grant them not merely voting rights and the right to education, employment, marriage and child adoption, but also legal recognition as a third gender (see www.newsonweb.com/chennaionline).

As authors such as Dennis Altman (1997, 2001) have argued, there is a growing consciousness of belonging to a single, 'global' gay (or sexual) community of people with apparently similar desires and practices. However, the incorporation of such highly diverse groups into 'the movement' is not entirely seamless. For instance, sexual health clinics and support groups might have been established for gay men to help make the difficult transition from MSM to a self-identified gay man, as a report on the first annual 'gay' conference stated (Yaarian 1999). Non-*hijra kothis* I spoke to valued the clinics for more pragmatic reasons – it was a means to 'treat STDs and get condoms'. For the *hijras*, however, the objective was to 'ask doctors how we can get a *chathi* [breasts] of course', as Sathi told me patiently, in answer to what was, in her mind, obviously a stupid question. While it made absolute sense for *hijras* to avail their 'right' to access the services offered to 'homosexuals' or gay men, their desires and manifest agendas in accessing this global discourse were not necessarily similar to those of other members in this sexual landscape. While *hijras* are no doubt entering the public domain and doing so through the invocation of 'rights', the ways in which this translates into political action is perhaps a little more fractured than is implied by an ethic of equal rights. And often, these fractures and fissures play themselves out in terms of greater marginalisation of *hijras* owing to their visible difference along axes of gender, sexuality, kinship and class.

This was made evident to me in 2005, when I visited one of the local Hyderabadi MSM organisations that *hijras* have begun to frequent at least a few afternoons a week – not because of a prescriptive affinity with the MSM community, but because it had an air cooler that helped to alleviate the unbearable heat of the Hyderabadi summer. I was witness to an exercise conducted by MSM field officers with three *nirvan hijras* ('operated' *hijras*) present. Asking one of the *hijras* (Saroja, the only *hijra* who could read and write Telugu) to draw a picture of herself – a picture that the field officer ended up finishing because she was not drawing quickly enough – the field officers then told her: 'Next to this picture write down all your *problems* that stem from being a *nirvan hijra*. Being *nirvan* has greater difficulties, no? So write down those difficulties and problems'. Implicit in such a statement is the sense of opprobrium associated with becoming *nirvan*, a condition that is implicitly juxtaposed against a dominant, non-*nirvan kothi* status. And, according to the MSM fieldworkers in this organisation, it is, unequivocally, the former category that has 'greater difficulties'; difficulties stemming explicitly from *hijras'* greater visibility, their sartorial preferences and their apparently debilitating *nirvan* condition (and implicitly their class position), as one of these staff members noted on the sheet when Saroja hesitated during the exercise.

Hijras *and the moral economy of* izzat

Importantly, as I note elsewhere (Reddy 2005), for *hijras* themselves, it is the value of *izzat* (rather than *sharm*) that is the central authenticating trope, especially for those *hijras* who are doubly marginalised – as *hijras* (in the social world), and as sex workers (in the *hijra* world).

Having joined the *hijra* community, an individual *hijra's izzat* is dependent in some measure on the ability to be an *asli* (real) *hijra*, a position acquired through the performance of various embodied acts within the arenas of kinship, (a)sexuality, sartoriality and religion. In the eyes of *hijras*, these acts include the avowal of particular *hijra* kinship relations such as the *guru-cela* (master–disciple) relationship, the adoption of particular modes of self-presentation whether through dress or 'ideal' (Muslim) religious practice, the maintenance of asexuality or sexual renunciation and the excision of genitalia, a *visible* corporeal symbol that signals their irreversible and authentic occupation of this category.

In all these acts, *hijras* implicitly or explicitly define themselves in opposition to the overly licentious (in their constructions) and much disparaged MSM or *gandus*, as they more commonly and pejoratively refer to these individuals. According to *hijras*, *gandus*, as men who enjoy anal sex, are defined not only by the *form* of their sexual desire, but more importantly, by its *excess*. As such, *gandus* are disparaged by *all hijras* – both the supposedly asexual *hijras* as well as those who are sexually active. In reaction to senior 'asexual' *hijra* claims about their inauthenticity, *hijra* sex workers argue that they are passing through a 'lifecycle', progressing from sexual prostitution to asexual ritual practice. They also profess a dislike of *indiscriminate* and excessive sexuality. As my *hijra* interlocutor, Munira, told me disparagingly: 'We don't do like these *gandus*. We just go to the station for a few hours in the evening, make some money and come back here; not like these *gandus* who want to go with men *all* the time!' Through all of these authenticating practices, *hijras* take pride in their very visible performance of sexual/gender transgression, and explicitly deride *kothis* for their invisible or secret (*gupt*) lives.

In this moral economy of desire and practice, *izzat* operates as a complex qualitative currency of moral worth, a means through which individual *hijras* strive to gain status; and it is by performing various 'authentic' *hijra* acts that this currency is traded. *Izzat*, in other words, operates as an (idealised) form of currency through which individual *hijras* can trade their respective position on the moral ladder of *hijra* value.

Implications/conclusions: sexual difference and the cosmopolitics of care

Given this brief sketch of the idioms and tensions animating *hijra* life, what do such refractions mean for *hijra* self-making, for constructions of 'community' and for a cosmopolitics and ethics of care? While I do not presume to have definitive answers to these questions, I want to end this chapter with a set of speculations on two fronts: the first, centred on the trope of *izzat* and *sharm* in the moral economy of care; and the second, related point, the mobilisation of sexual difference as a platform for recognition and action, and the implications of such mobilisation for conceptualisations of care in the social and material landscape of 'AIDS cosmopolitanism'.

Drawing on *hijras*' articulations of *izzat*, I argue for a retheorisation or refraction of this notion. Specifically, I call for an extension of its meaning beyond a unitary and coherent 'libidinised' frame (Gilmore 1987). Contrary to most analyses of honour/*izzat* in the South Asian literature that construct the notion as a communal and gendered/sexualised construct – a matter of sexual regulation, typically located in the body of women, for men to safeguard or preserve on behalf of the family or community – I argue that *hijras*' use of this notion of *izzat* is a more individualised (and arguably more commodified) register of moral value. Critically, I argue that *hijras*' understanding of this construct spills out of a purely eroticised framework to incorporate several dimensions of subjectivity not *entirely* subsumable under the rubric of gender/sexuality. The transaction or negotiation of relative status through the currency of *izzat* occurs not *merely* through sexualised exchanges, but also through practices located outside the domain of sexuality. In other words, the concept of *izzat* among *hijras* has a moral valence that derives strength precisely from its diffusion beyond the axis of sex/gender to encompass a range of other domains, including kinship, religion and corporeality, in addition to sexuality.

By contrast, in the public domain, it is through the idiom of *sharm* that *hijras* are commonly represented. By lifting their saris and publicly flaunting their lack of procreative potential (and shame) in the public's face, *hijras* are disrupting the regulation of sexuality in the public sphere. As such, they embody shamelessness and, by the mere threat of such exposure, can apparently communicate their lack of shame to the 'respectable' public.

Drawing on this belief, perhaps one of the more interesting and troubling developments in recent years has been the capitalisation on such shame. Lately, *hijras* have been employed by major credit card companies to threaten and intimidate customers into repaying their credit card debt by manipulating precisely this fear of *hijra* shame (see for example http://news.bbc.co.uk/1/hi/world/south-asia/ 332173.stm). Even more strikingly, the Patna Municipal Corporation recently hired *hijras* as tax collectors; revenue officials accompany *hijras* with tax records to settle outstanding arrears on the spot (AP, 10 November 2006). Such practices are, in a sense, public commodifications of shame, drawing on *hijras*' perceived 'reputations' in the public sphere (as public shamers extraordinaire). But while the commodity is *izzat* in the *hijra* subaltern imaginary, in the public cultural matrix, it is *sharm*. In this mirrored logic of exchange therefore, what gets traded are not only the moral registers of individual and social worth, but also their entrenchment within the domain of sexuality and stigmatised moral difference.

Following the early recognition of the HIV epidemic and subsequent flows of AIDS-related NGO capital into India, there has been, from the public health perspective, a seeming consolidation of identities as I have noted; an incorporation of sexual difference under the label MSM, a complex category that repudiates cultural difference in favour of a risk–behaviour model. It is the particular acts that men who have sex with men engage in and the risks associated with those acts that condition their inclusion within this category. Such a conceptualisation, as scholars and activists have repeatedly pointed out, takes into account neither the differential power inequalities nor the different moral economies of value embedded in this social landscape.

Partly in response to such critiques and contests over meaning – that is, with a growing recognition of the importance of the 'cultural' in development/public health discourse – as well as in direct response to the material politics of HIV funding, MSM (both as category and community) is showing distinct signs of wear in recent years. Not only has there been a proliferation of sexual identities in the domain of public health – including *kothi*, *hijra*, gay, MSM who are married, and 'double-decker', to name a few – all, importantly, laying claim to the MSM label, but differentiating themselves on cultural grounds in order to access greater resources, but the boundaries between these categories are becoming increasingly rigid as these various groups (and their public health interlocutors) have attempted to splinter off to form separate organisations to capitalise on such 'difference' and funding potential. Just a few years ago, in April 2004, a new initiative was floated in Hyderabad to set up a separate organisation for *nirvan hijras* – a new 'TG project' as one of the two MSM-identified non-*hijra* field staff associated with it referred to the initiative. When I asked him why he thought a separate organisation was needed, he replied: 'Because funding is there, no? And also it is easy to get the funding for this project because there is nothing like this for these people in Andhra'. Well intentioned as these projects might be, they invariably reproduce the hierarchies of gender, class and *sharm* (and the discriminatory practices stemming from these divisions), with 'these people' – the visibly 'othered' *hijras* – on the bottom rung of this ladder of respect/care.

Whether we attribute the shifting sexual landscape – this social formation of AIDS cosmopolitanism – to the politics of HIV-related funding, or as some scholars argue, to a neo-colonial sexual globalisation (Altman 2001), how do we understand this proliferation of categories, each predicated on emphasising and maintaining their sexual difference, even as they articulate these notions within the terms of (state and) public health-recognised discourse? What issues does such a politics of sexual difference raise for each of these 'communities' and for the *hijras*, in particular?

On the one hand, such mobilisations of sexual difference could merely *re*marginalise *hijras* in the spheres of politics, law and public health. In the domain of juridical politics for instance, the Madhya Pradesh High Court has deemed invalid the recent election of at least two *hijras* for seats reserved for women; *hijras* are not women, the court ruled. Perhaps for the first time since the *hijras'* incorporation into the colonial Criminal Tribes Act in 1871, their position has been publicly legislated in the courts, cementing or fixing their sexual/gendered difference more rigidly than their earlier location between the cracks of the post-/colonial Indian state. Further, as noted earlier, *hijras* themselves are moving the courts in Tamil Nadu to recognise them as civic citizens of the modern world; citizens of a different, 'third gendered' status. The irony, of course, is that such a lens of sexual difference allows for a certain visibility in mainstream society – the ostensible goal of an emancipatory discourse of rights – at the same time as it *fixes hijras'* location within this domain, often remarginalising them in the process.

In the domain of public health too, *hijras'* incorporation into the wider MSM rubric expressly criminalises their activity, bringing them under the purview of the anti-sodomy law. Even if they do form their own community outside this semantic/practical domain, they are constructed and accessed through the domain of HIV prevention, being ostensibly high risk for HIV on account of their 'criminal' sodomitical practices. Both in politics and in the field of public health, far from emancipating *hijras*, their mobilisation of sexual difference thus risks a further entrenchment within a criminalising, pathologising and marginalising framework.

On the other hand, if the examples provided here indicate anything, it is that these categories of difference (and subjectivity more generally) are not rigid domains but are shifting and constantly *becoming* in contexts of relationship – with each other, with NGOs, with the state. How then do we make sense of this domain and of the fluid if discrepant cosmopolitanisms (Clifford 1998) that structure patterns of subject formation and the differential provisions of care within this field of social relations? As I have suggested, *one* avenue or pathway of research (and activism) is to move beyond carving out sexuality as a separate arena, but to see it within a field of *social* difference. *Hijras* themselves provide the model here in terms of the ways in which they conceptualise their identity as beyond merely a *sexual* category. Although sex/gender is one, and perhaps even the most important aspect of their lives, *hijras* do not reduce their understanding to just this frame of analysis, articulating perhaps the best argument (and model) for a politics of *intersectionality* rather than a politics of identity – a framework that takes account of the multiple ways in which sexuality, gender class, caste, religion and kinship intersect with and construct each other in constituting difference.

Given the ways in which stigma plays itself out along these very faultlines, perhaps the most important avenues through which to speak to *hijra* stigma and marginalisation are: one, a collective mobilisation across various sites of difference, incorporating struggles for caste, class, gender and religious oppression within the bounds of 'sexual' oppression, as localised struggles for human rights – a 'pragmatic solidarity in response to structural violence' as Paul Farmer notes in a different context (2003: 220); and two, seeing the need for 'caring and being cared for' to invoke John Borneman's phrase (1998: 29), as vital to the wellbeing of *hijras* (and *all* humans), and fundamental to addressing stigma along the faultlines of social difference. In his paper, Borneman calls for a shift in the object of anthropological research – from regulative ideals for humanity (including and especially, kinship and marriage, the focus of his article), to an ontological process, 'a concern for the actual situations in which people experience the need to care and be cared for and to the political economies of their distribution' (1998: 30). Care, he notes, is the 'source and result of human creativity' and as such it is in foregrounding this ethic – and obligation (if not 'right' as Borneman argues) – that we can not only attend to questions of social justice but also better understand the 'diversity of relations in which caring is expressed and the power matrix in which they are assigned value' (1998: 584).

The lack of care extended to *hijras* can be seen as a violation of such an obligation, a symptom of deeper pathologies of power (Farmer 2003) that determine this social landscape of suffering. As Surekha, one of the few *hijra* sex workers remaining in Hyderabad indicated to me when I returned in the summer of 2005: 'These programmes-wogrammes are mostly for the *mogabatta kothulu* [the male-clothed *kothis*/MSM]. *Nirvan hijras*' lives and concerns are different. We can come here to this office and to the clinic and everything. But ultimately, who is going look after us, Gayatri?' This chapter offers a very preliminary attempt to take up the challenge posed by Surekha's question. It points at one small way by which attention to the local politics of *izzat* and *sharm* reveal the ways in which 'caring and being cared for' are articulated, shape and play themselves out in the cosmopolitanisms of *hijras* and their interlocutors in Hyderabad. Even as the answers to Cohen's question as to the kinds of ethics and care that are possible within these global conjunctures remain fraught – it is only in wrestling with such questions of ethics and care at the *local* level that concrete starting points can be delineated for better understanding the logics of self and 'other'-making in the contemporary cosmopolitan world.

Notes

1 This chapter is based on research conducted in the south Indian city of Hyderabad at various points between 1995 and 2005. It is a revised version of an article that was published in 2005 in the journal *Anthropology and Medicine*.
2 See Cohen 2006 for a problematisation (and historicisation) of the '*kothi* model'.

References

Altman, D. (1997) 'Global Gaze/Global Gays', *GLQ: A Journal of Lesbian and Gay Studies*, 3: 417–36.
Altman, D. (2001) *Global Sex*. Chicago: University of Chicago Press.
Bearak, B. (2001) 'Katni Journal: A Pox on Politicians', *New York Times on the Web*, 19 January 2001; available at www.nytimes.com/2001/01/19/world/19eunu.html
Bondopadhyay, A. (2002) 'State-Supported Oppression and Persecution of Sexual Minorities in India', *Pukaar: Journal of Naz Foundation International*, 38: 3–5.
Borneman, J. (1998) 'Caring and Being Cared For: Displacing Marriage, Kinship, Gender and Sexuality', in Faubion, J. (ed.) *The Ethics of Kinship*, Boston, MA: Rowman & Littlefield.
Clifford, J. (1998) 'Mixed Feeling', in Cheah, P. and Robbins, B. (eds) *Cosmopolitics: Thinking and Feeling Beyond the Nation*, Minneapolis: University of Minnesota Press.
Cohen, L. (2006) 'The Kothi Wars: AIDS Cosmopolitanism and the Morality of Classification', in Adams, V. and Pigg, S. (eds) *Sex and Development*, Durham, NC: Duke University Press.
Farmer, P. (2003) *Pathologies of Power: Health, Human Rights, and the New War on the Poor*, Berkeley: California University Press.
Gilmore, D. (1987) *Honor and Shame and the Unity of the Mediteranean*, Special Publication No. 22, Washington, DC: American Anthropological Association.

Kumta, S., Setia, H. R., Jerajana, H. R., Mathur, M. S., RaoKavi, A. and Lindan, C. P. (2002) 'Men who have Sex with Men (MSM) and Male-to-Female Transgender (TG) in Mumbai: A Critical Emerging Risk Group for HIV and STIs in India', paper presented at the XIV International AIDS Conference, Barcelona, Spain.

Narrain, A. (2004) *Queer: Despised Sexuality, Law and Social Change,* Bangalore: Books for Change.

Narrain, A. and Bhan, G. (eds) (2005) 'Introduction', in *Because I Have a Voice: Queer Politics in India,* New Delhi: Yoda Press.

National AIDS Control Office (2008) 'HIV Sentinel Surveillance and HIV Estimation in India 2007: A Technical Report', New Delhi: NACO, Ministry of Health and Human Welfare, Government of India.

People's Union for Civil Liberties (PUCL) (2003) 'Human Rights Violations Against the Transgender Community: A Study of Kothi and Hijra Sex Workers in Bangalore, India', report, Karnataka: PUCL.

Reddy, G. (2003) '"Men" "Who Would be Kings": Celibacy, Emasculation, and Re-Production of Hijras in Contemporary Indian Politics', *Social Research,* 70 (1): 163–98.

Reddy, G. (2005) *With Respect to Sex: Negotiating Hijra Identity in South India,* Chicago: University of Chicago Press.

Setia, M. S., Lindan, C., Jerajani, H. R., Kumta, S., Ekstrand, M., Mathur, M. *et al.* (2006) 'Men Who Have Sex with Men and Transgenders in Mumbai, India: An Emerging Risk Group for STIs and HIV', *Indian Journal of Dermatology, Venereology and Leprology,* 72 (6): 425–31.

Sharma, S. (1989) *Hijras: The Labelled Deviants,* New Delhi: Gian Publishing House.

Vyas, S. and Shingala, D. (1987) *The Life Style of the Eunuchs,* New Delhi: Anmol Publications.

Yaarian (1999) www.healthdev.org/viewmsg.aspx?msgid=95e297fc-bff9-4c10-9c0c-4c99be42d48b

12 Intersexuality, biomedical regulation and sexual rights in Brazil[1]

Paula Sandrine Machado

It was in the early stages of fieldwork at the hospital that a meeting was called for medical staff from different specialities to discuss the 'case' of a child born at the institution a few days previously. At that time, the team was still referring to the baby as 'Carolina's newborn'. A meeting of specialists had been called to deal with a 'case' of intersexuality – now known by the term disorder of sex development (DSD) in the medical sphere[2] – where the precise diagnosis and attribution of male or female sex to the baby was seen as especially complicated. The meeting was attended by two paediatric surgeons, a paediatric endocrinologist, a psychiatric intern, a geneticist, a genetics intern, a paediatric intern, a neonatologist, two medical students and me.

Factors considered relevant to a diagnosis were presented: data from physical examinations and tests to determine karyotype and hormone levels aimed to offer a more or less coherent picture, but at the same time indicated that other tests were required to fill in gaps concerning the diagnosis. In relation to the karyotype test, the geneticist reported that he could not 'see' clearly whether either the XX or the XY karyotype – considered respectively as the female and male karyotypes – were present. 'We can't say that it is Y', he stated, as 'none of the markers is indicative of Y'. The endocrinologist, contrariwise, pointed out that the 'gonads' were producing 'testosterone'.

The discussion continued and various opinions were offered regarding the child's 'biological condition' and the 'psychological aspects' of the mother, until one of the doctors surprised the group with the question, 'but why operate?' The question was received with a degree of shock and even impatience. Laughs and mutters could also be heard. After all, the team's concern was how best to intervene, which required the unequivocal definition of the baby's sex. The doctor's question sounded foolish in the context, because, the others remarked, 'how would the child live in the world without a defined sex?' This was precisely the decision they had come together to make.

This vignette, drawn from the fieldwork, raises at least two questions. First, it shows the complex clinical/surgical and social situation in which the medical staff had found themselves. Even though more or less established practices exist in the medical field for issues related to intersexuality, this particular case shows how some decisions can be very difficult to make and that all should ideally involve professionals trained in the different specialities. Second, the vignette shows that 'sex' often becomes an all-encompassing category, including everything that defines a person and makes them, in a sense, recognisable.

In relation to these two problems, this chapter analyses a number of issues relevant to the sociomedical management of intersexuality. The elements involved in decision making form an entangled complex net consisting of several different relational levels. These include: (1) the relations between the fields of knowledge involved (paediatrics/neonatology, paediatric endocrinology, paediatric surgery/ urology, genetics and psychology); (2) daily relations between the specialists (including, for example, team meetings, case discussions and exchanges of information); and (3) the relations established between the health professionals and the intersex people and their families. For the purposes of this analysis, I will focus mainly on the first of these levels, although it is important to note that the divisions between them are not stable and each level articulates with and involves the others.

Findings reported on here come from a qualitative, socioanthropological study conducted using ethnographic methodology in a hospital in southern Brazil. The principal investigation techniques were participant observation, informal interviews and semi-structured interviews. Data were collected in the paediatric surgery/ urology and paediatric endocrinology outpatient clinics, at meetings of relevant specialist teams and in discussions with health professionals of intersex 'cases' with less straightforward medical solutions. Semi-structured interviews were conducted with the relatives of medically 'diagnosed' intersex people under treatment by health professionals at the study hospital; the relatives of children 'diagnosed' during the course of the study; young people who had already undergone genital 'correction' surgery and/or hormonal treatment; and health professionals involved in decision making and treatment regarding intersexuality including a paediatric endocrinologist, paediatric surgeons, a geneticist, a paediatrician and psychologists.

It is important to note that none of the young intersex people or family members had any involvement in the intersex political movement, neither did they describe themselves or their children as intersex. In addition, although the medical literature mentioned 'intersex states', even the medical staff with whom I worked at the hospital rarely used the term 'intersex' among themselves and, as far as I could gather, never used it during consultation with intersex children or young people and their families. Instead, in the course of their everyday discussions the medical staff used the term 'ambiguous genitalia' among themselves when referring to certain conditions that they defined as intersex, although they stressed the importance of not doing so in front of the families, preferring the term 'incompletely formed genitalia'. I therefore use the terms intersex and intersexuality as reflexive choices by the researcher rather than as self-identified categories or ones commonly used by the people who participated in the study. I use the term intersex as defined by activist groups for two reasons: (1) it relativises the idea of intersexuality as pathology and (2) it broadens the range of reference beyond medical classifications without completely losing touch with them. The central idea of this definition is that of variation: that intersexuality includes a range of situations in which the body varies in relation to a culturally established male/female dichotomy (Cabral and Benzur 2005). These variations may include the anatomical appearance of internal and/ or external genital organs, as well as hormonal, gonadal and/or genetic characteristics.

Hide and seek: from 'the search for the sex' to the materialisation of gender

As described elsewhere (Machado 2005a, 2006), medical protocols in Brazil specify that the moment a baby is born with a genital anatomy considered 'ambiguous', a full team of specialists – endocrinologists, surgeons, paediatricians, geneticists, psychologists – should be activated in order to investigate the 'cause' of the condition, determine the 'diagnosis' and decide which 'corrective' modalities will be applied, be they surgical or hormonal. During this process, 'looking' is key to evaluating the best form of intervention. The surgeon's and endocrinologist's 'gaze', informed and supported by all the other collected information and opinions, will 'recognise' the best clinical or surgical management to be applied. Meanwhile, psychology will direct its 'gaze' towards the families of the children and their 'future wellbeing'. The psychologists may or may not be called at any given stage in the process, but their constant presence at meetings of the paediatric surgical team at the study hospital gives psychology significant weight as a backdrop for the decisions, be it through support to the team or through offering the necessary theoretical justification for early surgical intervention.

By analyzing the discourse of the medical practitioners who made up the empirical universe of the study, a general distinction could be made between cases that were considered by them to be 'simpler' or 'more difficult', based on the degree to which the baby's sex is easily discernible and/or that intervention is possible. On the basis of observations and interviews, cases are normally considered by doctors to be simpler if they satisfy at least one of the following criteria: (1) when it is judged that there is little or no chance of virilisation or masculinisation of the external genitalia, which leads to an assignation of female sex; and (2) when, despite the supposed visual 'genital ambiguity', a certain 'harmony' can be established by doctors between the different levels at which sex is located, such as when genetic characteristics considered female can be 'lined up' with female gonads (ovaries), female internal anatomy (such as the existence of uterus and fallopian tubes) and the possibility of reproduction.

Cases classified as congenital adrenal hyperplasia (CAH) in children with 46XX karyotype are not only the most frequent, but are also those regarded by the doctors as most straightforward with regard to sex assignation and choice of treatment. According to medical definitions in children with 46XX karyotype, CAH can lead to an increase in the size of external genital organs at birth or thereafter. Usually, the child will have reproductively functional uterus and ovaries. In such cases, there is usually no doubt for the doctors that female sex should be assigned and that the best approach is hormonal intervention (which is, in some cases, vital for the control of salt loss by the individual organism), and surgical intervention to reduce the size of the 'hypertrophied clitoris'. The most common medical argument is that the child in question is a 'normal woman' (or 'girl') with uterus and ovaries, the possibility of fertility, and the possibility of reconstruction of a vagina by surgical means.

Other 'cases' often classified as 'simple to resolve' were those described by the doctors as suffering from complete androgen insensitivity syndrome (CAIS). When referring to children born with karyotype 46XY but whose testosterone receptors do not respond. These 'cases' were unlikely to be diagnosed in the antenatal period or at birth, as the appearance of the external genitalia is considered 'standard female'.

The diagnosis is frequently made in adolescence, often when medical assistance is sought as a result of absence of menstruation or minimal breast development. The combination of the 'female appearance' of the external genitalia and the absence of 'peripheral testosterone response' – which means, in practice, that there is no 'development of the penis' or of 'male secondary sex characteristics', such as body hair growth and deepening voice – means that cases identified as CAIS raise no doubts for the doctors about the appropriateness of assigning 'female sex'.

In each of these two situations, there is also medical concern with the possibility of a 'virilisation of the brain' in female-assigned children who receive 'testosterone superstimulation' in the antenatal period. In this case, there is a further type of 'ambiguity' to be managed: namely a possible lack of 'harmonisation' between the 'corrected' anatomy and the assigned gender.

The cases regarded as 'difficult' are those that do not meet, or meet only partially, the criteria set out earlier. This category normally includes partial androgen insensitivity syndrome (PAIS) and mixed gonadal dysgenesis (MGD) XY, where difficulties can arise in making a 'precise' diagnosis and in deciding about sex assignation. It is interesting to note that both cases refer to situations where the main difficulty, in fact, is knowing whether the 'potential' for male sex can be more or less satisfactorily guaranteed by the intervention techniques. Guaranteeing fertility is of lesser significance, especially compared to the situation just described for CAH (in fact, fertility is even less present in these cases).

It could be argued that these situations are more difficult because 'ambiguity' is more evident and the genetic, hormonal and anatomical aspects are seen as being less 'harmonised', especially when there are only two sexes to choose from. In a more explicit and complex way, these 'cases' bring doctors face to face with the variability of sex and the different levels at which it can be located; paradoxically, such levels are defined by medicine itself: anatomical, hormonal, genetic, psychological, social and so on. As a result, categorising sex in an either/or framework becomes more difficult.

Making the decision

In order to reach decisions regarding intersexuality, a complex set of factors needs to be taken into account which includes the diagnosis, the appearance of the external genitalia (especially their size and 'structure'), the viability of surgical techniques, hormonal possibilities (for example, levels of testosterone, oestrogens and luteinising hormone) and potential for fertility. These factors, which are, in fact, considered in all the decisions, direct the issue simultaneously to biological and to sociocultural elements.

The most important factors when considering assignation of female sex are: reproductive capacity; anatomical possibility of constructing a vagina that could be penetrated by a penis; a vagina with the possibility of (hetero)sexual pleasure for the woman (which is associated with an attempt to maintain clitoral innervation); and a clitoris that is not 'too large' (Machado 2005a). For male sex, the following factors are emphasised: the possibility of constructing a penis that will develop to a size and erectile function regarded as 'adequate' for a man; the possibility of future sexual pleasure (which is associated with ejaculation); the possibility of 'satisfactorily penetrating' a vagina; and reproductive capacity (which is, in fact, almost non-existent when dealing with male assignation). There is also concern with the issue of 'urinating standing up', which is considered socially important for boys (Machado 2005a).

There is also a certain hierarchy assigned to the elements listed, in which the maintenance of a virile, 'penetrative' masculinity occupies a privileged place. In this calculation, it seems to be regarded as more serious for a man to have a smaller than 'standard' penis and/or no erectile function than for a woman to be infertile, since her 'femininity' does not appear to be threatened. In all cases, 'simple' or 'difficult', it can be seen that sex emerges as a 'medico-diagnostic category' (Machado 2005a) and that there is a concern with removing, as much as possible, or at least attenuating the 'male traits' identified in a 'female body' and vice versa.

Terms such as 'intersexual states', 'incompletely formed genitalia', 'micropenis', 'hypertrophied clitoris' and 'ambiguity' emerge as discursive categories that produce concrete normative effects on bodies, the most obvious being surgical intervention. The medical system, supported by psychological knowledge, thus constructs a narrative of the intersex body, constructing intersexuality as a difference that should be rendered invisible. This construction of meaning has significant consequences for the lives of intersex people and those around them.

The relationship between medicine and intersexuality puts into play two main regulatory and normalising processes: (1) ways of 'looking at the body' (through physical examination, for example, but also through techniques capable of investigating its 'invisible materiality', including chromosomes, genes, stages of embryological development and molecules); and (2) ways of 'measuring the body', using scales that seek to classify by means of a 'taxonomy of exclusion', where decisions specify that measures should fall within the mutually exclusive categories of male or female. Within this logic, it can be said that it is necessary to have a 'sufficiently large' penis to be seen as a 'true', 'complete' man, and a 'sufficiently small' clitoris to be seen as a 'true', 'complete' woman. In this context, the clitoris defined as 'hypertrophied' and the 'micropenis' become both a social and a health problem.

Recent advances in genetics and molecular biology have led to these fields being accorded more importance in the decision-making context, and the role of molecular biology in the medical management of intersexuality deserves a separate, more detailed discussion, especially after the publication of the 'Chicago Consensus', where the valorisation of genetics and molecular biology became quite clear (Lee *et al.* 2006). At this point, I want to highlight the fact that, with the development of genetic and molecular biology technology, it is not merely by means of discourse that the truth about the subject is extracted, but also through other mechanisms which, in the final analysis, do not depend on the subject. The entire body thereby 'confesses' its sex in each molecule, in each genetic sequence, examined and translated in letters and numbers such as DSD, 46XX, 46XY, SRY, SOX9, WT1 and so on. In this context, what I have called the 'sex code' (Machado 2008) emerges, under the linguistic and cognitive domain of the new genetics and molecular biology. The sex code constitutes another truth about the subject, one that is revealed through the body at the microscopic and molecular level.

In the course of the bodily 'regulations' and 'corrections' to which intersex children are subjected, one constant feature is the insufficiency of a model based on dichotomous sexual categories. The insufficiency of the binary sex operator is revealed not only through the process of the 'construction' of a sex by means of medical intervention, but also in the need to reaffirm it, either by means of further interventions (hormonal, surgical and/or psychotherapeutic) or other forms of social regulation, such as the family (Machado 2006). Constant effort is exerted to adapt intersex bodies to certain social expectations, such as fertility, potential for penetrative heterosexual sex and penis or clitoris size, as stated earlier. In this way, the normalising and regulatory processes put in place by medicine seek to 'find the sex' – male or female – in the body of the intersex child and at the same time are based on certain markers of 'wellbeing' and 'health' – be they physical and/or psychosocial – in the name of which medical interventions, such as surgery, are justified.

A difficult knot to untie: health, bioethics and sexual rights

The term 'bioethics' was first used in 1927 in an article by Fritz Jahr published in the German magazine *Kosmos* (Goldim 2006). Currently, and in a broad sense, bioethics can be considered as a field that seeks to deal in an interdisciplinary manner with the dilemmas raised in the area of health and biomedical research. As the term itself suggests, discussions related to this field of knowledge and action invariably presuppose a certain notion of *bios* (life) in relation to which an 'ethics' can be applied or defended. Feminist-inspired bioethics, which took shape in the 1990s, offers a trenchant critique of certain universalising tendencies within the discipline, opposing the use of universal principles decontextualised and disconnected from factors such as gender, social and cultural belonging (Diniz and Guilhem 2000).

Approached from a human rights perspective, sexuality first emerges in these debates within the context of reproductive rights but extends to the formulation of the idea of sexual rights (Rios 2006). This intersection between the spheres of rights and health, although important in many aspects and historical, political and social contexts, has problematic consequences in a number of fields (Corrêa and Ávila 2003), especially when dealing with issues beyond the scope of 'health', including issues related to intersexuality.

Decisions involving the management of intersex children are normally relegated to the sphere of bioethics and are neither immediately nor necessarily discussed in terms of the perspective of sexual rights as human rights. Among other reasons, this is due to the fact that bioethics has a direct commitment to the field of 'health' and intersexuality is frequently seen as an issue exclusive to this field.

One result of the presupposition that intersexuality is an exclusively medical issue is that, as Maffía and Cabral (2003) indicate, intervention techniques end up being problematised only in the sense of tools to be perfected. The difficulties or bodily consequences they cause are therefore seen as being related to 'the state of the technique', more or less 'sophisticated' at a given historical moment, rather than being seen in terms of the intervention itself. In this sense, debate tends to cover up the issue of whether or not intervention is even necessary.

In the context where I carried out fieldwork, it was not seen as inappropriate to submit the intersex body to interventions, to cuts and stitches, with the aim of 'correcting' it and registering the individual within a certain 'sociocultural intelligibility'. At the same time, however, it is the story of an intersex body that is cut, stitched and, sometimes, masked (Cabral 2006). The point at which an attempt is made to hide intersexuality as a possible corporality is also the point at which a body to be corrected appears, circumscribed by a medical language. This discourse contains both the promise of a cure, of the erasure of the signs of a particular sexual conformation and, also, the hope of instituting an expected 'coherence' between the assigned gender and the 'corrected' anatomy (Machado 2005b), with its implied heteronormative, homophobic and transphobic sociocultural traits.

In the context of medical decision making, debates about the 'technical' issues involved in the interventions thereby end up obscuring reflection on human rights. Cabral (2004) highlights a second problematic question that emerges in the sphere of sexual and reproductive rights: that of the presupposition of 'sexual difference' on which a certain notion of sexual citizenship is based. The intersex political movement and ethical and theoretical discussions around intersexuality also raise a challenge for the field of sexual rights as human rights and for bioethics, as they question the whole definition of humanity from which they spring: a humanity in which cultural diversity is established upon the presupposed truth of a two-sex division of the world. In this way, even though gender can be perceived as multiple, it ends up being anchored in two, and only two, sexes.

In this context, surgical intervention is generally regarded, by doctors as well as by many relatives of intersex people, as 'unavoidable', 'humanitarian' and 'humanising', since, from this perspective, the intervention seeks to register the body into what Cabral (2004) describes as a 'sexed subjectivity'. The fieldwork vignette with which I began this chapter clearly illustrates this point in the concern expressed by the medical team that the child – in this case, 'Carolina's newborn' – should not live in society '*without a defined sex*'. Here, 'sex' appears explicitly as that which allows access to social intelligibility and even to juridical existence (for instance, to obtain a baby's birth certificate, the parents must present a document from the hospital informing whether the sex is male or female).

Some final considerations

The discussion in this chapter has raised important questions when thinking about sexual rights as human rights. It also raises questions as to what constitutes 'health'. As regards intersexuality, in particular, this requires us to take into account the perceptions, definitions and demands of families, intersex people, political movements and other actors involved in decision making and in the comprehension of the meaning of 'health'. All these factors extend well beyond the realms of strictly medical and psychological criteria for decision making, challenging them and increasing their complexity.

By resignifying the polarised dichotomy of the categories of male and female, debate around intersexuality also points to the discussions of nature and nurture (so dear to anthropology) within the context of technological innovations and technical interventions on the body. This raises new questions concerning the relationship between sex and gender, in as much as it is the normative dichotomy of gender that shapes attempts to place bodies neatly in one of two, and only two, sexes.

Finally, there are issues related to biotechnology and the concrete, material effects of scientific discourse on the body. Specifically, and in relation to the medical and psychological management of intersex bodies, it is important to stress, to borrow from Suzanne Kessler (1998), that there are no 'neutral interventions', but rather the production of cultural effects. On the basis of – and beyond – the problematisations presented here, it is necessary to embrace the challenge of constructing a broader approach to sexual and reproductive rights as human rights, one which is not restricted to the notion of health as the locus for normative productions regarding bodies.

Notes

1 My thanks to Mauro Cabral for his invaluable commentaries and our stimulating discussions and to Daniela Riva Knauth for her enduring support and assistance in relation to this study.
2 August 2006 saw the publication of the *Consensus Statement on Management of Intersex Disorders*, also known as the 'Chicago Consensus', a medical consensus which suggests the use of the term disorders of sex development (DSD) in place of 'intersex' or 'intersexual states' (Lee *et al.* 2006).

References

Cabral, M. (2004) 'Ciudadanía (Trans)sexual', available at www.ciudadaniasexual.org/publicaciones/ganadores.htm (accessed January 2005).

Cabral, M. (2006) 'En Estado de Excepción: Intersexualidad e Intervenciones Sociomédicas', in Cáceres, C. F., Careaga, G., Frasca, T. and Pecheny, M. (eds) *Sexualidad, Estigma y Derechos Humanos. Desafíos para el Acceso a la Salud en América Latina*, Lima: FASPA/UPCH.

Cabral, M. and Benzur, G. (2005) 'Cuando digo Intersex. Un Diálogo Introductorio a la Intersexualidad', *Cadernos PAGU*, 24: 283–304.

Corrêa, S. and Ávila, M. B. (2003) 'Direitos Sexuais e Reprodutivos. Pauta Global e Percursos Brasileiros'. in Berquó, E. (ed.) *Sexo & Vida: Panorama da Saúde Reprodutiva no Brasil*, Campinas: Editora Unicamp.

Diniz, D. and Guilhem, D. (2000) 'Feminismo, Bioética e Vulnerabilidade', *Revista Estudos Feministas*, 8 (1): 237–44.

Goldim, J. R. (2006) 'Biotica: Origens e Complexidade', *Revista HCPA*, 26 (2): 86–92.

Kessler, S. (1998) *Lessons from the Intersexed*, New Brunswick, NJ: Rutgers University Press.

Lee, P. A., Houk, C. P., Ahmed, S. F., Hughes, I. A. *et al.* (2006) 'Consensus Statement on Management of Intersex Disorders', *Pediatrics*, 118: e488-e500.

Machado, P. S. (2005a) '"Quimeras" da Ciência: A Perspectiva de Profissionais da Saúde em Casos de Intersexo', *Revista Brasileira de Ciências Sociais*, 59: 67–80.

Machado, P. S. (2005b) 'O Sexo dos Anjos: O Olhar Sobre a Anatomia e a Produçãoo do Sexo (como se Fosse) Natural', *Cadernos PAGU*, 24: 249–81.

Machado, P. S. (2006) 'No Fio da Navalha: Reflexões em Torno da Interface entre Intersexualidade, (Bio)Ética e Direitos Humanos', in Grossi, M. P., Heilborn, M. L. and Machado, L. Z. (eds) *Antropologia e Direitos Humanos* 4, Blumenau: Nova Letra.

Machado, P. S. (2008) 'Intersexualidade e o "Consenso de Chicago": As Vicissitudes da Nomenclatura e suas Implicações Regulatórias', *Revista Brasileira de Ciências Sociais*, 23: 109–24.

Maffía, D. and Cabral, M. (2003) 'Los Sexos ¿Son o se Hacen?', in Maffía, D. (ed.) *Sexualidades Migrantes. Género y Transgénero*, Buenos Aires: Feminaria.

Rios, R. R. (2006) 'Para um Direito Democrático da Sexualidade', *Horizontes Antropológicos*, 26: 71–100.

13 Understanding sex between men in Senegal

Beyond current linguistic and discursive categories

Cheikh Ibrahima Niang

Condemnation of homosexuality on the grounds that it is alien to African tradition and religious teachings can be found in numerous statements by African heads of state. For example, Arap Moi, former president of Kenya, is recorded as having said: 'It is not right that a man should go with another man or a woman with another woman. It is against African tradition and Biblical teachings'. He added 'I will not shy away from warning Kenyans against the dangers of scourge', stating that 'Kenya has no room or time for homosexuals and lesbians' (Foreman 1999: 115).

Postcolonial expressions of opinion on homosexuality in Africa, however, often obscure the relation between colonialism and sexuality. Writers on the history of homosexuality have rarely focused on same-sex relations in the contexts of colonialism, and, when they do so, their focus is often on homosexual experiences between Europeans and local people in colonised countries (Aldrich 2003). What needs closer inquiry therefore are the forms of same-sex sexual relations that existed pre- and postcolonialism. An analysis of these practices and experiences needs integrating not only with later postcolonial analyses of homosexuality but also with a more general rethinking of sexuality throughout Africa (Anfred 2004; Thomas 2007).

Discourses on homosexuality in Africa are located within troubled epistemological paradigms in which basic assumptions about sex, sexuality and gender often go unchallenged in the light of anthropological findings (Oyěwùmí 1997) and recent advances in biological discourse and research (Fausto-Sterling 2000). Within this context, Moore (1994) has cautioned against reducing account of gender, culture and experience to their linguistic and cognitive elements; features which, she points out, should be understood as embodied in social and political processes. Instead, deeper questions need to be asked about the local descriptors applied to particular expressions of sexuality. How and through which metaphors and discursive expressions are sexual categories constructed, for example? Which discourses come to situate the wordings and legitimate practices, policies, gender politics and biopolitics? And what underlying histories, cultures, social relationships, social organisations and dynamics give their meaning to these discourses?

Goor-jigeen (men-women)

Since the nineteenth century, Western authors have offered descriptions of men dressed as women and male sex workers looking for male partners or dancing like women in the Senegalese cities of Saint-Louis and Dakar and in other parts of West Africa (Corre 1894; Crowder 1959; Werner 1993; Teunis 1996). Crowder (1959) among others noted the local use of the word *goor-jigeen* (man-woman in the Wolof language) to refer to those men.

It is important to note that, in the expression man-woman, the word woman is not used as an adjective but as a substantive. In fact, the expression is constituted by two substantives, the idea being that a particular type of man is *also* a woman. The term *goor-jigeen* does not imply or make reference to genital anatomy; other words are used for those who have both male and female genitals. There are also critical differences between the notion of *goor-jigeen* and homosexuality. In recent research on men's same-sex sexual relations in Senegal,[1] when the term *homosexuel* (the official language in Senegal is French) was used in questionnaires, Senegalese informants (particularly those born in colonial times) provided examples of Europeans they knew and who used to live in their town. None acknowledged having known or heard about a European *goor-jigeen* (man-woman).

Despite this, Western literature insists on misreading local realities. Authors such as Teunis (1996) for example have sought to construe the term *goor-jigeen* (which they translate by homosexuals) thus:

> Although these homosexuals are called *gordjiguène*, which is the Wolof-language term for 'man-woman', there are two kinds of men-women. Each one takes on a different role in sexual intercourse, which typically involves anal intercourse. The men who insert during intercourse are called the *yauss* (penetrators), and the men who receive are called the *oubi* (receivers).
>
> (Teunis 1996: 161)

But this is incorrect. In Wolof, there is no such inclusive category encompassing both categories of receptive and penetrative partner. The *goor-jigeen* is only associated with the receptive role. The person who occupies the top position is never identified as a *goor-jigeen*, but as a *goor* or man. The most usual way of referring to such a person is to call him a *faru goor-jigeen* (the male lover of a man-woman), a description that refers explicitly to the relationship *not* to an identity.

Etymologically, the *goor-jigeen* is defined as both a man and a woman, but socially, he belongs to the women's world. Sometimes, the expression *gooru jigeen yi* may be employed, meaning the 'the women's man', or a man who has become very attached to women. Words used to specify different categories of *goor-jigeen* often refer to the age of the person. As an adult, a *goor-jigeen* can be called *jeeg*. Generally speaking, a *jeeg* is a woman who is conscious of her sexual maturity. One of the highest positions that can be held by a *goor-jigeen* is that of '*ndeyale*', meaning: 'to be given the status of a mother'. A *goor-jigeen* may be awarded this position either by women in family ceremonies such as dancing parties or weddings or by other *goor-jigeen* in similar circumstances. Younger *goor-jigeen* usually call older ones *jeeg*, as a sign of respect, or *yaay* (mother or mummy) via an analogy to mother–daughter relationships. In return, an older *goor-jigeen* may call a younger one *nenne* (a word of affection used by mothers to refer to their babies). Reference to age is also present in the use of terms such as *mag* or *rakk* (respectively older and younger siblings). Very young *goor-jigeen* are called *janxx*, or virgins. This taxonomy reveals the systematic use of words designed to qualify women of various family, age and reproductive statuses. The family model reproduced by groups of *goor-jigeen* suggests a social unit consisting in females occupying various positions, and that also functions as a strong support group.

In the past, but less so in the present, *goor-jigeen* may also "marry" a *goorgi* taking that man as their *jëkër* or husband. Marriage does not necessary mean the couple live together in the same place; but this may happen in some cases (especially when the person referred to as the husband can afford to live in relative isolation from the local community). Marriage may also take place between a young *goor-jigeen* and an older one who takes on the role of the provider. Regardless of their type, *goor-jigeen* weddings are as much social events and an opportunity to construct ties between networks, than the consecration of a couple's life.

Performing social roles in the women's world

In the past, there were numerous woman-dominated spaces into which *goor-jigeen* were socially integrated. *Goor-jigeen* might become the companions of one or more *diriyanké*, women of high social position with a particular physical appearance (strong corpulence and big buttocks) and an associated sense of elegance and generosity. In women's ceremonies, long before the event starts, *goor-jigeen* used to provide advice to the organisers regarding dress and make-up. On the day of the ceremony, the *goor-jigeen* used to play the role of poets and musicians and spokespersons. They used to sing the organising ladies' praises, to recount their families' genealogy and to act as middlepersons between the organisers and other participants in the ceremony.

Within women's societies, *goor-jigeen* used to promote social prestige. They had a special role to play in gift giving (*teranga*), which used to occur in all collective ceremonies. Gift giving is part of a whole system of interactions which confer on their authors respect and social prestige within the group and community. *Goor-jigeen* also used to recite short poems or *taasu* that play an important role and social function in women's ceremonies (McNee 2000). Some decades ago, in the cities of Northern Senegal, *goor-jigeen* also used to organise traditional dances and ceremonies called *tannber* that were well attended by the whole community. Women's *tannber* success was ensured by the presence of *goor-jigeen*.

Numerous concepts organise the relationship between women and *goor-jigeen* at an interpersonal level. A *ndey dike* relationship generally takes the form of a long-term friendship between a *goor-jigeen* and a woman of status. Before cementing the relationship, however, the women will first want to know whether the *goor-jigeen* has a '*full*' or strong personality, and whether he/she has renowned friends. A *full* personality is seen as inspiring respect from other women, men and community members; it ensures that every time the woman concerned organises a ceremony she too will be well thought of. To celebrate a *ndey dike* relationship, the woman invites the *goor-jigeen* to her home and offers him presents (money, living-room furniture, material, kitchen utensils) in the presence of her kin and friends and the delegation that accompanies the *goor-jigeen*. In return, the *goor-jigeen* has to invite the lady and her friends to attend a festive ceremony organised at his home or in a house reserved for that event to thank her for her generosity.

Goor-jigeen also play important political roles alongside women. Lamine Guèye and the future President Senghor, the two main African political leaders in the period just prior to Senegalese independence were both very popular with the female electorate. They benefited from networks of female leaders capable of mobilising important masses of voters. Several of these women leaders – if not all of them

Table 13.1 Translation of *goor-jigeens'* songs during former President Senghor's political campaign

Sentences of the slogan	Literal translation	Language used and source for the translation
Ar watam	Come and have sexual intercourse [with] me	Pulaar/Fulfulde (Seydou 1998: 10, 768)
mbimi	I say	Pulaar/Fulfulde
xañ ma ci	Strike it inside me	Wolof

– were surrounded by networks of *goor-jigeen* who played decisive roles in social and political mobilisation. Tradition states that women and *goor-jigeen* together organised the triumphal entry of Senghor into the Senegalese city of Saint-Louis after his successful election campaign. He was reportedly welcomed by *goor-jigeen* singing '*Ar watam, mbimi xañ ma ci*', which in a coded language signifies 'Come and make love to me'. Encoding relies on the fact that some words of the slogan are spoken in Pulaar (a language that is not predominantly spoken in Saint-Louis; thus the meaning of those words are not understood by 'ordinary people') and the other ones in Wolof (the language of the majority of people in Saint-Louis), as shown in Table 13.1.

New naming categories

Unlike in the past, in modern-day Dakar, the word *goor-jigeen* is often considered demeaning and stigmatising. As one informant in a recent study I conducted stated:

> [T]he term *gor-jigeen* frightens us. When someone says it in our presence, it makes us shiver. The term is like the sound of a siren which we apprehend to be followed by insults, blows, or stones thrown at us by out-of-control mobs.
>
> (Niang *et al.* 2003: 505)

The value attached to the word seems to have changed in parallel with the rise of homophobic violence. The new word *ibbi* was said by *goor-jigeen* to be employed '*so as the outsider will not decode our messages nor identify our sexual inclinations*'. The introduction of this new term was accompanied by a whole set of changes in dressing and bodily expression. Nowadays, *goor-jigeen* avoid wearing women's dresses (at least in public), and have invented new codes of communication and ways of dressing that correspond both to the need to show conformity to norms and to the willingness to express their sexual identity.

Etymologically, the term *ibbi* is a corruption of the Wolof word *ubbi* which means to open. It refers to the opening of the anus to allow penetration during sexual intercourse. In opposition to the term *ibbi* is the word *yoos*, which is one among several terms used to refer to the partner who penetrates, designating a person (most usually the male client of female sex workers) who is essentially interested in brief sexual relationship in exchange of money. From the point of view of *ibbi*, the term *yoos* carries pejorative connotations, in the sense that a *yoos* cannot be considered a reliable person with whom a lasting relationship can be built. In the eyes of some sex workers, *yoos* lack prestige because of their instability and their incapacity to give sexual relations the time and space necessary to result in romance and attachment.

A *coof* is another type of male sexual partner of both women and *goor-jigeen*. *Coof* are distinguished by their wealth and their generous and distinguished manners. But this appellation too describes a temporary relationship. For longer-term and more durable partners, it is preferable to seek out a *far* (a male sexual partner) or a *goorgi* (literally an adult man or husband).

Men becoming women

Goor-jigeen may partially or entirely wear women's clothing, especially on occasions such as dances or when frequenting pick-up places for men. They may also dress as women when cooking or serving meals, or when participating in festive ceremonies. The adoption of female dress has strong resonance in Senegal where men may also become women when a woman's spirit or *rab* takes possession of that body, revealing itself through dance and in other ways (Zempleni 1968). Among the Lebu (the most ancient Wolof community in Dakar), the leader of *ndëp* ceremonies, that are meant to restore harmony following psychic, social or ecological disorder, is either a woman or a man who wears women's clothes and adopts the attitudes and manners characteristic of a woman. Some of the men involved as members of the *ndëp* rituals may have sex with other men (Niang *et al.* 2004) although there is an organised silence concerning their sexual lives.

Within the conceptual frameworks of many Senegalese languages, sexual categories (in particular man-woman) cannot be defined without referring back to a more inclusive category which encompasses both sexes. In Wolof, the basic inclusive categorical reference is that of *nit* whose radical has nothing in common with any of the terms referring to man or woman. *Nit* cannot even be qualified as masculine or feminine; it is improper to join to it an adjective that refers back to belonging to a sex. You cannot for example say *nit bu goor* (a human being of male sex), or *nit bu goor* (a human being of male sex); since *nit* (human being) is beyond sex. Instead, the notion of *nit* implies a whole set of concepts that include those associated with masculinity and femininity. The terms *goor* and *jigeen* (usually translated by man and woman) point out to both a sexual category and a position in initiatory routes, and to a status, social roles, attitudes, behaviours and concept embodiments that largely transcend reference to solely physical attributes.

Concepts of womanhood can be also found in the use of woman as a political metaphor. The state is often referred to as a mother, and the expression 'mother of twins', that is used when referring to the head of state, offers a model for claiming both social justice and political equity (the twins). Historically, the title *ndey ji reew* (literally mother of the country) that of the highest authority in the Lebu political system, prior to colonialism. The language of everyday social life is also full of metaphoric expressions giving men female attributes when they are performing specific social acts. For example a man may *boot* or 'carry people on his back' when he takes care of a large family or a community; he may *nampal* or breastfeed when he educates or transmits knowledge and he may *jur* or 'give birth' when indicating a kinship relationship.

Traditional Islam, which was constructed within the discursive context of these allegorical discourses, seems to have developed a relative tolerance towards *goor-*

jigeen, as documented in early ethnographic writings (Crowder 1959). Traditional Muslim leaders often stress repentance, which is to be encouraged and obtained before a *goor-jigeen* dies. The Koran is thereby interpreted as being in line with concepts of God's mercifulness and the promotion of social cohesion as the antithesis of social or interpersonal tensions. Some religious leaders we recently interviewed as part of unpublished fieldwork go so far as to condemn the use of physical violence against *goor-jigeen*, encouraging cursing and advice giving instead; this is consistent with Ben Naum (1933: 88, cited by Murray and Roscoe 1997: 89). In the Senegalese Muslim brotherhoods, the presence has been reported of effeminate men (some of whom are said to have been *goor-jigeen* when they were younger) who periodically carry out tasks traditionally ascribed to women, and men who sometimes dress as women. Some religious leaders wear clothes made of material designed for women's use, and a few are suspected of using cosmetic products more usually worn by women and *goor-jigeen*.

Religious brotherhoods have also developed the idea of return to 'normality', whereby *goor-jigeen*, having reached old age, make amends and are reintegrated into the religious community of their birth. Their homosexual lives are thereby placed in parenthesis before they die. *Goor-jigeen* who do not openly display their inclination, as well as those who make amends before dying, receive religious funerals at their death. If they fail to do so, they may be buried in a separate graveyard alongside the graves of those who committed suicide. But, in this respect as well, women are the surest and most faithful allies of the *goor-jigeen*. They are the ones who go behind the stage to lobby and advocate, so as to have male religious leaders change their position and authorise prayers and burials to conform with religious rites.

Rising homophobia

In recent decades, however, there has been a growth of violence and ill treatment towards sexual minorities. In January 2009, nine young men were sentenced to nine years' imprisonment by a Senegalese court in Dakar for 'unnatural sexual acts' and for the creation of an HIV/AIDS-prevention association that was construed by the authorities as being a criminal gang.[2]

Newspapers frequently run abusive and debasing headlines together with the images of people said to be homosexuals. In the content of these articles, *goor-jigeen* are frequently dealt with as second-class citizens. Such vilification often becomes a marketing device for raising newspaper sales. On private radio stations, broadcasts often take the form of phone-ins tantamount to inciting to violence. In 2008 the reporting of a 'homosexual marriage' by the Senegalese press (www.xibar.net/publication 2008) was followed by lynching and police arrests (www.pambazuka.org/fr/2008). Newspapers have reported cases of graves of deceased *goor-jigeen* being desecrated and corpses dragged into the streets, or cases of persons who were refused burial in the graveyards (www.jeuneafrique.com 2009).

In recent times, some *goor-jigeen* have been beaten up by crowds or assaulted in their homes without any legal action being taken against those responsible for that. The *goor-jigeen*'s traditional recreational places are frequently disturbed by stone throwing or acts of violence that systematically go unpunished. The *tannber* have practically disappeared from the festive landscape, due to the fear of assaults, whereas, until recently, they used to be a tradition in some districts of Dakar. *Goor-jigeen* complain about the fact that the police and the judiciary do little to ensure their security or do not sanction the damages done to them.

The origins of these changes are complex. In the 1960s, Senegal witnessed the rise of a discourse advocating moral regeneration as part of an ambitious nationalist project. In this context, police roundups of *goor-jigeen* and sex workers, and the harassment of unmarried women or women considered as being of dissolute morals became common. The security forces (both the police and the gendarmerie) acted as if the nation's defence had to include in the repression of elements symbolising lack of moral vigour and ideological purity. The *goor-jigeen* give accounts of those years as those of rains of burning stones (personal communication). They say they owed their salvation to the downfall of the then ruling regime and the return in force of a more tolerant political discourse. But the trauma endured engendered lack of trust in the political system.

Between 1964 and 1974, Senegal experienced single party rule (Diouf 2001). The disappearance of multiparty elections made irrelevant the need of women's organising power in voter mobilisation. The single party regime was a setback to women's political power, especially *jeeg* power. Female leaders (the *diriyanke*, the *diongoma* and the *jeeg*) disappeared from the political scene. With the lessening of such power in the political arena, the *goor-jigeen* felt the ground giving way beneath their feet. Between 1970–1980, the position of the *goor-jigeen* underwent a new assault, this time by fundamentalist Muslim – as opposed to more traditional forms of Islamic – pressures advocating moral purification. In several respects, this fundamentalist discourse has given legitimacy to the stigma and violence nowadays directed against the *goor-jigeen*. Political Islam, represented by religious political parties, has developed an openly homophobic discourse (Djamra 1984).

At its roots, however, homophobic violence expresses indeed violence against women and everything that is feminine. The *goor-jigeen*, whose femininity is made visible by the interpretation of bodily or behavioural indicators, are the ones who are hunted down, beaten up or harassed by mobs and the police. The *yoos* and the other sexual partners of the *goor-jigeen* remain unidentified and do not become the subjects of acts of violence. This leads to a new disciplining of the body and of appearance, aimed at suppressing demonstrations of femininity and devaluing cultural concepts and metaphors associated with women.

Conclusions

The study of the *goor-jigeen* highlights both, on the one hand, the need to question the validity of the predominant analytical models, the basic concepts, the approaches and the epistemological paradigms in which homosexuality and sexuality are conceptualised and, on another hand, the need for collecting and analyzing good quality cultural data using inventive and appropriate methods.

Within the traditional framework of Wolof culture in the cities of Saint-Louis and Dakar, the *goor-jigeen* used to hold prestigious positions within women's social organisations and used to share common multiple identities with the category of women defined through age and sex organising principles. The traditional situation of *goor-jigeen* coheres with concepts of men becoming women expressed through cross-dressing and the symbolism associated with clothing, and connected to spiritual constructs that confer on woman central ontological value. Traditional Islamic beliefs as well as beliefs relevant to traditional African religions developed forms of acceptance of the *goor-jigeen*, alongside formal doctrinal condemnation of homosexuality.

The adoption of the single-party system (1964–1974) was the starting point for new setbacks in women's political power and the decline of their alliance with the *goor-jigeen*, as well as the intensification of structural violence against the latter. The birth of new names and identities (such as *ibbi*) appeared as survival strategies in the face of homophobic violence. Current assaults against *goor-jigeen* can be seen as expressions of the politically motivated social control seeking to establish a male hegemony more in line with new fundamentalist religious discourses and the predominant culture of postcolonial political systems.

There is a convergence between the attacks against femininity and those against so-called homosexuals. These are cultural attacks as well, in so far as they deny the metaphors, the allegories and the concepts relating to the construction of womanhood as it appears in Wolof language and traditional beliefs. Therefore, the struggle for homosexuals' and any other people's human rights cannot do without a reappropriation of the cultural legacies of African societies.

Notes

1 The SAHARA Program, unpublished preliminary report of a study led by the SAHARA program on stigma and HIV, sponsored by DGIS and CIDA.
2 In Senegal, Article 319 of the Penal Code considers sexual acts between two individuals of same sex as a crime, punishable by up to five years' imprisonment, and by up to a one million franc fine. The law is written in French and reproduces concepts that are sometimes difficult – if not impossible – to translate in local languages. Senegalese law, for example, defines sexual acts between persons of the same sex as 'unnatural', yet the notion of there being an unnatural act is irrelevant to most local conceptions of sexuality. Official laws relating to homosexuality ignore local notions of pleasure and desire as a fundamental individual right, whereas in the local languages, the right to pleasure (if not harmful to others) is an inalienable principle, and in Wolof, the notion of pleasure is strongly associated with life.

References

Aldrich, R. (2003) *Colonialism and Homosexuality*, London: Routledge.

Anfred, S. (2004) *Re-thinking Sexualities in Africa*, Uppsala: The Nordic Africa Institute.

Corre, A. (1894) *L'Ethnographie Criminelle d'après les Observations et les Statistiques Judiciaires Recueillies dans les Colonies Françaises*, Paris: C. Reinwald.

Crowder, M. (1959) *Pagans and Politicians*, London: Hutchinson.

Diouf, M. (2001) *Histoire du Sénégal*, Paris: Maisonneuve & Larose.

Djamra Magazine (1984) 'Les Dossiers Noirs de la Dégradation Sociale au Sénégal No. 5', Dakar.

Fausto-Sterling, A. (2000) *Sexing the Body. Gender Politics and the Construction of Sexuality*, New York: Basic Books.

Foreman, M. (1999) *AIDS and Men. Taking Risks or Taking Responsibility*, London: Panos/Zed Books.

McNee, L. (2000) *Selfish Gifts. Senegalese Women: Autobiographical Discourses*, New York: University of New York Press.

Moore, H. L. (1994) 'A Passion for Difference: Essays in Anthropology and Gender', Bloomington: Indiana University Press.

Murray, S. O. and Roscoe, W. (1997) *Islamic Homosexualities, Culture, History and Literature*, New York: New York University Press.

Niang, C. I., Moreau, A. M., Bop, C., Compaore, C. and Diagne, M. (2004) 'Targeting Vulnerable Groups in National HIV/AIDS Programs: The Case of Men who have Sex with Men. Senegal, Burkina Faso, The Gambia', Washington, DC: World Bank. (African Region Human Development Working Paper Series No. 82)

Niang, C. I., Tabsoba, P., Weiss, E., Diagne, M., Niang, Y., Moreau, A. M. *et al.* (2003) 'It's Raining Stones: Stigma, Violence and HIV Vulnerability among Men who have Sex with Men in Dakar, Senegal', *Culture, Health and Sexuality*, 5 (6): 499–512.

Oyěwùmí, O. (1997) *The Invention of Women. Making an African Sense of Western Gender Discourses*, Minneapolis: University of Minnesota Press.

Seydou, C. (1998) *A Dictionary of Verb Roots in Fulfulde Dialects*, Paris: Karthala.

Teunis, N. (1996) 'Homosexuality in Dakar: Is the Bed the Heart of a Sexual Subculture?', *Journal of Gay, Lesbian and Bisexual Identity*, 1 (2): 153–69.

Thomas, C. (2007) *The Sexual Demon of Colonial Power. Pan-African Embodiment and Erotic Schemes of Empire*, Bloomington: Indiana University Press.

Werner, J.-F. (1993) *Marges, Sexe et Drogues à Dakar. Enquête Ethnographique*. Paris: Karthala.

Zempleni, A. (1968) 'L'Interprétation et la Thérapie Traditionnelles du Désordre Mental chez les Wolof et les Lebou (Sénégal)', Doctoral thesis in Psychology, University of Paris.

www.jeuneafrique.com. Sénégal. L'homophobie gagne du terrain. AFP (accessed 12 January 2009).

www.pambazuka.org/fr/ (accessed 15 February 2008).

www.xibar.net/publication (accessed 3 February 2008).

Part III

Reproductive and sexual health

14 Why a history of childhood sexuality?

Gail L. Hawkes and R. Danielle Egan

Currently in the USA, UK and Australia, the issue of childhood and sexuality is as controversial as it is fascinating. Popular and professional discourses on these two phenomena abound in the current furore about the 'sexualisation' of the child through visual representation, especially in advertising copy but also in artistic texts, – the content of which is assumed to be threatening and destructive of the essence of 'childness' – its innocence. A crucial, yet unaddressed social and political consequence of this popular manifestation is that the child operates in abstraction – as a categorical object instead of a subjective being and in so doing legitimates social and/or moral intervention by its further endangerment. The complexity of children's cultural, historical or subjective variability is obscured and silenced and this is particularly the case in discussions of sexuality.[1] Instead, in the first decade of the twenty-first century, and in contexts as diverse as US feminist psychology, the Australian political left and Girlguiding UK, discourses of the child remain, predominantly, discourses of protection.[2] But ensuring protection paradoxically ensures also the containment of children within intensifying surveillance and restriction, further affirming the dependence and helplessness of the child.

Although contemporary concerns about the sexuality of children tend to emphasise dangers in the life of the child as the result of cultural innovations (e.g. the internet), the problem of childhood sexuality has a long history. In this chapter, we will briefly address dominant ideas about childhood sexuality to demonstrate a key distinction between pathology and normality in nineteenth-century sexological writings in Europe. In particular, we focus on the work of the physician and sexologist Albert Moll who offered an especially provocative additional element in this process – an argument for the equal normalisation of active and agentic sexual children. We propose that his work theorised about, and presented empirical evidence for, the existence of a 'sexual life of the child' expressed in terms of childhood experience rather than adult judgment. As such, Moll's work offers a starting point from which perhaps to think more dispassionately about children and their sexuality as well as to contribute critically to contemporary discussions of sexualisation. Specifically, we suggest that a critical acknowledgment of agency in childhood sexuality could offer a way out of the contemporary ideological impasse that insists on protection of the child, while at the same time focusing on its perilous sexual potential.

Masturbation phobia and the compulsive body

Since the beginnings of the ideological distinctions between adulthood and child-hood in Europe and elsewhere, the moral, physical and sensual status of the child has been under debate and scrutiny. As Jordanova has claimed, even in the eight-eenth century 'children could be valued as aesthetic objects for their beauty and physical perfection – but they could equally be feared for their instinctual animal-like natures' (Jordanova: 1987: 6; O'Malley 2003: 79). 'Mixed feelings' (Porter 1982) prevailed in relation to adult sexuality in the eighteenth century, and this mixture of optimism and ambivalence is also evident in the conceptual twinning of the child with nature. However, this closeness to nature was not necessarily a positive attribute. For if the child is left in the condition in which it remains driven by its senses (in the state of nature) it will become a slave to its passions and pursue a life of self-indulgent misery (Buffon 1857: 56). Reason, acquired by education in the context of sensual experience, offered an antidote to the passions, which were them-selves viewed with ambivalence. For, on the one hand, it was through these experi-ences that the child was able to acquire self-control; on the other, left to rule the behaviour of the child, the passions could cause individual and social misery. Thus it was that the child of nature of the eighteenth century was still the child who required guidance and management, but through pedagogy of the mind not (at least directly) the body (Benzaquen 2004).

By the end of the eighteenth century, as Foucault details, a new discourse emerged around the parent/child relationship in the context of the 'somatisation' of the masturbating child (Foucault 2003). It was, he suggests, through the prism of what came to be called masturbation phobia (see Barker-Benfield 1976; see also Laqueur 2003; Darby 2005), that the body or the child was to be sexualised a very specific manner. The masturbating child was established within medical and quasi-medical discourses by the beginning of the nineteenth century as the autoeroticisa-tion of its body legitimated constant parental surveillance and the medical prescription of constraints or surgical intervention. Both strategies were considered to be a rational response to the problem of the diseased body – the offending or dis-eased part is cut out for the good of the whole. Children as young as a few months old were claimed to be capable of the compulsive and destructive habit of self-abuse, long before they could make any conscious choice. Accidental stimulation of the genitals led rapidly to compulsive repetition. The genitals of the child came to be the site of a double anxiety – as the source of unpredictable or accidental stimula-tion as well as a subsequent source of dangerous and consciously sought pleasures (Hodges 2005: 210). Constructed as simultaneously lacking the capacity for self-control or self-management, on the one hand, and as sensually combustible, on the other, the sexual child was recognised in masturbation phobia as the supreme unan-swerable proof of the compulsion and destructiveness of masturbation.

The unthinking autoerotic child

But this was not the only form in which the sexual child appeared in the profes-sional writings of the nineteenth century. Sexologists from Krafft-Ebing, to Ellis, Bloch and Forel identified the phenomenon of what Ellis was to name 'autoeroti-cism' (a term he invented in 1898) in infants and children, as well as adolescents and adults. 'Every physician conversant with nervous affections and diseases incident to childhood is aware of the fact that manifestations of the sexual instinct may occur in very young children' (Krafft-Ebing 1931: 48). Thus, Krafft-Ebing (in keeping with the other writings of sexology) distinguished between those children who accidentally came on the practice through external stimulation, inadvertent or intended, and those children whose behaviour manifested a precocious and pathological form of sexual development. This he refers to as 'premature manifestations of the sexual instinct' (ibid.: 56), and identified as a sign of a more generalised neuropsychiatric condition.

Ellis, in distinguishing 'autoeroticism' from dangerous compulsive behaviour, criticised the work of Tissot, Rousseau, Voltaire and Lallemand all of whom he accuses of exaggerating and universalising the effects of masturbation (Ellis 1921: 49–50). In his efforts to normalise autoeroticism, in the face of the still prevailing masturbation phobia, Ellis records numerous accounts from his own and other medical evidence for deliberate self-stimulation in children and adolescents that result in no physical or mental detriment. In his concern to report rather than to judge, Ellis perhaps unwittingly offers evidence for erotic agency in quite young children. He identifies what he terms 'accidental stimulation' of infants from clothes or servants; that leads in some cases to the formation of a compulsive habit. He distinguishes such behaviour in infants and young children from the conscious pursuit of sexual pleasure that he details in prepubescent and adolescent young people. He acknowledges that both girls and boys engage in autoerotic behaviour, but that the girls appear to be able to practise masturbation more frequently with less enervation. He quotes a correspondent who is a teacher to support his claim:

> My experience proved that many of the lads regarded masturbation as reprehensible; but their plea was 'everyone does it'. The greater number made no attempt to conceal the habit, they enlarged upon the pleasure of it; it was 'ever so much nicer than eating tarts', etc.
>
> (Ellis 1921: 241)

Iwan Bloch likewise distinguished between masturbation that is pathological (associated with neurotic manifestations) and normal autoeroticism, that begins before puberty 'autoeroticism is almost always a precursor of completely developed sexuality, and manifests itself a long time before puberty' (Bloch n.d.: 413). Being to 'a certain extent physiological in its manifestations', such activities are not considered pathological but a 'natural physiological masturbation' (ibid.: 410) that cannot be explained in terms of moral turpitude or criminality but of a 'premature development of sexual sensibility' (Bloch ibid). For Bloch, such sensibility in young children is part of a natural continuum, a claim he supports with reference to the animal world as well as 'primitive races' where masturbation is a 'popular custom' (ibid.: 411).

August Forel discusses the sexual child in the context of acquired sexual perversions that he sees primarily as the consequence of seduction or of corrupting influences. He comes closer to the discourse of hygiene when he proposes sex education as protection from such external influences, but, he cautions, 'in giving these explanations it is important not to awaken eroticism in the child by dwelling more than necessary on sexual topics' (Forel 1931: 485). In adding this caveat, Forel implicitly acknowledges the instability of the sexual child, simultaneously unawakened and excitable. But he identifies another pathological manifestation of sexuality in the child: what he calls a 'sexual paradox [...] the appearance of a sexual appetite, or even of love, at an abnormal age' (Forel 1931: 221). He offers a number of examples of children of seven and nine years, both boys and girls; who exhibit such behaviour (Forel 1931: 221), and who, he says, could be rehabilitated if they undertook rigorous retraining in special institutions. Here, precociously sexual children would be occupied from morning to night rendering them 'too tired than do else but sleep' (Forel 1931: 231). Demonstration of an active and self initiated sexuality in the child could not be ignored; nevertheless, in proposing reformatory cure, Forel was acknowledging that sexual paradox was not inherent but acquired.

The construction of the sexual child by these early sexologists differed from that found in masturbation phobia. But it was not a complete separation. All four writers agree on a normative distinction between autoeroticism and expressions of sexual perversion; where the common factor in the former was accidental and unconscious stimulus/response; and, in the latter, some evidence of conscious intention to re-experience the pleasurable sexual activity. Thus they continue to make a normative, if more covert, judgment based on the presence or absence of consciously sought erotic experience. Normal childhood sexuality is thereby understood and lacking in any sensibility or active engagement. Instead, it is characterised as being driven by an unconscious physiological response. It is this elision of any consciousness or agency in the construction of the sexual child that is directly challenged by the much less often discussed work *The Sexual Life of the Child* (Moll 1912).

The question of agency: Moll's sexual child

Like Sigmund Freud, Albert Moll was a physician trained in psychiatry. They were countrymen and contemporaries (Freud was six years older) and died in 1939 (on the same day). Both shared a conviction that the sexuality of the child had been hitherto ignored or misrepresented. However, Moll was critical of Freud's claims about manifestations of the sexual instinct and especially what Moll saw as Freud's claim that sexual experiences in the child predisposed to a range of neurotic and somatic disorders as adults. Moll's work, like Freud's, was empirically based, but he avoided dependence on 'pathological considerations', relying instead on the child-hood recollections of healthy individuals (Moll 1912: 15).

Moll's work is distinguished by its aim to gain scientific information that would end the silence about the 'sexual life of the child'.[3] Here, he is departing from what Foucault identified as the somatisation of childhood sexuality (Foucault 2003) by widening the exploratory lens to include subjective experience. He claims that in literature and history there was abundant evidence that prepubertal children were not just capable of, but habitually engaged in, forms of sexual expression that far exceeded the unconsciously and accidentally elicited autoeroticism recognised by his fellow sexologists. The crucial distinctive element was not somatic but affective. He lists the biographic recollections of Rousseau, Goethe, Dante, Byron, Napoleon and Flaubert, all of whom provide vivid accounts of physical and emotional engagement as children from the age of 8–10 years old (Moll 1912: 10). This evidence not-withstanding, Moll complains, 'this important question is handled in a casual or cursory manner. A thorough presentation of the subject has not, as far as my knowledge extends hitherto been attempted' (Moll 1912: 14). In retrospect, he was justi-fied in this claim for although his name is customarily included in a list of sexologists at the turn of the century, his argument, and its implications for a more systematic formulation of childhood sexuality, has remained largely on the margins, eclipsed by the more familiar work of Freud. We want to suggest that Moll offered the first normative recognition of a sexually agentic child: a scientifically based and empirically supported account of childhood sexuality that was not dependent on adult definitions for either its meaning or its legitimacy.

Like his fellow sexologists, Moll begins by identifying the 'sexual impulse' as a normal phenomenon. However, he immediately departs from their orthodoxy by claiming that the sexual impulse takes two observable forms: detumesence[4] and con-trectation.[5] The former comprises 'physical processes that take place in the sexual organs' (1912: 29). This he likens to the unconscious actions of, say, a horse or a cow that will stimulate its sexual organs to orgasm but with no especial object, person or thought in mind. The latter term, however, refers to feelings of emotional attachment and the need for physical intimacy that may or may not be directly related to the detumescent impulse.

In contrast to the somatic foundations of detumescence, contrectation expresses itself in a quest for physical intimacy driven by emotional attachment. Both ele-ments of the sexual impulse can occur independently of each other in all humans but especially, he argues, in the child. He offers examples from case studies to illus-trate that the child may even masturbate to ease the tumescence without making any connection, necessarily, between the experience of masturbation and orgasm and the object of its intimate attraction. He distinguishes between the two stages of childhood: whereas up to the age of seven, the detumescent impulse may come about from local stimulation and its relief may involve pleasure, the voluptuous acme and ejaculation do not occur until well into the second stage (8–14 years).[6] He is especially interesting when he offers examples of the range of connections pos-sible in children's contrectational relationships: these can be between the same age; the same sex or the opposite; between children and animals; between the child (male or female) and adults and/or older children; even between the child and its parents. These feelings may be intense and long-lasting, and may or may not express themselves also in tumescence and detumescence.

Here, Moll demonstrates the distinctive nature of his work: a dispassionate detached account of same and opposite sex attractions, and especially of what we would now call cross-generational sex. Additionally, he acknowledges intense emo-tional and psychosexual attachments between children and animals (1912: 137–8). Indeed it is this polymorphously perverse expression that brings him close to Freud's argument, yet he makes no comment about this connection, despite his obvious familiarity with Freud's *Three Essays on Sexuality*. Moll's work extends the boundaries of childhood sexuality beyond the passive body or the regulation and surveillance within the arenas of medicine or family (Foucault: 2003). His 'sexual impulse' includes elements that necessarily fall outside existing parameters of sci-entific inquiry as well as of those of social expectations, then, and arguably still now. These include emotion, conscious sensibility, erotic fantasy and the possibility of a spiritual as well as physical level of sexual expression.

His theory of the sexual impulse opens a space for an understanding of child-hood sexuality in its own terms. The disengagement of the physiological from the emotional and the psychic (in the imagination and fantasy) in childhood allows for the child to learn about its sexual sensibilities in terms much wider than simply physical stimulation and response. It is the child's experience that is the teacher, not the imparted and filtered knowledge of adults seen through their eyes, whether parents or professionals. However, we do not wish to overstate the revolutionary intentions of this turn-of-the-century physician: he also acknowledged the negative outcomes of precocious sexuality in children, and although an exponent of sexual enlightenment as an antidote held no misapprehensions about the effectiveness of this strategy on either component of the sexual impulse: 'It must not be supposed that their adaptation will immediately result in the disappearance of all unfavourable aspects of the sexual life'. We will not, he says turn children into 'little angels' (Moll 1912: 302). His theory does not, therefore, fully resolve, or render redundant, the ongoing anxieties about the management of unruly childhood sexuality.

Insights from the past

In the historical construction of childhood sexuality (see Egan and Hawkes 2009) children are distinguished by their 'incomplete status' sexually, a characteristic to be developed, carefully, under the watchful eyes of adults. Evidence of independently acquired or exercised eroticism has been constructed as at worst a corruption of innocence (Egan and Hawkes 2007, 2008) and at best distortion of healthy development (Hawkes and Egan 2008). In contemporary western culture, the question of whether or not children are normatively erotic, as opposed to having a 'sexual instinct', is currently hidden beneath a range of concerns about inappropriate exposure of the child to, or in, representations that are identified as sexualised by adults. Two recent examples can be found in the Bill Henson case in Australia, and in the claims expressed in the USA and UK that girls are psychologically damaged by Bratz dolls.

Our historical work thus far has presented evidence to support the claim that it is the features of sexual agency – most especially conscious choice and resistance – that underpin the associations of youthful sexual volition with individual danger and social disruption. These by now almost naturalised equations inhibit a dispassionate consideration of the child as a sexual agent: capable of independence from, and even resisting, the social expectations within which it is situated (Giddens 1984). Moll's work renders visible what remains normatively absent. The acknowledgement of the self-aware and agentically sexual child exposes the fictional protection offered by the existing boundaries that continue to frame childhood sexuality in terms of adult expectations.

Questions of sexual agency have been a key dynamic in the challenges to and revisions of constructions of the sexuality in relation to homosexual identity (for example, Weeks 2000); to young women (see for example, Holland *et al.* 2004) and most recently of older women (Loe 2004). It is noteworthy, however, that in certain respects these studies relate to what might be called marginal sexualities, and that of the child (as opposed to the adolescent) is arguably the most marginal of all. The deconstruction of prevailing discourses of childhood sexuality remains in its infancy, and the work of Moll, offered nearly a century ago introduces foundations for a new normative framework, one that offers the possibility of reconstructing a distinctive sexuality *for* and not *of* the child – one that does not conform to adult categories or adult preconceptions.

Notes

1 A historiography of childhood that claims its social construction has been in place, since the work of Philippe Aries in 1962. Similarly, historical analyses of adult sexualities have proliferated since the mid-twentieth century. But deconstructing discourses on childhood sexualities is only in its infancy, with the notable exception of Stevi Jackson in 1982 and, in more introductory theoretical framing by Foucault 1978.
2 www.abc.net.au/news/stories/2008/05/28/2257747.htm. www.girlguiding.org.uk/xq/asp/sID.628/qx/whoweare/article.asp
3 'Other writers, such as Freud, Bell and Kötscher, have contributed certain data towards the solution of these questions; no comprehensive study of the subject has hitherto been attempted' (Moll 1912: xii).
4 Reduction, subsidence or lessening of a swelling, especially the restoration of a swollen organ or part to normal size: http://medical-dictionary.thefreedictionary.com/detumescence.
5 The impulse to caress or embrace one of the opposite sex: http://cancerweb.ncl.ac.uk/cgi-bin/omd?contrectation
6 'During the undifferentiated period, it may happen that quite normal children exhibit homosexual excitement, whose importance is apt to be greatly over-estimated by their relatives and others [...] On the other hand, during the undifferentiated stage a boy may exhibit an inclination towards someone of the opposite sex [...] This inclination, whether homosexual or heterosexual, often leads to bodily acts [...] without the necessary occurrence of any manifestations on the part of the external genital organs, although such manifestations may at times ensue'. www.cerius.org/ref/book/Moll/chapter_iv.htm.

References

Aries, P. (1965) *Centuries of Childhood. A Social History of Family Life*, London: Vintage Books.

Barker-Benfield, G. J. (1976) *The Horrors of the Half-Known Life: Male Attitudes Towards Women and Sexuality in Nineteenth Century America*, New York: Harper & Row.

Benzaquen, A. (2004) 'Childhood, Identity and Human Science in the Enlightenment', *History Workshop Journal*, 57: 34–57.

Bloch, I. (n.d.) *The Sexual Life of Our Time in its Relations to Modern Civilization* (trans. M. Eden Paul), New York: Allied Book Company.

Buffon, G. L. L. (1857) *Buffon's Natural History of Man, the Globe, and of Quadrupeds, Volumes 1 and 2*, London: Leavitt & Allen.

Darby, R. (2003) 'The Masturbation Taboo and the Rise of Routine Male Circumcision: A Review of the Historiography', *Journal of Social History*, 36, Spring: 737–57.

Egan, R. D. and Hawkes, G. (2007) 'Producing the Prurient through the Pedagogy of Purity: Childhood Sexuality and the Social Purity Movement', *Journal of Historical Sociology*, 20 (4): 443–61.

Egan, R. D. and Hawkes, G. (2008) 'Imperiled and Perilous: Exploring the History of Childhood Sexuality', *Journal of Historical Sociology*, 22 (1): 355–67.

Egan, R. D. and Hawkes, G. (2010) *The Sexual Child in Modernity*, New York: Palgrave Macmillan.

Ellis, H. (1921) *Studies in the Psychology of Sex, Volume 1*, Philadelphia: F. A. Davis and Co.

Forel, A. (1931) *The Sexual Question. A Scientific, Psychological, Hygienic and Sociological Study*, New York: Physicians and Surgeons Book Company.

Foucault, M. (1978) *The History of Sexuality Volume 1: An Introduction*, London: Penguin.

Foucault, M. (2003) *Abnormal. Lectures at the Collège de France 1974–75*, New York: Picador.

Giddens, A. (1984) *Outline of the Theory of Structuration*, Cambridge: Polity Press.

Hawkes, G. and Egan, R. D. (2008) 'Developing the Sexual Child', *Journal of Historical Sociology*, 22 (1): 443–65.

Hodges, F. M. (2005) 'The Anti-masturbation Crusade in Antebellum American Medicine', *Journal of Sexual Medicine*, 2 (5): 722–31.

Holland, J., Ramazanolglu, C., Sharpe, S. and Thomson, R. (2004) *The Male in the Head: Young People, Heterosexuality and Power*, London: Tufnell Press.

Jackson, S. (1982) *Childhood and Sexuality*, Cambridge: Blackwell.

Jordanova, L. (1987) 'Children in History: Concepts of Nature and Society', in Scarre, G. (ed.) *Children, Parents and Politics*, Cambridge: Cambridge University Press.

Krafft-Ebing, R. V. (1931) *Psychopathia Sexualis with Especial Reference to Antipathic Sexual Instinct. A Medico-forensic Study*, London: Rebman.

Laqueur, T. W. (2003) *Solitary Sex: A Cultural History of Masturbation*, New York: Zone Books.

Loe, M. (2004) 'Sex and the Senior Woman: Pleasure and Danger in the Viagra Era', *Sexualities*, 7: 303–26.

Moll, A. (1912) *The Sexual Life of the Child* (trans. M. Eden Paul), London: Macmillan.

O'Malley, A. (2003) *The Making of the Modern Child: Children's Literature and Childhood in the Late Eighteenth Century*, New York and London: Routledge.

Porter, R. (1982) 'Mixed Feelings: The Enlightenment and Sexuality in Eighteenth-century Britain', in Boucé, P. G. (ed.) *Sexuality in Eighteenth-Century Britain*, Manchester: Manchester University Press.

15 From sexology to sexual health

Eli Coleman

A fundamental change has occurred in public health discourse over the last 20 years with the acknowledgement that sexual health is essential to overall health and well-being. This chapter examines this phenomenon and traces the origins of this transformation. It focuses in particular on how changes in understandings of sexuality have brought about a reorientation of clinical and professional practice, and how in particular the field of sexology has become transformed so as to engage with progressively broader health concerns.

Origins of the field of sexology

The field of sexology – defined as the interdisciplinary and scientific study of sexuality – was founded in Germany in the early part of the twentieth century. Iwan Bloch (1928) is credited with coining the term *Sexualwissenschaft* (sexology) (Haeberle 1983, n.d.). With his colleague Magnus Hirschfeld, Bloch published the first sexological journal, *Zeitschrift für Sexualwissenschaft*, in 1908 (Bloch 1928). In 1919, the first Institute for Sexology was founded at Humboldt University in Berlin, and in 1921 the first international sexological congress took place (Haeberle 1983, n.d.).

Sexology was born in a time of rapid social change fuelled by the women's emancipation movement and the Industrial Revolution. A basic principle of the emerging new field was that in order to understand the complexity of human sexuality, an interdisciplinary perspective was necessary. Medical science, which hitherto was a dominating discourse on sex, was viewed as a limited lens – and one that tended to view things from a pathological viewpoint. It is interesting to note, however, that most early pioneers in sexology were physicians (e.g. Albert Moll, Max Marcuse and Havelock Ellis; Bullough 1994), and the focus was often on understanding sexual variations and disorders (Krafft-Ebing 1908). However, for the most part what distinguished early sexology from medicine was its attempt to understand the normality and healthiness of a wide range of forms of sexual expression. In addition, the pioneers were sexual reformers fighting for sex education, access to care and sexual rights. Science was their tool for advocacy (Bullough 1978, 1994).

From Germany to the USA

After the destruction of the Hirschfeld Institute by the Nazis in 1933, the field of sexology was revitalised in the USA much to the credit of Alfred Kinsey and the publication of his famous studies (Kinsey *et al.* 1948; Kinsey *et al.* 1953). The Kinsey

Institute for Sex Research was founded in 1947 (The Kinsey Institute, n.d.). Twelve years later, the Society for the Scientific Study of Sex came into being. The interdisciplinary nature of this group is particularly notable, signalling a shift in the composition of the next generation of sexology pioneers. Albert Ellis, a psychologist, served as the society's first president. It is notable too that the Americans chose the terms 'sex research' and 'sexual science' over 'sexology'. This was a deliberate attempt to try to legitimise the scientific study of sexuality in science.

While Kinsey and Ellis were both sexual reformers, Ellis did not limit himself to the study of sexuality or teaching courses but was an avid lecturer and writer in popular forums. He had a major influence on the sexual revolution, publishing popular books such as *The Folklore of Sex* (1951), *The American Sexual Tragedy* (1954) and *Sex Without Guilt* (1958). These books illustrated his liberal sexual attitudes in the context of the very conservative times of the 1940s and 1950s. He testified in court on behalf of issues related to sexual rights and engaged in many other advocacy activities (Reiss and Ellis 2002).

The new era rekindled European sexology and spawned new centres around the world. The International Academy of Sex Research (note the use of the term *sex research*; www.iasr.org) was founded in 1974 by Richard Green from the State University of New York at Stony Brook. The first meeting was held there in 1975. The Association is still dominated by scientists from the USA, Canada and, less so, western Europe, but it does have a worldwide membership. Annual meetings generally rotate between North America and western Europe.

On an international level, sexology remained more dominated by physicians, as illustrated by the first World Congress of Medical Sexology which was held in Paris in 1974 (note the term *medical*). This forum resurrected the sexological congresses first organised by Hirschfeld and Moll. The World Association for Sexology (WAS) was founded in 1978 in Rome at the 3rd World Congress of Medical Sexology. The name of the World Congresses was changed to the World Congress of Sexology, which reflected a wider view of sexology. Male physicians and primarily clinicians led this organisation for most of its early history.

In the fertile environment of the budding sexual revolution of the 1960s and 1970s, sex research was revived and gained speed. This second sexual revolution focused on 'wellness' and self-actualisation. Publications by Kinsey (Kinsey *et al.* 1948; Kinsey *et al.* 1953), Masters and Johnson (1966, 1970), Gagnon and Simon (1973), Bell and Weinberg (1978) and others challenged the notion of what was considered sexually healthy or not. Kinsey in particular examined the nature of human sexual expression without attempting to find the roots of disease and dysfunction. As with the early German sexologists, an interdisciplinary approach was continued in an attempt to understand normal sexuality (Bullough 1978, 1994).

Sexology gains a foothold in public health

In the context of the sexual revolution of the 1960s and 1970s, and the revitalisation and growth of the sexology field worldwide, the World Health Organisation (WHO) held two expert consultations on the training and education of healthcare professionals in 1972 and 1974. Some of the most notable sexologists at the time attended for what was probably the first time that sexual scientists had been called on as experts to address a public health concern. As a result of these consultations, a technical document was published entitled *Education and Treatment in Human Sexuality: The Training of Health Professionals* (World Health Organisation 1975).

In developing this document, the authors recognised that training was needed to promote sexual health and wellbeing. They also recognised the need to advance knowledge by developing the field of sexology and disseminating knowledge through sexual resource centres around the world. As a first step towards promoting sexual health, the authors recognised the need to define sexual health. Until the WHO consultation, no definition had been constructed. In 1975 the World Health Organisation published the following definition of sexual health:

> Sexual health is the integration of the somatic, emotional, intellectual and social aspects of sexual being, in ways that are positively enriching and that enhance personality, communication and love.
>
> (WHO 1975)

In the next paragraph, the authors wrote, 'Fundamental to this concept is the right to sexual information and the right to pleasure'. The document went on to cite Mace *et al.* (1974), who described sexual health as having three basic elements: (1) the capacity to enjoy and control sexual and reproductive behaviour in accordance with a social and personal ethic; (2) a freedom from fear, shame, guilt, false beliefs and other psychological factors inhibiting sexual response and impairing sexual relationships; and (3) freedom from organic disorders, diseases and deficiencies that interfere with sexual and reproductive functions. The WHO document concluded:

> Thus the notion of sexual health implies a positive approach to human sexuality, and the purpose of sexual healthcare should be the enhancement of life and personal relationships and not merely counseling and care related to procreation or sexually transmitted diseases.
>
> (WHO 1975)

While the 1975 document had profound impact on the field of sexology, its influence in the sphere of public health was hardly palpable. It was not until 1986 that WHO took up the issue of sexual health again. In that year and the next, the European Region of WHO held two consultation meetings to clarify concepts of sexual health by (a) focusing on different groups of people within the region; (b) identifying factors contributing to sexual ill health and the means of promoting sexual health; (c) suggesting indicators that could be used to evaluate the effectiveness of programmes and policies by 2000; and (d) making recommendations for further steps forward (Langfeldt and Porter 1986; WHO Regional Office for Europe 1987). While a report was published from the 1986 meeting and a number of background papers were prepared for the 1987 consultation, no official report was ever published of this latter meeting.

In the expert consultation in 1987, participants expressed deep concern about the possibility or utility of defining sexual health. Gunter Schmidt, a German sexologist, was particularly critical of this effort. He said that sexual health implied certain norms for 'proper' sex that can be termed 'healthy'. Attempting to define sexual health risked propagating sexual norms disguised as medical truths (Schmidt 1987).

A new sexual revolution and the demand for a public health response

With the advent of HIV in the 1980s, new technological developments such as the internet, and further developments in the field of human sexuality such as biomedical advances and an understanding of the importance of gender and power analysis, a further sexual revolution began (Coleman 2000). Much like the revolution of the 1960s and 1970s, this revolution was fuelled by scientific advances, as well as by dramatic social and economic change (Coleman 2000; Inglehart 1997; Reiss 1990, 2001; Reiss and Reiss 1997).

The HIV pandemic and the new sexual revolution put pressure on health ministries to develop new approaches to sexual health promotion. The combined burden of HIV, increases in unwanted pregnancies, greater awareness of sexual violence and greater publicity about sexual dysfunctions and disorders, raised awareness of the need for better quality sexuality education and a more concerted approach to addressing sexuality problems. A new public health mandate began to emerge to address these issues (Coleman 1997, 2002, 2007).

In parallel, the term sexual health became incorporated in discourse at a public health level. The programme of action (POA) from the 1999 International Conference on Population and Development (ICPD) provided governments with guidance in addressing the sexual and reproductive health in a comprehensive, integrated manner. The document defined reproductive health as including sexual health, echoing the WHO 1975 definition of sexual health, 'the purpose of which is the enhancement of life and personal relations, and not merely counseling and care related to reproduction and sexually transmitted diseases' (United Nations 1994: para. 7.2). The POA also contained two important objectives pertaining to sexual health: (1) 'to promote adequate development of responsible sexuality, permitting relations of equity and mutual respect between the genders and contributing to improving the quality of life of individuals' (United Nations 1994: para. 7.36) and (2) 'to ensure that women and men have access to the information, education and services needed to achieve good sexual health and exercise their reproductive rights and responsibilities' (United Nations 1994: para. 7.36b).

This global effort as well as the general crisis of HIV stimulated the development of sexual health national strategies in Australia (Australian Institute of Health and Welfare 2000; England (Department of Health 2001); and the USA (US Surgeon General 2001). In Australia and England, strategies to promote sexual health were clearly tied to HIV prevention and the prevention of teenage pregnancy. In the USA, the Surgeon General took a somewhat broader sexual health approach.

With the passage of time, however, it became evident that the WHO 1975 definition needed to be revisited. The Pan American Health Organization (PAHO) responded by holding a regional consultation in 2000 in Antigua, Guatemala, in collaboration with the World Association for Sexology. For the first time, WAS was consulted to provide expert input, help organise the meeting and invite experts in the field. A regional strategy for sexual health promotion was developed. A new definition of sexual health was crafted (see PAHO 2000) that was crisper and more comprehensive than the original 1975 definition. This reaffirmed the concept of wellbeing and the absence of disease, dysfunction and infirmity. It also recognised that sexual rights were an essential condition for the attainment of sexual health.

WAS's involvement was critical in this respect. In 1999 it had issued a Declaration of Sexual Rights asserting that sexual health was contingent on society's efforts to protect, promote and preserve the sexual rights of every citizen (World Association for Sexology 1999) (see Box 15.1).

Box 15.1 WAS Declaration of Sexual Rights

Sexuality is an integral part of the personality of every human being. Its full development depends upon the satisfaction of basic human needs such as the desire for contact, intimacy, emotional expression, pleasure, tenderness and love.

Sexuality is constructed through the interaction between the individual and social structures. Full development of sexuality is essential for individual, interpersonal and societal well being.

Sexual rights are universal human rights based on the inherent freedom, dignity and equality of all human beings. Since health is a fundamental human right, so must sexual health be a basic human right. In order to assure that human beings and societies develop healthy sexuality, the following sexual rights must be recognised, promoted, respected and defended by all societies through all means. Sexual health is the result of an environment that recognises, respects and exercises these sexual rights.

1   **The right to sexual freedom.** Sexual freedom encompasses the possibility for individuals to express their full sexual potential. However, this excludes all forms of sexual coercion, exploitation and abuse at any time and situations in life.
2   **The right to sexual autonomy, sexual integrity and safety of the sexual body.** This right involves the ability to make autonomous decisions about one's sexual life within a context of one's own personal and social ethics. It also encompasses control and enjoyment of our own bodies free from torture, mutilation and violence of any sort.
3   **The right to sexual privacy.** This involves the right for individual decisions and behaviors about intimacy as long as they do not intrude on the sexual rights of others.
4   **The right to sexual equity.** This refers to freedom from all forms of discrimination regardless of sex, gender, sexual orientation, age, race, social class, religion or physical and emotional disability.
5   **The right to sexual pleasure.** Sexual pleasure, including autoeroticism, is a source of physical, psychological, intellectual and spiritual well being.
6   **The right to emotional sexual expression.** Sexual expression is more than erotic pleasure or sexual acts. Individuals have a right to express their sexuality through communication, touch, emotional expression and love.
7   **The right to sexually associate freely.** This means the possibility to marry or not, to divorce and to establish other types of responsible sexual associations.
8   **The right to make free and responsible reproductive choices.** This encompasses the right to decide whether or not to have children, the number and spacing of children and the right to full access to the means of fertility regulation.
9   **The right to sexual information based upon scientific inquiry.** This right implies that sexual information should be generated through the process of unencumbered and yet scientifically ethical inquiry, and disseminated in appropriate ways at all societal levels.
10 **The right to comprehensive sexuality education.** This is a lifelong process from birth throughout the lifecycle and should involve all social institutions.

11   **The right to sexual healthcare.** Sexual healthcare should be available for prevention and treatment of all sexual concerns, problems and disorders.

Sexual rights are fundamental and universal human rights.

Declaration of the 13th World Congress of Sexology, 1997, Valencia, Spain. Revised and approved
by the General Assembly of the World Association for Sexology (WAS) on 26 August 1999, during
the 14th World Congress of Sexology, Hong Kong, People's Republic of China.

Through pressure by the World Association for Sexology, the PAHO document and
the worldwide demand for a public health response to growing sexual health problems, WHO was challenged to revisit its own 1975 definition. Recognising the public
health imperative to develop strategies to promote sexual health on a global scale,
WHO together with WAS planned an expert consultation in 2002, in Geneva. A
range of experts were called on to grapple with the daunting task of finding
common ground from all the diverse regions, ideologies and values (WHO 2002a).
To everyone's surprise, there was remarkable consensus. A working group was commissioned to finalise a new definition of sexual health (and included new definitions of sex, sexuality and sexual rights (WHO 2002b)) (see Box 15.2).

Box 15.2 Sexual health

Sexual health is a state of physical, emotional, mental and social well-being related to
sexuality; it is not merely the absence of disease, dysfunction or infirmity. Sexual health
requires a positive and respectful approach to sexuality and sexual relationships, as well
as the possibility of having pleasurable and safe sexual experiences, free of coercion,
discrimination and violence. For sexual health to be attained and maintained, the
sexual rights of all persons must be respected, protected and fulfilled.

Working Definition, World Health Organisation, 2002. www.who.int/reproductive-health/topics/
gender-rights/defining-sexual-health.pdf

By way of follow up to the 2002 expert consultation, WHO established a new them-
atic work programme within one of its departments. Although sexual health had
been implicitly understood to be part of the reproductive health agenda, the emergence of HIV-, sexual- and gender-based violence, and the extent of sexual dysfunction (to name but a few of the developments over the past two decades), highlighted
the need to focus more explicitly on sexuality and the promotion of sexual health.
WHO developed a conceptual framework to guide this work, although this document remains as yet unpublished.

From sexology to sexual health: WAS changes its name

Meantime, WAS changed its name to the World Association for Sexual Health
(WAS) (retaining the acronym) in 2005. This change was a significant departure
and illustrates this chapter's theme, the transition from sexology to sexual health.
As WAS articulated its mission, there was a realisation that it was not only through
the promotion of sexology, but also of sexuality education, clinical work and advo-

cacy efforts that the association could be influential. By changing its name, WAS recognised that sexual health had come of age. The World Congress *of* Sexology changed its name as well and became the eighteenth World Congress *for* Sexual Health.

With its newly refined vision and mission, WAS launched an effort to make a declaration for the promotion of sexual health. It saw an opportunity to advance the sexual health agenda with the advent of the UN Millennium Development Goals (MDGs). A series of round tables at the World Congress in Montreal in July of 2005 developed the *Montreal Declaration: Sexual Health for the Millennium*. Ultimately, WAS revised and published Sexual Health for the Millennium: A Declaration and Technical Document (WAS 2008). WAS saw sexual health as central to the attainment of wellness and wellbeing, and the achievement of sustainable development and the implementation of the MDGs. Individuals and communities who experience sexual wellbeing are better positioned to contribute to the eradication of individual and societal poverty. By nurturing individual and social responsibility and equitable social interaction, the promotion of sexual health can and will foster the quality of life and the realisation of peace (WAS 2008).

More recent advances

In 2006 ministers of health from 48 African countries (later affirmed by the African heads of states) declared that the MDGs could not be achieved without more work on sexual and reproductive health and rights. In a historic declaration, they asserted that sexual health – beyond a venereological approach – was needed to combat poverty and promote human development. This included access to good quality sexual and reproductive health services, information and education related to sexuality, the protection of bodily integrity and the guarantee of sexual rights such as choice of sexual and marriage partners, childbearing and, ultimately, the right to pursue a satisfying, safe and pleasurable sexual life (African Union Commission 2006).

Two years later, in 2008, the Swedish International Development Cooperation Agency published a remarkable concept paper entitled *Sexuality: A Missing Dimension in Development* (Sida 2008). Taking up the issue of the MDGs, Sida affirmed the centrality and importance of promoting sexual health and rights in attaining these goals. The concept paper acknowledged that much work hitherto had focused on the problematic and negative aspects of sexuality and/or gender equality. The concept paper endorsed many of the sexual health principles outlined in the Maputo Plan of Action alongside a rights-based approach to sexual health. Sida committed itself to take a leading role internationally in the area of sexuality, and to supporting empowering approaches to sexuality in general and sexuality education in particular.

In the same year the International Planned Parenthood Federation (IPPF) published a declaration affirming sexual rights as a component of basic human rights (IPPF 2008). This was a significant development for this organisation. Putting the 's' into sexual and reproductive rights had hitherto been difficult for many organisations working in the field of reproductive health. The IPPF Declaration recognised that many expressions of sexuality are non-reproductive and that sexual rights cannot be subsumed under reproductive rights and reproductive health.

Yet another recent historic achievement was the recent declaration 'preventing through education' drafted and signed by ministers of health and education from Latin American and the Caribbean on the eve of the World AIDS Conference in Mexico City, 1 August 2008 (Ministers of Health and Education in Latin American and the Caribbean 2008). This declaration affirmed sexual rights as a basic human right, and the critical importance of comprehensive sexuality education as a strategic means of stemming the HIV pandemic. It was significant that this was a joint declaration made by ministers of health and education. While the discourse of sexual health had dominated the health sector, the issue of sexuality education is more current in education. There was recognition of the need for cooperative intersectoral strategies. Never before had regional policymakers embraced the concept of sexual health so completely.

Conclusion

From a slow beginning, there has been steady progress towards the development of a strategic and comprehensive approach to the promotion of sexual health. What began with the pioneering work of sexologists in the early part of the twentieth century, and a WHO technical document in 1975 has led to an increasing number of commitments, declarations, technical documents and concept papers. The term 'sexual health' is now widely used at a global level and is likely to have far reaching effects. Critically, something fundamental has shifted, and a new era has begun. Sexual health is now part of public policy discourse and is recognised as a key strategy to promoting health and wellbeing.

References

African Union Commission (2006) *Plan of Action on Sexual and Reproductive Health and Rights (Maputo Plan of Action)*, Addis Adaba: African Union Commission.

ANCARD Working Party on Indigenous Australians' Sexual Health (1997) *The National Indigenous Australians' Sexual Health Strategy 1996–97 to 1998–99: A Report of the ANCARD Working Party on Indigenous Australians' Sexual Health*, Canberra: Commonwealth Department of Health and Family Services.

Australian Institute of Health and Welfare (2000) *Australia's Health 2000: The 7th Biennial Report of the Australian Institute of Health and Welfare*, Canberra: AIHW; available at www.aihw. gov.au/publications/aus/ah00/ah00-c00a.pdf (accessed 23 May 2009).

Bell, A. and Weinberg, M. (1978) *Homosexualities: A Study of Diversity among Men and Women*, New York: Simon & Schuster.

Bloch, I. (1928) *The Sexual Life of Our Time in its Relations to Modern Civilisation* (trans. M. Eden Paul), London: Heinemann.

Bullough, V. (1978) *Sexual Variance in Society and History*, Chicago: University of Chicago.

Bullough, V. (1994) *Science in the Bedroom: A History of Sex Research*, New York: Basic Books.

Coleman, E. (1997) 'Promoting Sexual Health: The Challenges of the Present and Future', in Borras-Valls, J. J. and Perez-Conchillo, M. (eds) *Sexuality and Human Rights: Proceedings of the XIIIth World Congress of Sexology*, Valencia: Scientific Committee, Instituto de Sexologia y Psicoterapia Espill.

Coleman, E. (2000) 'Revolutionary Changes in Sexuality in the New Millennium: Sexual Health, Diversity and Sexual Rights', in Ng, E. M., Borras-Valls, J. J., Perez-Conchillo, M. and Coleman, E. (eds) *Sexuality in the New Millennium*, Bologna: Editrice Compositori.

Coleman, E. (2002) 'Promoting Sexual Health and Responsible Sexual Behavior: An Introduction', *Journal of Sex Research*, 39 (1): 3–6.

Coleman, E. (2007) 'Sexual Health: Definitions and Construct Development', in Tepper, M. and Owens, A. F. (eds) *Sexual Health, Volume 1: Psychological Foundations*, Westport, CT: Praeger.

Department of Health (2001) *National Strategy for Sexual Health and HIV*, London: Department of Health; available at www.dh.gov.uk/assetRoot/04/06/55/43/04065543.pdf (accessed 23 May 2009).

Ellis, A. (1951) *The Folklore of Sex*, New York: Doubleday.

Ellis, A. (1954) *The American Sexual Tragedy*, New York: Twayne.

Ellis, A. (1958) *Sex without Guilt*, New York: Lyle Stuart.

Gagnon, J. and Simon, W. (1973) *Sexual Conduct: The Social Sources of Human Sexuality*, Chicago: Aldine.

Haeberle, E. (1983) 'The Birth of Sexology: A Brief History in Documents', paper presented at the Sixth World Congress of Sexology, 22–27 May 1983, Washington, DC.

Haeberle, E. (n.d.) *History of Sexology*; Available at www2.hu-berlin.de/sexology/Entrance_Page/History_of_Sexology/ history_of_sexology.html (accessed 23 May 2009).

Inglehart, R. (1997) *Modernization and Postmodernization: Cultural, Economic, and Political change in 43 Societies*, Princeton: Princeton University Press.

International Planned Parenthood Association (2008) *Sexual Rights: An IPPF Declaration*, London: International Planned Parenthood Association.

Kinsey, A. C., Pomeroy, W. B. and Martin, C. E. (1948) *Sexual Behavior in the Human Male*, Philadelphia: W. B. Saunders.

Kinsey, A., Pomeroy, W., Martin, C. and Gephard, P. (1953) *Sexual Behavior in the Human Female*, Philadelphia: W. B. Saunders.

Kinsey Institute (n.d.) *History of the Institute*, Bloomington: Indiana University Press: available at www.kinseyinstitute.org/about/history.html (accessed 22 March 2009).

Krafft-Ebing, R. V. (1908) *Psychopathia Sexualis with Especial Reference to Contrary Sexual Instinct: A Medical Legal Study*, 7th edn (trans. C. G. Chaddock), Philadelphia: F. A. Davis.

Langfeldt, T. and Porter, M. (1986) *Sexuality and Family Planning: Report of A Consultation and Research Findings*, Copenhagen: World Health Organisation, Regional Office for Europe.

Mace, D. R., Bannerman, R. H. O. and Burton, J. (1974) *The Teaching of Human Sexuality in Schools for Health Professionals* Geneva: World Health Organisation (Public Health Paper No. 57).

Masters, W. H. and Johnson, V. E. (1966) *Human Sexual Response*, Boston: Little Brown.

Masters, W. H. and Johnson, V. E. (1970) *Human Sexual Inadequacy*, Boston: Little Brown.

Ministers of Health and Education in Latin America and the Caribbean (2008) 'Ministerial Declaration: 1st Meeting of Ministers of Health and Education to Stop HIV and STIs in Latin America and the Caribbean to Stop HIV and STIs: Preventing Through Education'; available at http://data.unaids.org/pub/BaseDocument/2008/20080801_minsterdeclaration_en pdf (accessed 23 May 2009).

Pan American Health Organization, Regional Office of the World Health Organisation (2000) *Promotion of Sexual Health: Recommendations for Action*, Washington, DC: PAHO; available at www.paho.org/English/HCP/HCA/PromotionSexualHealth.pdf (accessed 23 January 2009).

Reiss, I. L. (1990) *An End to Shame: Shaping Our Next Sexual Revolution*, Amherst, NY: Prometheus Books.

Reiss, I. L. (2001) 'Sexual Attitudes and Behavior', in Smelser, N. J. and Baltes, P. B. (eds) *International Encyclopedia of the Social and Behavioral Science*, New York: Elsevier.

Reiss, I. L. and Ellis, A. (2002) *At the Dawn of the Sexual Revolution: Reflections on a Dialogue*, Walnut Creek, CA: AltaMira Press.

Reiss, I. L. and Reiss, H. M. (1997) *Solving America's Sexual Crises*, Amherst, NY: Prometheus Books.

Saracci, R. (1997) 'The World Health Organization Needs to Reconsider its Definition of Health', *British Medical Journal*, 314 (7091): 1409–10.

Schmidt, G. (1987) 'Sexual Health within a Societal Context', in *Concepts of Sexual Health: Report of a Working Group*, Copenhagen: WHO Regional Office for Europe.

Sida (2008) *Sexuality: A Missing Dimension in Development*, Stockholm: Edita Communication AB; available at www.sida.se/sida/jsp/sida.jsp?d=118&a=40003&language=en_US&searchWords=sexuality%20a%20missing (accessed 23 May 2009).

United Nations (1994) *International Conference on Population and Development Programme of Action: Report of the International Conference on Population and Development*, Cairo; available at www.iisd.ca/cairo.html (accessed 23 May 2009).

US Surgeon General (2001) *The Surgeon General's Call to Action to Promote Sexual Health and Responsible Sexual Behavior*, Rockville, MD: Office of the Surgeon General; available at www.surgeongeneral.gov/library/sexualhealth (accessed 23 May 2009).

World Association for Sexual Health (1999) *Declaration of Sexual Rights*; available at www.worldsexology.org/about_sexualrights.asp (accessed 23 May 2009).

World Association for Sexual Health (2008) *Sexual Health for the Millennium Declaration*; available at www.worldsexology.org/doc/SEXUAL_HEALTH_FOR_THE_MILLENNIUM.pdf (accessed 23 May 2009).

World Health Organisation (1975) *Education and Treatment in Human Sexuality: The Training of Health Professionals* (Technical Report Series Nr. 572); available at www2.hu-berlin.de/sexology/ GESUND/ARCHIV/WHOR.HTM (accessed 23 January 2009).

World Health Organisation (2002a) 'Challenges in Sexual and Reproductive Health: Technical Consultation on Sexual Health', 28–31 January 2002; available at www.who.int/reproductive-health/publications/sexualhealth/defining_sh.pdf (accessed 23 May 2009).

World Health Organisation (2002b) *Sexual Health: Working Definitions*; available at www.who.int/reproductive-health/gender/sexual_health.html (accessed 23 May 2009).

World Health Organisation Regional Office for Europe (1987) *Concepts of Sexual Health: Report of a Working Group*; available at http://whqlibdoc.who.int/euro/-1993/EUR_ICP_MCH_521.pdf (accessed 23 January 2009).

16 Sexual and reproductive

Connections and disconnections in public health

Jane Cottingham

At one point during government negotiations on the Programme of Action of the International Conference on Population and Development (ICPD) in Cairo, 1994, someone suggested that the term 'sexual health' should be included in the definition of reproductive health. There was a flurry of activity. Representatives of the World Health Organisation (WHO) were asked whether an official definition of sexual health existed and urgent messages were sent back to Geneva for people to comb the archives. They identified one technical report on human sexuality, published in 1975, which provided the following definition:

> Sexual health is the integration of the somatic, emotional, intellectual, and social aspects of sexual being, in ways that are positively enriching and that enhance personality, communication, and love ... The notion of sexual health implies a positive approach to human sexuality, and the purpose of sexual healthcare should be the enhancement of life and personal relationships and not merely counselling and care related to procreation or sexuality transmitted diseases.
>
> (WHO 1975: Section 2.1)

It was the second part of this definition that was slightly amended for inclusion in the eventual ICPD Programme (United Nations 1994). Considering the importance now being attached to sexuality and sexual health, it is striking that, apparently, no further elaboration of the definition of sexual health took place in the 20-year period between the publication of the Technical Report and the ICPD Programme. And despite the fact that the ICPD Programme included sexual health in reproductive health, by far the lion's share of attention in policies and programmes following ICPD – at least in the developing world – continued to be given to the aspects of reproductive health that had been historically accepted: maternal and child health and family planning. At the level of international development assistance, sexual health as just defined has not been a target of support per se.

Why was this? There are several lines of argument that I will explore here. The first relates to the international political environment that influenced the entire casting of the ICPD Programme of Action. Growing concerns during the 1960s about the population explosion described in best-selling publications such as Paul Ehrlich's *The Population Bomb* (1968) and the Club of Rome's *Limits to Growth* (Meadows *et al.* 1972), led to an unprecedented investment during the end of the 1960s and the 1970s in population control through support to family planning programmes (Dixon-Mueller 1987). It was assumed that the substantial distribution of contraceptives to women in developing countries would inevitably have an impact on population growth. Large campaigns were often undertaken to sterilise women in some Latin American countries and both men and women in India, or to bring implantable contraceptives to women in Indonesia through 'safaris' in which buses were driven out to the rural areas and women rounded up for the insertions (Isis 1984). That these campaigns were often coercive started to be documented by the emerging international women's health movement (Hartmann 1987; Garcia-Moreno and Claro 1994), which led to a serious questioning of the impact of 'international development' on women's health and rights. Women's health advocates argued that women needed ways of regulating their fertility, yes, but this would only become acceptable when they knew they could go through pregnancy and child-birth safely, and have their children survive. Women's health and lives could not be reduced to stopping pregnancy occurring.

At about the same time, the first global estimates of maternal mortality appeared (AbouZahr and Royston 1991) showing that more than 500,000 women died each year in pregnancy. This hitherto unnamed scandal – women dying, not from a disease but in the act of producing life – was placed high on the international agenda of both the women's movement and the international development community. Thus, the ICPD Programme was seen as an essential platform for creating a major paradigm shift: from population control to reproductive health. The latter was formulated to be 'a state of complete physical, mental and social well-being and not merely the absence of disease or infirmity, in all matters relating to the reproductive system and to its functions and processes' (United Nations 1994: paragraph 7.2). The definition goes on to state that reproductive health:

> [T]herefore implies that people are able to have a satisfying and safe sex life and that they have the capability to reproduce and the freedom to decide if, when and how often to do so. Implicit in this last condition are the right of men and women to be informed and to have access to safe, effective, affordable and acceptable methods of family planning of their choice as well as other methods of their choice for regulation of fertility which are not against the law, and the right of access to appropriate healthcare services that will enable women to go safely through pregnancy and childbirth and provide couples with the best chance of having a healthy infant.
>
> (United Nations 1994: paragraph 7.2)

The following paragraph speaks of reproductive rights, also defined for the first time. It cannot be emphasised enough how essential this shift was for the health and rights of women as it provided for the first time an international mandate to focus on, and invest in, women's health far beyond their need for contraception and away from seeing them as agents of demographic change. It gave legitimacy to the Safe Mother-hood Initiative, launched in 1987, and a basis for action related to the overall improvement of primary healthcare, much of which provided reproductive health-related care. In the light of all this, it was almost inevitable that reproductive elements would take precedence over the 'satisfying and safe sex life' part of the definition, something which was much more complex. For the time being, pursuing the health and rights dimensions of reproduction to their full extent would take precedence.

The second line of argument relates to enormous prejudices and taboos related to talking about sexuality in nearly all cultures. Historically, public health has shied away from dealing with sexuality, leaving it rather to the domain of private, clinical medicine where only the problematic aspects of sexuality are of interest. Thus, sexual problems have been broadly labelled 'sexual dysfunctions', with an ever growing array of medication and other treatment, usually dispensed through the private sector. There is almost the implication here that problems related to sexuality are not legitimate health problems and should therefore only be dealt with, and paid for, in private as a luxury.

In the mid-1990s, however, when governments were struggling to understand what ICPD meant for their national policies and programmes, and when the HIV pandemic was beginning to make its horror felt to some extent, sexual behaviour became a legitimate topic of inquiry for public health. Yet reviews show that, far from focusing on the 'safe and satisfying' dimensions of sexuality, research into sexual behaviour was mainly conducted with a view to understanding (a) how coital frequency within marriage influences contraceptive use and vice versa; (b) how adolescent sexual activity and (lack of) contraceptive use are related to the risks of out-of-wedlock pregnancy and childbearing; and (c) how 'high-risk' sexual behaviours are related to the spread of sexually transmitted infections including HIV (Dixon-Mueller 1993). In other words, research into sexuality (and sexual health) was only useful insofar as it contributed to an increase in contraceptive use and a decrease in unintended pregnancies and sexually transmitted infections.

During this same period, there were almost no studies to examine the impact of contraception on sexual health, for instance, despite the fact that demographic surveys indicated that one of the main reasons women discontinued methods was for health concerns (Jain and Bruce 1989). In this sense, the population control imperative continued to have an impact, and the taboos could conveniently be left unexamined.

A third consideration – although not a legitimate argument for leaving out sexuality and sexual health from programmes and policies following ICPD – is that of measurement difficulties. In 1997, the first list of reproductive health indicators was developed by WHO and partner agencies (WHO 1997) using a certain number of criteria including scientific robustness, validity and reliability. They included elements for which health systems or national surveys were already gathering data, such as contraceptive prevalence, births attended by skilled health personnel, prevalence of low birth weight, maternal mortality ratio, perinatal mortality rate, availability of comprehensive obstetric care, etc. Of the 15 indicators, not one can be said to deal directly with sexual health and sexuality with the possible exception of reported prevalence in women of female genital mutilation. Others, such as the prevalence of infertility in women or the prevalence of urethritis in men, could be seen to be related to sexual *ill* health, but could certainly not be used to measure the 'satisfying and safe sex life' mentioned in the definition of reproductive health.

Four years later when the list was revised, the two indicators added in order to capture dimensions related to HIV – prevalence of HIV in pregnant women and knowledge of HIV-related prevention practices – did no better in reflecting dimensions related to sexuality and sexual health. On the other hand, it must be said that the concept of sexual health was vague and potentially all encompassing – 'the enhancement of life and personal relationships' – presenting an almost impossible challenge for measuring progress. It is only in the last two years that, at the international level, an attempt has been made to elaborate indicators for measuring sexual health (WHO forthcoming), through a process that is described further later.

In the larger international arena, then, the truly reproductive elements of reproductive health were given priority for at least a decade after ICPD. Yet, on a parallel but much lower key track, there was a movement to focus on sexual health within public health, at least in Europe. In 1987 the WHO Regional Office for Europe (EURO) convened a working group of 20 people to examine 'concepts of sexual health'. The purpose was to clarify the concepts of sexual health by considering a range of population groups, to identify factors contributing to sexual ill health and means of promoting sexual health and to suggest indicators that could be used to evaluate the effectiveness of programmes and policies and measure any general movement towards sexual health.

The report notes that sexuality had been recognised as an important aspect of health and that the European regional family planning programme had included it since 1984. Interestingly, the report notes that due to the range of individual, cultural, religious and social differences and the various patterns of lifestyles, social and gender roles, there could be no single definition of a sexually healthy individual. A definition, it goes on, would be normative, and restrictive and it would also not be feasible. The importance of laws and policies to underpin individuals' rights related to sexuality is highlighted:

> Some positive concept of individual needs, responsibilities and rights in the area of sexuality needs to be established in order that laws that repress human rights can be changed (such as those against homosexuality or abortion) and that policies may be implemented to reduce restrictions on sexual expression and enable services to be established to deal with sexual problems.
>
> (WHO Regional Office for Europe 1987: 8)

On the question of indicators, however, the report concludes that objective measures of sexual health are impossible (perhaps not surprisingly if no definition can be established), although measures of self-perception of sexual health may be valid. It posits that the only indicators possible must be related to the provision of information and reduction of discrimination, such as the existence of laws, regulations and government policies and government funding to promote public information about sexuality, the existence of educational programmes in schools that reflect the individuality and variability of human sexuality, and the existence of training programmes for educational, social and health professionals that also reflect this. Indeed, the greatest emphasis was given to the training of health professionals, particularly those dispensing family planning services, as they were considered likely to be one of the first sources of help for people with sexual problems.

The report is clear and concise, concluding with very specific recommendations relating to preventive as well as therapeutic services, the inclusion of sexuality in professional training courses and the need for community and policy action as well as research to shore up these efforts. Over 20 years later, the report remains utterly pertinent. Yet it appears that little action was taken as a result of this meeting, almost certainly as a result of it being a 'working group' report as opposed to a policy document brought to member states for their approval.

More than a decade later, in 2000, the Pan American Health Organization (PAHO, which also serves as the WHO Regional Office for the Americas) and the World Association for Sexology (WAS), convened a regional consultation to examine how to promote sexual health including the role of the health sector in the achievement and maintenance of sexual health. While the basic reflections around sexual health are very similar to those in the EURO document, the report emanating from the PAHO/WAS consultation is elaborated from an advocacy and policy standpoint, fuelled, among other things, by the HIV pandemic, which had barely been named at the time of the EURO meeting.

The recommendations here are more detailed and are presented in the form of goals, strategies and actions to promote sexual health. They include proposals to integrate sexual health into public health programmes, promote responsible sexual behaviour, provide comprehensive sexuality education to the population at large, provide education, training and support to professionals working in sexual health-related fields, provide access to comprehensive sexual healthcare services to the population and promote and sponsor research on sexuality and sexual health. This report can probably boast being the first international (albeit regional) policy document focusing exclusively on sexual health. It is being used widely throughout the region to promote sexual health.

Two more recent events have contributed towards greater articulation of the 'sexual' part of 'reproductive health'. First was an international consultation on sexual health organised in 2002 by WHO at the international level, in conjunction with WAS (WHO 2006). Its purpose was to discuss concepts and definitions, examine barriers to the promotion of sexual health and propose effective and appropriate strategies for such promotion. Unlike the EURO group in 1987, this consultation took up the challenge of defining sexual health and, in line with the PAHO 2000 report, described three other interrelated terms: sex, sexuality and sexual rights. These were deemed essential to the understanding of sexual health.

It is significant that, even in the Technical Report of 1975, the recognition of rights is seen as essential: 'Fundamental to this concept are the right to sexual information and the right to pleasure' (WHO 1975: Section 2.1). The 1987 EURO document also affirmed 'the rights and needs of individuals to be free from sexual exploitation and oppression by others' (WHO 1987: 19). The PAHO report states that 'since protection of health is a basic human right, it follows that sexual health involves sexual rights' (PAHO 2000: 10). The WHO report of the 2002 meeting anchors the definition of sexual rights in human rights documents, including UN human rights treaties such as the Convention on the Elimination of All Forms of Discrimination against Women and international consensus documents such as the Beijing Platform for Action of the Fourth World Conference on Women (United Nations 1995). The latter speaks, inter alia, of women's human rights as including their right to have control over, and decide freely and responsibly on matters related to their sexuality, including sexual and reproductive health, free of coercion, discrimination and violence.

The working definition of sexual health from the 2002 meeting makes clear that 'for sexual health to be attained and maintained, the sexual rights of all persons must be protected, respected and fulfilled' (WHO 2006: 5) Rape, FGM and persecution on the basis of sexual orientation or sexual practices not only lead to sexual ill health, but are also violations of the right to bodily integrity and to non-discrimination. Thus rights and health are taken to be inextricably linked, in the same way as reproductive rights were defined in the ICPD Programme, even though sexual rights per se were not (see also the chapter in this volume by Carmen Barroso). It was striking that both the PAHO and the WHO meeting reports gave specific focus to different sexualities, thus moving well beyond sexuality as some kind of subset of reproduction.

The second event was the adoption by the World Health Assembly in May 2004 of the WHO Global Reproductive Health Strategy. Despite its title, which was deliberately crafted to be aligned with the ICPD Programme of Action, the Strategy uses the term '*sexual and* reproductive health' throughout the main text. More significantly, it describes five core aspects of sexual and reproductive health, the fifth of which is *promoting sexual health* (WHO 2004). This represents a major move forward not only because it articulates much more clearly than the ICPD Programme the importance of sexual health along with all the other aspects – maternal and newborn health, family planning, eliminating unsafe abortion and combating sexually transmitted infections – but it has also necessitated the development of clear indicators for its measurement. These include indicators intended to capture, for instance, to what extent young people's first sexual experience is protected, consensual and without regret, as well as the more classic prevalence of female genital mutilation (WHO 2007, forthcoming).

Health sector indicators include the availability of service delivery standards and protocols in promoting sexual health, the proportion of the population who has ever received counselling on sexual health/sexuality and the availability of psychosexual services. Because the Strategy's key actions include creating supportive legislative and regulatory frameworks, indicators for sexual health also include a series of legal/policy indicators such as whether there is a law prohibiting discrimination including that based on sexual orientation, whether there is a law prohibiting sexual violence (including marital rape) and whether comprehensive sexuality education is mandatory. Information on these indicators may not necessarily be easy to collect, but their very existence in official WHO documents designed for use at national level will mean that serious monitoring of sexual health can begin, at least in some countries.

What conclusions can be drawn from these connections and disconnections between sexual health and reproductive health, sexuality and reproduction? The first is that the political environment plays a critical role in which issues are taken up and which are left aside. At ICPD, the women's health advocacy movement had considerable lobbying power, and at the time their main concern was to ensure that the concepts of reproductive health and gender equality were accepted. As with all strategies, choices usually have to be made, and the importance of the reproductive part meant that it had to take precedence over the sexual health part. One year later, at the Fourth World Conference on Women in Beijing, there was a powerful attempt to include 'sexual rights' in the Platform, but the opposition was too strong and despite the additional reference to women's human rights including their right to decide in matters relating to their sexuality, the ICPD language relating to reproductive health remained the dominant mandate, at least in the international health community.

The second conclusion also relates to strategy. Technical meetings such as the one in 1975 resulting in the WHO Technical Report and that in 1987 in EURO are all well and good. They bring important data and analysis to the table. They can raise and examine issues not previously dealt with. But recommendations from such meetings are likely to remain on desks or in cupboards if they are not backed up or complemented by a process to elaborate and implement policy. At the international level in public health, it is clear that the World Health Assembly carries great weight. The adoption of the Reproductive Health Strategy was done through a resolution which calls for a report on progress every two years. This means that all of the 'core aspects' – including promoting sexual health – can be highlighted and debated at high ministerial level on a regular basis. This is an essential piece in the continuing fight for recognition of sexuality and sexual health issues at national level.

At the same time, such initiatives within the United Nations mechanisms are unlikely to be successful unless accompanied by other initiatives at different levels, particularly by civil society. Throughout the period reviewed here, there has been a growing movement in civil society to have sexual health, sexuality and sexual rights named and recognised both nationally and internationally. It is almost certain that the HIV pandemic stimulated the huge activism for such recognition, and that the PAHO and WHO meetings were able to take place because of this. It is noteworthy, too, that the mid-2000s saw the development and publication of two international, NGO documents: the Yogyakarta Principles (2007) signed by over 20 key activists in the field of human rights, and the IPPF Sexual Rights Charter (2008) now being used across the Federation's members which cover the globe.

Finally, for policies to be taken up and implemented there must be measures of progress and accountability. It is a frequently cited truism that if things are not counted they will not be addressed. The development and use of indicators in the domains of sexuality and sexual health is absolutely critical to keeping sexuality, health and rights on the public health agenda for the foreseeable future.

References

AbouZahr, C. and Royston, E. (1991) *Maternal Mortality: A Global Factbook*, Geneva: WHO; abstract available at: www.popline.org/docs/1031/074640.html (accessed 24 January 2009).

Dixon-Mueller, R. (1987) 'U.S. International Population Policy and "the Woman Question"', *New York University Journal of International Law and Politics*, 20 (1): 143–67.

Dixon-Mueller, R. (1993) 'The Sexuality Connection in Reproductive Health', *Studies in Family Planning*, 24 (3): 269–82.

Ehrlich, P. (1968) *The Population Bomb*, New York: Ballatine Books.

Garcia-Moreno, C. and Claro, A. (1994) 'Challenges from the Women's Health Movement: Women's Rights versus Population Control', in Sen, G., Germain, A. and Chen, L. C. (eds) *Population Policies Reconsidered: Health, Empowerment and Rights*, Boston, MA: Harvard University Press.

Hartmann, B. (1987) *Reproductive Rights and Wrongs: The Global Politics of Population Control and Contraceptive Choice*, New York: Harper & Row.

IPPF (2008) 'Sexual Rights: An IPPF Declaration'; available at: www.apf.pt/cms/files/conteudos/file/SexualRightsIPPFdeclaration.pdf?PHPSESSID=5ca72b06632f81193b7049afa4f4eeaf (accessed 30 January 2009).

Isis (1984) *Women and Development: A Guide for Organization and Action*, Geneva: Isis Women's International and Information Service.

Jain, A. and Bruce, J. (1989) 'Quality: The Key to Success', *People*, 16 (4): 6–8.

Meadows, D. H. *et al.* (1972) *The Limits to Growth: A Report for the Club of Rome's Project on the Predicament of Mankind*, New York: Universe Books.

PAHO (2000) 'Promotion of Sexual Health: Recommendations for Action', Proceedings of a

Regional Consultation convened by the Pan American Health Organization and the World Health Organisation in Collaboration with the World Association for Sexology, Guatemala: PAHO; available at www.paho.org/english/hcp/hca/promotionsexualhealth.pdf (accessed 20 February 2009).

United Nations (1994) *Programme of Action of the International Conference on Population and Development*, New York: United Nations; available at www.un.org/popin/icpd/conference/offeng/poa.html (accessed 24 January 2009).

United Nations (1995) *Platform for Action of the Fourth World Conference on Women, Beijing, 1995*, New York: United Nations; available at www.un.org/womenwatch/daw/beijing/platform/index.html (accessed 25 January 2009).

WHO (1975) *Education and Treatment in Human Sexuality: The Training of Health Professionals*, Geneva: World Health Organisation (WHO Technical Report Series No. 572); available at: www2.hu-berlin.de/sexology/GESUND/ARCHIV/WHOR.HTM#N3 (accessed 24 January 2009).

WHO (1997) *Reproductive Health Indicators for Global Monitoring*, Report of an Interagency Technical Consultation, First Meeting, April 1997, Geneva: World Health Organisation; available at www.who.int/reproductive-health/publications/HRP_97_27/index.html (accessed 24 January 2009).

WHO (2001) *Reproductive Health Indicators for Global Monitoring*, Report of an Interagency Technical Consultation, Second Meeting, July 2000, Geneva: World Health Organisation; available at www.who.int/reproductive-health/publications/rhr_01_19/index.htm (accessed 24 January 2009).

WHO (2004) *Reproductive Health: A Global Strategy*, Geneva: World Health Organisation; available at www.who.int/reproductive-health/publications/strategy.pdf (accessed 24 January 2009).

WHO (2006) *Defining Sexual Health*, Report of a Meeting, January 2002. Geneva: World Health Organisation; available at www.who.int/reproductive-health/publications/sexual-health/index.html (accessed 24 January 2009).

WHO (2007) *National Level Monitoring of the Achievement of Universal Access to Reproductive Health. Conceptual and Practical Considerations and Related Indicators*, Geneva: World Health Organisation; available at www.who.int/reproductive-health/publications/universalaccess/index.html (accessed 24 January 2009).

WHO (forthcoming) *Measuring Sexual Health: Conceptual Considerations and Related Indicators*, Geneva: World Health Organisation.

WHO Regional Office for Europe (1987) *Concepts of Sexual Health*, Report of a Meeting in Copenhagen, May 1987, Copenhagen: World Health Organisation.

Yogyakarta Principles (2007) available at www.yogyakartaprinciples.org (accessed 30 January 2009).

17 Sex as 'risk of conception'?

Sexual frames within the family planning field

Jenny A. Higgins

Although family planning methods are expressly designed for use during sex, we know stunningly little about how contraceptive use affects sexual experiences and processes. As individuals, we tend to think of sex's potential for pleasure, for forming relationships and for building individual identities. However, as Kirsten Moore and Judith Helzner have argued, professional roles as family planning researchers and practitioners may demand that we instead tend to focus on the 'risk' and 'threat' of unwanted pregnancy, disease or sexual violence (Moore and Helzner 1996). Rather than presenting sex as a potentially enjoyable, affirming or generative experience, family planning discourse portrays sex at best as the sanitised 'exposure to the risk of conception'[1] or, at worst, the cause of unfortunate outcomes such as violence, STIs or unintended pregnancy (Dixon-Mueller 1993b). This tendency to de-emphasise sexual pleasure, desire and enjoyment is especially strong when it comes to women, toward whom family planning efforts are disproportionately directed.

In this chapter, I will further illustrate the sexually sanitised framework used within contemporary family planning research and programming, providing examples and suggesting some of the limitations and double standards of this framework. I also overview some of the well-intentioned causes of this 'pleasure deficit' (Higgins and Hirsch 2007). Perhaps surprisingly, roots reach back to the early feminist birth control movement and extend through far more recent international women's rights advocacy. In concluding, I suggest some possible reframings of sexuality within the field, drawing on some encouraging new research to light our way.

Sexual frames within current family planning discourse

Before providing some examples of the field's de-eroticised approach to sexuality, I want to define what I mean by 'family planning'. For the purposes of this chapter, my own definition closely resembles the one first advocated by Margaret Sanger and her pro-birth control compatriots in the early twentieth century – that is, the practice in which couples together, and sometimes women or men singly, have (or *prevent* having) the precise number of children they want, and when. Avoiding unplanned pregnancies is achieved in large part through the use of a vast array of available contraceptive methods, from hormone-based methods such as the pill or the patch, to barrier methods such as male and female condoms, to sterilisation, to periodic abstinence or lactational amenorrhea (the temporary infertility that can occur when a woman breastfeeds). Indeed, family planning is often used in the public lexicon as synonym for 'contraception', even though the phenomenon has far more expansive meanings.[2]

A final note on my definition of the field concerns the so-called 'targets' of family planning programmes – the people to whom contraceptive development and programming have been almost entirely directed. Of course, both women and men are involved in creating and preventing pregnancies. However, despite some long-stalled efforts on methods for men, contraceptives are overwhelmingly made for women's bodies, and pregnancy prevention has long been seen as women's domain (Watkins 1993). For the most part, the field portrays men as either uninterested in or incapable of participating in family planning in the same way as women. In many ways, this approach both reflects and perpetuates larger socially held beliefs about gender, sexuality and responsibility. For example, men's stronger and allegedly unchangeable sex drives undermine contraceptive efforts, whereas women's supposed greater sexual responsibility and relative lesser interest in sexual pleasure translate into contraceptive accountability.

On that note, I want to turn to examples of how the field's current framing of sexuality fails to acknowledge how contraceptive use is influenced by women's seeking of sexual enjoyment. Take, for example, the behavioural models used to explain women's contraceptive practices. Given that one of the field's central goals is to avert unwanted pregnancies, family planning practitioners are intent on understanding what helps explain contraceptive use (or non-use), method preference and continuation. The field's current behavioural models of contraceptive practices suggest that a woman's choice and consistent use of a particular method are related primarily to access, effectiveness, ease of use and the woman's desire to limit births. Models rarely consider how methods either enhance or detract from the sexual experience, even though methods are designed specifically for use during sex.

A lack of sex positivity also exists in the behavioural models used to explain unintended pregnancy.[3] The prevalence, health consequences and political salience of unintended pregnancy have made it a source of significant policy concern for several decades. Worldwide, an estimated 80 million of the 210 million pregnancies each year (approximately 40 per cent) are unplanned (WHO 2004), and the average woman will have at least one abortion in her lifetime (AGI 1999). In the USA, nearly half (48 per cent) of all pregnancies are unintended, giving the country one of the highest unintended pregnancy rates in the industrialised world (Finer and Henshaw 2006; Henshaw 1998). Most unintended pregnancies are caused by lack of contraceptive use, not by contraceptive failure (Henshaw 1998; Trussell *et al.* 1999). Current explanations for non-use generally pertain either to women's knowledge of or access to contraceptive services (or lack thereof), or gender-based power imbalances in sexual relationships, which can render women unwilling or unable to negotiate for contraceptive use with their male partners (Brown *et al.* 1995). Few family planning researchers have examined whether unprotected sex or pregnancy ambivalence may heighten sexual experience, or whether the romantic notion of creating a child with someone may deter contraceptive use. We know little about the emotional, physical and cognitive states that contribute to situations in which lack of contraceptive use is pleasurable or purposeful to women and men.

This dearth of sexuality in explaining unintended pregnancy is more striking when we compare it to research on men in parallel areas of public health. For example, the HIV/AIDS literature has examined ways in which sexual pleasure-seeking may sometimes motivate HIV risk taking among men who have sex with men (Dowsett 1996: Parker 1999; Parker *et al.* 2000). Deliberately unprotected anal sex, or barebacking, may be eroticised among certain men who have sex with men, even those who may be well aware of the attendant risk of HIV (Díaz 1999; Carballo-Dieguez and Bauermeister 2004; Shernoff 2005; Junge 2002). In some circumstances, riskier sex may be hotter or closer than protected sex; some men may also desire to share a disease with a loved one in order to facilitate closeness or connection. An unintended pregnancy is likely to carry even more potential for closeness, affirmation and connection. Yet we know next to nothing about how desire for a pregnancy or conception, even when a child is not wholly intended or wanted, shapes contraceptive practices.

Neither have individual contraceptive methods been studied or explored extensively for their effects on sexual experience, or how such sexual effects shape the ways in which people use these methods.[4] Hormone-based contraceptives (which include the pill, the patch, the ring, injectables), which are the most widely used reversible methods in many parts of the world, have not been systematically assessed for how they affect women's sexual pleasure, lubrication or ability to achieve orgasm.[5] Contraceptive researchers have thoroughly documented hormonal methods' effect on ovulation. Far fewer have demonstrated their effects on the peak in sexual interest that many women experience during ovulation (Anderson-Hunt *et al.* 1996; Dennerstein 1996).

In attention to the sexual aspects of hormonal methods for women is even more striking with juxtaposed to the attention afforded to sexuality within the arena of hormone-based methods under development for men. Research on male-based methods is strongly marked by concern for their effects on libido, sex drive and sexual functioning (Solomon *et al.* 2007; WHO 1982; Oudshoorn 2003). Contraceptive developers implicitly recognise that men's uptake of these new methods will be limited if their ability to experience pleasure is compromised.

Women's potential sexual resistance to male condoms has also been relatively unexplored. Family planning programmes, as well as HIV/AIDS and public health programmes more generally, often rely on women to ensure that male condoms are used, even though women do not wear male condoms. Research indicates that women may lack the power to press for condoms (Amaro 1995; Amaro *et al.* 2001; Worth 1989; Blanc 2001; Exner *et al.* 2003), and that even when women are able to negotiate for condom use, they may be disinclined to do so out of desire for sex that seems loving, trusting and intimate (Sobo 1995; Hirsch *et al.* 2002). However, we know relatively little about women's *sexual* experiences with male condoms, or how their condom practices may be shaped by sexual preferences or changes in sexual sensation enjoyment. In contrast, family planning research tends to assume that many men do not like using condoms because they curtail sexual sensation (Crosby *et al.* 2004; Thomsen *et al.* 2004; Khan *et al.* 2004; UNAIDS 2000) and that many men dislike using condoms – or outright refuse to wear them – because they reduce sexual pleasure (UNAIDS 2000).

Given that a sex-positive approach has been largely absent from contraceptive research, development or acceptability studies, it is no surprise that it also rarely features in contraceptive market and programming. Contraceptive advertisements and promotional materials tend to adhere to the rational actor model used frequently in public health, in which women supposedly weigh the economic and health costs

and benefits of various methods in making their contraceptive choice. Sexual benefits or detractions are rarely, if ever, included on these materials. Pamphlets and
advertisements tout methods' efficacy, convenience and non-contraceptive benefits
(e.g. acne improvement or menstrual lightening), but not their contribution to or
reduction of enjoyable and exciting sex.

Well-intentioned roots

Undoubtedly, sexual stereotypes fuel some of the pleasure deficits and sexual
double standards outlined earlier. Family planning discourse stems from a larger
cultural model in which men's greater sexual 'needs' and desires allegedly dictate
that men cannot or will not take responsibility for preventing pregnancy, whereas
women stereotypically have the ability to be more sensible and responsible –
perhaps due to their comparatively lesser sex drives (Tolman and Diamond 2001).
The current family planning approach to sexuality is also consistent with a number
of other prevailing policy discourses (e.g. sexual trafficking, child marriage and
women's rights in Afghanistan and Arabic countries), which describe women as
sexual victims rather than sexual agents and men's sexual behaviour as out of
control or unchangeable (Girard 2004). However, some far more well-intentioned
roots also underlie the pleasure deficit.

To start, it may be nearly impossible to devise a suitable universal definition for
healthy, pleasurable sexuality, given the deeply personal nature of sex and myriad
cultural and social influences on sexual desires, meanings and behaviours (Parker
and Aggleton 1999). In other words, it may be more straightforward, as well as more
pressing, for family planning researchers and policymakers to define threats to
women's sexuality than to operationalise those factors that maximise sexual enjoyment. This distinction between 'freedom from' phenomena such as violence and
sexual assault and 'freedom to' healthy, happy sex lives has been noted by Rosalind
Petchesky, who calls for a distinction between 'negative' (freedom *from*) and 'positive' (freedom *to*) sexual rights (Petchesky 1990; Petchesky *et al.* 1998).

A focus on negative sexual rights can be traced back to the earliest debates about
modern birth control in the USA and England. Whereas today we consider access to
contraception and abortion inextricably linked with feminism, many western feminists in the early 1900s were against contraception (Smith 1997; Gordon 1984). A
number of bourgeois Victorian women's advocates viewed birth control as only
leading women to further sublimate themselves to men's sexual desires (Banks
1981). In this context, contraception would give women less opportunity to avoid
unwanted sexual contact and was a step away from bodily integrity and social
emancipation.

Contraception was also feared to contribute to more philandering on men's
behalf. In bourgeois western sectors at this time, sex was not thought of as especially
enjoyable for socially privileged women (D'Emilio and Freedman 1988; Weeks
1981/1989). Several years later, even after concept of 'voluntary motherhood' had
gained widespread feminist appeal, Margaret Sanger and her colleagues continued
to distance themselves from the sexual aspects of birth control, even though sexual
emancipation may have been an underlying goal of many feminists of the time,
including Sanger herself (Tone 2001).[6] To win medical, governmental and public
approval, feminists and neo-Malthusians emphasised birth control's ability to reduce

maternal mortality and morbidity, slow the increase of poor and immigrant populations and '*strengthen the family* as a unit rather than *to free women*' (Dixon-Mueller
1993a: 42, emphasis in original). Indeed, particularly as feminists tried to enlist clinicians and policymakers to their cause, they were forced to emphasise the ways in
which contraception could control rather than liberate sexuality.

Many decades later, women's rights advocates continued a focus on negative
versus positive rights in relation to family planning. Beginning in the 1970s, feminists across the globe rallied against western countries' efforts to control population
growth in developing countries; they argued that these policies and programmes
were so intent on declining birth rates that they often vanquished women's individual rights to use or not use contraception as they wished (Dixon-Mueller 1993a;
Connelly 2008). To convince population planners to change their tactics, some feminists argued that one of the best ways to encourage smaller families was to help
women achieve social and sexual autonomy. A new body of research was born, documenting how threats to women's sexual self-determination could undermine their
ability to prevent pregnancies.

Thus, recent decades have witnessed a surfeit of work on *negative* sexuality in the
family planning field – how threats to women's sexual wellbeing can undermine
larger family planning goals, as well as (more recently) the prevention of HIV transmission. Feminist researchers have documented how gender-based violence (McCarraher *et al.* 2006; Pallitto and O'Campo 2004; Watts and Mayhew 2004; Stephenson
et al. 2006; El-Bassel *et al.* 2005), non-volitional sex (Kalmuss 2004; Doyal 1995) and
relationship power imbalances (Pulerwitz *et al.* 2002; Blanc 2001) can all sabotage
women's self-determination. In turn, the violation of women's sexual rights contributes to high rates of unintended pregnancy, HIV transmission and other forms of
reproductive morbidity and mortality (Finkler 1994; Doyal 1995).

Thus, the family planning field has long been marked by a focus on negative
versus positive sexual rights for women, even among those constituencies fighting
for gender equity. And to be sure, a sex-positive family planning agenda may be a
far less important feminist, social justice agenda item compared to issues such as
clean water, poverty reduction or deleterious globalisation policies and development practices. Some feminists have also warned that a focus on pleasure may also
inadvertently perpetuate gender inequality. At least one scholar has cautioned
against the promotion of a universal human right to pleasure, arguing that men's
demands for sexual pleasure could infringe on women's basic sexual rights (Oriel
2005).

Future directions and new sexual frames for the field

Despite these cautions, a growing body of work indicates the importance of pleasure
not only as an end in itself, but also as a critical part a complete understanding of
sexual and reproductive behaviours. In this concluding section, I highlight some of
the studies that show the importance of sex-positive work and suggest some new
framings for the future of the field.

Some investigations have examined contraceptive influences on sexual functioning, with results suggesting that women's contraceptive behaviours are shaped by
sexual acceptability and side effects. In a longitudinal study of new oral contraceptive users in the USA, for example, researchers found that a decrease in women's

libido and sexual enjoyment was strongly associated with discontinuation (Sanders *et al.* 2001). In a study of the features most likely to shape contraceptive method choice, women ranked 'lack of interference with sexual pleasure' as a 'very important consideration' as often as men did (30 per cent of men and 28 per cent of women) (Grady *et al.* 1999).

Similarly, in qualitative research on sexual pleasure and contraceptive use, the way contraceptives altered 'sexual aesthetics' (sensation, libido, lubrication, spontaneity and other sexual attributes) mattered to women and men equally and shaped both the choice of method and manner of use (Higgins and Hirsch 2008). However, gender and power influenced these aesthetics in striking ways. For example, women often disliked male condoms because they diminished their *partner's* pleasure, and thus their own. Women were often concerned about the sexual side effects of male condoms for their partners, whereas men expressed comparatively little concern about the sexual side effects of women's methods.

Indeed, burgeoning scholarship demonstrates a small but growing awareness that the ways male condoms feel sexually matter to women as well as men, often in gendered ways. One qualitative study from the UK (Holland *et al.* 1998) explored women's sexual experiences with male condoms, with attention to the pressures put on young men and women to conform to gender-appropriate sexual behaviours. In both this latter study and in a quantitative analysis of women at risk for HIV in New York City (Ehrhardt *et al.* 2002), those women who felt that condoms undermined their sexual pleasure were less likely to use them than women who did not report condom-related reductions in pleasure.

There have also been attempts to theorise and demonstrate pregnancy-associated pleasures and how they can stymie effective contraceptive use, even in the absence of desire for a child. At least one preliminary study has suggested that in the heat of the sexual moment, a couple's or individual's temporary desire for a pregnancy could lead to unprotected sex, even if a baby were not fully or rationally intended (Peacock *et al.* 2001). Likewise, US abortion clinic clients have sometime described a temporary surrender to the fantasy of a pregnancy (Higgins 2007). My own work has begun to explore the degree to which women and men find pleasure in the possibility of a pregnancy with a particular partner or at a particular moment, and how this can undermine contraceptive use (Higgins *et al.* 2008). For some respondents in this study, sex occasionally became a way to flirt with and eroticise pregnancy risk, often as an avenue for seeking ultimate closeness with one's partner. Aroused during sex by the idea of pregnancy, these respondents dispensed with contraceptives.

This study and others have also demonstrated a less direct, less strongly erotic relationship between pregnancy ambivalence and lack of contraceptive use. In some situations, although pregnancy is neither intended nor *not* intended, the notion of creating a baby can be compelling – a situation that could contribute to inconsistent contraceptive use (Higgins *et al.* 2008). This finding echoes the work of Stanford and colleagues, who have used the term 'passive procepting behaviour' to describe fecund couples who do not use contraceptives but are not trying to conceive (Stanford *et al.* 2000: 185). Along similar lines, one study of women found that half of coital events were unprotected, even among those respondents who reported they were committed to not getting pregnant (Bartz *et al.* 2007). Day-to-day factors such as respondents' daily assessments of partners' support and feelings of being in love could help predict lack of contraceptive use. Feeling loved and supported are two social benefits that can carry great weight in the heat of the sexual moment.

Taken together, the studies mentioned here indicate that pleasure seeking influences the ways in which contraceptives are used or not used. They suggest that, without a better understanding of how people seek sexual enjoyment, we will fail to have a complete picture of reproductive behaviours.

In particular, the last studies create the groundwork for a new framework that considers the ways in which unprotected sex can meet people's sexual, emotional and social needs, including sexual arousal and fulfilment, closeness and connection with their partner and a more emotionally and materially secure future. Given the existence of these needs, intermittent or nonexistent contraceptive use – practices that are consistently portrayed in the family planning field as failure to do something, an 'unmet need' for family planning or a health risk that rational people would want to avoid – may instead represent purposeful action.

One hopes that these studies are not so much exceptions to the field's pleasure deficit as much as harbingers of things to come. In constructing a new sexual frame for itself, the family planning field should continue to dispense with the rational actor model and consider myriad reasons why people engage in the sex that leads to pregnancy in the first place. Researchers and practitioners should attend to the ways in which both women *and* men's desires influence the ways in which sex happens, and thus, the ways in which pregnancies are either created or prevented. Finally, the field's most basic premises should build from the assumption that the way sex feels matters to women and, as a result, shapes contraceptive practices. Recognising and addressing the positive sexual aspects of people's lives will help us better understand and address not only people's risk behaviours, but also their wellbeing more generally.

Notes

1 For a small sampling of family planning and demographic literature that speaks of sex in this way, see Ali *et al.* 2003; Montgomery *et al.* 1998; Spira *et al.* 1985; Léridon 1977. Thanks to Susan Watkins (1993) and Jennifer S. Hirsch for bringing this issue to my attention.

2 For example, one could argue that 'family planning' encompasses communication between couples about their desired family size or the reproductive choices of those who cannot or chose not to have children through heterosexual intercourse – for example, gays, lesbians or infertile heterosexual couples who wish to become parents.

3 There is a great deal of disagreement on the definition of, precursors to, and even the usefulness of the concept of pregnancy 'intendedness'. For example, women often report being happy about an unintended pregnancy, and one-third of pregnancies resulting from contraceptive failures are subsequently classified as intended (Klerman 2000; Trussell *et al.* 1999). Despite these definition controversies, the pervasiveness of unsafe abortion worldwide serves as one persistently strong case for the social and health costs of unintended pregnancy for women.

4 I should note the two exceptions to this statement: both *microbicides* and *the female condom* have been explored much more fully than other methods in terms of their sexual dimensions. But both of these methods emerged from efforts to create female-controlled HIV prevention strategies rather than from within the family planning field.

5 Studies have been conducted of oral contraceptives' effects on women's libido, with decidedly mixed results (Davis and Castano 2004; Schaffir 2006; Gambrell *et al.* 1976). Some women report diminished sexual interest while taking the pill, whereas other women report no change or even increases in sexual interest.

6 Often and unfortunately, feminists also adopted popular eugenicist and racist arguments to further their cause – that is, suggesting that birth control could be used to control growing populations of African Americans and Irish, Italian and Jewish immigrants (Gordon 1976).

References

Alan Guttmacher Institute (1999) *Sharing Responsibility: Women, Society, and Abortion Worldwide*, New York: Alan Guttmacher Institute.

Ali, M. M., Cleland, J. G. and Shah, I. H. (2003) 'Trends in Reproductive Behavior among Young Single Women in Colombia and Peru: 1985–1999', *Demography*, 40: 659–73.

Amaro, H. (1995) 'Love, Sex, and Power: Considering Women's Realities in HIV Prevention', *American Psychologist*, 50: 437–47.

Amaro, H., Raj, A. and Reed, E. (2001) 'Women's Sexual Health: The Need for Feminist Analyses in Public Health in the decade of Behavior', *Psychology of Women Quarterly*, 25: 324–34.

Anderson-Hunt, M., Dennerstein, L. D., Hatton, L., Hunt, J., Mahony, J., Sargeant, D. *et al.* (1996) 'Hormones and Female Sexuality: Developing a Method for Research', in Zeidenstein, S. and Moore, K. (eds) *Learning about Sexuality: A Practical Beginning*, New York: The Population Council and The International Women's Health Coalition.

Banks, O. (1981) *Faces of Feminism: A Study of Feminism as a Social Movement*, Oxford: Martin Robertson.

Bartz, D., Shew, M., Ofner, S. and Fortenberry, J. D. (2007) 'Pregnancy Intentions and Contraceptive Behaviors among Adolescent Women: A Coital Event Level Analysis', *Journal of Adolescent Health*, 41: 271–76.

Blanc, A. (2001) 'The Effect of Power in Sexual Relationships on Sexual and Reproductive Health: An Examination of the Evidence', *Studies in Family Planning*, 32: 189–213.

Brown, S. S., Eisenberg, L. and IOM (1995) *The Best Intentions: Unintended Pregnancy and the Well-being of Children and Families*, Washington, DC: National Academy Press.

Carballo-Dieguez, A. and Bauermeister, J. (2004) ' "Barebacking": Intentional Condomless Anal Sex in HIV-risk Contexts. Reasons For and Against It', *Journal of Homosexuality*, 47: 1–16.

Connelly, M. J. (2008) *Fatal Misconception: The Struggle to Control World Population*, Cambridge, MA: Belknap.

Crosby, R. A., Graham, C. A., Yarber, W. L. and Sanders, S. A. (2004) 'If the Condom Fits, Wear it: A Qualitative Study of Young African-American Men', *Sexually Transmitted Infections*, 80: 306–9.

D'Emilio, J. and Freedman, E. B. (1988) *Intimate Matters: A History of Sexuality in America*, New York: Harper & Row.

Davis, A. R. and Castano, P. M. (2004) 'Oral Contraceptives and Libido in Women', *Annual Review of Sex Research*, 15: 297–320.

Dennerstein, L. (1996) 'Female Sexuality, the Menstrual Cycle, and the Pill', in Zeidenstein, S. and Moore, K. (eds) *Learning about Sexuality: A Practical Beginning*, New York: The Population Council and The International Women's Health Coalition.

Díaz, R. (1999) 'Trips to Fantasy Island: Contexts of Risk Sex for San Francisco Gay Men', *Sexualities*, 2: 89–112.

Dixon-Mueller, R. (1993a) *Population Policy and Women's Rights: Transforming Reproductive Choice*, Westport, CT: Praeger.

Dixon-Mueller, R. (1993b) 'The Sexuality Connection in Reproductive Health', *Studies in Family Planning*, 24: 269–82.

Dowsett, G. W. (1996) *Practicing Desire: Homosexual Sex in the Era of AIDS*, Stanford: Stanford University Press.

Doyal, L. (1995) *What makes Women Sick: Gender and the Political Economy of Health*, New Brunswick, NJ: Rutgers University Press.

Ehrhardt, A., Exner, T. M., Hoffman, S., Silberman, I., Yingling, S., Adams-Skinner, J. *et al.* (2002) 'HIV/STD Risk and Sexual Strategies among Women Family Planning Clients in New York: Project FIO', *AIDS and Behavior*, 6: 1–12.

El-Bassel, N., Gilbert, L., Wu, E., Go, H. and Hill, J. (2005) 'HIV and Intimate Partner Violence among Methadone-maintained Women in New York City', *Social Science & Medicine*, 61: 171–83.

Exner, T. M., Dworkin, S., Hoffman, S. and Ehrhardt, A. A. (2003) 'Beyond the Male Condom: The Evolution of Gender-specific HIV Interventions for Women', *Annual Review of Sex Research*, 14: 114–36.

Finer, L. B. and Henshaw, S. K. (2006) 'Disparities in Rates of Unintended Pregnancy in the United States, 1994 and 2001', *Perspectives on Sexual and Reproductive Health*, 38: 90–6.

Finkler, K. (1994) *Women in Pain: Gender and Morbidity in Mexico*, Philadelphia: University of Pennsylvania Press.

Gambrell, R. D., Jr., Bernard, D. M., Sanders, B. I., Vanderburg, N. and Buxton, S. J. (1976) 'Changes in Sexual Drives of Patients on Oral Contraceptives', *Journal of Reproductive Medicine*, 17: 165–71.

Girard, F. (2004) 'Global Implications of U.S. Domestic and international Policies on Sexuality, Columbia: International Working Group on Sexuality and Social Policy', Working Papers Center for Gender, Sexuality and Health, Mailman School of Public Health, Columbia University (IWGSSP Working Paper No. 1).

Gordon, L. (1976) *Woman's Body, Woman's Right: A Social History of Birth Control in America*, New York: Grossman.

Gordon, L. (1984) 'Voluntary Motherhood: The Beginnings of Feminist Birth Control Ideas', in Leavitt, J. W. (ed.) *Women and Health in America: Historical Readings*, Madison: University of Wisconsin Press.

Grady, W. R., Klepinger, D. H. and Nelson-Wally, A. (1999) 'Contraceptive Characteristics: The Perceptions and Priorities of Men and Women', *Family Planning Perspectives*, 31: 168–75.

Henshaw, S. K. (1998) 'Unintended Pregnancy in the United States', *Family Planning Perspectives*, 30: 24–9, 46.

Higgins, J. A. (2007) 'Sexy Feminisms and Sexual Health: Theorizing Heterosex, Pleasure, and Constraint for a Public Health Research Agenda', *Atlantis*, 31: 72–81.

Higgins, J. A. and Hirsch, J. S. (2007) 'The Pleasure Deficit: Revisiting the "Sexuality Connection" in Reproductive Health', *Perspectives on Sexual and Reproductive Health*, 39: 240–7.

Higgins, J. A. and Hirsch, J. S. (2008) 'Pleasure and Power: Incorporating Sexuality and Inequality into Research on Contraceptive Use and Unintended Pregnancy', *American Journal of Public Health*, 98: 1803–13.

Higgins, J. A., Hirsch, J. S. and Trussell, J. (2008) 'Pleasure, Prophylaxis, and Procreation: A Qualitative Analysis of Intermittent Contraceptive Use and Unintended Pregnancy', *Perspectives on Sexual and Reproductive Health*, 98: 130–7.

Hirsch, J. S., Higgins, J., Nathanson, C. A. and Bentley, P. (2002) 'Social Constructions of sexuality: the meanings of marital infidelity and STD/HIV risk in a Mexican Migrant Community', *American Journal of Public Health*, 92: 1227–37.

Holland, J., Ramazanoglu, C., Sharpe, S. and Thomson, R. (1998) *The Male in the Head: Young People, Heterosexuality and power*, London: Tufnell Press.

Junge, B. (2002) 'Bareback Sex, Risk, and Eroticism: Anthropological Themes (Re-)surfacing in the Post-AIDS Era', in Lewin, E. and Leap, W. L. (eds) *Out in Theory: The Emergence of Lesbian and Gay Anthropology*, Chicago: University of Illinois Press.

Kalmuss, D. (2004) 'Nonvolitional Sex and Sexual Health', *Archives of Sexual Behavior*, 33: 197–209.

Khan, S. I., Hudson-Rodd, N., Saggers, S., Bhuiyan, M. I. and Bhuiya, A. (2004) 'Safer Sex or Pleasurable Sex? Rethinking Condom Use in the AIDS Era', *Sexual Health*, 1: 217–25.

Klerman, L. V. (2000) 'The Intendedness of Pregnancy: A Concept in Transition', *Maternal and Child Health Journal*, 4: 155–62.

Léridon, H. (1977) *Human Fertility: The Basic Components*, Chicago: University of Chicago Press.

McCarraher, D. R., Martin, S. L. and Bailey, P. E. (2006) 'The Influence of Method-related Partner Violence on Covert Pill Use and Pill Discontinuation among Women living in La Paz, El Alto and Santa Cruz, Bolivia', *Journal of Biosocial Science*, 38: 169–86.

Montgomery, M., Cohen, B. and National Research Council (US) Committee on Population (1998) *From Death to Birth: Mortality Decline and Reproductive Change*, Washington, DC: National Academy Press.

Moore, K. and Helzner, J. F. (1996) *'What's Sex Got to do with It?': Challenges for Incorporating Sexuality into Family Planning Programs*, New York: The Population Council.

Oriel, J. (2005) 'Sexual Pleasure as a Human Right: Harmful or Helpful to Women in the Context of HIV/AIDS?', *Women's Studies International Forum*, 28: 392–404.

Oudshoorn, N. (2003) *The Male Pill: A Biography of a Technology in the Making*, Durham, NC: Duke University Press.

Pallitto, C. C. and O'Campo, P. (2004) 'The Relationship between Intimate Partner Violence and Unintended Pregnancy: Analysis of a National Sample from Colombia', *International Family Planning Perspectives*, 30: 165–73.

Parker, R. G. (1999) *Beneath the Equator: Cultures of Desire, Male Homosexuality, and Emerging Gay Communities in Brazil*, New York: Routledge.

Parker, R. G. and Aggleton, P. (1999) *Culture, Society and Sexuality: A Reader*, London: UCL Press.

Parker, R. G., Barbosa, R. M. and Aggleton, P. (2000) *Framing the Sexual Subject: The Politics of Gender, Sexuality, and Power*, Berkeley: University of California Press.

Peacock, N., Lahurd, K., Abicht, H., Gilliam, M., Kumar, A., Geller, S. *et al.* (2001) 'Exploring the Complexities of Pregnancy Intentions for African American Women', Annual Meeting of the American Public Health Association, Atlanta.

Petchesky, R. P. (1990) *Abortion and Woman's Choice: The State, Sexuality, and Reproductive Freedom*, Boston, MA: Northeastern University Press.

Petchesky, R. P., Judd, K. and IRRRAG (eds) (1998) *Negotiating Reproductive Rights: Women's Perspectives across Countries and Cultures*, New York: Zed Books.

Pulerwitz, J., Amaro, H., De Jong, W., Gortmaker, S. L. and Rudd, R. (2002) 'Relationship Power, Condom Use and HIV Risk among Women in the USA', *AIDS Care*, 14: 789–800.

Sanders, S. A., Graham, C. A., Bass, J. L. and Bancroft, J. (2001) 'A Prospective Study of the Effects of Oral Contraceptives on Sexuality and Well-being and their Relationship to Discontinuation', *Contraception*, 64: 51–8.

Schaffir, J. (2006) 'Hormonal Contraception and Sexual Desire: A Critical Review', *Journal of Sexual Marital Therapy*, 32: 305–14.

Shernoff, M. (2005) *Without Condoms: Unprotected Sex, Gay Men, and Barebacking*, New York: Routledge.

Smith, D. S. (1997) 'Family Limitation, Sexual Control, and Domestic Feminism in Victorian America', in Tone, A. (ed.) *Controlling Reproduction: An American History*, Wilmington, DL: SR Books.

Sobo, E. J. (1995) 'Finance, Romance, Social Support, and Condom Use among Impoverished Inner-city Women', *Human Organization*, 54: 115–28.

Solomon, H., Yount, K. M. and Mbizvo, M. T. (2007) ' "A Shot of His Own": The Acceptability of a Male Hormonal Contraceptive in Indonesia', *Culture, Health and Sexuality*, 9: 1–14.

Spira, N., Spira, A. and Schwartz, D. (1985) 'Fertility of Couples following Cessation of Contraception', *Journal of Biosocial Science*, 17: 281–90.

Stanford, J. B., Hobbs, R., Jameson, P., DeWitt, M. J. and Fischer, R. C. (2000) 'Defining Dimensions of Pregnancy Intendedness', *Maternal and Child Health Journal*, 4: 183–9.

Stephenson, R., Koenig, M. A. and Ahmed, S. (2006) 'Domestic Violence and Contraceptive Adoption in Uttar Pradesh, India', *Studies in Family Planning*, 37: 75–86.

Thomsen, S., Stalker, M. and Toroitich-Ruto, C. (2004) 'Fifty Ways to Leave your Rubber: How Men in Mombasa rationalise Unsafe Sex', *Sexually Transmitted Infections*, 80: 430–4.

Tolman, D. L. and Diamond, L. M. (2001) 'Desegregating Sexuality Research: Cultural and Biological Perspectives on Gender and Desire', *Annual Review of Sex Research*, 12: 33–74.

Tone, A. (2001) *Devices and Desires: A History of Contraceptives in America*, New York, Hill & Wang.

Trussell, J., Vaughan, B. and Stanford, J. B. (1999) 'Are all Contraceptive Failures Unintended Pregnancies? Evidence from the 1995 National Survey of Family Growth', *Family Planning Perspectives*, 31: 246–7, 260.

UNAIDS (2000) *Men and AIDS – A Gendered Approach*, Geneva: UNAIDS.

Watkins, S. C. (1993) 'If All We Knew about Women was what we Read in *Demography*, What would We Know?', *Demography*, 30: 551–77.

Watts, C. and Mayhew, S. (2004) 'Reproductive Health Services and Intimate Partner Violence: Shaping a Pragmatic Response in Sub-Saharan Africa', *International Family Planning Perspectives*, 30: 207–13.

Weeks, J. (1981/1989) *Sex, Politics, and Society: The Regulation of Sexuality since 1800*, New York: Longman.

WHO (1982) 'Hormonal Contraception for Men: Acceptability and Effects on Sexuality', World Health Organisation Task Force on Psychosocial Research in Family Planning, Special Programme of Research, Development and Research Training in Human Reproduction, *Studies in Family Planning*, 13: 328–42.

WHO (2004) *Unsafe Abortion: Global and Regional Estimates of the Incidence of Unsafe Abortion and Associated Mortality in 2000*, 4th edn, Geneva: World Health Organisation.

Worth, D. (1989) 'Sexual Decision-making and AIDS: Why Condom Promotion among Vulnerable Women is likely to Fail', *Studies in Family Planning*, 20: 297–307.

18 Teenage pregnancy

From sex to social pathology

Maria Luiza Heilborn and Cristiane S. Cabral

About 50 years ago, as a consequence of the introduction of the contraceptive pill, the process of separating sex from procreation began. This brought about important transformations in sexual and gender norms and behaviours. In particular, women's sexuality became less constrained once greater control over fertility could be achieved. Within the context of these social and sexual behavioural changes, the problem of 'teenage pregnancy' began to emerge. While some of the most heated debate has taken place in the north (the USA, Canada and Europe), moral panic and outrage concerning teenage pregnancy has also been evident in industrialising nations such as Brazil (Le Van 1998; Bonell 2004; Breheny and Stephens 2007). These concerns play to larger anxieties about 'adolescence' in general and young people's sexual behaviour in particular (Luker 1996; Schalet 2004).

Growing interest in teenage pregnancy in Brazil is linked to a number of different factors. First, there is the mistaken perception that a demographic explosion is underway, which is contradicted by the fact that census data show a significant *fall* in Brazilian fertility rate over the last 30 years – the current rate is of 1.8 newborns per woman, which is below the population replacement level (Ministério da Saúde 2008; Berquó and Cavenaghi 2005). Second, as a result of widespread social change, sexual experience independent of marriage is no longer the privilege of young men, and the moral value of female virginity has faded. Third, there have been major changes in conceptions of age and gender, which have redefined social aspirations and the nature of youth. Young people are expected to spend ever longer periods of time in education prior to entry into the labour market, leaving the parental home and (eventual) marriage (Galland 1997). Pregnancy is disruptive because it interrupts this process. Together, these three factors have contributed towards a social pathologisation of teenage conception and pregnancy in countries such as Brazil.

The data we will draw on in this chapter come from the Gravidez na Adolescência (GRAVAD) study.[1] This involved interviews with 4634 young people of both sexes aged 18–24 years in three Brazilian cities (Porto Alegre, Rio de Janeiro and Salvador) between 2001 and 2002. Findings from the study allowed us to question the reductionist and moralist frame in which teenage pregnancy is often constructed – one with stresses its supposedly abnormality and danger both for the individual(s) concerned and for society at large. The study also revealed that pregnancy in youth is a remarkable diverse phenomenon (Heilborn *et al.* 2006).

The social valorisation of schooling and the increasing professionalisation of the workforce, together with the belief that poverty might be controlled by limiting early childbirth together have nourished the portrayal of teenage pregnancy as a social pathology of epidemic dimensions. Brazilian public debates frequently associate teenage pregnancy with poverty and urban violence (Oliveira 2005; Heilborn *et al.* 2007), and they usually advocate population control to tackle all three of these problems at once.

Teenage pregnancy: does it result from early sexual initiation?

Prevailing representations portray young people as individuals whose sexual and emotional lives do not follow any rules and whose relationships are ephemeral, and lack depth and commitment (Reis 1993; Luker; 1996; Schalet 2004). The mainstream literature on youth often interprets pregnancy as an event that is unwanted, unplanned and associated with too active a sexual life (Camarano 1998; Leite *et al.* 2004; Le Van 1998; Kirby 1999). An alternative and more generous perspective sees teenage pregnancy as part of a process of learning about sexuality, emotions and relationships (Gagnon and Simon 1973; Bozon and Heilborn 2006).

Findings from the GRAVAD study point to the range of ways in which young people experience teenage pregnancy (Aquino *et al.* 2003). Although the percentages differ slightly across the three study sites, the general finding is that 29.6 per cent of women and 21.4 per cent of men had experienced an episode of pregnancy, whether it had reached term or not. The frequency of pregnancy before 15 years of age was, however, very low (1.6 per cent and 0.7 per cent for women and men, respectively).

It has frequently been suggested that earlier sexual initiation among young people leads to higher rates of pregnancy, such that as the number of sexually active young people increases, so too does the rate of pregnancy. In fact, recent data provided by the last demographic and health survey done in Brazil show that the percentage of women whose first sexual relation took place before the age of 16 years tripled in the course of one decade, rising from 11 per cent in 1996 to 33 per cent in 2006 (Ministério da Saúde 2008). Nevertheless, even taking into account the fact that sexual initiation for women happens at an earlier age than occurred in previous generations, it does not take place as early as commentators and pundits sometimes erroneously suggest.

By way of example, in 1999, for example, the Brazilian newspaper *O Globo* published a highly influential article by José Serra, then Minister of Health, with the suggestive title 'Child-Mothers'. In the story, Serra describes a situation in which girls at an age when it would be appropriate to be still playing with dolls, being victimised by precocious sexuality and motherhood. Obedient to a cliché-ridden, alarmist view of youth sexuality, the author blames the media and television soap operas for stimulating 'precocious erotisation, uninformed sexual initiation, and accidental and undesired pregnancy' (Serra 1999: 8). The Ministry of Health, he argues, should initiate a major campaign to change young people's behaviours.

In contrast to such alarmism, GRAVAD data reveal that half of young men had their first sexual experience at the median age of 16.2 years, while for women the median age was 17.9 years (Bozon and Heilborn 2006).

One new finding to emerge from the study was that for women to gain sexual experience prior to marriage is increasingly acceptable (Ministério da Saúde 2008). In the lives of young people there is an increasing distance between first sex and marriage. Young women's age at first sex has decreased by two years in the last two decades, while marriage is being postponed (Berquó 1998; Bozon 2003, 2005). A steady relationship is no longer the forerunner to marriage but has acquired a meaning in itself. It provides an opportunity to explore feelings and to learn about sexuality.

The median age of first sex for men varies little by region of residence, social group or colour/race. Men's behaviour tends to be relatively uniform, in line with strong cultural pressures to assert masculinity through early sexual experience. There is more variation among women, however, by origin and biographical characteristics. Those who come from the poorer sectors of society experience sexual initiation earlier. For both women and men, later sexual initiation is associated with prolonged schooling.

GRAVAD data also contradict the popular belief that sexual initiation among young black people takes place at an earlier age than among non-blacks. This belief is based on the social myth that equates the sexuality of indigenous peoples and blacks with spontaneity, sensuality and corporality – qualities that are also manifest in samba music and in soccer. There was no evidence for greater frequency of sex and earlier sexual initiation among blacks in our study.

Other interesting findings include the following. At first sex, men rarely have younger partners, while women usually have older and more experienced partners. Women tend to have their first sexual relationship with a *namorado* or steady boyfriend (86 per cent) or with their husband (4 per cent). Only 45 per cent of men, by way of contrast, have their first sexual experience with a *namorada* or regular girlfriend. It is more likely for them to begin their sexual life with a casual partner (48 per cent) or sex worker (5 per cent).

Importantly, the use of contraception is higher among young people whose sexual initiation occurs later. The frequency of using contraception also varies with education and is higher among those with more years of schooling. GRAVAD data reveal that contraceptive use varies from 54 per cent, among women with a low level of schooling, to 80 per cent among those with college education (similar data were also found in the 2006 Demographic Health Survey conducted in Brazil – Ministério da Saúde 2008). Gender differences are apparent when it comes to partners' previous sexual experience: 83 per cent of women's partners had prior sexual experience whereas this was true of only 57 per cent of men's partners.

Together, these data reveal that first sexual experiences for women and for men vary considerably, a fact that results in major differences in the ways in which they manage the use of contraception. Although an equivalent percentage of men and women (70 per cent) say they used some form of contraception at first sex, there is a decline in the regular use of contraceptives over time as partners acquire trust in each other. Likewise, the frequency of contraceptive use decreases in subsequent relationships decreases.

Comparing the findings across the three study sites, findings reveal that in Porto Alegre women tend to begin their sexual life with a partner relatively early at 17.2 years of age, use contraception more (79.6 per cent), have fewer abortions (2.1 per cent) and have lower rates of teenage pregnancy (27.7 per cent). This may reflect the broader social context. In comparison to the other studied cities, Porto Alegre has a strong education and public health system. In Salvador, a state capital with comparatively fewer public resources and a more impoverished population, women report later sexual initiation (at 18.4 years on average), use contraception less (62.9 per cent), have more early pregnancies (31.3 per cent) and have higher rates of abortion (7.7 per cent). Rio de Janeiro occupies an intermediate position. This evidence runs counter to the claim that teenage pregnancy is simply and directly associated with early sexual initiation.

Teenage pregnancy: relational and social contexts

Teenage pregnancy and parenting do not constitute the dominant experiences of young people in Brazil today. However, it is important to focus on them because contemporary debate concerning early sexual initiation and sexual activity in youth is still very passionate, even in a relatively open society such as Brazil. In developing a better appreciation of the issues at stake, it is important to recognise something of the diversity of young people's experiences. Teenage pregnancy can happen to teenage couples or to couples in which only one of the partners is a teenager. For some young people, it can mean the acquisition of adult status and lead to a renegotiation of roles within the family. For others, teenage pregnancy can be the fulfilment of a personal desire for individualisation and autonomy, a detour from a linear trajectory, an accident in the process of learning about sexuality and feelings, the constitution of a new conjugal unit, the repeat of family history and so on. It is impossible therefore to think of there being only one cause of teenage pregnancy.

Most usually, the relationship present when conception first takes place is preserved. For young women, pregnancy is usually with an older partner within the context of an ongoing relationship – either with a first sexual partner or with another stable partner. Men provide fewer reports of pregnancy, their partners tend to be of the same age, but when pregnancy happens it does so also within the context of a stable or regular relationship. In the GRAVAD data, relatively few instances are observed of teenage pregnancy being the result of sex with a casual partner. Nevertheless, this kind of stereotype abounds, with public representations of teenage motherhood most usually taking this form, stressing promiscuity and thoughtlessness.

Teenage pregnancy tends to be more frequent among the poorest sectors of society, although it also happens to young people with high levels of schooling and income. The occurrence of pregnancy before the age of 20 varied inversely with levels of schooling and income. The most significant contrast is found among women: the percentage of pregnancy among those whose family income is half of the minimum wage (53.8 per cent) is almost six times higher than the percentage observed among those with an income more than three minimum wages (9.7 per cent). Among lower class young people of a similar social background, those who continue to study or reach a higher level of schooling than their mothers show a lower rate of pregnancy (and close to the rate shown by very rich and schooled women). Clearly, claims that parenting is the sole destiny of poor youth need to be put into perspective.

Turning to variations by racial/ethnic group, pregnancy before the age of 20 years was more frequent among self-declared black (35.5 per cent) and *pardas* (mixed race) (34.8 per cent) than among white (23.4 per cent) women. No significant differences were found between the studied cities. It is important to note that these first two categories are also those with lower levels of income and schooling.

In the case of men, the percentages reporting teenage pregnancy were blacks (36.8 per cent), whites (15.8 per cent) and *pardos* (mixed race) (16.4 per cent).

In Brazil, there are many factors influencing young people's attendance at school, many of which occur before pregnancy. In the GRAVAD data, there is much evidence of discrepancies between chronological age and school grade, as well as dropouts (Almeida 2008). Overall, men and women are about equally affected. The situation is more disadvantageous for young people who live in Salvador, compared to residents of Rio de Janeiro and Porto Alegre. Young people of both sexes who are black, whose family monthly income is low and whose mothers have low levels of school education are the ones likely to be affected (Almeida 2008). Young women and men who experience problems at school are also likely to begin their sexual life earlier, and use contraceptive methods or protection less frequently at first sex.

One hidden dimension of teenage pregnancy is that of termination. According to Brazilian law, abortion is permitted in only two circumstances: when pregnancy results from rape, and when it jeopardises the life of the mother. Among GRAVAD interviewees, 6.2 per cent of women and 10 per cent of men who had experienced at least one episode of pregnancy opted for abortion (Menezes *et al.* 2006). Given its illegality and social disapproval, it is reasonable to believe that this is an underestimate of the number of abortions taking place. It is also important to recognise that reports of abortion are more frequent among young men and women with regular school careers (Almeida 2008).

Becoming a father, becoming a mother

Among young people overall three out of four pregnancies were carried to term. Among lower class men, paternity provides evidence of maturity and responsibility. The same is not true for middle- and upper-class men, among whom fatherhood holds little symbolic value. Among those who are poor, being a father encourages men to take on the role of provider (Cabral 2003), and strengthens the passage into adulthood. Work, home building and having children provide the bases for masculine emancipation from the family of origin, although families of birth may continue to provide aid. Young women from a similar background move from being daughters to being 'women' and 'mothers' (Carvalho 2007).

In the middle class, however, different processes take place (Heilborn *et al.* 2002). Here, the importance of personal development is likely to be stressed, alongside the challenges that teenage pregnancy poses. A more 'psychologised' discourse transforms parenting into a more subjective experience. In contrast to what takes place among members of the lower social classes, having a child is not a decisive factor in turning young parents into 'providers', 'heads of the family', 'housewives' and 'mothers', whereby their social identities are redefined (Cabral 2003; Costa 2002; Heilborn *et al.* 2002; Le Van 1998; Vilar and Gaspar 1999). For middle-class young people, the birth of a child is subordinate to continued forms of socialisation whereby leisure, schooling, the right to develop relationships and experimentation relating to sexuality and feelings continue to parallel the experience of parenting (Brandão 2005; Davies *et al.* 1999).

Nevertheless across all social classes, being a young mother or a young father can be a way of gaining social prestige. In the absence of other life projects, becoming a parent provides young men and women with the autonomy and status of being an 'adult', 'married', a 'mother' or a 'father'. This helps redefine their relations with their family of origin and opens up new horizons of relative independence (Carvalho 2007; Davies *et al.* 1999; Breheny and Stephens 2007).

What has changed with the birth of a child, however? According to GRAVAD data, almost half of pregnancies carried to term before the age of 20 years happened when the young person had already left school (Aquino *et al.* 2003, 2006) – 40.2 per cent of young women and 47.8 per cent of the men. Therefore, although it is not possible to deny categorically that pregnancy is one of the causes of school dropout, it is clearly not the only factor, neither is it the main factor leading to school abandonment. Many times, young people need to work, fail their exams, have a lack of interest in study, change their place of residence and so on.

The birth of the child produces a distribution of responsibility that follows prevailing gender expectations: all the indications are that young women remain at home and devote themselves to caring for the child (65 per cent of them did not work before giving birth and continue not to work during the child's first year), while young men have their role as provider reinforced. Few (14.2 per cent) remain out of the job market.

News of pregnancy is usually shared with grandmothers to be, and negotiations with the couple's family members takes place. Among young women, families tend to be happy with the news (40 per cent) and say that they will 'help take care of the baby' (18 per cent). Minorities of families suggest an abortion (11.3 per cent) or demand that the young people marry (7.7 per cent). Broadly similar responses are found among young men who reported their families having positive reactions (26 per cent), offering to help in taking care of the baby (25 per cent), suggesting an abortion (5 per cent) and demanding marriage (5 per cent).

Banishing a pregnant daughter from the family home, which was so common in the past, rarely happens nowadays (2.7 per cent) (Aquino *et al.* 2006). This change implies an important transformation in sexual morality and, consequently, in family and inter-generational relations. On the whole, families provide a very important source of support for the new couple, by incentivising the union, hosting the couple in their homes and contributing to the expenses and care for the child. Among lower class young people, family support can help alleviate social constraints; among middle-class young people, family support helps preserve educational projects (Heilborn *et al.* 2002).

Yet another factor, however, differentiates young men's and women's trajectories: namely, the constraints imposed to their sociability. With the advent of pregnancy, socialising with friends diminishes, particularly for women (73 per cent versus 40 per cent). The kind of motherhood young women from the lower social classes experience accentuates withdrawal into the domestic realm, with complaints of 'loneliness' and 'isolation' being frequent (Heilborn *et al.* 2002; Costa 2002). In the middle classes, young mothers are more restricted to the house than their partners, and the care of the child imposes further constraints on socialising with friends. However, compared to young working class women, middle-class young mothers can count on higher levels of social support (Heilborn *et al.* 2002; Brandão 2005).

Final remarks

Prevailing ideas about teenage pregnancy present negative images of young people and their lives. Public debate stresses juvenile irresponsibility, lack of parental authority and the absence of intergenerational dialogue, as the principal causes of teenage pregnancy. Against this background, this chapter suggests that the characterisation of teenage pregnancy as a social problem or a form of social pathology needs to be viewed with caution.

Importantly, teenage pregnancy does not occur equally across all social strata; it is more likely among young women with lower levels of education, and whose families have low cultural and economic capital. Becoming a mother can constitute an aspired social status for many young women in this stratum. Having said this, and contrary to the popular belief that teenage pregnancy is the result of poverty, it also takes place among young people from more privileged backgrounds who have better access to information, contraceptive methods and safe, although often illegal, forms of abortion.

Ultimately, then, teenage pregnancy is perhaps best understood not as an aberration or abnormality but as an event that may occur within the broader context of learning about sex, sexuality and relationships. Its occurrence and experience is structured by prevailing gender, class and racial/ethnic relations. Better understanding of this will benefit not only our understandings of young people and their needs, but also the programmes and interventions used to promote young people's sexual and reproductive health.

Note

1 The GRAVAD study was designed and implemented by Maria Luiza Heilborn the Universidade do Estado do Rio de Janeiro (UERJ), Michel Bozon of the Institut National d'Études Démographiques (INED), Estela Maria Aquino of the Universidade Federal da Bahia (UFBA) and Daniela Knauth from the Universidade Federal do Rio Grande do Sul (UFRGS). The main research findings were published in *O Aprendizado da Sexualidade: Reprodução e Trajetórias Sociais de Jovens Brasileiros*, edited by M. L. Heilborn, E. M. Aquino, M. Bozon and D. R. Knauth and published by Fiocruz/Garamond, Rio de Janeiro, in 2006.

References

Almeida, M. C. C. (2008) 'Gravidez na Adolescência e Escolaridade: Um Estudo em três Capitais Brasileiras', doctoral thesis, Instituto de Saúde Coletiva/Universidade Federal da Bahia.

Almeida, M. C. C., Aquino, E. M. L. and Barros, A. P. (2006) 'School Trajectory and Teenage Pregnancy in three Brazilian State Capitals', *Reports in Public Health*, 22 (Suppl.7): 1397–409.

Aquino, E. M. L., Almeida, M. C., Araújo, M. J. and Menezes, G. (2006) 'Gravidez na Adolescência: A Heterogeneidade Revelada', in Heilborn, M. L., Aquino, E. M. L., Bozon, M. and Knauth, D. R. (eds) *O Aprendizado da Sexualidade: Reprodução e Trajetórias Sociais de Jovens Brasileiros*, Rio de Janeiro: Garamond/Editora Fiocruz.

Aquino, E. M. L., Heilborn, M. L., Knauth, D. R., Bozon, M., Almeida, M. C. C., Araújo, M. J. *et al.* (2003) 'Adolescência e Reprodução no Brasil: A Heterogeneidade dos Perfis Sociais', *Cadernos de Saúde Pública*, 19: 377–88.

Berquó, E. (1998) 'Arranjos Familiares no Brasil: Uma Visão Demográfica', in *História da Vida Privada no Brasil. Contrastes da Intimidade Comtemporânea, Volume 4*, São Paulo: Companhia das Letras.

Berquó, E. and Cavenaghi, S. M. (2005) 'Increasing Adolescent and Youth Fertility in Brazil: A New Trend or a One-time Event?', paper presented at the Annual Meeting of the Population Association of America, Philadelphia, 30 March–2 April 2005. Session No. 151, Adolescent Fertility in Developing Countries; available at www.abep.nepo.unicamp.br/docs/ PopPobreza/BerquoElzaeCavenaghiSuzana.pdf (accessed 5 April 2009).

Bonell, C. (2004) 'Why is Teenage Pregnancy Conceptualized as a Social Problem? A Review of quantitative Research from the USA and UK', *Culture, Health and Sexuality*, 6 (3): 255–72.

Bozon, M. (2003) 'A quel Âge les Femmes et les Hommes commencent-ils leur Vie Sexuelle? Comparaisons Mondiales et Évolutions Récentes', *Population et Sociétés*, 391: 4.

Bozon, M. (2005) 'As Novas Formas de Entrada na Vida Sexual no Brasil e na América Latina', in Heilborn, M. L. *et al. Relações Familiares, Sexualidade e Ethos Religioso*, Rio de Janeiro: Garamond.

Bozon, M. and Heilborn, M. L. (2006) 'Iniciação à Sexualidade: Modos de Socialização, Interações de Gênero e Trajetórias Individuais', in Heilborn, M. L., Aquino, E. M. L., Bozon, M. and Knauth, D. R. (eds) *O Aprendizado da Sexualidade: Reprodução e Trajetórias Sociais de Jovens Brasileiros*, Rio de Janeiro: Garamond/Editora Fiocruz.

Brandão, E. R. (2005) 'Revelação da Gravidez na Adolescência em Famílias de Camadas Médias: Tensões e Dilemas', in Heilborn, M. L., Duarte, L. F. D., Peixoto, C. E. and Lins de Barros, M. (eds) *Família, Sexualidade e Ethos Religioso*, Rio de Janeiro: Garamond.

Breheny, M. and Stephens, C. (2007) 'Individual Responsibility and Social Constraint: The Construction of Adolescent Motherhood in Social Scientific Research', *Culture, Health and Sexuality*, 9 (4): 333–46.

Cabral, C. S. (2003) 'Contracepção e Gravidez na Adolescência na Perspectiva de Jovens Pais de uma Comunidade Favelada do Rio de Janeiro', *Cadernos de Saúde Pública*, 19 (Suppl. 2) : 283–92.

Camarano, A. A. (1998) 'Fecundidade e Anticoncepção da População Jovem', in Comissão Nacional de População e Desenvolvimento (CNPD) *Jovens Acontecendo na Trilha das Políticas Públicas, Volume 1*, Brasília (DF): CNPD.

Carvalho, J. E. C. (2007) 'How Can a Child be a Mother? Discourse on Teenage Pregnancy in a Brazilian Favela', *Culture, Health and Sexuality*, 9 (2): 109–20.

Costa, T. J. N. M. (2002) 'A Maternidade em Menores de 15 Anos em Juiz de Fora (MG): Uma Abordagem Socioantropológica', *Praia Vermelha. Estudos de Política e Teoria Social*, 7: 154–83.

Davies, L., McKinnon, M. and Rains, P. (1999) ' "On my Own": A new Discourse of Dependence and Independence from Teen Mothers', in Wong, J. and Checkland, D. (eds) *Teen Pregnancy and Parenting: Social and Ethical Issues*, Toronto: University of Toronto Press.

Gagnon, J. and Simon, W. (1973) *Sexual Conduct: The Social Sources of Human Sexuality*, Chicago: Aldine.

Galland, O. (1997) *Sociologie de la Jeunesse*. Paris: Armand Colin.

Heilborn, M. L., Aquino, E. M. L., Bozon, M. and Knauth, D. R. (eds) (2006) *O Aprendizado da Sexualidade: Reprodução e Trajetórias Sociais de Jovens Brasileiros*, Rio de Janeiro: Garamond/Editora Fiocruz.

Heilborn, M. L., Brandão, E. R. and Cabral, C. S. (2007) 'Teenage Pregnancy and Moral Panic in Brazil', *Culture, Health and* Sexuality, 9: 403–14.

Heilborn, M. L., Salem, T., Knauth, D. R., Aquino, E. M. L., Bozon, M., Rohden, F. *et al.* (2002) 'Aproximações Socioantropológicas sobre a Gravidez na Adolescência', *Horizontes Antropológicos*, 17 : 13–45.

Kirby, D. (1999) *Looking for Reasons Why: The Antecedents of Adolescent Sexual Risk-taking, Pregnancy, and Childbearing*, Washington, DC: National Campaign to Prevent Teen Pregnancy; available at www.popline.org/docs/1364/152782.html (accessed 10 March 2009).

Leite, I. C., Rodrigues, R. N. and Fonseca, M. C. (2004) 'Fatores Associados com o Comportamento Sexual e Reprodutivo entre Adolescentes das Regiões Sudeste e Nordeste do Brasil', *Reports in Public Health*, 20 (Suppl. 2): 474–81.

Le Van, C. (1998) *Les Grossesses à l'Adolescence: Normes Sociales, Réalités Vécues*, Paris: L'Harmattan.

Luker, K. (1996) *Dubious Conceptions: The Politics of Teenage Pregnancy*, Cambridge, MA: Harvard University Press.

Menezes, G., Aquino, E. M. L. and Silva, D. O. (2006) 'Induced Abortion during Youth: Social Inequalities in the Outcome of the First Pregnancy', *Reports in Public Health*, 22: 1431–46.

Ministério Da Saúde (2008) *PNDS 2006. Pesquisa Nacional de Demografia e Saúde da Criança e da Mulher*, Brasília: MS; São Paulo: CEBRAP.

Oliveira, J. C. (2005) *Perfil Socioeconômico da Maternidade nos Extremos do Período Reprodutivo*, Rio de Janeiro: IBGE, Diretoria de Pesquisas (DPE), Coordenação de População e Indicadores Sociais (COPIS).

Reis, A. O. A. (1993) 'O Discurso da Saúde Pública sobre a Adolescente Grávida: Avatares', (Tese de Doutorado em Saúde Coletiva), São Paulo: Universidade de São Paulo.

Schalet, A. (2004) 'Must we Fear Adolescent Sexuality?', *Medscape General Medicine*, 6: 4, 44.

Serra, J. (1999) 'Child-Mothers', *O Globo*, 15 August: 8.

Vilar, D. and Gaspar, A. M. (1999) 'Traços Redondos: A Gravidez em Mães Adolescentes', in Pais, J. M. (ed.) *Traços e Riscos de Vida. Uma Abordagem Qualitativa a Modos de Vida Juvenis*, Porto: Ambar.

World Health Organisation (WHO) (2001) *Sexual Relations among Young People in Developing Countries: Evidence from WHO Case Studies*. Geneva: World Health Organisation.

Part IV

How to have sex in an epidemic

19 Knowledge, power and HIV/AIDS

Research and the global response

Carlos F. Cáceres and Kane Race

Few events in the modern history of public health have elicited social consequences comparable to those of the HIV epidemic, and even fewer have had such dramatic effects on the way we think about and discuss sexuality. The HIV crisis has brought about dramatic changes in sexual cultures (Martin 1987; Evans *et al.* 1989), while simultaneously having a powerful impact on the health and social sciences (Patton 1990; Treichler 1988; Rosenbrock *et al.* 1999), the arts (Crimp 1988; Gott 1995), the women's and sexual diversity movements (Schneider and Stoller 1995; Jagose 1996) and the fields of both human and health rights (Mann and Tarantola 1998; Mann and Gruskin 1999; Petchesky 2003).

As several authors have argued (Watney 1987; Patton 1990; Epstein 1996; Sendziuk 2003), these processes of change were anything but consensual, and implied a complex chain of dialogue, negotiation and struggle involving a large number of institutions and constituencies. The source of disagreement varied with time: from the cause of the crisis, to the best forms of HIV prevention and care, to the responsibilities of the individual and government. Also in tension have been different forms of knowledge, which, based on their specific origin, producers and loyalties, called for contrasting courses of action. Rich understandings emerging from the community response have often been in tension with the scientific evidence (Watney 1990; Escoffier 1999; Rofes 1998; Kippax and Race 2003) posing problems for the consensual integration of knowledge, and reflecting epistemological positionings that are impossible to reconcile (Kippax 2003). While the need to move forward has pushed for solutions and helped to bring about consensus, evolving contexts constantly pose new and often unexpected tensions.

The goal of this chapter is to discuss how different epistemological positionings have determined specific forms of knowledge that have shaped the response to HIV, with a special focus on how this has affected both sexuality politics and the evolution of sexual cultures. We will also highlight a number of lessons learned from this analysis and suggest areas in which remaining gaps should be addressed to save time, energy and resources in the response to the epidemic and in the advance of sexual rights.

The emergence of HIV

While a detailed historical account of the emergence of HIV is beyond our focus and possibilities, an analysis of key elements in the history of the epidemic and the social response to it is crucial here. Early on, authors such as Susan Sontag (1989) were among the first to describe the powerful social meanings that AIDS had acquired: it was a deadly disease associated with painful deterioration of usually young bodies, but also affecting those on the margins of society, often on grounds of their sexuality. Interestingly, and regardless of the transmission routes taken by HIV in the 1970s, the epidemic was first recognised in the large urban centres of industrialised countries among members of the gay community, some of whose ideologists were still discussing the revolutionary potential of the gay lifestyles and mores. The early thesis of HIV being a sexually transmitted disease triggered a call for drastic changes in sexual behaviour, including condom use. It also mobilised the gay community and its allies to fight the crisis, while truncating ideological debate regarding the transgressive/liberating potential of gay culture (Crimp 2002). The significant decrease in unprotected anal sex observed among gay men of cities in the industrialised north during the first half of the 1980s is now recognised as a formidable achievement driven mostly out of the common sense knowledge of men who had (and enjoyed having) sex with other men, but who also realised how their practices could be linked to STI epidemics. It was this practical knowledge, in a community with high social capital, outraged and frightened by the crisis, that guided a major shift in this early history.

The identification of HIV in 1983 (Popovic *et al.* 1984) confirmed the infectious basis of the crisis. HIV was recognised as a lethal infectious disease with complex social causes as well as complex clinical and psychosocial manifestations. As a consequence, practitioners within a number of scientific fields became involved in the search for responses and solutions in an unprecedented fashion. They included professionals working in the basic sciences of virology and immunology, clinical medicine specialities, epidemiology, psychology and fields within the social sciences and cultural studies (Patton 1990; Stengers 1997). This heterogeneous 'expert' perspective interacted, on the one hand, with the needs of programme managers and decision makers, and, on the other hand with those of the community, which continued to play a key role particularly in asking for more resources, questioning international inequality in access to these, and especially calling for the accelerated search for a cure, for which they critiqued procedures for testing and approving new medicines (Epstein 1996). Such unprecedented community involvement significantly influenced the way in which the interaction with communities for now conceived of in health research and in other aspects of health policy, with concrete implications in what might stand as valid knowledge (Epstein 2007).

As the HIV epidemic gradually became visible in the rest of the world, including the Caribbean, Latin America, Asia and especially Africa, issues such as resources, economic and demographic consequences, human rights/health rights and north–south inequalities emerged, leading to an increasing number of professional fields becoming interested in HIV: economics, mathematical modelling, political science and the law (Petchesky 2003). Likewise, since the mid-1980s an official international response had started to take shape under the lead of the World Health Organisation, and one decade later the whole United Nations system would become involved through the creation of the Joint United Nations Programme on HIV/AIDS (UNAIDS) (Seckinelgin 2008).

The 'scientific response' and its social impact

While an in-depth analysis of disciplinary involvement and the power issues implicit in the scientific response to AIDS is also beyond the scope of this chapter, we will focus here on certain aspects that, reflecting distinct epistemological positioning of disciplinary bodies, had a direct impact on the formulation of a response to the epidemic in terms of (a) a discourse on causation, with moral implications; and (b) a prescription for a preventive response, particularly in relation to sexuality and sexual behaviour.

From the early 1980s until the mid-1990s, lack of effective treatment for HIV resulted in AIDS being seen as 'a death sentence' and a focus on primary prevention. Understanding of factors increasing the risk of HIV acquisition were largely defined by epidemiology, a discipline related historically to hygiene and tropical medicine, devoted to the study of the distribution and determinants of diseases. The first epidemiological studies compared persons diagnosed with AIDS with supposedly healthy controls, and suggested that specific risk factors included male homosexuality, haemophilia and injection drug use (Sonnabend *et al.* 1983). When HIV was later identified and a test became available to ascertain infection, studies were conducted to ascertain further the correlates of infection. Studies then identified unprotected anal and vaginal sex, high numbers of sex partners and sharing needles and equipment for drug use as key risk factors (Murray and Payne 1989).

In response to these findings, the first wave of science-led HIV prevention work aimed to modify 'high-risk behaviours', interpreted as the consequence of individual, rational decisions (Fishbein and Middlestadt 1989), and a number of prevention interventions were designed at this time by health psychologists and health educators. Over this same period, however, a significant tension emerged between those who advocated 'test and contain' strategies (i.e. the mass testing of 'high-risk' populations and restricting the movement and rights of infected individuals) and those who advocated community education, the protection of civil rights and anti-discrimination measures (Sendziuk 2003). The latter approach formed the basis of a new or 'social' public health, and came to be regarded as a more effective response to HIV (Rosenbrock *et al.* 2000; Kippax and Race 2003).

While in the past 50 years epidemiological theories and methods have become increasingly complex with the inclusion of multicausal frameworks and methods to study those frameworks, the use of more classical social theory (from which useful ideas could feed into causal models) in epidemiological reasoning has been very limited. In consequence, hypotheses about social phenomena or social determinants have often been poorly articulated in epidemiological and surveillance studies (Kippax and Race 2003). When theories were utilised, they were often highly individualistic. Social cognitive theories, for example, used to guide behavioural interventions also presumed empowered individuals making decisions based on rational choices, and disregarded the extent to which individuals either did not decide what they did sexually or did not have a chance to so decide given power imbalances with partners or broader conditions of vulnerability (Ingham *et al.* 1992; Kippax and Crawford 1993; Paicheler 2000). The limited impact that many programmes based on such models have had in the epidemic, as revealed both by research and programme evaluation (Cáceres 2000a) has led to a consensus about the insufficiency of individual models of sexual risk behaviour and behaviour change and has triggered the growth of other approaches that take a social/ structural perspective.

During the early 1990s an alternative paradigm began to emerge: significant interest began to be placed on ethnographic inquiry in an effort to describe sexual cultures under the assumption that (a) the specificities of sexual cultures implied the need to tailor behaviour change goals to each culture, and (b) approaches that changed cultural norms were needed to effective behaviour change (Cáceres 2000a). While this approach had some utility, the need was identified to go beyond a largely apolitical view of culture and recognise issues of power and inequality which, together with cultural meanings, play an important role in defining sexual practices across societies. This led to the development of a framework that has been central in understanding the difficulties experienced by prevention programs: that of *vulnerability*. This concept highlighted the structural inequalities that posed fundamental barriers to behaviour change: from limited access to resources, to gender power imbalances, to the exclusion of sexual and ethnic minorities. Vulnerability analysis has become a key element in international discourse on HIV since the late 1990s (Parker *et al.* 2000; Aggleton 2004), leading to efforts to mainstream the HIV response beyond the health sector, and justifying a multisectoral response (UNAIDS 1998).

While concepts of vulnerability have been powerful as an anchor to political commitment, their implications for response planning have been less clear. Conditions of vulnerability tend to be broad based, involve several factors simultaneously, and are not easily reducible to explanation within a single conceptual framework. While 'interventions' for vulnerability reduction have been implemented (Cáceres 2000b), the principle has never become generalised as such. Moreover, the practice of positioning certain (usually already marginalised) groups as vulnerable has drawn criticism to the extent that it failed to recognise the agency of such groups, shoring up support for paternalistic strategies, while leaving the practices of more dominant groups (such as heterosexual men) largely unexamined (Brown 2000; Waldby *et al.* 1993).

The onset of the new century was marked by increasing concern for universal access to the combination antiretroviral treatment that had become accessible in higher income countries in the mid-1990s and which transformed the disease into a chronic, treatable condition. A landmark meeting of the United Nations General Assembly in 2001 focused on AIDS led to new global commitments and established the goal of universal access to prevention and treatment as a human rights issue (Petchesky 2003). In consequence, new resources have been made available through so-called global HIV initiatives (Bernstein and Sessions 2007) with a clear focus on scaling up antiretroviral therapy. Since the mid-2000s, however, renewed attention has been given to HIV-prevention goals after it became clear that universal access to treatment would not be sustainable if high levels of infection continued to take place. In this new focus on prevention, however, novel elements emerged as well.

First, in programmes funded by the US President's Emergency Programme for AIDS Relief (PEPFAR), the focus was put on 'ABC', **a**bstinence, **b**e faithful and (if all else fails) use **c**ondoms. Such an approach was received with scepticism and regret by the international community given its overemphasis on A and B, being regarded as a controversial formula not supported by evidence (Collins *et al.* 2008). Second, adequate access to HIV prevention by 'key populations' (a term opted for to avoid the paternalistic flavour of 'vulnerable groups') began to be debated, with an increasing emphasis on a strengthened human rights discourse. Concern was expressed about the need to amend laws penalising homosexual behaviour, sex work or drug use, and to end violations of human rights towards the groups involved, not only because these pose structural barriers to prevention and care, but also for the sake of human rights per se. Third, new emphasis was given to biomedical prevention, encompassing preventive vaccines, post- and pre-exposure oral prophylaxis, microbicides and diaphragms, male circumcision and strategies based on the diagnosis and treatment of other STIs (Padian *et al.* 2008). While some concern was expressed about the re-emergence of a quest for 'magic bullets' in the biomedical field, recent failures of progress in these strategies have led to a call for a 'combination prevention' approach in which biomedical, behavioural and social/ structural prevention strategies are combined to maximum effect (Coates *et al.* 2008).

Productive exchanges and debates have also taken place between epidemiology and the social sciences. Social scientific approaches understand sex as a social practice, shaped and constructed in social contexts. A crucial concern within such approaches is how particular practices are given meaning and interpreted by those involved. This emphasis differs considerably from epidemiological understanding, which tends to focus mainly on enumerating sexual behaviours and disease incidence and correlating these items with individual variables. The focus on meanings and contexts found in social approaches is perhaps better able to position members of affected populations as agents, actively grappling with sexual and health understandings (Kippax and Race 2003). Such an approach has been particularly significant in identifying the changing HIV-prevention strategies or 'prevention ethics' devised by affected populations (Race 2003). These include the practice of 'negotiated safety' where regular but non-monogamous partners of HIV-negative status dispense with condoms in the context of the relationship but maintain condom use in sex outside the relationship (Kippax *et al.* 1993). This practice, which was first identified among gay men in countries such as Australia, was initially invisible from a conventional epidemiological perspective, which measured safety in terms of condom use only.

Transformations in sexuality and impact on stakeholders

What have been the effects of HIV-prevention work on sexual behaviours during the past 25 years? There is no simple answer, but among gay and other homosexually active men in most parts of the world there were significant reductions in unprotected anal sex with non-stable partners, particularly during the 1980s and 1990s (Evans *et al.* 1989). Over the past decade, however, changes seem to be occurring towards lower levels of condom use, reflecting the development of new risk reduction strategies, including serosorting, role selection, selective protection ('negotiated safety') and withdrawal before ejaculation (Van de Ven *et al.* 2002; Race 2003; Elford 2006). Among non-gay identified homosexually active men, practices have varied largely depending on education, access to services and feasibility of controlling the conditions in which they had sex (Cáceres *et al.* 2008a, 2008b). Among heterosexually active populations, condom use between stable partners has rarely become an established norm, even among serodiscordant couples (Grunseit *et al.*

1997), but has in some countries become more accepted with casual partners and especially with sex workers (Cáceres 2004).

And how have different constituencies been affected in this process? First, the different academic disciplines within the HIV field have experienced robust development over the past 20 years, not only because of need, but also because of increased resources. Likewise, HIV-related social movements have experienced transformations not thought of before the advent of AIDS. Concern to limit the sexual transmission of HIV has forced society to confront issues such as sexual diversity that were silenced beforehand. It has also helped legitimise academic work on sexuality. While early discourses were often unsympathetic to non-conventional sexualities, both the need to confront realities and renewed consciousness about the right to diversity has opened an unprecedented space for the discussion of sexuality and gender, and for the central inclusion of women's and lesbian/gay organisations in such discussion. This occurred first in higher income countries but has since extended to the rest of the world, including countries where homosexuality is still illegal (Petchesky 2003). Finally, a human rights perspective has become central in international HIV work, with a strong commitment to community building among people living with HIV (Mann and Tarantola 1998; Mann and Gruskin 1999).

Epilogue: how to produce knowledge at the crossroads of distinct streams of disciplinary power

This historical review of the social response to AIDS with a focus on sexuality and sexual constituencies has sought to illustrate the impact that the epidemic had on the way people think about, discuss and have sex. It has also attempted to describe key processes involved in that transformation, influenced by a changing discourse on sexuality which departed from an epidemiological perspective but has later been informed by views from the social sciences, human rights and affected communities themselves. A short account such as that which can be provided here inevitably simplifies a complex process full of contradictions, inconsistencies and partial certitudes. It does, however, stress the importance of different groups of stakeholders and their privileged discourses, based on power and authority, as well as on access to resources.

While the global response to HIV has brought greater commitment towards universal access and unprecedented resource mobilisation, the history recounted here illustrates how often contradictory discourses around HIV prevention can emerge, which have their origins in somewhat different understandings of social and human reality. While consensus building is often presumed necessary for global policy development, different stakeholders' positions are not equal. For example, the authority of epidemiology and biomedicine to articulate strategies for HIV-related behaviour change could not be questioned until their insufficiency became progressively clear. And despite some progress in multidisciplinary work, experience in cross-discipline collaboration remains limited; models requiring the instrumental involvement of social scientists to meet the goals set by biomedical scientists and epidemiologists remain more typical. Disagreements go far beyond epistemological perspectives, however, since new actors represent a broader array of interests. For example, pharmaceutical companies have become powerful stakeholders in HIV prevention now that a number of biomedical prevention strategies are being tested.

Research demonstrating the effectiveness of their products may lead to the large-scale use of antiretroviral medications in prevention, with major consequences for the future funding of sexual health programmes (Rosengarten 2009). Other actors too (e.g. academic groups, development agencies, activist organisations and others) often have competing interests beyond the epistemological realm.

Foucault (1978) was among the first to highlight how, in the nineteenth century, sexuality became the subject of a proliferation of discourses. The advent of HIV generated, and continues to generate, sexual prescriptions and pedagogies that reflect deeply held beliefs about sex and the sexual, but has also led to the emergence of new stakeholders and new notions of actorship. Out of 'disaster' (Altman 1988), the epidemic has transformed sex in a fundamental way, and has given a voice to many who did not have one before. This, in turn, has had many positive consequences – in research, in international relations and in perspectives on citizenship and rights. But this history will remain in progress until the epidemic comes to a close. Lessons to be learned from this process are numerous, and they point to the importance of truly horizontal transdisciplinary work, community involvement, transparency, accountability and real political will.

References

Aggleton, P. (2004) 'Sexuality, HIV Prevention, Vulnerability and Risk', *Journal of Psychology & Human Sexuality*, 16 (1): 1–13.

Altman, D. (1988) 'Legitimation through Disaster: AIDS and the Gay Movement', in Fee, E. and Fox, D. (eds) *AIDS: The Burdens of History*, Berkeley: University of California Press.

Bernstein, M. and Sessions, M. (2007) 'A Trickle or a Flood: Commitments and Disbursements for HIV/AIDS from the GFATM, PEPFAR and the World Bank's Multi-Country AIDS Program', Washington, DC: Center for Global Development.

Brown, T. (2000) 'AIDS, Risk and Social Governance', *Social Science and Medicine*, 50: 1273–84.

Cáceres, C. (2000a) 'The Production of Knowledge in the AIDS Era: Some Opportunities and Challenges', in Parker, R., Barbosa, R. and Aggleton, P. (eds) *Framing the Sexual Subject: The Politics of Gender, Sexuality and Power*, Berkeley: University of California Press.

Cáceres, C. (2000b) 'Relevant Social Dimensions for the Prevention of HIV/AIDS in Latin America and the Caribbean', in Izazola, J. (ed.) *A Multi-disciplinary Review of HIV/AIDS. Relevant Aspects for Decision-making in Latin America and the Caribbean*, Mexico City: FUNSALUD.

Cáceres, C. (2004) 'Intervenciones para la Prevención del VIH e ITS en América Latina y Caribe: Una Revisión de la Experiencia Regional', *Cadernos de Saúde Pública* 20 (6): 1466–83.

Cáceres, C. F., Aggleton, P. and Galea, J. (2008a) 'Sexual Diversity, Social Inclusion and HIV/AIDS', *AIDS*, 22 (Suppl. 2): S45–S55.

Cáceres, C. F., Konda, K. A., Segura, E. and Kyera, R. (2008b) 'Epidemiology of Male Same-sex Behaviour and Associated Sexual Health Indicators in Low and Middle-income Countries: 2003–2007 Estimates', *Sexually Transmitted Infections*, 84 (Suppl. 1): i49–i56.

Coates, T. J., Richter, L. and Cáceres, C. (2008) 'Behavioural Strategies to Reduce HIV Transmission: How to Make them work Better', *Lancet*, 372 (9639): 669–84.

Collins, C., Coates, T. J. and Curran, J. (2008) 'Moving beyond the Alphabet Soup of HIV Prevention', *AIDS*, 22 (Suppl. 2): S5–S8.

Crimp, D. (ed.) (1988) *AIDS: Cultural Analysis/Cultural Activism*, Cambridge, MA: MIT Press.

Crimp, D. (2002) *Melancholia and Moralism: Essays on AIDS and Queer Politics*, Cambridge, MA: MIT Press.

Elford, J. (2006) 'Changing Patterns of Sexual Behaviour in the Era of Highly Active Antiretroviral Therapy', *Current Opinion in Infectious Diseases*, 19 (1): 26–32.

Epstein, S. (1996) *Impure Science: AIDS, Activism and the Politics of Knowledge*, Berkeley and Los Angeles: University of California Press.

Epstein, S. (2007) *Inclusion: The Politics of Difference in Medical Research*, Chicago: University of Chicago Press.

Escoffier, J. (1999) 'The Invention of Safer Sex: Vernacular Knowledge, Gay Politics and HIV Prevention', *Berkeley Journal of Sociology*, 43: 1–30.

Evans, B., McLean, K., Dawson, S., Teece, S., Bond, R., MacRae, L. *et al.* (1989) 'Trends in Sexual Behaviour and Risk Factors for HIV Infection among Homosexual Men, 1984–7', *British Medical Journal*, 289: 215–18.

Fishbein, M. and Middlestadt, S. E. (1989) 'Using the Theory of Reasoned Action as a Framework for Understanding and Changing AIDS-related Behaviors', in Mays, V. M., Albee, G. W. and Schneider, S. F. (eds) *Primary Prevention of AIDS*, New York: Sage.

Foucault, M. (1978) *The History of Sexuality*, New York: Pantheon Books.

Gott, T. (1995) *Don't Leave Me This Way: Art in the Age of AIDS*, Canberra: National Gallery of Australia.

Grunseit, A., Kippax, S., Aggleton, P., Baldo, M. and Slutkin, G. (1997) 'Sexuality Education and Young People's Sexual Behaviour: A Review of Studies', *Journal of Adolescent Research*, 2 (4): 421–53.

Ingham, R., Woodcock, A. and Stenner, K. (1992) 'The Limitations of Rational Decision-making Models as Applied to Young People's Sexual Behaviour', in Aggleton, P., Davies, P. and Hart, G. (eds) *AIDS: Rights, Risk and Reason*, London: Falmer Press.

Jagose, A. (1996) *Queer Theory*, Melbourne: Melbourne University Press.

Kippax, S. (2003) 'Sexual Health Interventions are Unsuitable for Experimental Evaluation', in Stephenson, J., Imrie, J. and Bonell, C. (eds) *Effective Sexual Health Interventions: Issues in Experimental Evaluation*, Oxford: Oxford University Press.

Kippax, S. and Crawford, J. (1993) 'Flaws in the Theory of Reasoned Action', in Terry, D. J., Gallois, C. and McCamish, M. M. (eds) *The Theory of Reasoned Action: Its Applications to AIDS-preventive Behaviour*, Oxford: Pergamon.

Kippax, S. and Race, K. (2003) 'Sustaining Safe Practice: Twenty Years On', *Social Science and Medicine*, 57: 1–12.

Kippax, S., Crawford, J., Davis, M., Rodden, P. and Dowsett, G. (1993) 'Sustaining Safe Sex: A Longitudinal Study of a Sample of Homosexual Men', *AIDS*, 7: 257–63.

Mann, J. and Gruskin, S. (1999) *Health and Human Rights: A Reader*, New York and London: Routledge.

Mann, J. and Tarantola, D. (1998) 'Responding to HIV/AIDS: A Historical Perspective', *Health and Human Rights*, 2 (4): 5–8.

Martin, J. L. (1987) 'The Impact of AIDS on Gay Male Sexual Behavior Patterns in New York City', *American Journal of Public Health*, 77 (5): 578–81.

Murray, S. and Payne, K. (1989) 'The Social Classification of AIDS in American Epidemiology', *Medical Anthropology*, 10: 115–28.

Padian, N., Buvé, A., Balkus, J., Serwadda, D. and Cates, W. (2008) 'Biomedical Interventions to Prevent HIV Infection: Evidence, Challenges, and Way Forward', *Lancet*, 372 (9638): 585–99.

Paicheler, G. (2000) 'Understanding Risk Management', in Moatti, J. P., Souteyrand, Y., Prieur, A., Sandfort, T. and Aggleton, P. (eds) *AIDS in Europe: New Challenges for the Social Sciences*, London and New York: Routledge.

Parker, R. G., Easton, D. and Klein, C. (2000) 'Structural Barriers and Facilitators in HIV Prevention: A Review of International Research', *AIDS*, 14 (Suppl. 1): S22-S32.

Patton, C. (1990) *Inventing AIDS*, New York: Routledge.

Petchesky, R. (2003) *Global Prescriptions: Gendering Health and Human Rights*, London: Zed Books.

Popovic, M., Sarngadharan, M. G., Read, E. and Gallo, R. C. (1984) 'Detection, Isolation, and

Continuous Production of Cytopathic Retroviruses (HTLV-III) from Patients with AIDS and Pre-AIDS', *Science*, 224: 497–500.

Race, K. (2003) 'Revaluation of Risk among Gay Men', *AIDS Education and Prevention*, 15 (4): 369–81.

Rofes, E. (1998) *Dry Bones Breathe: Gay Men Creating Post-AIDS Identities and Cultures*, New York and London: Harrington Park Press.

Rosenbrock, R., Dubois-Arber, F., Moers, M., Pinell, P., Schaeffer, D. and Setbon, M. (2000) 'The Normalization of AIDS in Western European Countries' *Social Science and Medicine*, 50: 1607–29.

Rosenbrock, R., Schaeffer, D., Dubois-Arber, F., Moers, M., Pinell, P., Setbon, M. *et al.* (1999) *The AIDS Policy Cycle in Western Europe: From Exceptionalism to Normalization*, Berlin: Research Unit, Public Health Policy.

Rosengarten, M. (2009) *HIV Interventions: Biomedicine and the Traffic between Information and Flesh*, Washington: University of Washington Press.

Schneider, B. and Stoller, N. E. (eds) (1995) *Women Resisting AIDS: Feminist Strategies of Empowerment*, Philadelphia: Temple University Press.

Seckinelgin, H. (2008) *International Politics of HIV/AIDS*, New York: Routledge.

Sendziuk, P. (2003) *Learning to Trust: Australian responses to AIDS*, Sydney: University of New South Wales Press.

Sonnabend, J., Witkin, S. and Purtilo, D. (1983) 'Acquired Immunodeficiency Syndrome, Opportunistic Infections and Malignancies in Male Homosexuals: A Hypothesis of Etiologic Factors in Pathogenesis', *Journal of the American Medical Association*, 249: 2370–4.

Sontag, S. (1989) *AIDS and its Metaphors*, New York: Farrar, Straus, & Giroux.

Stall, R. D., Coates, T. J. and Hoff, C. (1988) 'Behavioral Risk Reduction for HIV Infection among Gay and Bisexual Men. A Review of Results from the United States', *American Psychologist*, 43: 878–5.

Stengers, I. (1997) *Power and Invention: Situating Science*, Minneapolis and London: Minnesota University Press.

Treichler, P. (1988) 'An Epidemic of Signification', in Crimp, D. (ed.) *AIDS: Cultural Analysis/Cultural Activism*, Cambridge, MA: MIT Press.

UNAIDS (1998) *Expanding the Global Response to HIV/AIDS Through Focused Action: Reducing Risk and Vulnerability: Definitions, Rationale and Pathways*, Geneva: UNAIDS; available at www.un.org.kh/unaids/pdfs/una98e1.pdf (accessed 14 February 2009).

Van de Ven, P., Kippax, S., Crawford, J., Rawstorne, P., Prestage, G., Grulich, A. *et al.* (2002) 'In a Minority of Gay Men, Sexual Risk Practice Indicates Strategic Positioning for Perceived Risk Reduction rather than Unbridled Sex', *AIDS Care*, 14: 471–80.

Waldby, C., Kippax, S. and Crawford, J. (1993) 'Cordon Sanitaire: "Clean" and "Unclean" Women in the AIDS Discourse of Young Men', in Aggleton, P., Davies, P. and Hart, G. (eds) *AIDS: Facing the Second Decade*, London: Falmer Press.

Watney, S. (1987) *Policing Desire: Pornography, AIDS and the Media*, London: Methuen.

Watney, S. (1990) 'Safer Sex as Community Practice', in Aggleton, P., Davies, P. and Hart, G. (eds) *AIDS: Individual, Cultural and Policy Dimensions*, London: Falmer Press.

20 Safe sex

It's not as simple as ABC

Susan Kippax

HIV is a blood-borne virus transmitted by sexual practice, particularly penetrative intercourse (vaginal or anal) with an HIV-infected person; by the sharing of HIV-contaminated needles and syringes; from an HIV-positive mother to her child during birth and breast feeding; and via the transfusion of HIV-infected blood and blood products. It is estimated that over 25 million people have died of AIDS and 33 million people are living with HIV, with 95 per cent living in low/middle income countries (UNAIDS 2007; Cohen *et al.* 2008). In 2007 2.5 million people became infected with HIV, while 2.1 million people died of AIDS (UNAIDS 2007). Each year, prevalence has increased as new infections outstrip the number of deaths. So although the global incidence rate is thought to have peaked, the absolute number of HIV infections continues to grow (UNAIDS 2007).

In response to what is a growing global crisis, questions have been raised concerning the efficacy and effectiveness of HIV prevention efforts, particularly those addressing sexual transmission. As sexual transmission accounts for the majority of HIV infections, this chapter focuses on HIV prevention with reference to sexual practice, that is, on the promotion of 'safe sex'. Why has safe sex been so difficult to achieve?

HIV-prevention 'failure' is a function of at least three factors: the promotion of non-efficacious or ineffective HIV-prevention strategies; the ineffective promotion efficacious strategies; and a failure to address the sociocultural and political factors driving/producing sexual risk. The first two factors are to a large extent a function of the third: the failure to address the sociocultural and political contexts in which sexual practice and associated sexual risk is enacted, and HIV-prevention education is positioned. In order to address these questions I focus on the social aspects of HIV prevention and in particular on the difference between sexual 'behaviour' and sexual 'practice'.

First, however, it is necessary to distinguish between *efficacy* and *effectiveness*. Many public health researchers appear to confuse or conflate the two (e.g. see Potts *et al.* 2008). Effectiveness is different from efficacy in important ways. Aral and Peterman (1998) define efficacy as 'the improvement in health outcome achieved in a research setting, in expert hands, under ideal circumstances' and they define effectiveness as 'the impact an intervention achieves in the real world, under resource constraints, in entire populations, or in specified subgroups of a population' (p. 33). So while effectiveness is the improvement in a health outcome in the real world, efficacy refers to whether, under ideal conditions, a particular prevention tool works. So, for example, condoms when used correctly and consistently under clinical trial conditions prevent HIV transmission in 95 per cent of cases, in real life their effectiveness falls somewhat short of 95 per cent – because in real life they are not always used and, when used, they are sometimes not used properly.

Prevention strategies

What 'tools' or prevention strategies do we have to prevent or, at least, reduce the likelihood of the sexual transmission of HIV? Among those currently advocated, the most common 'behavioural' prevention tools are the **ABC**: **a**bstinence from sex or the delay of sexual initiation/debut, **b**eing faithful to one partner/practising monogamy and **c**ondom use.

Others although not advocated by many have nonetheless been adopted by some and these include: the practice of serosorting, i.e. engaging in unprotected sex only with those believed to be the same HIV serostatus as oneself; and withdrawal before ejaculation.

More recently there has been a push to promote so-called 'biomedical' prevention strategies. They are so named to distinguish them from behavioural strategies such as those just listed, however, with the exception of male circumcision, most biomedical prevention strategies require behavioural change of some sort. Current biomedical strategies include: microbicide use, treatment of sexually transmissible diseases, male circumcision, use of antiretroviral therapy used as pre-exposure prophylaxis and use of antiretroviral therapy to reduce viral load in individuals living with HIV.

Abstinence is 100 per cent efficacious – in the sense that, if practised, HIV cannot be sexually transmitted. Similarly, if lifelong monogamy is practised by both HIV-negative sexual partners, then it, too, is 100 per cent efficacious. Condoms, when properly and consistently used, are around 95 per cent efficacious (Pinkerton and Abramson 1997). However, withdrawal has been shown not to have reliable efficacy and serosorting is efficacious only under certain conditions (see later discussion of 'negotiated safety') (Zablotska *et al.* 2009; Jin *et al.* 2009). Male circumcision has been shown to be around 50–55 per cent efficacious in preventing HIV transmission from women to men (Nagelkerke *et al.* 2007), while evidence for the efficacy of treating sexually transmissible infections (STIs) continues to be debated and there is growing evidence that its impact on HIV control appears to be minimal (Potts *et al.* 2008). While the efficacy of antiretroviral therapy for the prevention of mother-to-child transmission is proven (Sperling *et al.* 1996) the efficacy of pre-exposure prophylaxis with reference to sexual transmission remains uncertain as does the efficacy of microbicides and efficacy trials are ongoing. There is ongoing debate about the efficacy of using antiretroviral therapy to reduce viral load and hence prevent or reduce the likelihood of sexual HIV transmission between serodiscordant partners (Garnett and Gazzard 2008; Vernazza *et al.* 2008; Wilson *et al.* 2008).

So at the time of writing, with reference to the sexual transmission of HIV *efficacious* prevention tools available are abstinence, being faithful, consistent condom use and, to a lesser degree, male circumcision. There is no vaccine and at present the efficacy of microbicides and pre-exposure prophylaxis has not been shown.

Compared with efficacious prevention tools, there are fewer effective prevention tools and the clarity of evidence is diminished. This is because effectiveness cannot be assessed under ideal conditions but rather is concerned with the social, political and economic conditions of people's everyday lives and the place that sex occupies within individual lives and communities. There is no evidence that abstinence is effective and little evidence that delaying sexual initiation works – at least in the industrialised world (Grunseit *et al.* 1997; Weaver *et al.* 2005).

The evidence with regard to the effectiveness of monogamy (being faithful) is very patchy and debate continues. While a range of factors, which include the practice of zero grazing (fidelity) and condom use, appears to have reduced HIV transmission in Uganda (Shelton *et al.* 2004; Epstein 2007; Potts *et al.* 2008), fidelity is more a fiction than a fact of adult sexual life (Holtzman and McLeroy 2007). Many men have extramarital sex: sociocultural structures produce the desire for sexual reputation among men exacerbating gender inequality and giving rise to infidelity in married men – in Mexico (Hirsch *et al.* 2007) and in Papua New Guinea (Wardlow 2007). In the context of no condom use, extramarital sex leaves wives (even if faithful themselves) vulnerable to HIV, for example, married women in some African countries (Smith 2007) and in India (Holtzman and McLeroy 2007). Infidelity in men and women and concurrent sexual partnering is often the outcome of economic need which results in forced migration for work. For example, about 35 per cent of all documented HIV cases in the Philippines are among returning overseas workers, as were 42 per cent of new cases recorded in 2006 (CARAM 2007).

Studies have shown that prevention programmes advocating condom use have been associated with a 50 to 90 per cent effectiveness in both high income as well as low and middle income countries (Auerbach 2006; Noar 2008). For example, there is evidence that condom use is effective in lowering HIV incidence among gay men in Australia (Kippax and Race 2003; Bowtell 2005) and among sex workers in Thailand (Hanenberg *et al.* 1994) and India (Evans and Lambert 2008). But it is also true to say that in much of the world their use is neither widespread nor consistent (Global HIV Prevention Working Group 2008).

Whether male circumcision is effective or not remains to be seen and some researchers have argued that recent evidence indicates that the protective claims are overstated (Myers and Myers 2007). On the basis of an analysis of a cross-sectional national household-based community survey in South Africa carried out in 2002, Connolly *et al.* concluded that 'male circumcision does not appear to be protective against HIV infection among men in South Africa' (Connolly *et al.* 2008: 793). Certainly, time is needed to assess the impact of circumcision in the real world and, in particular, to assess whether male circumcision inhibits condom use.

So with reference to *effectiveness*, we can say that condom use lowers HIV incidence in some countries and contexts, but not in others, and that while reduction in number of partners in general and fidelity in particular have an impact on HIV infection rates at the population level to slow the HIV epidemic, fidelity does not protect all individuals. More evidence is needed with reference to male circumcision.

In general, with regard to behavioural change, according to the available evidence, strategies that prove to be effective are likely to pursue a combination of behaviour change strategies – condom use and reduction in number of partners (Rutherford 2008). Furthermore, as I shall describe later, they are likely to be effective only if these 'safe' sex strategies are promoted in such a way as to engage the communities and sub-populations at risk so as to enable normative as well as individual change (Global HIV Prevention Working Group 2008).

Social aspects of prevention

The major reason for the unevenness of the effectiveness of HIV prevention strategies and the lack of clarity with regard to evidence of effectiveness when compared with efficacy, is that the practices that comprise the prevention strategies – condom use, 'being faithful' – are cultural practices par excellence. Male circumcision, too, albeit in a somewhat different way, is a cultural practice linked in many societies to initiation rites associated with manhood (Aggleton 2007). Furthermore, because effectiveness, unlike efficacy, refers to health improvement in the real world, it is dependent to some degree on how these strategies – fidelity, condom use and male circumcision are promoted and, in turn, understood and taken up by those whose attend to the health promotion messages.

Practices are socially produced: they are behaviours that are organised and patterned by culture. They cannot be sensibly understood as the behaviour of individuals. The forms sexual behaviour takes are, to a large degree, organised by the sociocultural, economic and political structures in which they are situated and produced (Kippax 2003). The practices that give rise to HIV infection/transmission or contribute to the likelihood of transmission are, to some extent, under the control of those individuals who engage in sexual activity. These individuals are thus open to social transformation and change, via education, health promotion and HIV prevention campaigns, where the information contained within is actively appropriated not simply passively imbibed (Stephenson and Kippax 2006; Kippax 2008).

Practice not behaviour

While sexual behaviour may be similar across time and place, sexual practice differs. There are only a small number of sexual behaviours in which two or more people can engage: vaginal and anal intercourse; oral-genital sex (fellatio) and oral-anal sex, a number of more esoteric behaviours, such as sadomasochism, as well as a range of behaviours that involve touching, mutual masturbatory behaviours. Sexual practice, by way of contrast, is more fluid: it takes on a number of forms. It is enacted in marriage or regular relationships, concurrent partnering, sex work, casual sexual encounters; it involves sexual initiation, changes of regular partner, group sex, rape and so on. In real life, people do not engage in sexual behaviours – penis-in-vagina or penis-in-anus – rather they enact sexual practices: they 'make love', 'have a one night stand', 'lose their virginity' or reassert their sexuality. They act for pleasure, for money, for control. In response to sexual desire, they communicate their love to one another and build intimacy and trust.

Practices are socially produced; they are behaviours that are organised and patterned by culture and organised with reference to normative understandings or discourses: they have meaning (Kippax 2003). As many researchers have pointed out, the most powerful influences on human sexuality are social norms – morals, taboos, laws, beliefs – that regulate and govern its expression. The scale of the regional diversity in sexual practice is matched only by the range of cultural constraints on practice (Wellings *et al.* 2006).

What is in need of modification is sexual practice and in order to do that prevention experts need to engage with the social and cultural forms that give rise to it.

They also need to understand that the HIV prevention strategies that are being promoted, such as condom use and fidelity and male circumcision, are themselves practices. How people respond to the promotion of each of these, especially whether they adopt them or not, will vary depending on how the promoted prevention strategies are understood with reference to people's sexual relationships and sexual practices. For example, the introduction of condoms into the marriage bed is a very different act from suggesting they might be used with a casual sexual partner. What do people understand by 'faithfulness'? While some clearly understand monogamy as 'lifelong', others – particularly those in countries with high income, read 'fidelity' as serial monogamy, and for others in stable concurrent relationships, fidelity will have a different understanding.

Uses of health information

Prevention information is not passively imbibed by individuals but is actively taken up (appropriated) through talk and collective action within given social and structural contexts in order to acquire meaning. The advice of public health workers, doctors and nurses, is not simply accepted passively. Indeed unless prevention information is actively taken up it is unlikely to be effective. To illustrate: the majority of gay men in high income countries have regulated their sexual practice depending on the interpersonal context – regular, casual encounter; in terms of whether they are HIV positive or HIV negative; and in terms of the prevailing cultural or community norms that are generally responsive to current medical knowledge. This knowledge, however, is not simply accepted but appropriated in ways that can best support intimacy and pleasure, love and desire in gay communities – and as well reduce risk of HIV transmission. Findings from studies of gay men in Australia demonstrate the ways in which gay men have developed a number of risk-reduction strategies over time in response to changing community norms that, in turn, have changed in response to changing medical knowledge (Kippax and Race 2003).

The strategies used by gay men in Australia include condom use and most gay men use condoms consistently – at least with casual sexual partners (Imrie and Frankland 2008). Gay men, however, also fashioned other harm-reduction strategies for themselves; strategies that allowed them to dispense with condoms under certain conditions. These strategies include: negotiated safety (a strategy of dispensing with condoms within HIV seroconcordant-negative regular relationships under certain conditions – one of which includes monogamy) (Kippax *et al.* 1993; Kippax *et al.* 1997); positive-positive sex (a strategy of dispensing with condoms when two HIV-positive men engage in sex) (Prestage *et al.* 2001); strategic positioning (a strategy for discordant couples in which the HIV-positive man takes up the receptive position in anal sex) (Van de Ven *et al.* 2002); and, to a lesser extent, reliance on undetectable viral load (a strategy of dispensing with condoms when one's sexual partner has 'undetectable' viral load) (Van de Ven *et al.* 2005). All these strategies carry some risk – but most of them do reduce risk to a greater or lesser extent (Jin *et al.* 2009).

All these strategies – with the exception of condom use, rely on knowledge of HIV status. Their adoption is dependent on: the interpersonal nature of the relationship (regular/casual) and whether the sexual partnership is seroconcordant (both of the same HIV status) or not; the social and cultural contexts of the sex ('marital bed', beat, sauna, sex club, sex party); and the prevailing cultural or community norms associated with HIV prevention, which are informed by HIV-prevention campaigns and programmes as well as current medical knowledge. These strategies came from community, from community members appropriating medical knowledge as well as from 'folk' knowledges that emerge as affected community members seek to reduce the likelihood of HIV transmission.

Community members are not isolated individuals but are persons connected through complex webs of social relationships. The strategies, the effective and sustainable strategies, came from within – from the bottom up not the top down. While mass media campaigns, targeted campaigns, peer-based education, school-based sex education and voluntary counselling and testing are all important sources of information and skills, the safe sex messages will not be taken up or if taken up not sustained unless the strategies being promoted and advocated are strategies that make sense to those to whom they are targeted. Political and community support of the prevention strategies are indispensable for an effective and sustained response to HIV (Kippax 2006). Communities (of gay men, of sex workers, of young people) must appropriate the health promotion messages and make them their own.

Conclusions

Effective HIV prevention needs to address the local and specific circumstances of the populations and communities it seeks to engage in 'safe' sex. It should also aim to affect multiple determinants of human practice – including individual knowledge, interpersonal relationships, community and societal norms (Global HIV Prevention Working Group 2008). Essential ingredients of HIV-prevention success are political and hence public acknowledgement of people's sexual lives and a detailed understanding of the ways in which risk is locally produced via social and cultural drivers. Like Australia, Brazil encouraged open discussion of HIV and supported frank public awareness campaigns as well as campaigns and prevention programmes targeting gay men and sex workers, condom promotion and school-based HIV education. As a result, condom use increased by almost 50 per cent among sexually active adults between 1998 and 2005 and HIV prevalence was maintained at a low level among sex workers (Global HIV Prevention Working Group 2008). Other success stories in Thailand and Uganda similarly illustrate the importance of working with communities at risk and engaging and supporting their efforts to reduce their own risk. Global success is dependent on local initiatives: HIV prevention must engage and build on local responses.

Social theorists agree that individual behaviour is always mediated and structured by social relationships, which are, in turn, traversed by important differences in community, social status, class and other structural differences such as sexuality and age. Individual behaviour is always contextual, always socially embedded. HIV prevention that does not engage with the social is likely to fail. Safe sex is not as simple as ABC – but many countries and communities using comprehensive, public and realistic prevention programmes that both take account of the social production of sexual practice and are politically supported have promoted it effectively.

References

Aggleton, P. (2007) '"Just a Snip?" A Social History of Male Circumcision', *Reproductive Health Matters*, 15: 15–21.

Aral, S. O. and Peterman, T. A (1998) 'Do We Know the Effectiveness of Behavioural Interventions?', *Lancet*, 351 (Suppl. 111): 33–6.

Auerbach, J. D. (2006) 'Overview of Effective and Promising Interventions to Prevent HIV Infection', in Ross, D. A., Dick, B. and Ferguson, J. (eds) *Preventing HIV/AIDS in Young People: A Systematic Review of Evidence from Developing Countries*, Geneva: WHO (WHO Technical Report Series No. 938).

Bowtell, W. (2005) *Australia's Response to HIV/AIDS: 1982–2005*, Sydney: Lowy Institute for Health Policy.

CARAM (2007) *State of Health of Migrants*, Kuala Lumpur. CARAM Asia.

Cohen, M. S., Hellmann, N., Levy, J. A., DeCock, K. and Lange, J. (2008) 'The Spread, Treatment, and Prevention of HIV-1: Evolution of a Global Pandemic', *Journal of Clinical Investigation*, 118: 1244–54.

Connolly, C., Simbayi, L., Shanmugam, R. and Nqeketo, A. (2008) 'Male Circumcision and its Relationship to HIV Infection in South Africa: Results of a National Survey in 2002', *South African Medical Journal*, 98: 789–94.

Epstein, H. (2007) *The Invisible Cure: Africa, the West, and the Fight Against AIDS*, New York: Farrar, Straus, & Giroux.

Evans, C. and Lambert, H. (2008) 'The Limits of Behaviour Change Theory: Condom Use and Contexts of HIV Risk in the Kolkata Sex Industry', *Culture, Health and Sexuality*, 10: 27–42.

Garnett, G. P. and Gazzard, B. (2008) 'Risk of HIV Transmission in Discordant Couples', *Lancet*, 372: 270–1.

Global HIV Prevention Working Group (2008) *Behavior Change and HIV Prevention: [Re]Considerations for the 21st Century*, Bill and Melinda Gates Foundation and the Henry J. Kaiser Family Foundation; available at www.GlobalHIVPrevention.org.

Grunseit, A., Kippax, Susan, Aggleton, P., Baldo, M. and Slutkin, G. (1997) 'Sexuality Education and Young People's Sexual Behaviour: A Review of Studies', *Journal of Adolescent Research*, 2 (4): 421–53.

Hanenberg, R. S., Rojanapithayakorn, W., Kunasol, P. and Sokal, D. C. (1994) 'Impact of Thailand's HIV Control Programmes as Indicated by the Decline in Sexually Transmitted Diseases', *Lancet*, 344: 243–5.

Hirsch, J. S., Meneses, S., Thompson, B. and Negroni, M. (2007) 'The Inevitability of Infidelity: Sexual Reputation, Social Geographies, and Marital Risk in Rural Mexico', *American Journal of Public Health*, 97: 986–96.

Holtzman, D. and McLeroy, K. R. (2007) 'Fiction or Fidelity: The Moral Economy of HIV Risk', *American Journal of Public Health*, 97: 971.

Imrie, J. and Frankland, A. (2008) *HIV/AIDS, Hepatitis and Sexually Transmissible Infections in Australia: Annual Report of Trends in Behaviour 2008*, Sydney: National Centre in HIV Social Research, University of New South Wales.

Jin, F., Crawford, J., Prestage, G., Zablotska, I., Imrie, J., Kippax, S. *et al.* (2009) 'Unprotected Anal Intercourse, Risk Reduction Behaviours, and Subsequent HIV Infection in a Cohort of Homosexual Men', *AIDS*, 23: 243–52.

Kippax, S. (2003) 'Sexual Health Interventions are Unsuitable for Experimental Evaluation', in Stephenson, J. M., Imrie, J. and Bonell, C. (eds) *Effective Sexual Health Interventions: Issues In Experimental Evaluation*, Oxford: Oxford University Press.

Kippax, S. (2006) 'A Public Health Dilemma: A Testing Question', *AIDS Care*, 18: 230–5.

Kippax, S. (2008) 'Understanding and Integrating the Structural and Biomedical Determinants of HIV Infection: A Way Forward for Prevention', *Current Opinion in HIV and AIDS*, 3: 489–94.

Kippax, S. and Race, K. (2003) 'Sustaining Safe Practice: Twenty Years On', *Social Science & Medicine*, 57: 1–12.

Kippax, S., Crawford, J., Davis, M., Rodden, P. and Dowsett, G. W. (1993) 'Sustaining Safe Sex: A Longitudinal Study of a Sample of Homosexual Men, *AIDS*, 7: 257–63.

Kippax, S., Noble, J., Prestage, G., Crawford, J. M., Campbell, D., Baxter, D. *et al.* (1997) 'Sexual Negotiation in the "AIDS Era": Negotiated Safety Revisited', *AIDS*, 11 (2): 191–7.

Myers, A. and Myers, J. (2007) 'Male Circumcision – A New Hope?', *South African Medical Journal*, 97: 338–41.

Nagelkerke, N. J. D., Moses, S., de Vlas, S. J. and Bailey, R. C. (2007) 'Modelling the Public Health Impact of Male Circumcision for HIV Prevention in High-prevalence Areas in Africa', *BMC for Infectious Diseases*, 7: 16.

Noar, S. M. (2008) 'Behavioural Interventions to reduce HIV-related Sexual Risk Behavior: Review and Synthesis of Meta-analytic Evidence', *AIDS and Behavior*, 3: 335–53.

Pinkerton, S. D. and Abramson, P. R. (1997) 'Effectiveness of Condoms in Preventing HIV Transmission', *Social Science & Medicine*, 44: 1303–12.

Potts, M., Halperin, D., Kirby, D., Swidler, A., Marseille, E., Klausner, J. D. *et al.* (2008) 'Reassessing HIV Prevention', *Science*, 320: 749–50.

Prestage, G., Van de Ven, P., Grulich, A., Kippax, S., McInnes, D. and Hendry, O. (2001) 'Gay Men's Casual Sex Encounters: Discussing HIV and using Condoms', *AIDS Care*, 13: 277–84.

Rutherford, G. (2008) 'Condoms in Concentrated and Generalised HIV Epidemics', *Lancet*, 372: 275–6.

Shelton, J. D., Halperin D. T., Nantulya V., Potts, M., Gayle, H. D. and Holmes, K. K. (2004) 'Partner Reduction is Crucial for Balanced "ABC" Approach to HIV Prevention', *British Medical Journal*, 328: 891–3.

Smith, D. J. (2007) 'Modern Marriage, Men's Extramarital Sex, and HIV Risk in Southeastern Nigeria', *American Journal of Public Health*, 97: 997–1005.

Sperling, R. S., Shapiro, D. E., Coombs, R. W., Todd, J. A., Herman, S. A., McSherry, G. D. *et al.* (1996) 'Maternal Viral Load, Zidovudine Treatment, and the Risk of HIV Transmission of Human Immunodeficiency Virus Type 1 from Mother to Infant', *New England Journal of Medicine*, 335: 1621–9.

Stephenson, N. and Kippax, S. (2006) 'Transfiguring Relations: Theorizing Political Change in the Everyday', *Theory & Psychology*, 16: 391–415.

UNAIDS (2007) *AIDS Epidemic Update: December 2007*; available at http//:www.unaids.org/en/KnowledgeCentre/HIVData/EpiUpdateArchive/2007 (accessed 5 May 2008).

Van de Ven, P., Kippax, S., Crawford, J., Rawstorne, P., Prestage, G., Grulich, A. *et al.* (2002) 'In a Minority of Gay Men, Sexual Risk Practice indicates Strategic Positioning for perceived Risk Reduction rather than Unbridled Sex', *AIDS Care*, 14 (4): 471–80.

Van de Ven, P., Mao, L., Fogarty, A., Rawstorne, P., Crawford, J., Prestage, G. *et al.* (2005) 'Undetectable Viral Load is associated with Sexual Risk Taking in HIV Serodiscordant Gay Couples in Sydney', *AIDS*, 19: 179–84.

Vernazza, P., Hirschel, B., Bernasconi, E. and Flepp, M. (2008) 'Les Personnes Seropositives ne souffrant d'aucune autre MST et suivant un Traitement Antiretroviral Efficace ne transmettent pas le VIH par Voie Sexuelle', *Bulletin des Médecins Suisses*, 89: 165–9.

Wardlow, H. (2007) 'Men's Extramarital Sexuality in rural Papua New Guinea', *American Journal of Public Health*, 97: 1006–14.

Weaver, H., Smith, G. and Kippax, S. (2005) 'School-based Sex Education Policies and Indicators of Sexual Health among Young People: A Comparison of the Netherlands, France, Australia and the United States', *Sex Education*, 5 (2): 171–88.

Wellings, K., Collumbien, M., Slaymaker, E., Singh, S., Hodges, Z., Patel, D. *et al.* (2006) 'Sexual Behaviour in context: A Global Perspective', *Lancet,* 368: 1706–28.

Wilson, D. P., Law, M. G., Grulich, A. E., Cooper, D. A. and Kaldor, J. M. (2008) 'Relation between HIV Viral Load and Infectiousness: A Model-based Analysis', *Lancet*, 372: 314–20.

Zablotska, I., Imrie, J., Prestage, G., Crawford, J., Rawstorne, P., Grulich, A. *et al.* (2009) 'Gay Men's current Practice of HIV Seroconcordant Unprotected Anal Intercourse: Serosorting or Seroguessing?', *AIDS Care*, 21: 501–10.

21 Exporting moralities

Dennis Altman

> The religious right is not simply a religious movement or a political movement; it has also, and above all, been a sexual movement. Nowhere has this been more evident than in the way the U.S. government's involvement in the project of HIV/AIDS prevention globally was invested with a sexually conservative agenda from the very beginning.
>
> (Herzog: 159)

For 20 years, a standard critique of US government responses to the HIV pandemic has been that it revealed a puritan distaste for sex, shown in the reluctance to support measures, such as condom promotion and support for gay and sex worker groups, which were a staple of the response in at least some other western countries. Many liked to point to the divergence between the US response and that of, say, Switzerland, the Netherlands and Australia as evidence of a significant cultural difference, rather as, several decades later, it became fashionable to juxtapose US and European values. The idea that 'America is from Mars, Europe from Venus', which was the name of an academic conference in Berkeley in 2006, became the popularised version of Robert Kagan's (2003) more fundamental claim for growing divergence across the Atlantic. Kagan does not write of matters sexual, but he might well have used issues such as gay marriage and sex education to demonstrate his claims for a growing cultural gap.

The role of the USA in helping define, frame and finance the global response to HIV and AIDS far outweighs that of any other country, and the religious right has undoubtedly had a considerable influence on this response. At the same time, other forces have been prominent in supporting rather different responses, such as strong support for emerging gay groups and programmes directed at male to male sex. While it is easy to point to the sex-negative aspects of official US policy, this too easily ignores the larger cultural, social and political impact of very different influences from within the USA. More important, it becomes an alibi for other governments that show equal distaste for recognising the sexual transmission of HIV, but who largely escape scrutiny because so much hostility is focused on the USA.

From its discovery, through the illnesses of young gay men on the two coasts in 1981, the USA has been central to global developments around the new epidemic, which in many places was originally conceptualised as an 'American' disease, such that in Japan and the Philippines gay bars and saunas originally banned westerners as if they carried contamination with them. An American disease perhaps? – but also one associated with globalisation, both in its spread and the responses to the epidemic. HIV was carried across military, trade and tourist routes, and even if the theory that a certain Quebecois air steward was Patient Zero, and somehow the source, an imaginary Adam, of all other infections, is fanciful (Shilts 1987), it took the multitudinous movements of the late twentieth century to ensure HIV quickly reached almost all parts of the world. Whatever the aetiology of the disease it spread quickly, the virus transmitted through sexual intercourse, shared needles and contaminated blood. We sometimes forget that one of the most seriously affected groups were people with haemophilia, many of whom died from HIV in blood that had been donated as a public service by men who were quite unaware of any danger.

The impact of the USA is reflected in both the dominance of biomedical science and the encouragement of political activism. The USA funds and carries out the majority of international biomedical research, and despite the early battle over whether the French discovered HIV ahead of the Americans, US-based researchers have dominated the field (Epstein 1996). Programmes against HIV/AIDS have become the means to spread certain discourses and identities, especially those connected with sex, so that western concepts such as 'men who have sex with men' and 'sex workers' have become part of the universal language of AIDS. It is important to remember that it was gay organisations across the world, beginning with the Gay Men's Health Crisis in New York City, that pioneered what would become the most effective mobilisation for prevention, namely peer-based education and information that accepted rather than prohibited a wide range of sexual behaviours and sought to give people the means to reduce the risk of HIV transmission, not change their desires (Altman 1985; Patton 1985).

AIDS is an excellent example of the globalisation of US-based epistemologies: even the dissident views of President Mbeki were fuelled by the US scientist, Peter Duesberg. The international language of the epidemic is largely North American, and its symbols – the red ribbon; the Memorial Quilt; the idea of the involvement of People with AIDS – have grown out of the US domestic response. Indeed, HIV demonstrates Connell's (2006) argument that the discourses of globalisation are disproportionately those of the North Atlantic. US influence is exerted through a range of institutions, including foundations, universities, pharmaceutical companies, church groups and development organisations, which are often working at apparent cross purposes. Yet in some ways their collective efforts involve an inevitable Americanisation, recalling Joseph Nye's term 'coercive democratisation' (Nye 2006).

US influence on the global pandemic is symbolised by treatment activism inspired by ACT UP, by programmes of monogamy and abstinence, often linked to evangelical Christianity, and by celebrities from Elizabeth Taylor and Richard Gere to Bill Clinton and Bill Gates. One might note the irony that, despite so many signs of US leadership, the major international conferences on AIDS have not been held in that country for 18 years because of the ban, shared with only a few other countries, on admitting people with HIV. This does not mean, of course, that the USA is absent from such meetings. At a planning meeting for the regional AIDS conference held in Sri Lanka in 2006 the names suggested by the local committee for plenary speakers were almost invariably those of people working in the USA; at a similar meeting in Mexico City two years later there were arguments in the programme committee about how far concerns around the US agenda should drive the global debate.

For the first decade of the new pandemic, the USA viewed the epidemic almost entirely through a domestic prism, one which associated the disease with the life-style excesses of gay men and drug users. When President Reagan's Surgeon General, Everett Koop, urged the promotion of condoms and clean needles in his 1986 report to the President, he was denounced by evangelical leaders who objected to any programmes they saw as condoning immorality (Lindsay 2007). HIV/AIDS was mobilised as a rhetorical weapon in attacks on gay rights and, more recently, as a new argument for sexual abstinence, which became an important part of right-wing fundamentalism in the 1990s (Girard 2004). Legislatures have increasingly mandated abstinence as a key part of sex education in schools, with no apparent impact on either the amount of sexual behaviour among teenagers or their rates of pregnancy and STIs. The impact on education is rather akin to that which notions of intelligent design have had on high school biology, with their confusion of ideology with science (Perrotta 2007).

Debate about HIV and AIDS policies, especially attitudes to sex work, abstinence and harm minimisation, has become a lodestone for the larger cultural and political divide in US politics. Expanding access to prevention often means clashes with existing laws and mores and acrimonious debate about sexual behaviours and needle use. Thus the early governmental response in cities such as San Francisco and New York was to close gay bathhouses, rather than, as was true elsewhere, regarding them as sites for prevention intervention. Ironically, more conservative jurisdictions ignored the issue, so that today the most active gay saunas in the USA seem to exist in conservative centres such as Orlando, Dallas and Indianapolis. To cultural conservatives, AIDS appeared the ultimate justification for their attacks on the sexual liberation movements of the 1970s, and morality rather than public health dominated much of the public debate about how best to respond to the new illness.

All religions exercise complex rules and prohibitions around sexuality, and the dominant traditions of monotheistic faiths has been to preach abstinence outside marriage, even while allowing men varying degrees of latitude within marriage. In the USA, the state promotion of abstinence is, however, a feature of the past decade, and a response to a growing hostility to all forms of extramarital sex among certain religious groups. Thus, True Love Waits, an international Christian group focused on teenagers and college students, was created in April 1993 and has organised large-scale rallies and promotions. Pledges to remain virgins until marriage, father/daughter nights and rallies featuring high-profile celebrities have helped make 'abstinence' the most surprising of all sexual movements.

US response to the global epidemic

Given the initial responses of the Reagan and Bush administrations, and the fairly timid moves under Clinton, the willingness of George W. Bush to embrace HIV/AIDS is seemingly surprising. In a front page article in the *New York Times* at the beginning of his last year in office, Sherry Stolberg suggested that President Bush's support for international efforts against AIDS might be his 'most lasting bipartisan achievement' (Stolberg 2008). Before his selection as Vice Presidential candidate, Senator Jo Biden was quoted as saying Bush's support for large-scale programmes against AIDS was 'bold and unexpected, and I believe historians may regard it as his finest hour' (Kane 2008). In the process of claiming global leadership on AIDS, the USA has also tried to impose a particular brand of sexual morality.

The new disease saw a rapid mobilisation of international responses, first through the World Health Organisation (WHO) then through a new agency, UNAIDS, which expanded on the work of the Global Programme on AIDS within WHO. The USA supported the creation of this new agency, but was not particularly central in the process. As awareness of the scale of the epidemic grew, there was a cautious engagement under Clinton, who has become far more committed to the issue since he left office. Vice President Al Gore and Clinton's UN Ambassador Richard Holbrooke played a significant role in putting HIV and AIDS on the agenda of the Security Council, which held its first ever debate on a health issue in January 2000. A cynic might note that it was a convenient issue for Al Gore, then beginning his own presidential campaign, as it allowed him to reach out to two important Democratic constituencies, African-American and gay.

The Security Council debate was followed a year later by a special meeting of the United Nations General Assembly, in which the USA under the new president adopted a cautious position on both prevention and treatment access. Indeed, the final statement released by a coalition of most civil society representatives in New York signalled out the Bush Administration for criticism: 'The United States was particularly damaging to the prospects for a strong declaration. Throughout the negotiations they moved time and again to weaken language on HIV prevention, low-cost drugs and trade agreements and to eliminate commitments on targets for funding and treatment. It's death by diplomacy, said Eric Sawyer, veteran activist and 25-year survivor of HIV/AIDS' (Global Network 2006). Specifically, the USA joined with conservative Islamic nations in refusing to name sex workers, men who have sex with men and drug users as particularly at risk. The new Global Fund to Fight AIDS, Tuberculosis and Malaria owed a great deal to advocacy by US academic experts in public health and development, especially Jeffrey Sachs, but it was the UN Secretary General, not the president of the USA, who took the political lead in its establishment, neither was the USA particularly generous in its initial pledges (Davis and Fort 2004).

However, over the coming years President Bush greatly increased bilateral assistance for AIDS programmes, and total US public and private expenditure on AIDS programmes and research now amounts to over half of all global spending on the epidemic. The Gates Foundation is a bigger donor to the Global Fund than countries such as the Netherlands and Australia. Pressure from the original stakeholders, such as gay organisations and some African-Americans, for US involvement was reinforced by the religious right, who developed considerable interest in the issue. The USA has become central in defining new paradigms and responses to the epidemic as the Bush administration has made the issue theirs, and cloaked it with a particular moral agenda.

International responses

There is a temptation to attribute too much to overt US influence. Yes, the US government has fostered a set of policies that seemed rather different to the sex-positive attitudes preferred by most community organisations and public health experts. But while it is easy to establish the ways in which this has affected US programmes and funding, it is less clear that these are a dominant factor in accounting for over two decades of denial and neglect in many parts of the world, including countries where there has been no American support for HIV programmes. Note the leap in Elizabeth Pisani's (2008: 160) recent comment that: 'We created the "HIV is a development" mantra because neither African leaders nor the international public health establishment wanted to talk about sex in Africa. It became the cement in Kofi Annan's wall of silence. We've exported that cement to countries where leaders don't want to talk about drug injection, or commercial sex, or anal sex.' Her last sentence seems to deny the central role of national leaders that is pointed to in the first sentence: how could 'we' export a 'cement' that was already in place?

Much of the rest of the world took its cues about the new epidemic from the USA, but developed responses that built on local cultural, social and political factors. Thus Sweden also closed its gay saunas in the early stages of the epidemic and has since criminalised the purchasing of sex (although with a feminist justification), while across the Oresund Denmark accepted that sex venues were better seen as opportunities to reach people at risk of infection. Few other western countries adopted US ideologies of sexual abstinence or refusal to recognise gay organisations. Indeed, in much of the western world the mobilisation of gay communities around the epidemic provided a source of government funding and recognition (Altman 1988, 2001).

In other parts of the world the response was far patchier, Thailand, partly due to pressures from the charismatic Meechai Viravaidya and his Population and Community Development Association, developed the 100 per cent condom programme, aimed not at ending sex work but at ensuring all commercial sex involved the use of condoms. While that programme has been criticised by a number of sex worker activists, it did accept the impossibility of preventing commercial sex, and made the promotion of condoms widespread in Thailand. In Uganda, there was an emphasis on zero grazing, namely the reduction of sexual partners plus use of condoms (Epstein 2007). Above all, in Brazil, which stands out as the model response in most areas among all middle income countries, there was extensive support for peer education and empowerment programmes among people whose sexual behaviour made them most vulnerable to infection, namely homosexual men and sex workers.

But for most of this history of the epidemic these were exceptions, and Brazil, Thailand, Uganda, sometimes with the addition of Senegal and Cambodia, became endlessly cited as examples of effective prevention programmes. (Except for Brazil, there was a real failure in these 'model' countries to recognise needle users and same sex attracted men in targeted prevention efforts.) In most of the world sex was ignored, and the denial of sexual reality for which the USA is so often blamed was based more on local religious and cultural prohibitions than on any efforts by US officials.

Uganda is the most interesting example, because during the past few years there has been a move away from the original emphasis on zero grazing to a stress on abstinence and monogamy. It is easy to attribute this to the influence of US evangelism, but this would deny the role of Ugandan church and political leaders, who have been very shrewd in lobbying the government to win support for programmes that are as much a product of local as of imported moralism.[1] It is an easy resort to neo-colonial analysis to simply attribute the campaign against condom use, and the denunciation of homosexuality and pornography to US money and influence.

Clearly Uganda was particularly susceptible to born-again Christian revivalism, but equally African fundamentalism is also impacting on American Christianity, most clearly in the very bitter splits within the Anglican/Episcopalian Church worldwide, where the USA has been far more progressive on issues such as women and gay priests than their African counterparts. Globalisation is not simply a matter of transferring ideas from the rich world to the poor.

Precisely because HIV prevention involves personal behaviours that are often heavily stigmatised and regulated in the name of religion, tradition and morality, it becomes a major arena for clashes. No one opposes access to treatments in the name of religion, but demands that HIV programmes empower sex workers or homosexual men are guaranteed to provoke opposition. A regional UN-sponsored workshop on homosexuality and AIDS in New Delhi in 2006 had to be identified as being on male sexual health to avoid these sensitivities, and most African governments continue to foster the myth that homosexuality is intrinsically 'non-African'. It is not US pressure that maintains antiquated UK laws criminalizing homosexuality in a majority of former colonies, even though all public health evidence suggests they increase the difficulties of doing effective sexual health promotion. Academic attention to rising religiosity rarely reflects on how this may impact on HIV and AIDS, although both Catholic and Islamic opposition to condoms is a critical factor.

Even allowing for the stated precepts of PEPFAR, the overall impact of the USA globally has been to increased awareness of and willingness to discuss sexuality. The impact of US film and television has been to open up once taboo topics, in ways that anyone who has travelled will recognise. From my early experience of being told by a young Malaysian that he knew all about AIDS from the US telemovie, *An Early Frost*, through to watching episodes of *Sex and the City* in Zagreb and *Will and Grace* in Johannesburg, I have been made aware of the extent to which the global imaginary reflects certain American views, in which the dominant portrayal of sex is far removed from that extolled by the abstinence movement.

The Christian right are strong proponents of a free market economy, and despite crusades against pornography it is difficult for them to square their religious views with the realities that sexuality fuels much of American advertising and consumerism. The moralities that the USA exports are as much those of Wisteria Lane in *Desperate Housewives* and *Beverley Hills 90210* as they are those of fundamentalist churches and abstinence movements.

Towards a new consensus? 'Combination prevention'

Despite the apparent influence of the religious right in AIDS programming, there is an evolving US response that combines both a moral and a scientific vision, summed up in the move towards what is called 'prevention science'. Recent international discourses on HIV prevention stress the idea of combining biomedical techniques with behavioural changes, but the language usually employed is remarkably free from references to sexual pleasure, adventure or experimentation (Pebody and Cairns 2008).

This is a vision that places less emphasis on empowerment and social activism, more on developing new technologies of prevention that both enshrine expertise and seemingly avoid complex moral issues. In 2007 apparent evidence that male circumcision slowed the rate of HIV infections was seized on by a coalition of scientists and international bodies to argue that this practice should be central to HIV prevention efforts. Those who suggested there were complex social and cultural forces that would make this ineffective and possibly dangerous (because it would encourage men to ignore condoms) were brushed aside. The possibility of reconciling science and religious moralism is now the dominant motif of many international HIV policies, and from outside the USA there is a common project of 'Americanising' the epidemic that unites apparently very different approaches.

During the past decade there has been a growing emphasis on biomedical interventions as a means of prevention (e.g. microbicides; male circumcision; vaccine development), resulting in concerns that the emphasis on biomedical expertise is at the expense of community mobilisation and empowerment. Too narrow an emphasis on the technologies of prevention leads to the problems identified by an unnamed source from Guyana: 'Priority prevention issues for the international consultancy firms which dominate the HIV/AIDS programmes in Guyana are not the national issues noted above [i.e. poverty and sexual violence], but the global technical prevention factors of condoms, testing and safe blood. Domestic actors have failed to resist imported formulae or even to articulate an alternative path' (personal communication).

There is a paradox in the AIDS world, where there are simultaneous pressures for empowering those most directly affected and for increasing biomedical control of prevention programmes rather than seeing them as community owned and directed. The radical vision of much early HIV and AIDS work, which reflected the 'health for all' movement that was articulated in the Alma Ata Declaration of 1978, seems increasingly imperilled (Epstein and Kim 2007). At the same time much of the international discourse on HIV has stressed the involvement of those affected and infected, and there have been attempts to assure this, including a strong 'community' presence on the board of the Global Fund and the inclusion of affected communities in delegations to UNGASS meetings. This creates demands for programmes to be participatory and community owned, but also ongoing debate whether apparent gains for representation and accountability disguise the creation of a new industry of professional experts (Scalway 2003).

There is some evidence that the US view of the epidemic is becoming more dominant in international discourses around HIV than was the case in earlier periods. Thus, a major session on prevention at the 2008 International Conference on AIDS, organised by the *Lancet*, included three speakers from the USA but none from Asia or Africa. This is clearest in opposition to sex work, where activists allege that UNAIDS has moved significantly closer to the official US position that equates all cases of prostitution to sex trafficking, and therefore denies the possibility of sex work as something in which people might choose to engage (NSWP Coordinated Response to UNAIDS Draft Guidance on Sex Work 2008).

But US attitudes have shifted as well, and there is tacit support from officials for programmes reaching homosexual men and supporting various harm reduction initiatives for drug users. What unites much of this approach is an emphasis on top-down expertise, and a colonisation of prevention by experts based in biomedicine. This is exemplified in a report from the International AIDS Vaccine Initiative, where prevention is defined almost entirely in biomedical terms (vaccine trials; pre-exposure prophylaxis; male circumcision; microbicides) with little attention paid to community education and 'safer sex' programmes (McEnery 2008).

Under the Obama administration there is, perhaps, likely to be somewhat less emphasis on religious ideology, more on scientific expertise. But the lessons of successful grassroots programmes that linked HIV prevention to empowerment and community norms seem to be forgotten in the rush to link biomedical research more tightly to prevention. The moralities that are being exported still reflect an emphasis on individual rather than social behaviour, but increasingly use the language of science rather than religion. What both approaches share is a reluctance to speak openly of sex, which becomes remarkably invisible in the new language of prevention technologies. When AIDS first emerged as a political issue quarter of a century ago, it was widely seen as requiring a new openness and awareness of the varieties of human sexuality. The combined pressures of moralism and biomedicine risk denying the eroticism and pleasures of sex in favour of an emphasis on risk and danger.

References

Altman, D. (1985) *AIDS in the Mind of America*, New York: Doubleday.

Altman, D. (1988) 'Legitimacy through Disaster', in Fox, D. and Fee, E. (eds) *AIDS: The Burdens of History*, Berkeley: University of California.

Altman, D. (2001) *Global Sex*, Chicago: Chicago University Press.

Connell, R. W. (2006) 'Northern Theory: The Political Geography of Social Theory', *Theory & Society*, 35: 237–64.

Davis, P. and Fort, M. (2004) 'The Battle against Global AID', in Fort, M., Mercer, M. and Gish, O. (eds) *Sickness and Wealth*, Cambridge, MA: South End Press.

Epstein, H. (2007) *The Invisible Cure*, New York: Farrar Strauss.

Epstein, H. and Kim, J. (2007) 'AIDS and the Power of Women', *New York Review of Books*, 5: 39–41.

Epstein, S. (1996) *Impure Science: AIDS, Activism, and the Politics of Knowledge*, Berkeley: University of California Press.

Girard, F. (2004) 'Global Implications of U.S. Domestic and International Policies on Sexuality', New York: Columbia University Press. (IWGGSP Working Paper No. 1)

Global Network of People Living with AIDS (2006) 'Civil Society declares UNGASS a Failure'; available at www.gnpplus.net/content/view/1249/77 (accessed 29 January 2009).

Herzog, D. (2008) *Sex in Crisis*, New York: Basic Books.

Kagan, R. (2003) *Of Paradise and Power: America and Europe in the New World Order*, New York: Knopf.

Kane, P. (2008) 'Senate Agrees to $50 Billion AIDS Plan', *Washington Post*, 17 July: A02.

Lindsay, D. (2007) *Faith in the Halls of Power*, New York: Oxford University Press.

McEnery, R. (2008) 'HIV Prevention Research', *IAVI Report*, 12: 4.

MacQuarrie, B. (2005) 'Pastor Rivets many without Politics', *Boston Globe*, 11 October.

Network of Sex Worker Projects Coordinated Response to UNAIDS Draft Guidance on Sex Work (2008) 'Revised Statement'; available at www.nswp.org/safety/unaids-response/ (accessed 1 January 2009).

Nye, J. (2006) 'Transformational Leadership and U.S. Grand Strategy', *Foreign Affairs*, July/August: 139–48.

Pankhurst, J. (2002) 'The Ugandan Success Story?', *Lancet*, 360: 78–80.

Patton, C. (1985) *Sex and Germs*, Boston, MA: South End Press.

Pebody, R. and Cairns, G. (2008) 'Prevention – There will be no Magic Bullet, we need "Combination Prevention,"' *AIDSMAP News*, 6 August: 1–3.

Perrotta, T. (2007) *The Abstinence Teacher*, New York: St. Martin's Press.

Pisani, E. (2008) *The Wisdom of Whores*, London: Granta.

Scalway, T. (2003) *'Missing the Message?' Twenty Years of Learning from HIV/AIDS*, London: Panos.

Shilts, R. (1987) *And The Band Played On*, New York: St. Martins Press.

Stolberg, G. (2008) 'In Global Battle on AIDS, Bush Creates Legacy', *New York Times*, 5 January.

22 'Bareback' – definitions and identity[1]

Constructs' limitation for HIV-prevention research

Alex Carballo-Diéguez, Ana Ventuneac, José Bauermeister, Gary W. Dowsett, Curtis Dolezal, Robert H. Remien, Iván C. Balán and Matthew S. Rowe

The term 'bareback' appeared in the gay press in the mid-1990s referring to intentional condomless anal intercourse, mainly among HIV-infected gay men (Gendin 1997). However, by the time Silverstein and Picano published *The Joy of Gay Sex* (2003), bareback was defined simply as condomless gay sex. Researchers who saw the need to operationalise the term chose 'intentional condomless anal intercourse in HIV-risk contexts' (Carballo-Diéguez and Bauermeister 2004; Suarez and Miller 2001), noting two key elements – intention and risk – that might distinguish the term from other less precise definitions. Others defined it as: 'intentional anal sex without a condom with someone other than a primary partner' (Mansergh *et al.* 2002); 'intentionally seeking or engaging in unprotected anal sex among HIV-positive gay men' (Elford *et al.* 2007); 'intentional unprotected anal intercourse regardless of serostatus or partner type' (Halkitis *et al.* 2003, Tomso 2004); or any 'sex that occurs without the protection provided by a condom', not limited to gay men (Gauthier and Forsyth 1999).

Lacking a standard definition of, and consensus on, the role that intentionality of condomless sex and HIV-transmission risk (or lack of it) play in bareback sex, some researchers went back to the sources, i.e. asking gay men what bareback sex means. Brief surveys, sometimes no longer than five minutes, were administered online or to community samples asking respondents to define bareback sex or presenting scenarios with degrees of intentionality (Halkitis 2007; Huebner *et al.* 2006). Yet respondents were not asked to describe their understanding of the term, and the HIV status of protagonists was not included. As a result, proportions of respondents endorsing different definitions vary widely. Given this definitional imprecision, there is difficulty in comparing findings and developing evidence-based prevention responses.

Researchers have also tackled a related topic: *bareback identity* (Halkitis *et al.* 2005; Wolitski 2005). Based on the idea of a distinct bareback identity, studies have compared individuals who identify as barebackers with those who do not (Halkitis *et al.* 2005; Halkitis 2007). However, the operationalisation of the term 'barebacker' as identity is also not clear in the literature. Our Frontiers in Prevention study was designed to explore the perspective of men who report engaging in bareback sex on the meaning of bareback sex, which words besides 'bareback' are used to name the practice and whether respondents identify as barebackers. Furthermore, we sought to redefine the term within a conceptual model that could orient future work.

In the first phase of the work, we identified the six most popular free internet sites used by men in New York City to meet other men interested in barebacking (see Carballo-Diéguez *et al.* 2006; Dowsett *et al.* 2008). Next, between April 2005 and March 2006, we recruited adult men who self-identified as a barebacker or as someone who practises barebacking ('Are you into bareback, or do you consider yourself a barebacker?'); had had intentional, condomless, anal intercourse with a man met over the internet; and use at least one of the internet sites identified in the first phase of the study. Men were recruited exclusively through these internet sites in approximately equal numbers of European Americans (EA), African Americans (AA), Latinos/Hispanics (LH) and Asian/Pacific Islanders (API). We also stratified the sample to include about two-thirds who reported both being HIV negative and having had unprotected receptive anal intercourse in the previous year. Qualifying individuals were invited to attend face-to-face interviews conducted by one of three psychologists on the research team. (For more details on recruitment, methods and data analysis, see Carballo-Diéguez *et al.* 2009.) The interviews lasted about two hours, and respondents were compensated with US$50 for their time.

Participants were 120 men, of whom 31 reported being HIV infected. Their average age was 34 with HIV-infected men being, on average, seven years older and earning about US$10,000 less per year than uninfected men. Respondents had, on average, two years of college education. Thirty-five per cent were European American, 31 per cent Latino/Hispanic, 28 per cent African American and 17 per cent Asian/Pacific Islander. Most of the respondents self-identified as gay. The men had had, on average, between 13 and 14 sexual partners in the previous two months, and they practised unprotected anal intercourse frequently.

Defining bareback

Lack of condom use

I: If I were to ask you for a dictionary definition of bareback sex, what would you say?

R: Sex without condoms.

I: Is there anything else in the definition or just that?

R: Just that.

(Mark, male, EA, HIV+, 43 years)

Lack of condom use was often the first and the only element mentioned. Sometimes, this was referred to as 'flesh on flesh' or 'latex-free' sex. Some defined it without reference to any type of sex and encompassing both heterosexual and homosexual acts:

R: In the sexual context, this means, um, just not using a condom, and having intercourse, whether anal, vaginal or, or oral. Not using a condom.

(Darryl, male, AA, HIV−, 33 years)

At other times, definitions were restricted to anal intercourse without condoms and to sex among men only, for which some respondents considered that intrarectal ejaculation should also be included in the definition:

R: A person who not only gets – has sex without using a condom but who also lets a guy come inside his anus or whatever you want to call it … That's what the true barebacker [is] in my book.

(Sergio, male, LH, HIV–, 24 years)

Last, respondents sometimes noted the words 'natural' and 'intimate' as key to their definition:

R: [sighs] Dictionary definition of bareback sex. Hmm. Wow. [laughter] Uh, the nitty gritty, the ultimate feeling of intimacy between two people … The way sex was meant to be … I consider it being truly intimate with somebody. There's no barriers … It feels so much better than a condom.

(Bernard, male, AA, HIV–, 25 years)

Intentionality

A few individuals spontaneously included intention not to use condoms as a required element of the definition:

R: I would say, the deliberate-less, the deliberate condom-less act of sexual intercourse, especially anal, um, what would you say? With the intent of enhanced pleasure.

(Wayne, male, EA, HIV+, 32 years)

However, most respondents did not mention intention. Therefore, we asked: 'If two guys are having sex with condoms and the condom breaks, would you call that barebacking?' About one-third of the respondents rejected this and, instead, introduced into the definition intention to have condomless sex or lack of intention to protect (not necessarily the same thing). This was referred to, for example, as 'prior agreement not to use condoms', or 'knowledge' or 'awareness that no condoms were used'. About one-third of respondents, however, qualified the 'condom breakage' scenario:

R: No, that's – no. Not if they don't realise it or they're, you know, I think if they realise it breaks and they choose to go without, then yeah, then it is barebacking.

(Daniel, male, EA, HIV+, 45 years)

Therefore, the intentionality was brought into the definition by the failure to stop having intercourse at the point of becoming aware that the condom broke. This nuance was not, however, without its reservations:

R: Technically, I guess, briefly, unless they don't pull out or if they continue, then yeah. But barebacking is usually a conscious choice. But I understand that is kind of complicating the situation. But if the condom breaks, then no, I don't think so, because I think that barebacking isn't by accident. It's a conscious choice, unless the person's fucked up and doesn't know what you're doing.

(Paul, male, EA, HIV–, 31 years)

Awareness of risk

Some respondents volunteered that bareback sex was risky:

R: Um. [pause] Condomless, unprotected sex, with knowing, with the knowledge
   that you could be having sex with men who have sexually transmitted diseases,
   or who don't know their HIV status or who are HIV positive.

(José Luis, male, LH, HIV–, 25 years)

To explore the issue of risk further, we asked: 'If two people are HIV negative and
monogamous, and they decided that they're going to have sex without condoms,
would you call that bareback or not?' Many respondents said they would consider
this bareback sex. Other respondents stated that condomless sex between an uninfected monogamous couple should not be considered bareback sex:

R: That's not bareback ... [I: 'Why not?'] It's not because these two guys are in a
   relationship. They're in a monogamous relationship. They love each other.
   They're both HIV negative. They know their status. They've – it's natural, I
   mean, for the gay world ... But it's just natural for them to have sex without a
   condom, if they know neither one has HIV or has an STD or whatever, and
   they're not sleeping around on each other.

(Albert, male, AA, HIV–, 41 years)

In other words, were it not for HIV and AIDS, condomless sex would not only be
the norm among gay men, it would not even be considered an issue.

Some ethnic minority respondents said that bareback was a term used by 'white
folks', whereas:

R: Oh, black guys, you know, mostly just say 'raw', you know, or 'skin-to-skin'
   [laughs].

(Courtney, male, AA, HIV–, 29 years)

There were richer metaphors too:

R: 'Raw dog', 'raw sex', um, 'I wanna flood your hole', um, a lot of fusion of hip-hop
   language, you know, applied to, to the sexual terms, um ... 'I'm going to give
   you nutt', as opposed to, um, 'I'm going to give you my load'. So, what 'cum'
   meant – well, rather, 'cum' and 'load' is analogous to 'nutt', n-u-t-t, for Black
   and Latino men. The word 'nasty' is used, you know.

(José Luis, male, LH, HIV–, 25 years)

Other words or phrases used were 'uninhibited', 'natural', 'pig', 'unwrapped',
'uncovered', 'unprotected', 'raunchy' and 'down and dirty'. A few respondents used
the word 'freak'. One Latino respondent even used *crudo*, the literal translation of
'raw' in Spanish.

'Seeding' and 'breeding' were terms that appeared to denote ejaculation:

I: What other words do you use for barebacking?

R: 'Raw'. And 'bareback'. They're the only two now. I mean, you see guys using euphemisms, but they usually refer to transmission of HIV. 'Breed me', 'seed me', give me the 'taint'. So they really go beyond that definition. Anything beyond 'raw' and 'bareback', it means fucking bareback with someone you know to be HIV positive.

(Peter, male, EA, HIV–, 53 years)

This is an important distinction. 'Bug chasing' and 'gift giving' are terms related to bareback sex that have caused much media fervour. These terms did not arise spontaneously in the interviews, and when probed, many respondents did not know about them and simply inferred their meaning:

R: Bug chasers! Ah, yes. Those poor, deluded people who romanticise getting HIV.

(Fernando, male, LH, HIV+, 35 years)

Bareback identity

When we asked respondents if they considered themselves barebackers, most replies focused on condomless sexual practices. Based on that, men responded either affirmatively or negatively or qualified how the term would apply to them. A few respondents queried whether having condomless sex sufficed to define someone as *being* one thing or another.

About one-third of the respondents labelled themselves as barebackers – more often HIV-positive men:

I: Do you think of yourself as a barebacker?

R: Yes.

I: Is that an identity?

R: That's an identity. That's the truth. The truth … is the light. So I'm a barebacker, baby. And I ain't going to sugar-coat [it] – I'm a barebacker [singing], I'm a barebacker! [laughter] […] I feel … it, it, it gives me a sense of empowerment, so to speak. I feel good about [that] shit. Yeah, I like the ass, I like to fuck, and I like to get fucked. You know, and I like to be explicit. And I can get to the exact nature of what I'm about, so it empowers me. Barebacker, huh? You know, that is that term.

(Ricky, male, AA, HIV+, 38 years)

About one-quarter of respondents rejected labelling themselves as barebackers. At times, this was related to the stigma associated with the behaviour, particularly for HIV-negative men:

I: What keeps you from considering yourself that?

R: I guess just the stigma attached to it. The stigma and – I'm not going to have bareback sex with every guy I meet. That's why I don't consider myself a barebacker.

(Philip, male, API, HIV–, 26 years)

Others said they did not consider themselves barebackers because they 'did try to use condoms' or it was not 'the biggest part of my sexual experience' or because labelling oneself as such would make others think, 'Oh, sure, he's a barebacker, so he'll accept my dick inside him'.

A few respondents said that the label applied to them only partially or sometimes. Some contradicted themselves in trying to explain why:

I: Do you consider yourself a barebacker?

R: Sixty percent of the times, yes, I do […] I do … my best to practise safe sex, but once, you know, I meet a certain person or – it's like – it's like something that will go off in me that I'll be, like wow, I would just love to feel him inside, you know? Or I would just love to run up in them and – stuff like that.

(D'Angelo, male, AA, HIV–, 29 years)

One uninfected Latino young man reasoned that he was only 40 per cent a barebacker because that was the proportion of times he had condomless sex with strangers, whereas the other 60 per cent of the time he did it with people he knew.

Discussion

Our methodology for this part of our study relied exclusively on qualitative interviews so as to gain a deeper understanding of the phenomenon of barebacking without imposing preconceived notions. Since we specifically recruited men who identified as barebacker or someone who practises barebacking, and furthermore, someone who had had intentional, condomless, anal intercourse with a man or men met over the internet, we expected some consensus in their accounts. Instead, responses varied widely, including among ethnic minority men.

We did not define 'bareback' for respondents, but they were in broad agreement that bareback refers to intercourse without condoms. This would seem to support investigators who reported that the colloquial term originally used mainly for HIV-infected individuals may have lost its early specificity (Halkitis 2007). However, generalisation has not occurred; we found much variation among respondents in the interpretation of everything beyond this initial phrasing. Our findings reveal pitfalls in considering bareback as a simple reference to condomless sex and to question the validity of some research undertaken thus far.

Moreover, the reification of barebacker from one who practises a behaviour to one who has a specific identity has exacerbated the confusion. Our respondents eloquently argued for and against the barebacker label. For some, identifying as barebacker might be interpreted as defiance of mores that restrict sexual freedom, but it is doubtful that it functions as the organising principle for a sexual identity. For others, the label was an uncomfortable one that they either rejected outwardly or accepted partially with different rationalisations to explain their views. There was evidence that stigma associated with intentionally having unprotected anal sex affected HIV-negative men in different ways from HIV-positive men.

Yet, it is more complex than that. In fact, there was no single definition embraced by all men, and assertions from researchers or practitioners that there is a prevailing community-held consensus on what bareback means are not supported by these men, the very ones practising bareback sex regularly enough to anticipate consensus.

Neither was there evidence of an overwhelming uptake or positioning of barebacker as a dominant or functional identity. These findings pose challenges for research and HIV prevention.

First, we focus on research implications. Researchers are not simply reflecting larger confusion existing among gay men or in gay community discourse; researchers have played a part in creating this confusion. As Junge (2002) argues, noting Farmer's (1996) call for a critical epistemology of emerging infectious disease:

> Farmer (1996) has focused particularly on how publication of AIDS research in peer-reviewed scholarly journals provides a site of discursive production wherein choices in lexical representation may reinforce stigmatising or essentialising conceptualizations of certain populations.
>
> (Junge 2002: 196)

Researchers, in arguing for a certain take on barebacking, bolstered by certain data, are involved in a discursive practise that exercises *constructive* power over the phenomenon – no research merely 'reports'. As Tomso (2004) argues:

> [B]ug chasing and barebacking exist as *phenomena* [emphasis in the original] largely because of what Foucault would call the constitutive, disciplinary operation of scientific, activist, and popular discourses about them. This is to say that those who are currently investigating and writing about these phenomena, as much so if not more than the men whose sexual lives are the subjects of these investigations, are epistemologically accountable for the emergence of bug chasing and barebacking as social 'problems'.
>
> (Tomso 2004: 88–9)

Second, we must note the interaction between researchers and our findings, with those responsible for designing and delivering HIV prevention. For researchers are not the only ones responsible; other social actors are involved too – activists, advocates, educators, commentators, the media and anyone else who proclaims on the issue. Within this interaction, the men who bareback lose their voice and the right to constitute bareback as it pertains to *their* lives. This can lead, inter alia, to a barebacker becoming a stigmatised 'other', an outcome that conceals rather than reveals the nature of the phenomenon and related prevention complexities.

Supporting evidence-based prevention is a central purpose of this project – called 'Frontiers in Prevention'. We believe the idea of bareback needs to be reconceptualised to focus public health discourse and inform its practice. However, Huebner *et al.* (2006) warn:

> Studies that fail to define barebacking for participants might be inquiring about any number of behaviours, depending on each participant's individual understanding of the term. Additionally, even studies that do define the expression might encounter problems among participants who understand barebacking differently and ignore researcher definitions when responding. Even if participants can be compelled to suspend their own understanding of the term and to report about barebacking as defined by researchers, the external validity of such

research is questionable given that definitions are constructed in the study that might not exist in the real world.

(Huebner *et al.* 2006: 70)

Yet, if no attempt is made to clarify this definition of barebacking, then confusion will continue, research incomparability will grow and evidence-based prevention will be even less possible.

Therefore, we propose an operationalisation of terms graphically presented in Figure 22.1. We distinguish condomless anal intercourse that is intentional from that which is unintentional, as well as those acts that carry risk for primary infection from those that do not. We think it useful to distinguish *intentional condomless intercourse in HIV risk contexts* (our preferred definition of bareback, quadrant I) from other condomless sex that may involve risk of primary infection but is accidental, unintentional or non-consensual (quadrant II), and from condomless sex that is risk free, whether intentional or not, such as between monogamous seronegative individuals or those non-monogamous couples who practise 'negotiated safety' (Kippax *et al.* 1993) (quadrants III and IV). We think that a specific focus is offered by quadrant I, which includes condomless anal intercourse that is intentional and may result in primary transmission of HIV, whether it is called 'barebacking' or not, and whether its practitioners identify as 'barebackers' or not. This category includes 'strategic positioning' (whether the infected partner takes the receptive role with a partner of the opposite status) irrespective of intrarectal ejaculation, which may further qualify the risk. The issue of awareness of appreciable risk is central to this category – the risk calculus is done and condomless sex proceeds anyway.

The usefulness of this typology lies in its capacity to focus attention where the epidemiological importance lies. By definition, behaviours in quadrants III and IV carry no epidemiological importance from the perspective of primary HIV transmission. HIV prevention education is still needed in these cases – mistakes can be made, judgement can be poor – but it needs a different kind of education. This includes strategies that stimulate correct and consistent condom use as well as strategies for dispensing with condoms in certain situations and after clear precautions,

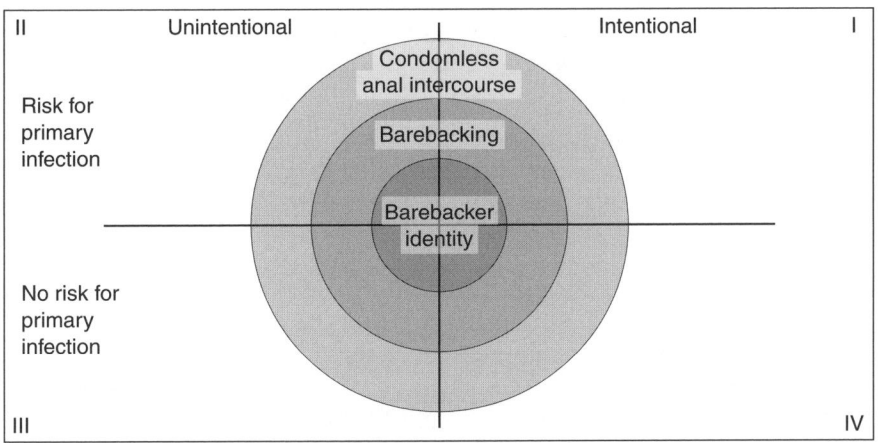

Figure 22.1 Bareback deconstruction.

e.g. sequential HIV testing, negotiated safety, serosorting and HIV-seroconcordant monogamy.

Quadrant II includes a well-known cluster of prevention problems that HIV prevention researchers and educators have uncovered and grappled with as the epidemic progressed and which have enhanced epidemiological importance. Adam (2005) details some of the behaviours to be included in this category but not in the bareback group:

> [B]arebacking is distinguishable from the wider range of unplanned, episodic, unprotected sexual encounters that men in interviews attribute to a variety of circumstances such as: a resolution to erectile difficulties experienced with condoms, through momentary lapses and trade-offs, out of personal turmoil and depression, or as a by-product of strategies of disclosure and intuiting safety.
>
> (Adam 2005: 334)

There is increased risk of primary infection here, but the risks arise from a very different set of circumstances from the other categories and warrant their own prevention agenda, e.g. post-exposure prophylaxis.

This leaves quadrant I as a clear – although not entirely new – target in which the condomless anal intercourse with appreciable risk that may result in new infection is intentional. This is the category we call 'bareback', and we believe the use of that term should be restricted to this category, first by researchers and subsequently by practitioners. It is this specificity that will lead to targeted prevention responses, ones that may not always be condom focused, such as risk reduction (Suarez and Miller 2001), strategic positioning (Kippax and Race 2003), microbicide use when it becomes available (Carballo-Diéguez *et al.* 2007), pre-exposure prophylaxis (Nodin *et al.* 2008) or others.

Barker *et al.* (2007) argue that there is a 'non-equivalence' between barebacking and unprotected anal intercourse in HIV epidemiology. Furthermore, it behoves researchers not to muddy the waters for both research and for the development of targeted HIV prevention or related health promotion with imprecise or inapplicable usage of the term 'bareback' for all sex acts in all four categories.

Our typology acknowledges that some gay men regard all condomless anal intercourse as bareback; others say not *all* condomless intercourse is bareback; and there are those who use the term merely as shorthand. Nonetheless, our typology prevents the confounding of prevention education targeting in deploying any overarching notion of barebacking that cannot offer sufficient specificity. It recognises that while all who call themselves barebackers practise barebacking, not all who engage in barebacking call themselves barebackers. Most importantly, our typology maintains a focus on *contextualised sexual behaviour* by focusing on the many kinds of 'relational nexus' (Riggs 2006) that are negotiated by men in sex (sometimes correctly, sometimes incorrectly in terms of HIV), rather than reifying risk as a single characteristic of individual personalities or psyches. After all, as Junge (2002) points out, a couple having condomless sex may include one partner who does it intentionally and another who is unaware of the situation or is responding to pressure. It is the sexual *relations* between people and how these influence behaviour – rather than the terms adopted or identity – which may, or may not, facilitate primary HIV infection. Such sexual events may be understood as belonging in different categories at the same time and so require different approaches to prevention.

There is heuristic value in focusing scientific inquiry on bareback internet sites, on sex clubs that sponsor bareback events or offer bareback rooms, and on serosorting networks that facilitate condomless intercourse. However, in developing evidence-based prevention focused on the terms 'barebacking' or 'barebackers', the target of these efforts would be less than specific and quite dispersed unless the definition is restricted as our typology suggests. Moreover, if norms concerning condom use relax, e.g. with the increased effectiveness of highly active antiretroviral therapies, and as the use and meaning of the term is unevenly distributed, the word 'bareback' may fade from being useful in understanding what is driving the epidemic in the USA – and maybe elsewhere. Until that happens, the focused usage we suggest may reduce the current confusion.

Our study has some limitations. It focused on a moving target – the use of a vernacular term – but one that is also discursively constructed in research. Our conclusions are likely to be time bound by where the debate is to date and should be considered with caution. The use of qualitative methods precludes generalisations to all gay men. Our findings may also be affected by sample specificity and may not reflect what is currently happening outside the USA or among all men who engage in intentional condomless sex in risk contexts. Clearly, there is more to discover about the contribution of serostatus and ethnicity and of 'bug chasing' and 'gift giving', but space limitations have prevented us from exploring that here.

Nevertheless, our findings emphasise the importance for researchers, as a start, to define and operationalise the terms we use carefully to reduce confusion. This is important if the evidence offered by researchers is to help prevention workers develop programmes where bareback sex may be implicated.

Note

1 This research was supported by a grant from the United States National Institute of Mental Health (R01 MH69333); Principal Investigator: Alex Carballo-Diéguez).

References

Adam, B. D. (2005) 'Constructing the Neoliberal Sexual Actor: Responsibility and Care of the Self in the Discourse of Barebackers', *Culture, Health and Sexuality*, 7: 333–46.

Barker, M., Hagger-Johnson, G., Hegarty, P., Hutchison, C. and Riggs, D. (2007) 'Responses from the Lesbian and Gay Psychology Section to Crossley's 'Making Sense of "Barebacking" (Commentary)', *British Journal of Social Psychology*, 46: 667–77.

Carballo-Diéguez, A. and Bauermeister, J. (2004) ' "Barebacking": Intentional Condomless Anal Sex in HIV-risk Contexts. Reasons For and Against It', *Journal of Homosexuality*, 47: 1–16.

Carballo-Diéguez, A., Dowsett, G. W., Ventuneac, A., Remien, R. H., Balán, I., Dolezal, C. *et al.* (2006) 'Cybercartography of Popular Internet Sites Used by New York City MSM Interested in Bareback Sex', *AIDS Education & Prevention*, 18: 475–89.

Carballo-Diéguez, A., Exner, T., Dolezal, C., Pickard, R., Lin, P. and Mayer, K. L. (2007) 'Rectal Microbicide Acceptability: Results of a Volume Escalation Trial', *Sexually Transmitted Diseases*, 34: 224–9.

Carballo-Diéguez, A., Ventuneac, A., Bauermeister, J., Dowsett, G., Dolezal, C., Remien, R. *et al.*

(2009) 'Is "Bareback" a Useful Construct from a Primary HIV-prevention Perspective? Definitions, Identity, and Research', *Culture, Health and Sexuality*, 11 (1): 51–65.

Dowsett, G. W., Williams, H., Ventuneac, A. and Carballo-Diéguez, A. (2008) ' "Taking it Like a Man": Masculinity and Barebacking Online', *Sexualities*, 11: 137–57.

Elford, J., Bolding, G., Davis, M., Sherr, L. and Hart, G. (2007) 'Barebacking among HIV-positive Gay Men in London', *Sexually Transmitted Diseases*, 34: 93–8.

Farmer, P. (1996) 'Social Inequalities and Emerging Infectious Diseases', *Emerging Infectious Diseases*, 2: 259–69.

Gauthier, D. K. and Forsyth, C. J. (1999) 'Bareback Sex, Bug Chasers, and the Gift of Death', *Deviant Behavior*, 20: 85–100.

Gendin, S. (1997) 'Skin-on-skin Sex – Been There, Done That, Want More', *POZ Magazine*, available at www.poz.com/articles/241_12394.shtml/ (accessed 07 June 2008).

Halkitis, P. N. (2007) 'Behavioral Patterns, Identity, and Health Characteristics of Self-identified Barebackers: Implications for HIV Prevention and Intervention', *Journal of LGBT Health Research*, 3: 37–48.

Halkitis, P. N., Parsons, J. T. and Wilton, L. (2003) 'Barebacking among Gay and Bisexual Men in New York City: Explanations for the Emergence of Intentional Unsafe Behavior', *Archives of Sexual Behavior*, 32: 351–7.

Halkitis, P. N., Wilton, L., Wolitski, R. J., Parsons, J. T., Hoffe, C. C. and Bimbi, D. S. (2005) 'Barebacking Identity among HIV-positive Gay and Bisexual Men: Demographic, Psychological, and Behavioral Correlates', *AIDS*, 19: S27–S35.

Huebner, D. M., Proescholdbell, R. J. and Nemeroff, C. J. (2006) 'Do Gay and Bisexual Men Share Researchers' Definitions of Barebacking?', *Journal of Psychology & Human Sexuality*, 18: 67–77.

Junge, B. (2002) 'Bareback Sex, Risk, and Eroticism: Anthropological Themes (Re-) Surfacing in the Post-AIDS Era', in Lewin, E. and Leap, W. (eds) *Out in Theory: The Emergence of Lesbian and Gay Anthropology*, Urbana and Chicago: University of Illinois Press.

Kippax, S. and Race, K. (2003) 'Sustaining Safe Practice: Twenty Years On', *Social Science and Medicine*, 57: 1–12.

Kippax, S., Crawford, J., Davis, M., Rodden, P. and Dowsett, G. W. (1993) 'Sustaining Safe Sex: A Longitudinal Study of a Sample of Homosexual Men', *AIDS*, 7: 257–63.

Mansergh, G., Marks, G., Colfax, G. N., Guzman, R., Rader, M. and Buchbinder, S. (2002) ' "Barebacking" in a Diverse Sample of Men who have Sex with Men', *AIDS*, 16: 653–9.

Nodin, N., Carballo-Diéguez, A., Ventuneac, A., Balán, I. and Remien, R. H. (2008) 'Knowledge and Acceptability of Alternative HIV Prevention Bio-medical Products among MSM who Bareback', *AIDS Care*, 20 (1): 106–15.

Riggs, D. W. (2006) ' "Serosameness" or "Serodifference"? Resisting Polarized Discourses of Identity and Relationality in the Context of HIV', *Sexualities*, 9: 409–22.

Silverstein, C. and Picano, F. (2003) *The Joy of Gay Sex*, New York: HarperCollins.

Suarez, T. and Miller, J. (2001) 'Negotiating Risks in Context: A Perspective on Unprotected Anal Intercourse and Barebacking among Men who have Sex with Men – Where Do We Go from Here?', *Archives of Sexual Behavior*, 30: 287–300.

Tomso, G. (2004) 'Bug Chasing, Barebacking, and the Risks of Care', *Literature & Medicine*, 23: 88–111; Discussion, 128–33.

Wolitski, R. J. (2005) 'The Emergence of Barebacking among Gay and Bisexual Men in the United States: A Public Health Perspective', *Journal of Gay & Lesbian Psychotherapy*, 9: 9–34.

23 Sex under the influence of crystal meth

The experience of Latino gay men in San Francisco

Rafael M. Díaz

During the past 15 years, particularly within gay communities in the USA, there has been a dramatic and troubling increase in the use of (so-called) 'club drugs', including methamphetamine – hereafter *crystal meth* – a toxic and highly addictive stimulant with well-documented neuropsychological dysfunctions and psychiatric problems related to its use (Colfax and Guzman 2006; Díaz 2007; Fernandez *et al.* 2007; Rippeth *et al.* 2004; Wang *et al.* 2004). A comprehensive review of the literature on drug use among gay/bisexual men, published in 2001, reported prevalence rates of crystal meth use among gay men ranging from 5–25 per cent in different samples as well as increases in emergency room admissions and in the number of gay men seeking psychological and medical help for crystal meth-related problems (Halkitis *et al.* 2001). The most recent data on Latino gay men in San Francisco, derived from two different random samples (time/location sampling and respondent-driven sampling), show an increase in crystal meth use from 14 per cent in 2001 (Díaz 2006) to 19 per cent in 2004 (Ramirez-Valles *et al.* 2008).

The fact that crystal meth use appears as a powerful predictor of unprotected sexual practices and HIV seroconversion has led experts in the field refer to crystal meth use as the 'second' epidemic, and as 'intertwining' epidemics when referring to crystal meth use and HIV (Stall and Purcell 2000). However, while a strong correlation between crystal meth use and HIV risk is clearly documented, the reasons that explain such relationship are poorly understood. There is little understanding about how the use of crystal meth changes sexual behaviour, the subjective sexual experience of users or the context of sexual activity in ways that may increase the probability of HIV transmission. In addition, there is little analysis on how cultural norms and expectations (within US gay communities) regarding what constitutes 'good' or 'great' sex may pressure some gay men to consume stimulants, and in particular crystal meth, with potential detriment to their health and wellbeing.

Based on data from a study of drug using Latino gay men in San Francisco, this chapter presents a qualitative descriptive analysis of perceived sexual effects under the influence of crystal meth. The study involved men who self-identified as Latino/Hispanic or by any Latin American nationality, whose self-identified sexual orientation was other than heterosexual, and who lived in the San Francisco Bay Area at the time of the study. As part of the inclusion criteria, men had to report current use of illicit drugs and the practice of unprotected anal intercourse at least once during the previous six months.

Approach

The study, sponsored by the US National Institute on Drug Abuse, was designed to provide a rich description (both qualitative and quantitative) of drug use among Latino gay men in the San Francisco Bay Area, with a particular focus on stimulant (crystal meth, cocaine and crack) use and its relation to HIV risk behaviour. The study was conducted in three different phases involving both qualitative and quantitative methods (see Díaz 2007 for more study details); this chapter reports findings only from the qualitative study.

Seventy drug-using Latino gay men (50 of them crystal meth users) who reported at least one instance of unprotected anal intercourse in the last six months were interviewed in a two-hour qualitative semi-structured interview. Beyond a detailed qualitative description of both drug use and sexual activity (including behaviour, social contexts and subjective meanings), the interview elicited narratives on specific episodes of drug use with and without sexual activity, and narratives on episodes of sex under the influence of drugs, with and without condom use. In this chapter, only qualitative data on 'sexual effects' are reported. Sexual effects of crystal meth were defined as any kind of sexual change subjectively experienced by the user while under the influence of crystal meth.

The qualitative interviews conducted during the first phase of the study were transcribed, coded and analysed in content with the aim of creating an exhaustive list of 'sexual effects' under the influence of crystal meth. I searched systematically for sexual effects of crystal meth on the interview transcriptions, particularly on text that was coded as the intersection of two different coding categories: 'Effects of drug use' and 'Descriptions of sex and sexual activity'. Particular attention was paid to text that emerged within the narratives of sexual episodes and also text that was coded under 'Perceived connections between sex and drugs'. The 20 different men quoted in this chapter are given fictitious names; a list of their demographic characteristics, including age, occupation, country of birth and HIV status is given after each name.

Perceived sexual effects

Hot, horny and not satisfied

The majority of participants agreed that a major reason for using stimulants was to alleviate their exhaustion with work, forget their problems and find renewed energy to participate in social activities and nightlife. However, they also drew an emphatic distinction between the two powerful stimulants they were most familiar with: cocaine and crystal meth. When talking about cocaine, they emphasised the renewed energy for socialising with friends; when talking about crystal meth, all of them mentioned an unusually strong, increased and prolonged desire to have sex:

> Cocaine is more for relaxing, for party, dancing. But crystal is for sex. To get nasty for hours and hours and hours.
>
> (Gabriel, 37 years old, social worker, born in Puerto Rico, HIV+)

For some men, this sexual effect of crystal meth seemed to happen almost instantaneously, as if a 'sex button' was turned on and men felt sexually aroused very shortly after consuming the drug:

I said 'Okay' and I used it. I felt very, at that moment, I felt very, very, how can I say it ... well, I was turned on, because of the drug I used ... I got excited, I got sexually excited, I mean I got an instant erection. And it was something, well, that hadn't ever happen to me before.

(Fernando, 26 years old, construction worker, born in Mexico, HIV–)

Even though many men described feeling euphoric with the increased energy and stimulating effects of the drug, increased sexual arousal appeared to be the most common and predominant subjective experience of crystal meth users:

If I take that drug, nine times out of ten it's going to incite an emotion in me, and I'm going to go out and actively seek some sexual partners ... My mood didn't really change, but I think my, yeah, somewhere in there it activated, you know, the horny button, somewhere in there. But my mood was still the same. It was more of a mental thing ... Like my mind wanted, you know, that dick or that you know, sexual contact. My emotions were still the same. I felt fine.

(Roberto, 33 years old, hairstylist, born in the USA, HIV–)

The sexual arousal was accompanied by a strong sensation of body heat, including a heating up of the skin, genitals and anus, the relevant body parts for sexual activity:

I felt like it rushed to my brain, I felt my skin get hot and I felt the desire to have sex with whoever was around.

(Raul, 35 years old, cosmetologist, born in Mexico, HIV+)

Depending on the product and quality it can be a euphoric rush. You can feel it in your ass, in your balls, where it heats them up all of a sudden. That's also when you shoot it up, you can feel it that way. Or if it's quality stuff, you feel your asshole get hot and like on fire. Or your balls kind of get that way, depending on what you're focused on.

(Angel, 40 years old, unemployed (on disability government assistance), born in the USA, HIV+)

By the same token, while men truly enjoyed the pleasures of strong sexual arousal, the fact that the arousal was unusually prolonged in time, and not diminished after orgasm, often resulted in some degree of tension and discomfort. Men reported still being sexually aroused right after having sex, or when tired after a night filled with sexual activity. Many men spoke of being so sexually hungry that they had to masturbate several times in an attempt to find sexual satisfaction:

I got up and ate something. I went back to sleep, I felt bad. I had a horrible hangover, but I still was aroused ... I was tired but aroused at the same time, I mean, every thought seemed to turn into wanting to have sex ... Sexually, physically, I mean extremely euphoric: I want to keep having sex, I want to do this, I want to do that, I'm telling you I was extremely sexually aroused. I masturbated three times that day.

(Fernando)

It is perhaps no surprise that for many, such prolonged states of arousal were often experienced as tension and dissatisfaction:

> I am running around looking for ass, or I'm not running around, just looking at ass. And I start like getting all like built up like you know, sexual energy, but not really like sexual, like tension.
>
> (Armando, 27 years old, shipping and receiving clerk, born in the USA, HIV–)

> It was hours and hours of wanting to be satisfied but not being able to be.
>
> (Roberto)

> On crystal meth you don't satisfy, you know, it's just like that need, you know, that urge for sex that you never satisfy.
>
> (Rodolfo, 39 years old, hairstylist, born in Nicaragua, HIV+)

> With drugs you start degenerating and you no longer are satisfied with one person … you want another and you want more and you want them all at the same time.
>
> (Raul)

> Makes me very interested in performing sexual activities, very interested. I just don't know why I walk around with all of this hunger, physical hunger. And I don't usually act on it. I mean I'll, I'll go home and think about stuff and masturbate.
>
> (Luis, 36 years old, legal assistant, born in the USA, HIV–)

Better sex or just longer?

Men described sex as being more intense, more passionate and more focused, as evidence by the following interaction between the interviewer and Martin (35 years old, health worker, born in Central America (specific country not disclosed), HIV negative) as well as in the subsequent quote from Ismael:

INTERVIEWER: Did you feel the effects of the drugs while you were having sex?
MARTIN: Oh yeah.
INTERVIEWER: What did you feel?
MARTIN: I felt very good. I enjoyed it and I felt like a very nice sensation in your body. You feel very good. Everything pretty much feels like … in a different motion. The sensation is … lasts longer and you feel more passionate, more connected and more sexual. You feel very good about what you're doing.
The intensity, it makes me feel incredibly well. Yes, the focusing on the sex, the focusing means unity in all that time when you are having sex … when I'm having sex under those circumstances there's nothing else to think about.
(Ismael, 40 years old, unemployed, on disability government assistance, born in Mexico, HIV+)

But more often than not, when sex was described as better or 'incredible', the description was qualified in terms of the length and/or frequency of sexual activity:

It's more passionate. It's more … [pause] … longer! It's like eight hours of sex!
(Alberto, 39 years old, unemployed, on disability government assistance, born
in the USA, HIV+)

I told my roommate, 'Hey listen, I did this and that, and I felt good. I have never
tried that … It's incredible, you can have sex for a long time' … I wanted to do
it again. I remembered what it was to have sex with that person for 4 or 5 hours
and I wanted to do it again … I wanted to be having that kind of sex, that prolonged sex all night long or all afternoon long.

(Fernando)

I feel like invincible, you have so much energy, you can do anything…you can
have a hard-on that goes for six hours, you know what I mean?
(Rodrigo, 44 years old, restaurant waiter, born in Cuba, HIV+)

When I had sex, I would have sex three times at night, three times in the day, I
will keep having sex during the day and … there would be no limit.
(Miguel, 43 years old, unemployed, on temporary general government
assistance, born in Mexico, HIV+)

Thus, even though it was generally agreed that sex was experienced so much more
intensely when under the influence of crystal meth, it was not clear from the narratives whether sex was actually better, more pleasurable or simply that it lasted
longer, or could be had more often under a state of prolonged arousal.

The multiple meanings of disinhibition

Study participants generally agreed that they felt sexually uninhibited when under
the influence of crystal meth. Disinhibition, however, meant different things for different men. Meanings of disinhibition ranged from a general feeling of relaxation
and freedom in sexual situations to a willingness to perform sexual acts that were
seen as risky, 'kinky' or forbidden when they were not under the influence of the
drug. For some, the experienced disinhibition took them to situations where they
felt a loss of control.

For many men, crystal meth produced a general feeling of sexual freedom – physical and psychological – that afforded a more comfortable sexual experience. Physical relaxation, particularly of the anus muscles, was often welcome for men who
tend to experience pain during receptive anal intercourse when not under the influence of substances. The following interaction between the interviewer and a somewhat shy and sexually inhibited participant – Rafael (34 years old, restaurant worker,
born in Mexico, HIV+) – describes the benefits of anal muscle relaxation under the
influence of crystal meth. Note the underlying meaning of the text, even though the
word 'anus' or other equivalents ('ass', 'butt') are not explicitly mentioned:

INTERVIEWER: And what did the speed feel like?
RAFAEL: It felt good. It helped me to relax when it comes to – you know, when it
came to the sex part.
INTERVIEWER: It helped you relax?

RAFAEL: Yeah.

INTERVIEWER: How so?

RAFAEL: Mm, I ... very tight person. You know, not uptight. You know, tight within my ... Maybe by stress or –

INTERVIEWER: You mean physically tight?

RAFAEL: Yeah.

INTERVIEWER: And it helped you loosen up?

RAFAEL: Yeah.

INTERVIEWER: And that was good for sex?

RAFAEL: It was great, yeah.

INTERVIEWER: How?

RAFAEL: Well, it was, you know, you just, you just relax and enjoy – you know, enjoy it.

INTERVIEWER: Enjoy what?

RAFAEL: Enjoy you know, the performance of it.

More typically, the perceived disinhibition was experienced as a willingness to do or go to places men would not normally do or go to when not using the drug. Some spoke about daring fantasies that they could enact with a new sense of courage under the influence of crystal meth: 'You can be wild and wish I could have a third buddy here and a great time... I'll tie you up and all those wild fantasies come up' (Martin). But more often than not, the narratives indicated that most men have a set of personal limits regarding sexual activity – limits about acts, persons and places – but that limits were trespassed when under the influence of crystal meth. Typically, the limits had to do with some kind of sexual activity that was seen as 'kinky' or 'hardcore', but sometimes they referred to trespassing limits around safer sex:

> It definitely puts you in a mindset where you feel safe enough to go somewhere where you shouldn't normally go, whether you're, you're going to be the bottom or you're going to be the top or you're going to be dominant, you're going to be this or you're going to have sex with different men all night at a sex club ... When I do speed or recreational dugs, it leads me to not use condoms. It gives you a false sense of what you are doing like, you know, say you do it with somebody and you're in a close environment, it makes you relax with that person. It lets all your fears go away and so you don't use condoms and maybe the sex, the sex is a little rougher and a little more dangerous.
>
> (Antonio, 37 years old, self-employed small business accountant, born in the USA, HIV+)

Not infrequently the disinhibition felt like a new sense of liberation, power and aggressiveness in the sexual domain, perhaps in reaction to having in the past felt guilty or ashamed about sexuality or sexual body parts:

> I become even more hardcore. Sexual risks and inhibitions are totally gone. I become empowered in feeling, like, I can take on the world or anyone that fucked with me. It can be an euphoric rush. You can feel it in your ass, in your

balls, where it heats them up all of a sudden. It did help me explore my ass at one point when I refused to even think I had an ass.

(Angel)

It is important to note that, with few exceptions, men spoke not about being forced by the drug to trespass previously set limits. Rather, they spoke about a place they wanted to go to (or acts they wanted to do), but did not dare to for one reason or another. With crystal meth, they found a new sense of courage and safety that allowed them to do or go to those places. Thus, for the majority of those interviewed, particularly for those with less frequent use, there was a sense of personal agency rather than a sense of losing control under the influence of crystal meth:

Speed will take you there when you want to go there, you are like, like it gives you an excuse to like be freer with yourself which is a good thing, but I mean then it does, definitely does take you to the area where you can be unsafe too.

(Antonio)

For a selected few, however, the experience was one of loss of agency and control:

It can really make you do things that I wouldn't, I can lose a little self-control, in what I do and how far I go.

(Armando)

I got real high and I got really horny, so horny that it was out of control. It was very out of control. It's like I could have fucked forever.

(Cesar, 29 years old, sales clerk, born in the USA, HIV–)

Negative sexual side-effects

Throughout the interviews, men often spoke of negative side effects of crystal meth use on their sexual lives. The negative effects ranged from loss of erection ability to damaging their genitals as a result of repeated and prolonged sexual activity:

I couldn't get nobody, and I couldn't get an erection any more, I was so sore that, I kept playing with myself at home, and I rubbed it so sore, it became raw, that's how bad it was. It didn't feel good afterward.
(Juan, 36 years old, unemployed (on public assistance), born in the USA, HIV+)

Speed makes you horny, but the thing is you can't fuck for too long. Sometimes you get red and like swollen … on your genitals, on your dick or your pussy or whatever, your booty hole. You just fuck for so long, it gets raw.
(Ricardo, 23 years old, textile librarian, born in the USA, HIV+)

It was also clear from the narratives that the intense sexual appetite and the frequent and prolonged sexual activity were not conducive to intimate and warm connections with sexual partners. In most cases, sex under the influence of crystal meth was described as different from intimate, romantic encounters. For many, crystal meth was an obstacle to socialising or to the kinds of interactions that build relationships. The descriptions of sexual episodes were mostly focused on the physicality of the sexual experience, mostly on its intense and prolonged nature, with many descriptions portraying sexual partners simply as objects of sexual satisfaction:

> I have a lot of sexual energy and I'm just, I'm just looking at men like they are pieces of meat.
>
> (Armando)

> It's funny because I probably have a better time, chance, if I really like someone, being nice to them and talking them into like going out to dinner or whatever. Under the influence of drugs I don't know what to say, I stumble, I'm nervous, and all I think about is sexual gratification and wanting this person, wanting to use this person for sexual gratification.
>
> (Luis)

> I get horny, you know, and I just want to bust a nut. I don't want no fucking hi's no bye's, no conversation. I want to go in there, I want to bust a nut. I'm going to leave you know. I don't want no relationship, I don't want no fucking friendly conversation. I don't want breakfast, I don't want dinner. I don't want nothing, you know. All I want to do is give my cock a wash after I'm done.
>
> (Ramon, 32 years, assistant manager, born in the USA, HIV–)

For most of the participants, consistent with research findings to date, there was a clear connection between the use of crystal meth and sexual practices that could lead to HIV transmission:

> When I do crystal, because of the higher sex drive that it arouses within me, I'm more apt to have unsafe sex when I'm on that particular drug … the few times I have slipped up has been primarily because of that drug.
>
> (Roberto)

We interviewed some men who were, at the time of the study, in recovery from frequent and dependent use of crystal meth in their recent past. Those men spoke about the great sex they had under the influence, particularly at beginning stages of use or at times of moderate use. But those men looked back at their sexual experience under crystal meth as being 'not real sex' or 'clouded' by the drug. Some expressed that they have learned to have 'even better sex' without the drug:

> I used to think that I felt the sensation of having sex better with drugs, but I've learned to feel it even better without drugs, and I don't mean to say – I enjoy it both ways – but I prefer it not with drugs, because again your mind gets clouded. And I don't want to go back to the same old behaviour with drugs and what it can do – I'm tired of that kind of madness.
>
> (Ignacio, 36 years old, administrative assistant, born in the USA, HIV–)

Discussion

The qualitative findings described in this chapter allow a closer look at the subjective experiences of a group of Latino gay men in San Francisco who engage in sexual activity under the influence of crystal meth. The findings reveal the presence of very strong sexual effects while under the influence of this powerful stimulant, in particular, unusually prolonged states of sexual arousal and prolonged sexual activity.

The use of crystal meth is clearly related to men's desire to enhance their sexual experience, and users report not only intensely pleasurable sexual activity but also sex that is freer, less inhibited and more focused away from mental distractions. There are also pronounced effects of crystal meth use on anal sex, not only because the drug relaxes the sphincter muscles but also because men experience a set of warm physical sensations around their anus that help them recognise it as an organ of sexual pleasure. Notably, while many men described engaging in receptive anal sex for its pleasurable sensations, very few spoke of it as a substitute for insertive penetrative sex when experiencing erection problems, as is commonly assumed.

It is commonly believed that a major drawback of crystal meth use is its interference with erectile function, and some men indeed spoke about it, but more often than not they spoke of having 'instant' erections that 'lasted for hours'. The narratives, however, revealed other sexual effects of crystal meth that can be considered uncomfortable or detrimental to men's sexual health, wellbeing and pleasure; some of these negative sexual effects are seldom documented in the literature. For example, men spoke not only about the pleasures of prolonged sexual arousal and activity, but also reported that the increased and prolonged arousal (sometimes labelled as 'hunger') was often experienced as a source of tension and discomfort that could not be easily alleviated.

Men spoke about the need to masturbate multiple times in an attempt to satisfy a sexual hunger that did not go away, to the point of physically damaging their penises. They spoke of a sexual desire that could not be easily satisfied and were at times self-deprecatory when they portrayed themselves as compulsively cruising the streets or the internet in search of sexual satisfaction. In addition, men spoke of how the intense states of sexual arousal interfered with different social and interpersonal aspects of sexual encounters, indicating that the extreme focus on sexual satisfaction did not allow interactions that were more cordial, intimate or caring for the other person(s).

The changes of perception that occur when under the influence of crystal meth tend to be subjectively experienced as liberation from sexual taboos and as an increased sense of comfort and safety in sexual activity. At the same time, most men recognised that a drug-induced sense of safety could backfire by placing them in situations of danger, including a higher risk for HIV transmission. Some of them spoke of an extreme aspect of disinhibition that was experienced as a loss of sexual control, but at present it is not clear whether the perceived lack of control is related to a larger trend towards more frequent and dependent patterns of drug use and abuse. A remaining research question is how the generally positive experience of disinhibition can develop into an experience of loss of control under the influence of crystal meth. Research is needed particularly to understand how occasional use turns into patterns of use that can be considered addictive and accompanied by a general perceived loss of control. Regardless whether they reported loss of control or not, the majority of men in the sample acknowledged that they were more willing to act sexually unsafe (unprotected), with a false sense of power, invulnerability and safety that the drug provided.

Most men reported a sense of personal agency to their crystal meth use throughout the in-depth interviews, suggesting that the drug allowed them to do things they would like to do sexually or go to sexual places they would like to go, but find difficult to do without it. For many, the drug allows them to engage in different types of sex acts and explore different sexual situations, that they have labelled as 'kinky', 'hardcore', 'raunchy' or 'dirty'. The narratives suggest that this stimulant drug might be particularly useful for men who tend to be sexually shy, inhibited or who experience sexual shame and discomfort for reasons related perhaps to their socialisation in a homophobic, hetero-normative society. Also, because many gay men, including Latinos, come to San Francisco for a sense of sexual freedom and openness about their homosexuality, it is possible that many of these men use the drug in order to fit into a sexual culture that in general terms frowns on sexual inhibition. It is imperative, therefore, that we as gay men engage in a critical reflection about the complex relationships between our experiences of homophobia and our patterns of drug use. Moreover, we must critically observe and analyse elements of our sexual cultures that can be, for some, a bridge to sexual liberation, while for others a path of social and cultural conformity that can be ultimately self-destructive.

References

Colfax, G. and Guzman, R. (2006) 'Club Drugs and HIV Infection: A Review', *Clinical Infectious Diseases*, 42: 1463–9.

Díaz, R. M. (2006) 'Fabulous Effects, Disastrous Consequences – Stimulant Use among Latino Gay Men in San Francisco', invited presentation for the First Annual Crystal Meth Summit, sponsored by the Latino Commission on AIDS at the Mailman School of Public Health, Columbia University.

Díaz, R. M. (2007) 'Methamphetamine Use and its Relation to HIV Risk: Data from Latino Gay Men', in Meyer, I. and Northridge, M. E. (eds) *The Health of Sexual Minorities: Public Health Perspectives on Lesbian, Gay, Bisexual, and Transgender Populations*, New York: Springer.

Fernandez, M. I., Bowen, G. S., Warren, J. C., Ibanez, G. E., Hernandez, N., Harper, G. W. and Prado, G. (2007) '"Crystal Methamphetamine": A Source of Added Sexual Risk for Hispanic Men who have Sex with Men?', *Drug and Alcohol Dependence*, 86: 245–52.

Halkitis, P. N., Parsons, J. T. and Stirratt, M. J. (2001) 'A Double Epidemic: Crystal Methamphetamine Drug Use in Relation to HIV Transmission among Gay Men', *Journal of Homosexuality*, 41 (2): 17–35.

Ramirez-Valles, J., Garcia, D., Campbell, R., Díaz, R. M. and Heckathorn, D. (2008) 'HIV Infection, Sexual Risk, and Substance Use among Latino Gay and Bisexual Men and Transgender Persons', *American Journal of Public Health*, 98: 1036–42.

Reback, C. J. and Grella, C. E. (1999) 'HIV Risk Behaviors of Gay and Bisexual Male Methamphetamine Users contacted through Street Outreach', *Journal of Drug Issues*, 29: 155–66.

Rippeth, J. D., Heaton, R. K., Carey, C. L., Marcotte, T. D., Moore, D. J., Gonzalez, R. *et al.* (2004) 'Methamphetamine Dependence increases the Risk of Neuropsychological Impairment in HIV Infected Persons', *Journal of the International Neuropsychological Society*, 10 (1): 1–14.

Stall, R. and Purcell, D. W. (2000) 'Intertwining Epidemics: A Review of Research on Substance Use among Men who have Sex with Men and its Connection to the AIDS Epidemic', *AIDS and Behavior*, 4 (2): 181–92.

Wang, G. J., Volkow, N. D., Chang, L., Miller, E., Sedler, M., Hitzemann, R. *et al.* (2004) 'Partial Recovery of Brain Metabolism in Methamphetamine Abusers after Protracted Abstinence', *American Journal of Psychiatry*, 61 (2): 242–8.

Part V
The choreography of sex

24 Stripping

The embodiment and creation of sexualised fantasy

Katherine Frank

Strip clubs catering specifically to heterosexual men are a popular form of entertainment in the USA. The clubs range from neighbourhood bars to high-end entertainment complexes known as gentleman's clubs, and may offer an array of services – stage dancing, table dancing or lap dancing, extended conversation opportunities with dancers, food and beverages and televised sports events. Upper-tier gentleman's clubs may provide conference or VIP rooms to draw a business crowd; many of these clubs are marketed to middle class customers as 'classy' venues featuring refined entertainers, differentiated from the clubs one would find in a red-light district.

It makes sense that strip clubs should multiply in the USA during the last several decades, alongside the panic about HIV/AIDS and fears about the dissolution of the family. The process of upscaling in strip clubs, with a promise of 'clean' and respectable interactions, alleviates fears about contamination and disease that escalated around prostitution. There are numerous other social changes that may be influencing this rapid increase in strip clubs in the USA as well: the increased presence of women in the workforce, a continued backlash against feminism and the idea of 'political correctness', ongoing and concerted marketing efforts to sexualise and masculinise particular forms of consumption ('sports, beer and women', for example), changing patterns of mobility that have influenced dating practices and the formation of intimate partnerships, renewed commitments to monogamy for certain groups of married men, and changes in the nature of work that involve more out-of-town travel for business and thus more anonymous opportunities to purchase commodified sexualised services, to name just a few.

I began researching strip clubs in 1995 and worked as an exotic dancer off and on for six years during this time. In the period 1997–8 I conducted fieldwork in five strip clubs in a fairly large southeastern city that I call Laurelton by seeking employment as a nude entertainer. As strip clubs are highly stratified in terms of 'classiness', I selected sites ranging from the most prestigious clubs in the city (offering valet parking, luxurious atmospheres, expensive lighting and sound systems, dozens of dancers on multiple stages, etc.) to lower tier 'dive' bars (dimly lit, sparsely furnished and located in red-light districts or simply known as smaller neighbourhood venues). Although the degree of nudity varies in strip clubs around the country, Laurelton laws allowed the dancers to strip completely. Dancers were required to perform onstage for tips; they were also, however, expected to circulate among the customers to sell 'private' table dances. Depending on the rules and layout of the club, the dancer might disrobe on a customer's table so that he could view her from below, on the floor between his legs while he was seated or in front of his chair on a slightly raised platform. A club might have between one and four stages with dancers on each, and any number of nude women might be performing among the audience at any given time. In addition to my fieldwork, over the past decade I have continued to observe in strip clubs around the country and to interview both customers and dancers.

A focus on bodily exposure distinguishes strip clubs from other types of bars and nightclubs (although this boundary may be eroding somewhat with some of the increasingly risqué fashions for women) and the focus on sexualised looking in a *public* atmosphere differentiates strip clubs from many other forms of adult entertainment such as pornography, prostitution or oral or manual release in a massage parlour. Yet, the desire to visit strip clubs is more than just a desire to passively observe women's bodies, even for the most voyeuristic of customers. There are many ways to potentially 'see' naked women – peeping, viewing pornography, reading medical texts or developing intimate relationships with them, for example. These visits, then, must also be seen as a desire to have a particular kind of *experience* rooted in the complex network of relationships between 'home', 'work' and 'away', an experience that I have elsewhere analysed as 'touristic' (Frank 2002a).

Although a strip club may be a space of touristic leisure for the male customers, it is, first and foremost, a workplace for the dancers. Granted, stripping may be a means of rebellion for young women in addition to being a lucrative job, especially for those in the middle classes (Frank 2002b; Johnson 1999). However, the fact remains that the parties to the transactions are coming to the encounters with different purposes. These different purposes and meanings are not rooted in essential gender differences; rather, they are informed by labour relations as well as social positionings (including, but not limited to gender). Certainly the categories of worker and leisure seeker are not absolute: customers may conduct business activities at strip clubs, for example, and most customers are also workers in other arenas. Likewise, there may be some dancers for whom stripping feels more like leisure than work, at least on certain days, and a large component of the job involves engaging in practices associated with leisure – drinking alcohol, dining, conversing, flirting, having fun (or at least appearing to) and, especially, being undressed. Yet in the immediacy of the encounter, the money nearly always flows in one direction – from the customer to the dancer (until the dancer is asked to pay the establishment a cut of her earnings). Further, even though a man may conduct forms of business on the premises, it is precisely because this space is inherently 'not work' that it has been chosen. Thus, while one or both of the participants to any transaction may be 'playing' at any given time, this play is firmly situated within a larger framework of cultural and economic relations. It is within this framework that the dancers' bodily revelations and performances of identity become meaningful, and hence profitable, both for themselves and for the clubs.

The relationship of nudity to forms of power and control has long been bolstered by the regulation of bodily exposure by state and local governments in the USA, as well as the ways that those regulations are proposed, implemented and debated in public forums. Although I do not have space here to detail the development of modern exotic dance out of other entertainment forms such as vaudeville, burlesque or cabaret shows, it is important to realise that the history of striptease is shaped by the history of regulation and the conflicts surrounding sexualised displays and behaviours in US public culture. Distinctions made between art and obscenity, lewd or acceptable behaviour or moral or immoral forms or representations of sexuality can be seen as ongoing arguments that are carried out in legal forums, academic treatises, public culture and the media and living rooms around the country. Frequently what is indecent in one decade is commonplace in the next (think of the scandal over the bodily exposure of famous burlesque star Lydia Thompson in the late nineteenth century – she wore *tights* and made them visible to an audience) (Allen 1991), yet that does not mean that the transgressions of the day are perceived any less seriously by their participants or treated less harshly.

Regulations against striptease have often been justified in the name of social control and public safety. Such public safety campaigns can also be seen as reflecting a social class bias, with working-class or lower tier forms of entertainment being penalised more harshly than those designated 'art' and enjoyed by relatively privileged audiences (Foley 2002; Hanna 1999b; etc.). Striptease is seen as dangerous and socially disruptive by conservative segments of the population and thousands of taxpayer and private dollars are spent in attempts to eradicate strip clubs in communities across the nation. Because of their lingering working class associations, and the persistent, often erroneous belief that they are indelibly linked to prostitution, crime and other 'negative secondary effects', strip clubs have already been subject to more severe regulations than other kinds of entertainment, and some municipalities have attempted to use restrictive regulations to close down adult businesses altogether: requiring extremely bright lighting, prohibiting tipping, requiring bikinis or cocktail dresses at all times, stipulating excessive distance rules to separate the entertainers and the customers, etc. (Hanna 1999a). In 2000, despite a lack of sound evidence that strip clubs cause negative secondary effects, the Supreme Court upheld legislation regulating exotic dance in the city of Erie, Pennsylvania, ruling that 'nude public dancing itself is immoral' (Foley 2002: 3).

The intricacies of the many battles fought in locales across the country throughout the twentieth century would be impossible to detail here, as would the complexities of the justifications that continue to be given for regulating, harassing, shutting down or allowing venues that offer the display of sexualised female bodies to their patrons. Instead, it is important to realise that regulation and scandal does not just repress unruly 'natural' desires in the name of civilisation and order, but actually helps to create and shape those desires (Foucault 1978).

Nudity has an assortment of sometimes conflicting meanings, including but not limited to: innocence, naturalness, authenticity, vulnerability, sexual power, truth, revelations of one's inner self, humiliation, degradation, a lack of self-respect, immorality, sexual accessibility and a prelude to sexual activity. *Public* nudity is embedded in a host of additional symbolic and emotional meanings, again often ambivalent and frequently revolving around issues of power and control. The use of stripping an individual of his or her clothes as a form of military action, punitive measure or means of humiliation is widely understood as a means of exercising power. At the same time, people who willingly or purposefully shed their clothes in public are often criminalised or stigmatised and seen as dangerous (powerful?) or pathological – 'trenchcoaters', streakers, nudists, strippers.

Prohibitions on nudity have long been seen as part of the repression of natural sexuality and the body by society, both in academic theories and in folk understandings; thus, nudity can appear as transgressive, even dangerous to the civilised order.

Patrons of strip clubs, being subjects to and of the same discourses as other individuals, also bring ideas about nudity as transgressive, dangerous and liberating to their visits to strip clubs and their encounters with dancers. The notion that strip clubs were somehow an expression of a transcultural, transhistorical 'natural' male sexuality that was repressed in everyday life was important to many of the customers. Similarly, the idea that strip clubs were places in which one was at risk for physical or moral contamination was also motivating and eroticised for the regular customers. Customers sometimes described themselves as 'adventurers', dancers as 'brave' and 'wild', and strip clubs themselves as places 'outside of the law' (Frank 2002a).

In strip clubs, customers also bring their own sexual histories to the transactions, as well as their beliefs about gender, sexuality and consumption. Although few of the customers claimed to be religious, and overwhelmingly expressed support for the dancers' right to disrobe and the 'naturalness' of such an act, their enthusiasm usually waned when they were asked how they would feel if it were a wife or daughter onstage. Many of the regular customers were married to women who had more conservative views about nudity and sexuality than they did. Some customers stated that they were never allowed to look at the bodies of their wives or partners, even during sex – in these cases, nudity might be fascinating, awe inspiring or even upsetting. Even for those men who did have access to private revelations of the female body, the fact that they were paying for live, public performances meant that there were additional emotional layers enwrapping their interpretations of their encounters – mixtures of shame, anxiety, excitement and desire. If it is true that 'there is no apprehension of the body of the other without a corresponding (re)vision of one's own' (Phelan 1993: 171), some of the pleasure in these commodified encounters arises from complicated, and concurrent, fantasies of security (rooted in the ritualised performances of sexual difference that unfold in the clubs) and fantasies of rupture or transgression (rooted in the feelings of degradation, vulnerability and freedom that many of the customers felt would accompany their own public nudity) (see Frank 2002a).

Perniola writes that in the figurative arts, 'eroticism appears as a relationship between clothing and nudity'. That is, eroticism is 'conditional on the possibility of movement – transit – from one state to the other' (1989: 237). This is so in a strip club as well – although perhaps a few customers would still be titillated if the dancers took the stage already nude – but with an added, *gendered* transit as dancers also move between categories and potentialities, performing as 'fantasy girls' who may be simultaneously, or alternatively, virgins and whores (Egan 2003). Although costumes are variable, ranging from the dominatrix to the schoolgirl, two themes continue to reappear in dancers' self-presentations and adornments: sexual availability/knowledge and innocence/untouchability. These themes emerge in a paradoxical relationship to each other – no dancer is actually sexually available within the confines of the club (or we are no longer talking about stripping) and no dancer is innocent in all social circles when her transgressions (disrobing in public and for money) become known.

Terrence Turner discusses the Kayapo of the Amazon, who exhibit an elaborate code of bodily adornment despite the fact that they do not wear clothing (lip plugs, penis sheaths, beads, body painting, plucked eyebrows, head shaving, etc.) and writes: '[T] apparently naked savage is as fully covered in a fabric of cultural meaning as the most elaborately draped Victorian lady or gentleman' (1980: 115).

Dancers, in this sense that Turner is referring to, are probably less naked than the rest of us under our clothes. One of the first things that a new dancer learns is how to adorn, present and move her body in ways that are legal, profitable and comfortable. Dancers continually modified their skin through grooming (cleansing, hair removal, texturising of the skin) makeup, scents and tanning. Hair has deeply symbolic meanings in many cultural systems (see Obeyesekere 1981; Rooks 1996; Turner 1980; etc.) and may become meaningful in different times and places through colour, length, style and so forth. The hair on the head, as well as the hair elsewhere on the body, is connected to gender systems in the USA: women are expected to remove hair from their legs, armpits, bikini line and face, for example, yet long hair on the head is generally associated with femininity. Longer hair has the advantage of being able to highlight particular body parts – it can be pulled in front to hide and then reveal the breasts; in a rear view pose it can brush the top of the buttocks; it can conceal or emphasise the eyes. Hair colour may also be used to send signals to customers and is associated with particular looks and personalities – the bubbly or sexy blonde, the exotic brunette, the feisty redhead. Although wilder styles and colours were found at the lower tier clubs, particularly among younger dancers, the upper-tier clubs tended to be more standardised. Dancers almost always conformed to the expectation of hair removal on the body, or were penalised for not doing so by the management or customers. In addition to removing leg and underarm hair, in the nude clubs most dancers also removed all of the pubic hair from the labia.

Accessorising the body did not stop at the skin or the hair, of course, and numerous kinds of plastic surgery are undergone by dancers perfecting their look: breast implants, breast lifts or reductions, lip injections, nose jobs, liposuction, tummy tucks, labia standardisation, etc. Other kinds of body modification included tattoos and piercings, especially tongue and clitoral piercings, and were increasingly common in the younger dancers (something that many of the older male customers commented on as marking a difference from their generation). While breast augmentations and other kinds of standardising surgeries usually served to enhance a woman's value in the industry, tattoos and piercings did not necessarily do so. Dancers also modified their bodies for the job through dieting and physical training such as working out and bodybuilding.

Although nudity itself has been referred to as the 'primal costume' (Lewin 1984), there are few, if any, dancers who do not continue to fashion their nude bodies through accessories like high heels, boots, boas, jewellery, makeup or other specialised or theme costuming options. Performance theorist Katherine Liepe-Levinson writes that, for strippers, 'Costumes are environments for bodies, and like the interior design of theatres, they not only frame those bodies, but also engage the wearers and viewers in environmental reciprocities with cultural symbols of gender and desire' (1998: 137). Costumes help shape customer perceptions of dancers as they mingle with the audience, and thus sometimes influence which customers a dancer will interact with on a given night. Further, even as a dancer undresses, her body may retain traces of her outfit and garner complex valuations of classy or 'trashy' associated with particular kinds of adornment and the way that she wears them.

Dancers often appropriated standard cultural fantasies in their self-presentations and often self-consciously mixed behavioural patterns with symbolic fashion choices.

Some women designed their approach to customers based on the bimbo stereotype – bubbly, giggly and light hearted – and might wear bikinis, brightly coloured clingy gowns or theme costumes depending on the rules of the club. Similarly, some dancers presented themselves as the girl next door – as students, friends or even possible lovers (although only in fantasy), and might wear cut-off shorts and tank tops, sundresses or 'tasteful' gowns. Others took up the position of bad girl – dressing in black and leather, talking dirty, promising dominance or adventure. Still others switched approaches depending on mood, type of customer and what the other dancers were doing that evening. One would rarely find a whole club of dominatrixes because the customer base usually would not support it; by the same token, one might find any number of plaid-skirted schoolgirls circulating among the audience. Sometimes costumes were chosen to fit body types – a small breasted woman, for example, might have a more difficult time pulling off the 'sexy secretary' than one who was literally spilling out of her business suit. Although the schoolgirl look was profitable for dancers with a wide range of body types, for different reasons, a very flat-chested or young looking dancer might be advised to try out the look. Many dancers also avoided particular looks that they found physically or morally uncomfortable. Some did not like little girl looks, for example, while others would not wear items associated with S&M.

An aesthetics of feminine excess (Waggoner 1997) works well in the sex industry, as everything can be overdone as a means of generating attention: necklines can plunge, skirt lengths can rise. Makeup can be exaggerated. Fetish boots might have platform heels and rise eight inches from the floor. Dancers may employ signs of wealth and glamour, and costumes can be extravagantly accessorised in a manner far too opulent (or trashy) for the average middle-class woman. How these signs are read by the customers varies, although is often patterned by the setting. In everyday life, of course, generating too much attention can be risky or annoying for women and the clubs could thus offer a safe place in which to try out forbidden looks or movements (Frank 2002b; Johnson 1999).

Over the last few decades, strip clubs have become ever more interactive and derive a great deal of their erotic charge from the promise of highly personalised encounters through the sale of table or lap dances. Unlike the burlesque shows of earlier years (Allen 1991), the highly choreographed Parisian striptease written about by Roland Barthes (1957) or the spectacular topless revues found in tourist locations such as Las Vegas, 'house'[1] dancers working in contemporary gentleman's clubs usually mingle with the audience members individually, possibly spending more time conversing or dancing at a single customer's table than in disrobing on stage. This increased interpersonal interaction requires new strategies on the part of the dancers for generating and maintaining customer interest, often involving performances of authenticity ('You're different from the other customers, I'll tell you my real name') and revelations of self ('Let's get to know each other') (see Frank 1998).

In a piece on Parisian striptease, Barthes writes that it is based on the fundamental contradiction that woman is 'desexualised at the very moment when she is stripped naked' (1957: 84). The classic props used in striptease, he argues, ensure that the nakedness that follows the woman's act is 'no longer a part of a further, genuine undressing'. Instead, it 'remains itself unreal, smooth and enclosed like a beautiful slippery object' (1957: 85). The dance routine is also a barrier to the true

erotic for Barthes – as through a series of ritualistic gestures it hides the very nakedness that it is supposed to reveal. Professional stripteasers 'wrap themselves in the
miraculous ease which constantly clothes them, makes them remote, gives them the
icy indifference of skillful practitioners, haughtily taking refuge in the sureness of
their technique' (1957: 86). He notes, however, that eroticism resurfaces in the
amateur contest, where beginners undress 'without resorting or resorting very clum-
sily to magic, which unquestionably restores to the spectacle its erotic power'. With
'no feathers or furs' and 'few disguises as a starting point – gauche steps, unsatisfactory dancing, girls constantly threatened by immobility, and above all by a "technical" awkwardness (the resistance of briefs, dress or bra)', amateurs are denied 'the
alibi of art and the refuge of being an object', which gives their disrobing an 'unexpected importance' (1957: 86). Barthes, of course, is discussing striptease that took
the form of elaborate costuming and lengthy stage shows which included little
contact between the stripper and the individual members of the audience. Nevertheless, the popularity of amateur contests in contemporary strip clubs, the allure of
'new girls' and the customers' confessed dislike of professionalism all support
Barthes' contentions, at least in part.

What Barthes perhaps did not realise, or what has perhaps changed since he
wrote, is that some dancers have themselves become mythologists of sorts – self-
consciously fashioning ways to produce an illusion of further unveiling in a room
where any number of women may simultaneously be nude. Such a strategy, of
course, does not work for every woman; neither does every woman need or want to
use it – there are some customers, after all, for whom nudity itself is thrilling enough
to compel financial generosity or who enjoy the spectacular rather than the individualised parts of the experience. Yet, such 'intentional' unveilings could indeed be
profitable and dancers use a number of strategies to produce such intimate expo-
sures – telling stories about their personal lives, feigning or summoning up attraction for the customer or embarrassment about being undressed in front of him or
providing customers with real names or cell phone numbers, for example (Frank
1998). Dancers also sometimes crafted mistakes in their performance or attire to
appear inexperienced or new.

The lack of 'professionalism' exhibited by dancers new to the business implied to
some men that they would not be as skilled at manipulating men out of their money.
To others, it seemed to provide a tension between purity and defilement which was
particularly exciting. Contrariwise, there were certainly interactions that made
dancers feel uncomfortably exposed, emotionally or physically, although the particularities varied for different women and boundaries were maintained in a variety of
ways. Some dancers found regulars too emotionally draining to deal with, for
example, and instead sought out quick encounters with men that they did not
intend to see again. Customers sometimes used financial incentives to lure dancers
across their boundaries of propriety or privacy. Women with the most financial need
would find themselves more vulnerable to such requests.

A tension between purity and defilement also played out through customer talk
about beauty. One frequently given justification by men for their visits to strip clubs
is that 'all men like to look at beautiful women' or that 'women's bodies are works
of art'. The appreciation of female beauty, then, was sometimes given as a justification for visiting the upper-tier clubs where the dancers were supposedly 'prettier'.
Men who were travelling or visiting with business associates would also often choose

the upscale clubs because of their reputation for beautiful women (reputations earned through vigorous marketing and timely photo spreads in magazines like *Playboy's Guide to Men's Clubs*) and because these clubs were seen as providing the most opportunity to impress friends or clients. Dancers at the lower tier clubs were sometimes referred to in a derogatory way as 'whores' and described as 'overweight, tattooed, and not very bright'. As symbols of conspicuous consumption in the clubs, beautiful women could also maintain the respectability and class status of the *men* who spent time with them. Just as the differentiation of a high-art nude from a centrefold in aesthetic terms can sometimes differentiate the *consumers* of each, an encounter with a beautiful woman could serve to partly legitimate a stigmatised behaviour in the strip club: a man could claim to be enjoying her in a purely aesthetic manner, which is generally seen as more respectable than looking at her for the purpose of pornographic (masturbatory) fantasy. This claim, however, is often made to balance out the 'obscene' body with which a customer is also faced with in such a scenario.

Beauty should not be seen simply as a 'natural' occurrence, however, for it is implicated in other social systems. Although a certain degree of physical attractiveness and athleticism may be a job prerequisite for working in a strip club (unless there is an extreme shortage of women willing to work as dancers), hierarchies within the industry are affected by social class. Skeggs writes that 'physical attractiveness may work as a form of capital (corporeal capital)' but also as a form of class privilege (1997: 102). Class privilege in attractiveness may also take the form of specialised knowledge and tools, as well as the resources to procure them. Women who have the most options as far as where they work, which customers they interact with, what kinds of service they are interested in performing and for retiring from the sex industry when they decide to do so, are usually those who are able to conform to middle-class standards of appearance (and sometimes also of behaviour, comportment and interaction).

Some dancers at every club enhanced their appearances through techniques such as hair extensions, plastic surgeries, year-round tanning, etc. Access to such techniques, however, as well as the quality of the results, was connected to social class and economic assets. Even the application of stage makeup and accessorising one's costume carried with it certain kinds of cultural capital as well as learned skill and financial flexibility. Cultural capital could also influence dancers' interactions outside the club, especially knowledge of the appropriate level of sexualised comportment and appearance for different situations. Women who had large implants or kept up a 'stripper look' or behaviour in other spheres could face harassment because of this decision and because of their visibility as women who transgressed expected codes of feminine display. Customers distinguished between dancers who they found attractive in the club and dancers that they would find attractive in other spheres as well – the girl you could 'take home to mom', the 'girl next door'.

Strip clubs are a contemporary form of adult entertainment and the performances and interactions that unfold inside must be understood in their political, economic, historical and cultural contexts. Strippers cater to the sexualised fantasies of their customers, and their various styles of adornment, comportment, movement and interpersonal engagement draw on both personal and cultural systems of meaning in complex ways.

Note

1 House dancers are regular employees of the clubs in which they work (or independent contractors, depending on the state). Feature dancers, by way of contrast, have travelling acts, pornographic credentials and receive special billing from the clubs.

References

Allen, R. C. (1991) *Horrible Prettiness: Burlesque and American Culture*, Chapel Hill: University of North Carolina Press.

Barthes, R. (1957/1972) *Mythologies*, New York: Hill & Wang.

Egan, D. (2003) 'Eroticism, Commodification and Gender: Exploring Exotic Dance in the United States', *Sexualities*, 6 (1), 105–14.

Foley, B. (2002) 'Naked Politics: Erie, PA v the Kandyland Club', *NWSA Journal*, 14 (2), 1–17.

Foucault, M. (1978) *The History of Sexuality, Volume I: An Introduction*, New York: Vintage Books.

Frank, K. (1998) 'The Production of Identity and the Negotiation of Intimacy in a "Gentleman's Club"', *Sexualities*, 1 (2), 175–202.

Frank, K. (2002a) *G-Strings and Sympathy: Strip Club Regulars and Male Desire*, Durham, NC: Duke University Press.

Frank, K. (2002b) 'Stripping, Starving, and Other Ambiguous Pleasures', in Johnson, M. L. (ed.), *Jane Sexes It Up: True Confessions of Feminist Desire*, New York: Four Walls, Eight Windows.

Hanna, J. L. (1999a) 'Toying With the Striptease Dancer and the First Amendment', in Reifel, S. (ed.) *Play and Culture Studies, Volume 2*, Stamford, CT: Ablex.

Hanna, J. L. (1999b) 'The Naked Truth', *Exotic Dancer Bulletin*, 4 (2): 138.

Johnson, M. L. (1999) 'Pole Work: Autoethnography of a Strip Club', in Dank, B. and Refinetti, R. (eds) *Sex Work & Sex Workers: Sexuality & Culture, Volume 2*, New Brunswick: Transaction Publishers.

Lewin, L. (1984) *Naked is the Best Disguise: My Life as a Stripper*, New York: William Morrow and Company, Inc.

Liepe-Levinson, K. (1998) 'Striptease: Desire, Mimetic Jeopardy, and Performing Spectators', *The Drama Review*, 42 (2), 9–37.

Obeyesekere, G. (1981) *Medusa's Hair: An Essay on Personal Symbols and Religious Experience*, Chicago: University of Chicago Press.

Perniola, M. (1989) 'Between Clothing and Nudity', pp. 237–65 in M. Fehrer (ed.), *Fragments for a History of the Human Body*. New York: Zone.

Phelan, P. (1993) *Unmarked: The Politics of Performance*, New York: Routledge.

Rooks, N. M. (1996) *Hair Raising: Beauty, Culture, and African American Women*, New Brunswick, NJ: Rutgers University Press.

Skeggs, B. (1997) *Formations of Class and Gender: Becoming Respectable*, London: Sage.

Turner, T. (1980) 'The Social Skin', in Cherfas, J. and Lewin, R. (eds) *Not Work Alone: A Cross-Cultural View of Activities Superfluous to Survival*, Beverly Hills, CA: Sage.

Waggoner, C. E. (1997) 'The Emancipatory Potential of Feminine Masquerade in Mary Kay Cosmetics', *Text and Performance Quarterly*, 17: 256–72.

25 Flirting, erotic interactions and sexual choreography among urban youth

Hip-hop in New York City[1]

Miguel Muñoz-Laboy and Richard Parker

For young people around the world, engagement in or disengagement from cultural narratives of masculinity and femininity forms an important backdrop for their own constructions of the meanings of sexuality, sexual behaviour and health risk. Although the emerging literature on young people's sexualities points towards the importance of social spaces in the development of young people's sexualities and gender ideologies, remarkably few studies have sought to explore the specific mechanisms through which the social and cultural construction of gender and sexuality might provide a meaningful context for the fuller understanding of their sexual practices and expressions, and gendered, sexual and reproductive health scripts.

Hip-hop culture is a key social medium in and through which many young men and women of colour (particularly in the USA, but also increasingly in other societies) construct their gender and sexuality (Kitwana 2002; Collins 2005; Watkins 2005). While it is certainly not the only important medium in this regard, it has nonetheless taken on increasing salience in recent years as it has been taken up and reproduced through the mass communications, fashion and the cultural and entertainment industries. Sexism, homophobia and violence are among the traits commonly associated with hip-hop in the popular media. Thus, it is not surprising to find an emerging research literature that has begun to identify relationships between listening to hip-hop modalities and increments in health risk behaviour among young people (Martino *et al.* 2006). By way of contrast, some scholars have deconstructed societal beliefs about hip-hop and have pointed out how many of these so-called facts about hip-hop are heavily influenced by the positions of those in social power to make such claims (Rivera 2003).

This chapter focuses on the hip-hop club scene with the intention of unpacking narratives of gender from the perspective of young men and women, and exploring how these relate to their sexual experiences. Our approach required 'listening' to young people's perceptions and interpretations of the ways in which the social structures of the hip-hop club scene intersect within the realm of sexual intimacy. Specifically, in this chapter, we will describe how young men and women negotiate gender relations on the dance floor of hip-hop clubs, the boundaries that govern such relations and how these dance encounters translate or not into sexual encounters. To explore these issues, we conducted a three-year ethnographic study (see Muñoz-Laboy *et al.* 2007 for information on the research design). The first part of this chapter will focus on the dance floor, gendered courtship, boundaries and transitions to sex. The second part of the chapter will contextualise these findings in relation to broader issues of sexuality, space and health.

The hip-hop club

Dancing in hip-hop clubs presents an opportunity for young men and young women to perform gender roles, sexual assertiveness and sexual appeal. The context of dancing to hip-hop, reggae, rap and reggaeton provides an opportunity for young men and women to get physically close to friends or other young people with whom they have not previously interacted. Reggaeton is a type of music that integrates reggae music with mixing and rap lyrics. Thus, the dance floors of hip-hop clubs turn into a competitive space where getting attention and being close to women is the goal for young men. For members of both sexes, the key aspect to compete in this space is dancing ability. Young men have to be smooth and show both confidence and competence in dancing to avoid rejection. To avoid rejection, young men also cannot get physically close to women on the dance floor unless they receive some form of cue from the female partner that getting close is permitted. Getting close to women is not only a motivation for dancing but it is the norm in the performance of reggaeton. For example Tony said that 'there's only one way to dance reggaeton and hip-hop, you have to dance close' (Tony, Hispanic, straight, 20 years old). Thus, dancing close and the performance aspect of dancing acquire relevant value for gender relations in the space of clubs.

Many young men see women's dancing as a way of calling attention to themselves, but for most young men being the best dancer is not as important as dancing at an acceptable level so that they can get close to women. Getting closer and 'grinding'[2] are consistent motivations when dancing with girls for almost all the young men in the study. From young women's perspectives, dancing in hip-hop clubs to hip-hop music styles was about having fun. One group of the women, however, equated dancing to hip-hop, reggae, etc., to sexual performance and sexual appeal. Jenn for example saw dancing and sex as similar behaviours:

> When I was dancing before I had sex I would dance all the stuff and be like whatever, and everybody would say sex is like dancing. If you know how to grind you'll know how to ride. I never thought it was true but when I did it I was like 'oh, I get it'.
>
> (Jenn, Dominican-Cuban, straight, 16 years old)

Jenn's experience thus provided her with 'proof' of the fact that this type of dancing served as a kind of simulation of sex. The phrase, 'if you know how to grind, you know how to ride', refers to the ability of moving the hips while performing vaginal (and/or anal) intercourse on top of a sexual partner. This captures the essence of the erotic value that showing sexual appeal on the dance floor has for these young women. Although most times the ability to grind did not translate directly into the sexual encounters in the lives of the young women, it was the ability to grind that was the key component of competition on the floor. This creates tremendous pressures for young women in the study to demonstrate their sexual womanhood through dancing. Similarly, young men were under constant pressures to present themselves as good dancers as a way of asserting aspects of their masculinity.

The courtship of dancing

The performance of gender and sexuality that takes place on the dance floors of the hip-hop clubs is enmeshed within the context of an elaborate set of cultural rules – a veritable etiquette of gendered scripts for appropriate male and female conduct. Within this etiquette, special emphasis is given to what might be described as 'the courtship of dancing'. Yet anyone expecting to find traditional courtship etiquette of old (or of some sectors of white, middle-class US society even today) will undoubtedly be surprised to encounter the rules of courtship operating in the hip-hop club scene. Asking girls to dance is not the 'correct' strategy in the hip-hop club. As Priscilla points out, 'at parties these days, they don't ask to dance, they just grab you up and dance' (Priscilla, Puerto Rican, heterosexual, 20 years old). Omar's strategy (Hispanic-Puerto Rican-Dominican, straight, 19 years old) was one of 'cutting in', and not asking and simply starting to dance was a consistent strategy among the men in the study (e.g. 'In a party I just grab a girl and just dance', Hector, Hispanic-Dominican, straight, 18 years old).

Some young men complement this dominant strategy with additional approaches that they believe make them more appealing to women on the dance floor. Carlos did not take the initiative with women. He caught their attention by actively ignoring them. Carlos explicitly used this approach in hip-hop clubs as well as other social spaces such as school. His approach was based on the notion that he should not demand attention, 'playing hard to get' (ignoring and treating young women with indifference and disinterest) until they approach him, making it clear that they demonstrated interest in him first. When Carlos was in his early teens he got rejected 'pretty badly' while trying to speak to a girl. Now he wants to avoid rejection by creating a demand for himself. This is an approach that many young men in his social environment use.

Hector's approach to getting attention is in opposition to Carlos'. He calls attention to himself through his dancing: 'I'm a show off so I have to make myself stand out ... If I want her I'm going to do everything to make sure she notices me' (Hispanic-Dominican, straight, 18 years old). Playing hard to get, being funny or calling attention by displaying dancing skills are not unique strategies to the hip-hop scene and reflect more common strategies of heterosexual men to get women's attentions (e.g. Seal and Ehrhardt 2003). However, when these scripts are deployed in the street or the school, for example, the desired outcome cannot necessarily be assessed by others. In the hip-hop dance floor, a successful outcome of the attention strategy is immediately assessed by whether or not the young woman dances with the young man. Thus, these scripts get reworked in the hip-hop club with the additional pressure of peers monitoring the success of the young man's actions.

Establishing and transgressing boundaries

While dancing close and grinding characterise the hip-hop club social scene, we now turn to another social trait of the courtship of dancing in the hip-hop scene: the establishment of boundaries on the dance floor, together with various, culturally defined, modes of transgressing these boundaries. Young women are the gatekeepers of dancing boundaries in the hip-hop scene. Even though most dances in hip-hop clubs involve grinding, particularly those that are derivative from reggae, there are levels of physical closeness that young men cannot cross. Young women's accounts on dancing boundaries reflect the control that they try to exert while dancing. Some women feel that they are in control of the level of physical closeness and that they can simply walk away if the dancing partner does not respect their boundaries.

One way of avoiding problems with men on the dance floor is through demonstrating 'a level of understanding' with respect to boundaries while dancing. Developing this is something that some young men, like Adrian, are aware of. He labelled this understanding as an issue of women's comfort. Since getting physically close to women is perceived as a natural positive outcome for young men, this notion of comfort presumes that young men's comfort while dancing is a non-issue. Young women control the boundaries and men have to be aware of the signs to not 'cross the lines'. And yet their roles as men are to skilfully push the boundaries while on the dance floor. As most of the young men also pointed out, balancing dancing boundaries becomes complicated if the dancers are drinking or getting high and 'people's judgment gets clouded'.

There is a specific type of young adult men in the club scenes with whom young women maintain their vigilance. These are men whose sexual interest is clear and goes beyond the erotic aspect of dancing. Jessica captures this concern in the following quote:

> Touching your butt is normal in hip-hop, that's like reggae. That's normal, because you're grinding against the guys so what did you expect would happen? But everything else, there's no need for that ... you know who to dance with; you know who's really a pervert and who's not.
>
> (Jessica, Dominican, straight, 16 years old)

Aware that this man had a crush on her, Jessica was able to exert control over the situation by shifting from dancing to getting something to drink. Jessica characterised certain types of men as 'perverts'. Jessica and other young women in the study define 'perverts' as those men who are too focused on getting or maintaining erections while dancing or too eager to grind on young women. Carmen's definition of a pervert on the dance floor included:

> Men grabbing me or lifting me up. I don't like men grinding on me, or when men are hard and want to dance all over me. I don't engage in dancing with guys who display those things. If a guy comes over to dance with me to continue his erection or to build an erection it's a turn off and I'm done.
>
> (Carmen, Hispanic, straight, 23 years old)

Young women in the hip-hop scene who are turned off by such male advances can limit how physically close men get to them. In the study, young women were consistently vigilant about maintaining control over their bodies and space. Men's physical impositions on the dance floor often led to negative feelings among young women. Eva expressed that when men come behind her she sometimes feels 'violated because they don't ask for my permission ... I tell them "get the fuck off my ass"' (Eva, black, straight, 15 years old). In the context of the clubs, many young women blame other women or themselves for the verbal attacks that they received from men on the dance floor as a result of trying to protect their boundaries.

As many of the young women expressed their vigilance to preserve these boundaries, their ability to control was also viewed as a source of power. For some, being able to control the grinding and getting young men erect was viewed as a 'fun' thing to do, simply as a part of dancing to this type of music. This perspective on grinding illustrates a larger position among the young women in the study: the reversal of who has control over courtship in the hip-hop scene. Some young women go beyond grinding to become something of the 'aggressor' in seeking men's attention. A few months prior to being interviewed, Linda (Latina, straight, 16 years old) made a bet with her girlfriends about playing 'the more dominant role, acting how guys act towards females in the club'. Now, when Linda and her friends go to the club and see a guy they like walk by, they grab his arms. This 'is very shocking to them, it's like "why you touching me, you're a lady, guys are supposed to do that."' Reversing the expected roles of men on the dance floor and taking the aggressive performance becomes a source of enjoyment for Linda and her girlfriends. Through this form of transgression, Linda becomes closer to her peers while collectively realising the actual flexibility of apparent normative gender roles on the dance floor.

As mentioned earlier, getting physically close to girls is a strong motivation for young men to dance at hip-hop clubs. Additional expectations are constantly present on the dance floor. These are sequential and include determining: whether or not the other person likes you; will there be 'making out' or heavy petting after dancing; will dancing in the club lead to continuing the making out someplace else; will there be sex involved; will they meet again socially after dancing tonight or will a relationship develop?

Young men consistently pointed to the 'fact' that girls show whether they like them or not through their expressions while dancing, which can be very confusing at times given that grinding is one of the key and most common moves in dancing reggae-type songs. However, men see the number of songs danced to together as a better indicator of a girl's interest in a boy. Between two to five songs were common points that young men mentioned as indicators of young women liking them. 'Asking' a woman to dance also symbolises young men's interest in the young woman. Dancing with a girl on repeated occasions shows more interest.

All the study participants have transitioned from the dance floor to an intimate sexual encounter with a dance partner they liked at least one time. When we asked the reasons for this, both the young men and women stressed the erotic value and sexually charged environment of dancing in the hip-hop scene. 'Dancing is like dry sex', said Kenneth (black, heterosexual, 16 years old). Grinding is considered a symbol of the value of sex in the hip-hop scene. Young women in the study agree with this position. Diana, like most of the young women in the study, told us that dancing to hip-hop and reggae songs is about sex: 'Sometimes a boy is standing on the wall and a girl is in front of him with her back to him and she grinds on him' (Diana, African-American, straight, 16 years old).

Eric met his last girlfriend in school, but it was through dancing that they got to know how much they like each other. Eric sees dancing like 'sex on the dance floor'. He continues: 'My girl, I kiss her around her neck, give her my moves. Play my dick around or something. They always like that stuff' (Eric, African-American, straight, 18 years old). Eric's perspective reminds us of the young women's earlier discussions about the tensions between having dancing boundaries and transgressing those boundaries. Do young men like Eric expect to have sex after dancing? Most have the expectation or the hope that this is a possibility.

José explains to us the transitioning property of grinding. He says:

> When you're dancing close on somebody and kind of those agreements are made, those nonverbal, its OK for you to get close to me, it's OK for you to touch me, it's OK for me to touch you, it's OK for my face to get close to your face, it's OK you know if she kiss me on the dance floor, it's like whoa, where is this going? And we be dancing the whole night, we dance for this amount of time and then, I see you later on, and we started dancing again and the party is winding down and it's, like, what's up, we can take this party someplace else, we can go to my house, or your house or wherever else we're going. Because at that point its not about, oh I want to share some time with you and talk to you, it's that we've gone this route, we've been close on each other, we want to take it a step further, and it's not going to happen on the dance floor ... Everything that happens in the club sets the stage. If you gonna take advantage of that, or go that route, its setting the stage. It's setting the stage for people to meet each other, get close to each other, get drunk, get high, or whatever people do, and hook up.
>
> (José, Dominican-Puerto Rican, straight, 17 years old)

The main idea is that it is at a club where young people can set the stage for what happens next. Thus, if thought through carefully, there are constant opportunities for transitioning from the club to a sexual scene. In fact, among this sexually active sample of young men and women, sexual networking is deeply embedded in the social spaces of the hip-hop club scene. Among the young men and women that we have interviewed (n=45), 74.4 per cent had experienced oral sex, 86.0 per cent had had vaginal intercourse and 25.6 per cent had had anal intercourse. Almost two-thirds (62.8 per cent) had between one and nine partners with whom they had vaginal intercourse, while 20.9 per cent had 10 or more lifetime partners with whom they had vaginal intercourse. Although grinding and dancing did not always lead to sex, the young men felt the pressures of the sexualised dance floor environment and of the current hip-hop 'hook up' scene. Although in the last two months 23.8 per cent did not have sexual intercourse, 11.9 per cent had at least one sexual encounter and 64.3 per cent had two or more sexual encounters. These accounts point to the pressures of having sex that many teens confront nowadays in multiple social environments (including the hip-hop club scene). Fears of not having condoms at the moment of having sex, or simply the fear of admitting not wanting to have (unprotected) sex, are real concerns for young men in the hip-hop club scene.

The hip-hop scene and young people's sexuality

Hip-hop dancing mimics the act of sex, where the man either stands against the wall or lays down on the ground and the women dance on top of him (Hutchinson 1999). This is particularly true in the reggaeton modality of hip-hop where 'the one thing every rising Reggaeton star must have to be noticed is a troupe of toned, hot and barely dressed female dancers gyrating behind them' (Chaplin 2006).

Yet precisely because the relationship between hip-hop genres and sexual relations is so clear, both to participants in hip-hop culture as well as to a wide range of outside observers, it is also imperative to avoid unintentionally demonising such cultural forms as somehow responsible for sexual risk. Pressures to sexualised interactions with other youth on the hip-hop dance floor may well be present in the interpretations that youth make of the visual imagery of the people dancing in the club, of hip-hop music videos and their lyrics and so on. But not all young people have sex in their minds as the outcome of going to the clubs – most are thinking just about 'having a good time' or about 'having fun' in the midst of social and economic circumstances that permit all too little relaxation, pleasure and enjoyment in their lives. Beyond that, going from the dance floor to having sex is a route that it is hardly unique to the hip-hop club scene, and that has been observed just as centrally in several other studies in rock concerts, raves, techno clubs and so on (see, for example, Kelly 2005, 2007).

In few contexts is the need for more nuanced, culturally sensitive readings more evident than in relation to the sexual meanings that are produced and reproduced in the world of hip-hop cultures. It is precisely because of their apparent contradictory quality – at once reproducing highly traditional and even reactionary sexual styles, while at the same time offering a space for deeply rooted cultural critiques that call these traditional styles into question – that the world of hip-hop escapes easy readings or superficial interpretations. On the one hand, hip-hop club dancing is an intrinsically gendered experience that, as our research demonstrates, reproduces gender power inequalities and unequal gender identities in systematic and predictable ways. Young men in our study, for example, experienced their masculinities through the ways of dancing with women and the game on the dance floor. Grinding and *perreo* (a term invented in reggaeton that refers to the main mode of dancing, i.e. doggie style) consist of the man mimicking the penetrating of a woman or the woman thrusting or riding a man.

In this sense, our findings seem to reproduce those of writers such as Joseph Pereira, who documented how sex in reggaeton is often portrayed as 'hammering' (*martillando*), and the penis as a hammer (*martillo*), reinforcing that only vigorous and violent movement satisfies the young women (Pereira 1998), and of Wayne Marshall, who has described the rise of reggaeton as a new modality in hip-hop styles that has taken the oppression of women to a new level, with a strong focus on male domination and control of women (Marshall 2006; see also Totten 2003).

Indeed, it is also particularly relevant to understand that rap, reggaeton and other hip-hop lyrics contain an archive of cultural and historical references that provide, through their multiple resonances, an oral history of contemporary African-American and Latino experience. It is essential to acknowledge that this history is present not only in the explicit narratives of the lyrics but in the highly textured form of their constructions and in the manner of their performance. That is, certain hip-hop recordings are both a representation of experience as well as an interpretative reading of that experience, a form of critique. They function, like other cultural formations and systems, both as 'models of' and 'models for' reality – like cultural 'blueprints' that the young women and men invested and engaged in hip-hop culture use to make sense of their realities (see Geertz 1973).

The complex nature of the form has led Cornel West (1999) to argue that: '[B]lack rap music is primarily the musical expression of the paradoxical cry of desperation and celebration of the black underclass and poor working class, a cry that openly acknowledges and confronts the wave of personal cold-heartedness, criminal cruelty and existential hopelessness in the black ghettos of Afro-America' (West 1999: 482). The interweaving of despair and celebration remains characteristic of the hip-hop cultures being produced by youth in the inner cities of the USA.

Notes

1 This chapter draws on material that was previously published in 'The Hip-Hop Club Scene: Gender, Grinding and Sex', *Culture, Health and Sexuality*, 9 (6): 615–28, 2007. It is reproduced here with permission.
2 Grinding is a type of dance move that resembles sexual acts that involve thrusting. Usually one partner is behind another while grinding.

References

Chaplin, J. (2006) 'For San Juan Youth, Reggaeton Rules the Night', *Cultured Traveler*, 8: 1–5.
Collins, P. H. (2005) *Black Sexual Politics: African Americans, Gender, and the New Racism*, New York: Routledge.
Geertz, C. (1973) *Interpretation of Cultures*, New York: Basic Books.
Hutchinson, J. (1999) 'The Hip Hop Generation: African American Male–Female Relationships in a Nightclub Setting', *Journal of Black Studies*, 30: 62–84.
Kelly, B. (2005) 'Conceptions of Risk in the Lives of Club Drug Using Youth', *Substance Use and Misuse*, 40 (9–10): 1443–59.
Kelly, B. (2007) 'Club Drug Use and Risk Management among "Bridge and Tunnel" Youth', *Journal of Drug Issues*, 37 (2): 425–44.
Kitwana, B. (2002) *The Hip Hop Generation: Young Blacks and the Crisis in African American Culture*, New York: Basic Books.
Marshall, W. (2006) 'The Rise of Reggaeton: From Daddy Yankee to Tengo Calderon, and Beyond', *The Phoenix*, 1–4l.
Martino, S., Collins, R., Elliott, M., Strachman, A., Kanouse, D. and Berry, S. (2006) 'Exposure to Degrading versus Nondegrading Music Lyrics and Sexual Behaviour among Youth', *Pediatrics*, 118 (2): e430–e441.
Muñoz-Laboy, M., Weinstein, H. and Parker, R. (2007) 'Hip-Hop Club Scene: Gender, Grinding and Sex', *Culture, Health and Sexuality*, 9 (6): 615–28.
Pereira, J. (1998) 'Translation or Transformation: Gender in Hispanic Reggae', *Social and Economic Studies*, 47: 79–88.
Rivera, R. Z. (2003) *New York Ricans from the Hip Hop Zone*, New York: Palgrave Macmillan.
Seal, D. and Ehrhardt, A. (2003) 'Masculinity and Urban Men: Perceived Scripts for Courtship, Romantic, and Sexual Interactions with Women', *Culture, Health and Sexuality*, 5 (4): 295–319.
Totten, M. (2003) 'Girlfriend Abuse as a Form of Masculinity Construction among Violent, Marginal Male Youth', *Men and Masculinities*, 6 (1): 70–92.
Watkins, S. (2005) *Hip-Hop Matters: Politics, Popular Culture and the Struggle for the Soul of a Movement*, Boston, MA: Beacon Press.
West, C. (1999) *Cornel West Reader*, New York: Basic Civitas Books.

26 Passionate uprisings[1]

Young people, sexuality and politics in post-revolutionary Iran

Pardis Mahdavi

> Over the past several decades, so it is said, a sexual revolution has occurred; and revolutionary hopes have been pinned to sexuality by many thinkers for whom it represents a potential realm of freedom, unsullied by the limits of present day civilisation.
>
> (Giddens 1993: 1)

> In Iran, all things related to sex had a door, a closed one. Now we, this generation, are opening them one by one. Pregnancy outside of marriage? Open it. Teenage sexual feelings? Open that door. Masturbation? Open it. Now the young people are trying to figure out what to do with all these opening doors.
>
> (Khodi, male, 23)

> In Iran, sex is in fashion. Luxury is in style. How do we live our lives in the Islamic Republic? We go out to a party, go for drinks at someone's house, order some food, drink a little, dance a little, go have sex. Then get up and repeat your routine the next day!
>
> (Ladan, female, 25)

This is a story about the children of the Islamic Revolution who now occupy a particular social, cultural, political and sexual space in urban Tehran. The study, conducted between 2000 and 2007, focused on emerging Iranian young adult culture in Tehran, describing and analysing the meaning and significance of young Tehranis' 'transgressive' sexual and social behaviours in relation to Iran's current sociopolitical climate. Research focused on sexual and social practices, as well as the daily experiences of young people (aged 18–25) in contemporary Iran. How do young adults understand and enact their erotic and sexual lives within the laws and restrictions of the Islamic Republic? Findings suggest that urban young adults in Tehran are constructing and embodying what they call a sexual revolution[2] in response to social and political changes.

Iran has experienced major economic, demographic, political and social changes in the last 30 years. The young people that this study focused on are literally 'children of the revolution' as they were born to a nation in the throes of revolution (Islamic), war (with Iraq) and shifts in economic power (oil boom followed by sanctions). According to scholars such as Janet Afary (personal communication 2006) or Kaveh Basmenji (2005), the nation's younger generation has been affected by the Islamic Republic's free education policies and its successful national literacy campaign. Ironically, these education policies have created an educated and highly politicised youth with voting rights (age 16 currently) many of whom are ready and willing to express their dissent. The body has become a major battleground in the Islamic Republic, seen in legislation and heavy punishment regulating Islamic dress and death sentences for 'sexual deviants' (those convicted of adultery or homosexuality). Many young adults argue that they are now using their bodies and sexualities to speak back to what they view as a repressive regime; they refer to their behaviour as a sexual revolution (*enqelab-e-jensi*). Consequently, a new sexual culture is emerging among Iranian young adults that requires further investigation.

Urban young adults who comprise the majority of Iran's population (70 per cent of Iran's population is under the age of 30) (Esposito and Ramazani 2001) are highly mobile, highly educated (84 per cent of young Tehranis are currently enrolled in university or are university graduates with 65 per cent of these graduates being women) and underemployed (there is a 45 per cent unemployment rate among this age group) (Basmenji 2005). Many are also highly dissatisfied with the current regime. Through in-depth research that looks at often overlooked elements such as style (Hebdige 1991), daily lives, sexual practices and health and education infrastructure, it may be possible to illuminate the ways in which young people in Tehran interact with their social, political and economic environment and express their dissatisfaction with their current situation. Can current changes in sexual behaviour among the young people of Iran be seen as an alternative form of substitution for the forbidden political activism?

Backdrop to the sexual revolution

Today, the Islamic Republic of Iran (IRI) is a country in transition. This transition is as much political and socioeconomic as it is demographic. Iran is theoretically a democratic theocracy, governed by Islamic law or sharia. Sharia, as interpreted by the clerics in power, mandates among other things, that women and men should interact minimally before marriage; and that women should be covered in 'proper' Islamic dress (ideally a cloak from head to toe, hiding any bodily shape). Much of Islamic law also seeks to legislate on social, sexual and familial behaviours through the language of morality. Ideas of *mahram* and *na-mahram* referring to those who are potential marriage partners (*mahram*) and those who are not (*na-mahram*) are part of state rhetoric (Haeri 1989) and have been discussed in religious spaces, public gatherings (at mosques) and in private settings such as the home. Some of the religious and moral rhetoric coming from the state is also reproduced by the family (for more religious young people) while other families (most usually non-religious) often contradict the harsh rules imposed by sharia. In accordance with sharia, heterosocial interactions between unmarried or unrelated men and women are forbidden and punishable by lashings and imprisonment; sex before marriage and extramarital sex is also punishable, however, the point is that in recent years there has been very little evidence of these arrests; further evidence that the youth movement is affecting change.

The Islamic authorities demand sexual and social modesty and dedication to living an Islamist lifestyle. This entails the strict enforcement of Islamic performative rituals (including prayer five times a day, Koran recitation and observance of the holy months of Ramadan[3] and Moharram[4]) as well as refraining from alcohol consumption, contact with members of the opposite sex prior to marriage, social gatherings and dancing. 'They tell us "go pray, five times a day, go visit the shrine of the prophets, observe your fasts," ' noted one 23-year-old young man from Tehran, 'but they don't tell us why. They teach us how to prepare for prayer over and over, but never for practical daily interaction! Why?' Many urban young adults throughout the social landscape increasingly reject Islamist social restrictions as they feel that religion has been forced on them without choice, and see their social behaviour (including style of dress, sociality and interactions) as political statements. Among some young people in Iran (mostly from the secular middle and upper middle classes), youthful rebellion represents counter discourses to revolutionary ideas about sexual purity, the good Islamic body and gender segregation, as well as the expression of dissidence.

Their behaviour, seemingly found on a lesser scale in young adult cultures in many countries, is understood and described by informants as rebellious or dissident. It is vital to look at the many layers of what young people are challenging, including what they perceive as tradition versus their perceptions of modernity, their parents, the authorities, sharia or the regime. Employing the notion that modernity is increasingly expressed in the transformation of gender relations (Hirsch 2003) or in the transformation of intimacy (Giddens 1993) in modernising societies, some young Iranians seem to find it easier to negotiate their everyday interactions and intimate relations than to negotiate changes in the state. For some of these young people, gender and social relations are a place to talk about citizenship. Many may be reacting to questions of citizenship through intimacy and intimate relations. In this way, young people perceive themselves acting out a sexual and social revolution in their daily lives on the streets of Tehran.

Methodology

Most of the fieldwork for this study took place during the summers of 2000, 2002, 2004, 2005 and 2007. The bulk of the data was collected when I moved to Tehran for the duration of 2004 and part of 2005. Participant observation was conducted in cafés, public parks, malls, parties, gyms, dance classes and local squares where young people tended to gather. I also worked as a volunteer in two drop-in centres and one needle exchange, served on the board of an anthropology journal at Tehran university and conducted archival work at the Ministry of Health, the Ministry of Education and several other government agencies (such as the state welfare organisation). I conducted 110 in-depth qualitative interviews (digitally recorded) with urban young Iranians (18–25), both men and women of varying socioeconomic classes, but with an emphasis on young people living in certain parts of town. Additionally, I interviewed and observed 30 service providers including doctors, nurses, counsellors and teachers, as well as 30 parents of young people.

Findings

Prior to the post-election fallout in 2009, the population of Iran was painted as religious and compliant with the theocratic regime by western media and in the international community. On my return from Iran in September 2002, I interviewed a UN official. 'Boys and girls (in Iran) have no need for reproductive healthcare services until they are engaged as no one engages in sexual relations prior to that moment', she said. I recognised that as a member of the UN, the officer was prohibited from openly criticising the regime, but, I thought to myself, if she could put on a veil that would turn her into a young Iranian partygoer, the following is what she might find.

Her face flushed, Yasaman Houtri,[5] 19, looks around the crowded Tehran apartment that at the moment resembles a cross between a US college party and a curtained bordello. She takes a sip of her Russian vodka martini. 'The difference between you young people in the west and us here in Iran is really very simple: when you want to have fun you go out, and when you want to pray and be spiritual you stay in. In Iran, when we want to pray and be spiritual we go out, when we want to have fun we go in.' Persian pop music blares from large speakers and everywhere there are pairs of flirting, drinking teenagers. Yasaman glances over at her best friend who is tucked away neatly under a boy on a nearby couch. The dimly lit room is filled with other young couples who are occupied in the same activity. As she sits down, Yasaman's purple miniskirt is pushed up so high that she catches the attention of a boy across the way. She shrugs and nonchalantly lights a cigarette after handing one to me.

Soon, Yasaman will leave her friend's house party. Like the other girls, most of whom she goes to school with, she will carefully don a navy blue hejab to cover her hair, and wrap a long flowing coat over her skirt and sweater. On the street, accompanied by a male friend, she will keep her eyes lowered, carefully blending into the streams of young people moving along Tehran's busy city streets in the centre of town. Like thousands of urban young people in Iran, Yasaman's public and private worlds could not be more different. But she and her friends have been making deliberate attempts to unite public and private comportment.

Hundreds of miles away from the capital, a group of girls and boys gather in Mashad, a religious city and important pilgrimage site in Shi'ite Islam. Everyone piles into the car of a young man named Siamak, who turns up the latest single from Usher that he has bootlegged from the USA. He starts driving and everyone is talking and laughing and explaining to me that our destination is one of the hottest spots in Mashad for people to meet each other. As Siamak rounds a corner, he spots some members of the *komiteh* (the Iranian morality police) and shouts for everyone to duck as he drives past them. He turns the music down and we dive beneath the seats so that only the boys remain seen. The girls giggle and scream and take another puff of the miniature hookah that holds remnants of opium, hash and marijuana.

On the surface it may seem to casual observers that boys and girls do not interact much or talk about sex before marriage. However, most of the young people I interviewed were unmarried and were either engaged in sexual relations, or had been at one time or another with a boyfriend/girlfriend or acquaintance. The majority of informants have been sexually active prior to marriage (some described their sexual activities primarily in terms of casual sex, while others indicated long-term monogamous sexual relationships, but it is important to note that even premarital sex with a long-term partner is still illegal, and thus would still be considered an act of rebellion), and of the married young adults whom I interviewed (20), more than half were engaged in sexual relations outside their marriage. It is interesting to note that according to anthropologists at Tehran University, the average age of marriage in Tehran is 26 for women and 29 for men (and in recent years ideals of companionate marriage have become popular among many urban Iranian couples, although some continue to marry at the suggestion of parents or family members), while the average age of first intercourse among this population is 16 for women and 15 for men. Therefore, there exists a 10-year period in which women and men are engaging in sexual relations illegally (before marriage) without access to information or treatment for potential risks they may incur while being sexually active.

According to informants, sexual relations and experiences are not limited to members of the opposite sex as many of the young adults indicated that they engage in same-sex sexual activity (both men and women). Some of this is attributed to the construction of homosociality in a gender-segregated context as very few of these young adults identified as gay or lesbian (Najmabadi 2005). Most of the young adults noted that they were not heterosexual or homosexual, but rather sexual. They noted that their sexual interaction with members of the same sex was just an extension of same-sex love and friendship, and a different level of intimacy (Halperin 1990; Katz 1990). Notions of romantic love in both heterosexual and homosexual relationships were present and often discussed, as several informants were involved in long-term relationships with people with whom they were 'in love.'

Discussion

The prevailing social and political system may have produced the sexual and social underworld of Iranian youth in many ways, and indeed, informants indicated different reasons for engaging in what they called the 'sexual revolution.' Some informants indicated that they were mobilising a sexual and social revolution to speak back to a regime they were unhappy with; many noted that because the regime was so overly focused on their bodies, physical appearance, moral code and sexualities, that they were using these very tools to speak back to their oppressors (although this would not be considered revolutionary in a Foucauldian context, the young adults defined it this way for themselves). Others admitted to being frustrated with tradition and cultural norms that mandated that they live constricted lives.

Leila Somagh, a 19-year-old Iranian girl living in Tehran, pointed out what she considers to be one of the most obvious flaws of the system, and an issue that is unique to the Islamic Republic: 'We are not supposed to be seen in public with a man, otherwise we go to jail. That means no dinner dates, no walks in the park, and no movie theatres. So what do we do? We go straight to his house, and what do we do there? I'll let you figure that one out; there is a room and a bed, and not much more. Do you see the problem?' According to Leila, and several other young women, because men and women cannot be seen in public, they skip the 'normal' procedures of a few dinner dates before intimacy. Therefore, boys and girls become intimate more quickly, and often more carelessly. Additionally, there is the problem that Leila alludes to of space. Many young people live with their parents and thus resort to engaging in sexual relations while their parents are away at work, visiting relatives or friends or out of town. According to many of the men with whom I spoke, oftentimes one member of a group of male friends has a private apartment, and this space is then shared among friends who 'sign up' for one to two hour blocks with their sexual partners. Still other young people utilise abandoned ware-houses and back alleys for various sexual encounters.

Young men have also been raised to be hypersensitive to young women. Reza Amiri, a 27-year-old Iranian man, describes his frustration at the authorities for turning the Iranian men into 'sex-starved animals.' He thinks that the Islamists in the regime deserve to be betrayed. 'They are so sick you know. They want us not to even think about girls, and what does that result in? Incessant planning and schem-ing about how to get girls! See in London or Paris, you go to a pub and girls are all around, and no one pays them that much attention. In Tehran, a girl brushes past you at the park, and you go crazy! Desire fills the two of you and you can't wait to go somewhere secretly and just get it out!' Reza is ashamed of his peers because he says that sometimes their judgement is clouded with desire. When asked if he feels that he is going against his religion by engaging in premarital sexual activity in extreme forms, his reply is a firm negative. He looks at me and quotes one of the holiest imams of Shi'ite Islam. 'Way back when, someone asked Imam Hossien if it is bad to take off a woman's clothes and just stare at her. The Imam told him that in fact he would be honouring the prophet if he partook in this activity. The man then pushed further and further, asking if petting was bad, then oral sex and finally coitus. The imam continued to tell the man that these things were in fact very *ba hall* (Farsi slang term roughly translating to cool)'. Reza smiles at me, 'you see, in fact we are honouring the Imam!' he says sarcastically.

Some possible implications

The level of risk that young people face with regards to the regime is high, but many of my informants indicated that this was a risk they were willing to take, and a pun-ishment that they were willing to face to advance their social causes. Other inform-ants noted that having grown up under the blanket of the current regime, they had developed an expertise in avoiding the *komiteh*, bribing their way out of situations (on rare occasions as more often than not the morality police loathe the rich young kids and inflict harsher punishment on them if offered a bribe) or tackling them head on.

Many of the health risks that the young adults are exposing themselves to are unknown by them as most reveal that they are uninformed about the consequences of unprotected sex, poly-drug use, multiple partners, abortion, self-administered contraceptive pills and other potential risk behaviours. Because premarital sex is forbidden under the current regime, efforts to disseminate information on family planning, harm reduction and sex education are minimal and reserved often for couples who are engaged to be married. Young adults who are not yet engaged (or who do not plan to be) do not have access to the information they need to perhaps make better informed decisions about their behaviours.

Very few informants reported using condoms or some form of contraception (not necessarily protection against STIs) and this condom usage was not 100 per cent of the time. When asked about the reasons behind their lack of usage, most answered that they were embarrassed to go to a pharmacy for fear of being 'found out.' Many women noted that as unmarried young adults they did not have access to oral contraceptives (such as birth control pills or the morning after pill which is occasionally dispensed at pharmacies without requiring a marriage license, although this is illegal), and if they did, many indicated that they were fearful of purchasing these lest their parents or family members discover them. Many of the young women said that going to a pharmacy to purchase such items (which were often quite expensive) made them vulnerable to being seen in public procuring items that would indicate their sexual activity. Most informants were deterred by the social risks (and costs) of being caught attempting to purchase contraceptives like condoms or the morning after pill, and thus did not feel that these were options available to them.

Additionally, several female informants revealed that because they did not have access to birth control, many had to rely on abortion in the case that they did get pregnant before marriage. Some of these young women reported going to expensive doctors uptown and paying high prices to 'get rid of their problem.' Other informants who did not have the means to access these high priced doctors relied on other methods such as purchasing animal abortion pills from the black market on Nasser Khosro Avenue. Many reported that their experiences taking these were horrifying, and some older informants noted that they were now facing reproductive difficulties because of their histories using these unidentified medications.

When informants were asked about STIs, most could not even name one. Many knew about HIV (but knew of it only in its other form: AIDS), but felt that they were not at high risk for contracting the virus. Many indicated, however, that they were concerned about pregnancy and the potential for contracting other diseases, which they felt uneasy about, but knew very little about. Most noted that they felt high levels of anxiety about their sexual relations, but did not know what avenues to turn to in order to procure support or information.

Currently, formal, codified knowledge about sexuality is transmitted only to women and girls through classes on puberty and menstruation provided at the elementary level, followed by a short course (only offered to women) about family planning at the university level, and supplemented by prenuptial courses provided for men and women separately (however these are only provided once couples decide to get married). The content of these courses varies, as does their utility. Of the 20 married interviewees in my sample, only one indicated that the course had been helpful, but she quickly added that it was information she would have appreciated once she became sexually active, rather than once she decided to get married.

Over the course of the fieldwork I did find several drop-in centres and areas where young people could receive free counselling about sex, drugs and harm reduction. Most of these were utilised by young, married couples who had taken their prenuptial counselling courses at these sites. Although the counsellors were very open minded and indicated that they were open to distributing information to unmarried young people, none of my unmarried informants knew about these centres or counsellors. There seemed to be a distinct gap between the service providers and the young people whom they were trying to serve. The young adults were sceptical of the providers or were uninformed of this option, and the providers were frustrated at interacting with the young people only when it was 'too late' according to them.

Conclusion

The sexual revolution described by many informants is not solely centred on casual sex, multiple partners or group sex. Rather, the sexual revolution they believe they are engaging in is also about changing sexual discourses, pushing the limits with regards to restrictions on social behaviours (such as style of dress, youth congregation, drinking and dancing) and attacking the fabric of morality under which the regime seeks to govern its citizens. In 2009, the post-election fallout resulted in weeks of protests, led by the youth against members of the morality police as well as conservative President Ahmadinejad's regime. Young people, fed up with at least 20 years of the regime's focus on social activities, rather than improving high unemployment or faulty infrastructure, took to the streets to take the youth movement a step further than the sexual revolution, making a political revolution inspired by the developing youth movement.

This study aimed to assess and unpack the sexual and social revolution that young Tehranis claim to be enacting. Throughout my time in Iran, I heard hundreds of young people use the phrase 'sexual revolution' in reference to changes taking place in Tehran. Key informants reminded me that wearing tight *monteaus* and head scarves that revealed highlighted hair was more than a fashion statement, and more than being a part of a globalised youth culture. They emphasised that changes in style were about codes and speaking to a regime that would only hear these signals. Their style and attempts to embody a sexual revolution, they told me, was their way of speaking back to the regime, to the morality police who had made them suffer for so long, and to other potential members of the revolution.

During my time in the field, I struggled with whether changes in fashion (which were the external indicators of the sexual revolution according to my informants) and sexuality could be revolutionary. I wondered if wearing a Gucci headscarf, drinking a martini and having lots of boyfriends was about opposing the Islamic Republic or about peer pressure. Certainly, some of my informants purchased and displayed designer wear in order to 'fit in' with their friends, or because they saw themselves as part of an affluent and stylish elite. Several informants told me that they wore makeup or highlighted their hair because they liked how it made them look; they emphasised that it made them more desirable. Most of my informants repeatedly told me, however, as they layered their makeup before going to class in order to outwit morality police who would insist on wiping down their faces before entering school grounds, that wearing makeup or certain types of Islamic dress was also about making a statement. Many of the goods that young Tehranis demanded were sold on the black market which made them desirable. If these goods were openly sold and easily accessible, they would no longer be seen as symbolic of a changing young adult culture. One informant made reference to certain kinds of tennis shoe. She said that because running shoes like Nike or Reebok were only sold on the black market, these were among the most desirable. She emphasised that these sneakers were more eye catching to the morality police than the plain tennis shoes sold in bazaars across the city. 'But', she added, 'I don't think they look that nice. Once they become copied and available everywhere, no one will want them'. Thus the black market itself creates a certain economy that is folded into young people's social revolution.

Throughout my fieldwork, I also struggled to understand the changes in sexual and social behaviour and their significance. After several years of field research, it became apparent that the changes taking place among young Tehranis are not ephemeral and that they have meaning and significance both to informants, as well as to the members of the regime and morality police who obsessively patrol, police and punish them. Many key informants reminded me that because wearing a DKNY headscarf or being in a car with their boyfriend could get them arrested, this headscarf was more than a label, and their boyfriend was more than a passing amusement; these behaviours are a threat to the social and moral order affecting all aspects of the Islamic Republic.

The results of fieldwork raise a lot of questions. I continue to struggle with the impact, meaning and future of sexual revolution in Iran. The changes taking place among urban young adults in Iran are many. The young people seem to be using their bodies to make social and political statements against what they view as a repressive regime. However, although the young adults have made great strides in attaining greater social freedoms and more attention and respect from authorities, the battle between the young Tehranis and members of the Islamist regime still rages. Unfortunately, due to the risks that accompany their social behaviours, most of the casualties will be among young people if education and information is not distributed and disseminated to them quickly. We must remember that the youth of today are the future of Iran tomorrow.

Notes

1 I would like to thank Carole Vance, without whose enduring support this research would not have been possible. I would also like to thank, Lila Abu-Lughod, Lynn Freedman and Shahla Haeri and Rebecca Young for helping me to better the work in all its forms. The research for this study would not have been possible without the financial support from the Woodrow Wilson Women's Health Fellowship, the Cordier Fellowship, a National Development and Research Institute behavioural science training fellowship and the Institute for Social and Economic Research and Policy fellowship programme.
2 Sexual revolution is defined by the young people concerned as changes in sexual and social behaviours and discourse as a means of reaction to state controls. In other words, because the current regime exercises its powers through enforcing a certain type of morality, young people seek to attack the regime by attacking the fabric of morality through which the regime maintains its power. Young people feel that by engaging in what the regime terms 'immoral' activities such as premarital sex, they are subversively attacking the regime and destabilising it on a daily basis.
3 Holy month of fasting.
4 Holy month of mourning.
5 Note that names have been changed to protect the identity of the interviewees.

References

Basmenji, K. (2005) *Tehran Blues: How Iranian Youth Rebelled Against Iran's Founding Fathers*, London: Saqi Books.

Esposito, J. L. and Ramazani, R. K. (2001) *Iran at the Crossroads*, New York and Basingstoke: Palgrave.

Giddens, A. (1993) *The Transformation of Intimacy*, Stanford: Stanford University Press.

Haeri, S. (1989) *Law of Desire: Temporary Marriage in Shi'i Iran*, Syracuse: Syracuse University Press.

Halperin, D. M. (1990) *One Hundred Years of Homosexuality and Other Essays on Greek Love*, New York: Routledge.

Hebdige, D. (1991) *Subculture: The Meaning of Style*, London: Routledge.

Hirsch, J. S. (2003) *A Courtship after Marriage: Sexuality and Love in Mexican Transnational Families*, Berkeley: University of California Press.

Katz, J. (1990) 'The Invention of Heterosexuality', *Socialist Review*, 20 (1): 7–34.

Najmabadi, A. (2005) *Women with Moustaches and Men without Beards: Gender and Sexual Anxieties of Iranian Modernity*, Berkeley: University of California Press.

27 Tourism and the body

Embodiment and sexual performance among Dominican male sex workers

Mark B. Padilla

As in many parts of the world, the tourism industry in the Caribbean is becoming an increasingly pervasive and all consuming force. In the Dominican Republic, the Caribbean country where the ethnographic research that informs this chapter was conducted, fully one-quarter of the country's GDP comes from tourism, and this single industry provides jobs for about one out of every five Dominicans, who cater to the more than three million international tourists who enter the country annually (Padilla 2007c). As a medical anthropologist, my work for the past several years has been oriented toward understanding the economic, social and health consequences of the tourism industry in the Dominican Republic. The lens through which I have done this is to examine men who are informally employed in tourism areas, and who have a history of intimate sexual and romantic exchanges with both male and female tourists.

Although these men have experience with sexual-economic exchanges, they often do not think of themselves as 'sex workers'. As I discussed in detail in my recent book *Caribbean Pleasure Industry* – based on ethnographic data from a three-year study in two Dominican cities – most of these men describe themselves as 'normal men' (*hombres normales*), are frequently married or intimately involved with women, often have children and use the local identities of *bugarron* or *sanky panky* to describe themselves (Padilla 2007c). Based on historical and ethnographic sources of evidence, I argue that these sexual identities have roots in particularly Dominican cultural expressions of sexuality, but they have also been incorporated into and redefined by the tourism industry since the 1970s. Through an increasingly diversified global sex tourism economy, local sexual identities have become global commodities as they have become incorporated into tourist sexual experiences and fantasies of Caribbean sexuality. For local people, they have become instruments not only for the enactment of intimate sexual pleasures, but for access to material securities and opportunities for social advancement, transnational marriage, remittances and immigration.

While many of these opportunities are often more mythic than real (see Brennan 2004), the tourism industry – and particularly the possibility of establishing instrumental relationships with wealthy foreigners – has become the repository for dreams of an elusive economic security. In a declining national economy that relies on cheap, exploited, unskilled and disenfranchised labourers, bodies and sexual practices have become ways in which informal tourism workers function as erotic entrepreneurs, generating what I have described as a 'marketable fantasy' in an attempt to respond as productive agents to the shifting constraints of a weak and dependent economy (Padilla 2007c).

Yet the creation of a marketable fantasy is not simply a one-way process of 'performing' for the tourist for profit, but also can involve the establishment of long-term intimate relationships described by both participants as 'love' or 'affection', and occasionally leading to marriage or sustained relational commitments. Thus, the rapid shift to a tourism-based economy not only affects the material conditions of society, but reverberates in the most basic ways people experience relational and sexual intimacy. Perhaps more provocatively, it affects how individuals use and understand their bodies and body parts, which is one of the primary arguments of this chapter.

The intention of much of my work in the Dominican Republic has been to understand how political-economic changes related to the intensification of the Caribbean tourism industry and other neoliberal development policies have influenced the enactment of local sexualities. In an attempt to investigate this linkage ethnographically, I have focused most of my research on the sexual exchanges between local Dominican men and foreign gay tourists, which are much more common than the literature on 'beach boys' in the Caribbean would imply, but which present social and emotional challenges for these men. As I argue in this chapter, the engagements with gay foreigners can lead to embodied moments of inter- and intrapersonal tension in which the material, cultural and emotional investments of sex workers and clients must be worked out and negotiated in the symbolically charged uses of genitals and orifices. In this chapter, I consider bodies and body parts as key sites for the analysis of the *embodiment of tourism*, and seek to use men's narratives of sexual encounters with tourists to examine how practices of sexuality are embedded in wider material and symbolic contexts.

As a medical anthropologist also working in HIV prevention, this approach is critical to understanding linkages between tourism and HIV. In the Caribbean, a growing body of evidence suggests that the tourism industry is associated with the emergence of local HIV epidemics and shapes vulnerabilities among those who work in tourism settings.[1] While some suggestive epidemiological evidence suggests a correlation between tourism dependence and HIV prevalence throughout the Caribbean, there is no research by which to specify or describe the mechanisms through which this association may or may not occur. Therefore, a critical question for HIV research in the region is: How might the structure of the tourism industry as it is embodied and experienced influence HIV-related vulnerabilities for specific individuals and groups? Answering this question requires ethnographic research that examines the contextualised, embedded nature of sexual practices in tourism areas.

Background

My ethnographic work consisted of three years of research in two cities in the Dominican Republic: Santo Domingo (the capital and largest urban centre in the country) and Boca Chica (a small tourist town about 30 kilometres to the east). In Santo Domingo – now home to three million people in the metropolitan area – sex work is an active and visible feature of the social landscape, especially in the many lower class *barrios* and in the more heavily touristic areas, such as the *Zona Colonial*. Non-governmental organisations (NGOs) and activists working with female sex workers in the Dominican Republic estimate there are nearly 300,000 women who are employed in the sex industry domestically, and another 300,000 working abroad – dramatic numbers given a national population of only 9.3 million (Padilla 2007c). Similar estimates have not been made of male sex workers, who have no organisational representation of any kind, are more independently employed, and have not been incorporated into HIV/AIDS prevention or treatment services. Boca Chica – which until relatively recently was a quiet beach town adjacent to the small community of sugar cane workers at *Batey Andrés* is now inundated with hotels and resorts catering to an international clientele. The town has been prioritised by the Dominican Secretary of Tourism as one of the five main 'tourism poles' in the country, motivating in part recent government investments in the highway linking Boca Chica to the nearby international airport, where most foreign tourists enter the country. It is also considered a 'must-see' on the travel itinerary of many tourists who come to the region primarily for sex, and is known in the Dominican Republic as a *zona caliente* (a hot zone) for prostitution.

Conducted through my affiliation with the local NGO *Amigos Siempre Amigos* – which has nearly 20 years' experience working on HIV prevention among gay-identified men – this project involved the combination of various research methods, including a large-sample social, behavioural and demographic survey with 200 male sex workers, focus groups, 98 in-depth interviews and extensive participant observation in male sex work sites. The research focused on two local categories of sex workers – *bugarrones* and *sanky pankies* – terms which overlap in meaning but which also express certain conceptual distinctions. *Bugarrón* is a term with a longer sociolinguistic history extending back to at least the nineteenth century, is used throughout the Hispanic Caribbean and is closely associated in actual discourse with sexual-economic exchanges between men. My research has also attempted to demonstrate that the social category of *bugarron* is a broader or superordinate category of Dominican homoeroticism, of which *sanky panky* is a specific subtype or example. The men I interviewed defined *bugarrón* in relation to three qualities: (1) he is 'the one who presents himself as the "macho" in the relationship'; (2) he is *stereotypically* the insertive partner in anal sex; and (3) he often accepts money or gifts from other men in exchange for sex. The *bugarrón* is also similar in many overall features to the identities *mayate* in Mexico and the *michê* in Brazil, as described in prior ethnographic accounts in those countries (Kulick 1998; Parker 1999; Prieur 1998), and has a deeper historical trajectory than the term *sanky panky*.

The figure of the *sanky panky* emerged during the country's historical transition to a tourism-based economy in the 1970s and 1980s. The term is a linguistic Dominicanisation that derives from the English phrase 'hanky panky', and came into vogue to describe the beach boys that have grown in number in direct proportion to the rising volume of tourists entering the country. *Sanky pankies* bear a certain resemblance to the phenomenon of the 'Rent-a-Dred' in Jamaica (Campbell *et al.* 1999), often wearing dreadlocks and catering more explicitly to the racialised stereotypes of Caribbean men that emphasise youth, hypermasculinity, athleticism and dark skin.

The general stereotype of *sankies* in Dominican society is that their sex work is primarily oriented toward foreign women, and indeed this interpretation is in accordance with their outward gender performance and public persona. Nevertheless, in my study, both *bugarrones* and *sanky pankies* commonly reported sexual encounters with male clients, despite social stereotypes to the contrary. It should be stressed that the identities of *bugarron* and *sanky panky* are not stable aspects of personhood, but rather are highly fluid, situational and performative. An example of this is the fact that some of my informants who self-identified as *bugarrones* in Santo Domingo would go to Boca Chica on the weekend to *sanquipanquiar* (to *sanky panky*). Similar constructions were used in converting *bugarron* to *bugarroniar*, linguistically signalling the action of performing a *bugarron* role, rather than assuming a stable sexual identity.

The seduction of tourism

With this general context in mind, it is useful to turn to the case of one of my key informants, Ricardo, who was aged 33 when I met him, and who had many years of experience in the industry. 'Ricardo' was an influential *maipiolo* (roughly, a pimp), partly because he was proficient in conversational English, and began what he described as the first 'agency' of male sex workers catering to a gay tourist clientele in Santo Domingo. Ricardo's childhood, until his early adolescence, began outside the small town of San Francisco de Macorís, in what he calls a 'humble' rural home.

When he was 14 the situation at home became, in his words, 'intolerable' (*insoportable*), due to the lack of work in his home town that made providing for him and his three siblings a constant stress on his parents, and an easy rationalisation for abuse by his father. As a result, Ricardo decided to head out for Santo Domingo, bartering some of his possessions for a ride to the capital city along the southern coastal highway. Ricardo's move to Santo Domingo required him to live with his aunt in a sprawling *barrio* of the capital city, Villa Mella, where there is an active sex work industry catering to both tourists and locals. While attending high school, Ricardo gradually got involved with *la gente mala* (or bad people), began using drugs and was 'seduced' (*seducido*), in his words, by the urban night life he encountered in Villa Mella. His first contact with the possibility of sex work occurred at age 15, when a friend – a self-identified *bugarrón* – took him to a gay disco frequented by many foreign tourists. This disco, a site of much participant observation during my first months of fieldwork, was closed in 2000 after a horrific multiple murder occurred there in full view of the clientele, and was covered extensively in the national press. Ricardo recalled:

> The person who took me [to the disco] explained to me, 'Look, a lot of American guys come here. Here they pay you. You have a good piece [*pedazo*, meaning penis] between your legs. With that you can make a lot of money'. So, he educated me in what the search [*la búsqueda* or sex work] is, because he had been in that environment and he knew how things worked there... [In friend's voice:] 'I'm going to take you to a place like this and like that, where you're going to be able to get money easily, things that you like, and you're not going to have to do anything disgusting [*asqueroso*] either'.

With this introduction, Ricardo began regularly engaging in sex-for-money exchanges, specialising in providing sexual services to male tourists, but also serving women on occasion. His friendships with gay business owners and wealthy foreign clients placed him in an ideal position from which to broker contacts between local men and tourists. As he described, his growing awareness of his social status in the world of international sex work convinced him to begin what he called an 'agency' of sex workers to serve foreign visitors. Ricardo explained:

> Well, the American queens [*las locas americanas*, meaning gay men] started to visit me at my house. They [the tourists] began with the *bugarrones* that I know from my generation, and from the [old] disco [a gay bar that closed in 1999]. They have the ability to get the expensive tennis shoes, the jewellery, the clothes … And so [the *bugarrones*] come to me and they say, Look, are you Ricardo? I'm so-and-so, I go to such-and-such gym, I don't drink, I don't use drugs, I'm in the university, things are really hard, I *like* doing this. Help me. So I think, I look at the economic situation like it is… and the idea occurs to me, I say, Well, these boys who look good, young, and look good, that don't have vices, and the queens come to me because they trust me, so why don't I start an agency? And so through one I got another, and through that one another, and I got 25 guys… And if I had my way I'd have 75 or 100 sex workers [*trabajadores sexuales*] here right now.

While Ricardo is a more dramatic case than most due to his level of professionalisation, as well as his use of terminology such as 'sex worker' (which is itself influenced by his incorporation into HIV-prevention efforts by the NGO with which I was affiliated), several aspects of his narrative are instructive, representing larger patterns in men's experiences of tourism labour. As with Ricardo, most of the men in the study emphasised the lack of options available in their natal areas, which motivated in part their movement to the city or to coastal resort towns, where they were gradually socialised into the sex industry. For example, approximately three-quarters of the sex workers in Boca Chica had immigrated to one of the two research sites, often for the purpose of finding work related to the tourism industry.

The important point about these migrations is that they are almost exclusively motivated by the country's development of coastal tourism enclaves, which are essentially clusters of hotels, resorts, bars, restaurants and shops in 'pristine' areas of coastline prioritised by historically recent development initiatives, and typically include adjacent communities of migrant Dominicans who provide the service labour for these tourism businesses (Padilla 2007c). Many of these labourers return regularly to their home communities or move away during the low tourism season, creating circular or complex internal migratory pathways. As with Ricardo, many of the participants in the research had not planned or sought out to engage in sexual-economic exchanges; it simply presented itself organically as an option for income generation in the pervasively opportunistic and diversified informal economy of tourism areas. Often, as in Ricardo's case, men were often introduced into the informal sex economy or learned about how to negotiate or consummate a deal through peers who were familiar with the tourism area and sexual exchanges. Social peers or co-workers therefore become conduits of information about how to use sexuality and eroticism as a means for making a living, illustrating how tourism areas function to situationally normalise 'deviant' sexual behaviours and identities through a resocialisation process. In the experience of many of the men I interviewed, however, this resocialisation did not function to entirely destigmatise sexual practices or sex-for-money exchanges, but to temporarily rationalise or justify them *in spite of* their 'bad' moral or social consequences.

Tourism areas were therefore perceived as ambivalent spaces, borderlands that blurred the boundary between 'normal' and 'bad' expressions of sexuality and sexual behaviour. One participant, Martin, described this quality of tourism areas when he remarked as follows in an interview: 'Here in Boca Chica one opens up a lot … Any person that works here *opens up* because that person has to … Sometimes a situation makes one do things, not so much for money, but tourism makes many things outside of the normal'.

Indeed, in this study, the quality of being 'outside of the normal' in tourism areas was connected to the fact that sexual encounters with foreigners were widely perceived as a potential source of 'easy money' (*dinero fácil*) within the tourism economy. For example, in Boca Chica, the economic benefits of instrumental exchanges were so pervasively understood that it created an environment in which the strategic use of sexuality was almost an expectation, even if explicit discourse about it was not always encouraged. In light of the high male unemployment and the shrinking options for men's labour, sexual-economic exchanges in the tourism industry provided a rational means to make ends meet that many men viewed as less exploitative and more economically viable than other options available to them, few of which had the income potential of sex-for-money exchanges. Additionally, many men possessed a talent for 'emotion work', or the ability to connect socially with clients, establish trust and rapport and effectively use interpersonal relations to leverage income (Hochschild 1979).

The best illustration of this is sex workers' awareness of the material benefits of sustained romantic relationships with tourists, which were perceived as means to a more generalised material security. In interviews, men explained that they often preferred such relationships because they can provide larger gifts or remittances that exceed the value of direct sex-for-money exchanges or casual encounters, and therefore have the greatest potential to influence overall economic stability. Men described these intimate relationships as possessing four interrelated qualities: they involve less explicit forms of exchange; they often include non-monetary compensation or payments 'in kind'; material benefits often take the form of 'gifts' or 'help' rather than rationalised payments for sex; and exchanges are often framed within a notion of partnership, intimacy, affection or love.

Constructing the marketable fantasy

Given the importance of intimate exchanges with foreigners as a means to make ends meet, participants' interactions with tourists had high stakes, resulting in performative interactions aimed at the construction of what I referred to earlier as a marketable fantasy. That is, for an encounter to be consummated, men sought to provide tourists with erotic experiences that were perceived as authentic, both conforming to tourist fantasies of Dominican masculinity and reconstructing those fantasies through the interaction itself. In producing this fantasy, local men cultivated a remarkable ability to deploy their masculinity and sexuality in ways that maximised their desirability. This required, first and foremost, a performance of *difference*, since the Dominican sex tourism economy functions, fundamentally, through the commodification of sexually exoticised differences. In tourists' stories, Dominican *bugarrones* are described as 'real men', more masculine or 'macho' and more 'natural' than men in their home countries (Padilla 2007a, 2007b), reflecting colonial assumptions about black sexuality that have been described by other scholars of Caribbean sex work such as Kempadoo (1999) and O'Connell Davidson (1996).

In order to produce a marketable fantasy consistent with these expectations, sex workers must learn to deploy their masculinity and sexuality in ways that maximise their desirability. As an expression of this, *bugarrones* often emphasised how Dominican men's bodies were fundamentally 'different' from those of their clients. Men claimed that Dominican men's bodies were 'stronger', more masculine or more capable of physical endurance than the 'weaker' bodies of the foreigners who visited their country. 'Many *gringos* don't have bodies like us – stronger, hotter', 21-year-old Antonio commented in an interview. 'Here we are strong. We are real men'. Similarly, Marcos, aged 21, explained that he was often nervous when he had sex with tourists, since their bodies were so 'weak' and 'fragile' 'that it feels like they're going to break'. Such narratives of physical differences were also implicitly or explicitly embedded in presumed racial differences that were expressed in distinctly sexualised bodies.

Rafael, a 43-year-old, highly experienced sex worker who made most of his money by connecting clients with sex workers, explained that one of the requests he commonly had from clients was to find the 'darkest, ugliest, smelliest, *prieto* [black man]'.[2] The fact that Rafael had an established relationship with a specific local sex worker to satisfy such requests not only reiterates that the global sex trade is fundamentally racialised, but also reminds us that sex workers possess a sophisticated understanding of these racial discourses and deploy them instrumentally to make a living in the tourism economy. By deploying racial and sexual stereotypes through such performances of masculinity, these men become subjects in their own commodification.

These bodily performances, however, were not without limits. In understanding how men deployed their bodies in the tourism area, it is critical to emphasise that one of the characteristics most consistently expressed by these men is that they do not participate in passive sexual acts, particularly receptive anal sex. In discussing sexual acts, many men emphasised that they were *hombres de verdad* (true men) or *hombres normales* (normal men), phrases intended to communicate not only that they were not *maricones* (or fags), but that they engaged exclusively in penetrative sexual practices with their male partners. Twenty-two-year-old Julio, a *bugarron* in Santo Domingo, for example, observed: 'I'm not homosexual, not bisexual, not anything. I consider myself a man always in sex. Always the man. Nothing more'. Julio's references to being 'always a man', in addition to reflecting a notion of normative masculinity and disavowing homosexuality, are references to his presumed 'manliness' in bed, communicating that he is the penetrative partner who is only insertive during sex with men, not the symbolic 'woman' (or *maricón*) who is penetrated. While it is clear that sex workers' behaviour cannot be stereotyped into the unrealistically fixed categories of *activo* and *pasivo* that have unfortunately dominated much of the literature on Latin American homoeroticism, one of the characteristics most consistently expressed by these men, and which is a critical feature of their gendered practices, is that they do not participate in passive sexual acts, particularly receptive anal sex, with their male clients. This reverberated throughout the interviews and functioned as a way to establish sociosexual boundaries between sex workers and the *maricones* who are symbolically feminised vis-à-vis their penetrable bodies.

Occasionally these sociosexual boundaries are challenged in the negotiation of sexual exchanges. When I inquired whether he had ever been asked to engage in receptive anal sex, Alfonso, a 26 year old in Santo Domingo, told a story of an incident in which he had protected his masculinity despite a client's persistent attempts to manipulate him financially into adopting a passive sexual role:

> Once a foreigner offered me 500 dollars for me to penetrate him, and later he told me – after I penetrated him – 'I'm going to give you 500 dollars more now for me to penetrate you', he told me. And he took out the 500 and put them in my hand and I said 'I don't let myself get fucked in the ass [*no me dejo dar por el culo*]'.... And the fag [*el pájaro*] said, 'Okay, that's fine, no problem. Come by tomorrow'. And I came back the next day like normal, for me to give it to him, and he wanted to give it to me! He handed me the money again, but I gave the 500 back. But I didn't let myself be penetrated! I never want to be penetrated. Because I'm going to tell you the truth: I'm not a *maricón*. I 'look for life'[3] out of necessity, but I don't feel anything back there. Here in front, around my dick, yes. It gets hard as soon as they put a hand on it, right away. But for them to penetrate me?! No, I don't feel anything back there.

Alfonso's narrative offers insight into the bodily boundaries and taboos that are established through gender definitions that organise sexual-economic exchanges with tourists but also can create bodily challenges to sex workers when material interests defy these boundaries. But his narrative also offers insight into the symbolic boundaries that envelope sexuality and the ways that participation in sexual-economic exchanges can create phenomenological challenges to *bugarrones* and *sanky pankies* as they navigate the precarious terrain of the tourism industry. The anxiety provoked by these moments of bodily boundary maintenance are an expression of the shame that is symbolically distributed in the body, since many of these men, drawing on Dominican cultural models that equate sexual passivity with the *maricón*, have constructed their sense of masculinity around a penetrative notion of self.[4] These men's insistence on bodily boundary maintenance provided a means to maintain masculine dignity in the course of their work and to construct sexual differences that are marketable in the tourism economy.

Conclusion: discovering the touristic body

In medical anthropology, *embodiment* has become a term of increasing theoretical discussion, reflecting a general turn in the social sciences toward the reassessment of the body not as a natural phenomenon with an objective biological essence, but as a *social* phenomenon that mediates individual experience and the organisation of human societies (Scheper-Hughes and Lock 1987; Scheper-Hughes 1993). Bodies, in this framework, are examined as the instruments of both exploitation and resistance in the context of social hierarchy. As such, bodies provide a highly productive unit of analysis for conceptualising how local and global inequalities are manifested and contested in and through individual experience.

Approaches to embodiment provide a useful synergy with one of the dominant frameworks in tourism studies: authenticity. According to Dean MacCannell, tourists express their status as modern workers and consumers through their experiences of 'authentic' local cultures, creating a market for the performance or 'staging' of difference (MacCannell 1976). As the successful performance of authenticity is often directly related to material success in the provision of tourism services, local tourism workers benefit from their ability to meet tourists' expectations for authentic experiences. This chapter has made a parallel argument in relation to the sex tourism economy. In the case of sex tourism, embodied practices of gender and sexuality become tools by which local men and women are able to stage authenticity through the production of a marketable fantasy. But in the case of sexual or erotic commodities, fantasies and the material inequalities that frame them are worked out in and through bodies and body parts, with myriad consequences for how local people understand and embody tourism.

Ethnographic research seeking to explain the linkages between the tourism economy and the embodied performances of locals is more than simply theoretical. While a variety of epidemiological and behavioural studies have suggested a linkage between tourism dependence and the HIV epidemic in the Caribbean, there is a near total lack of contextualised ethnographic projects aimed at understanding how tourism, as a broad set of social and economic processes, may be linked to sexual practices. Tourism-oriented HIV initiatives in the Caribbean – the region now showing the highest HIV prevalence rates outside sub-Saharan Africa – should be informed by nuanced analyses of how the micro-practices of sexuality are linked to the performative needs of the growing tourism economy. What are the valued attributes of 'authentic' sexual performance in Caribbean tourism environments? What are the cultural and material parameters of sexual performance that shape the behaviours and meanings of sexual practices? Answering such questions would assist greatly in understanding how HIV risk is shaped by the tourism economy, providing an evidence base for describing the social patterning of sexual practices and HIV-related risk behaviours in specific vulnerable populations, such as sex workers.

Notes

1 For example, a geographical association appears to exist between those Caribbean islands with the greatest economic dependence on tourism and the adult population prevalence of HIV on specific islands, an association that has been commented on by the Caribbean Epidemiological Centre in Trinidad (Camara 2001). In the Dominican Republic, studies among men who have sex with men (MSM) (De Moya and Garcia 1996, 1998; Padilla 2007c), female sex workers (Kerrigan *et al.* 2003) and hotel/resort employees (CEPROSH 1997; Forsythe *et al.* 1998) have found high rates of sexual contact and sexual risk behaviours with foreign tourists.
2 *Prieto* is a Dominican race term that is often employed disparagingly to refer to darker skinned persons or those with more pronounced Afro-Caribbean features (see Howard 2001).
3 'Looking for life', or *buscándose la vida*, is a local phrase in the Dominican Republic often used by sex workers to describe how they make a living. It connotes the ad hoc and flexible income generation activities in which informally employed sex workers engage (Padilla 2007c).
4 See Octavio Paz for a classic discussion of this phallic symbolism – embodied in the figure of the *chignon* – which Paz claims is a fundamental features of masculinity and sexuality in Mexico (Paz 1985). For a parallel discussion on Dominican men, see De Moya (2003).

References

Brennan, D. (2004) *What's Love Got to Do With It? Transnational Desires and Sex Tourism in the Dominican Republic*, Durham: Duke University Press.

Camara, B. (2001) *20 Years of the HIV/AIDS Epidemic in the Caribbean*, Port of Spain, Trinidad: CAREC-SPSTI.

Campbell, S., Perkins, A. and Mohammed, P. (1999) ' "Come to Jamaica and Feel Alright": Tourism and the Sex Trade', in Kempadoo, K. (ed.) *Sun, Sex, and Gold: Tourism and Sex Work in the Caribbean*, New York: Rowman & Littlefield.

CEPROSH (1997) *Proyecto Hotelero*, Puerto Plata, Dominican Republic: Centro de Promoción y Solidaridad Humana.

De Moya, E. A. (2003) 'Power Games and Totalitarian Masculinity in the Dominican Republic', in Reddock, R. E. (ed.) *Interrogating Caribbean Masculinities: Theoretical and Empirical Analyses*, Kingston: University of the West Indies Press.

De Moya, E. A. and Garcia, R. (1996) 'AIDS and the Enigma of Bisexuality in the Dominican Republic', in Aggleton, P. (ed.) *Bisexualities and AIDS: International Perspectives*, Bristol, PA: Taylor & Francis.

De Moya, E. A. and Garcia, R. (1998) 'Three Decades of Male Sex Work in Santo Domingo', in Aggleton, P. (ed.) *Men Who Sell Sex: International Perspectives on Male Prostitution and AIDS*, London: Taylor & Francis.

Forsythe, S., Hasbun, J. and Butler de Lister, M. (1998) 'Protecting Paradise: Tourism and AIDS in the Dominican Republic', *Health Policy & Planning*, 13 (3): 277–86.

Hochschild, A. R. (1979) 'Emotion Work, Feeling Rules and Social Structure', *American Journal of Sociology*, 85 (3): 551–75.

Howard, D. (2001) *Coloring the Nation: Race and Ethnicity in the Dominican Republic*, Boulder, CO: Lynne Rienner.

Kempadoo, K. (ed.) (1999) *Sun, Sex and Gold: Tourism and Sex Work in the Caribbean*, New York: Rowman & Littlefield.

Kerrigan, D., Ellen, J. M., Moreno, L., Rosario, S., Katz, J., Celentano, D. D. *et al.* (2003) 'Environmental-structural Factors Significantly Associated with Condom Use among Female Sex Workers in the Dominican Republic', *AIDS*, 17: 415–23.

Kulick, D. (1998) *Travestí: Sex, Gender and Culture among Brazilian Transgendered Prostitutes*, Chicago: University of Chicago Press.

MacCannell, D. (1976) *The Tourist: A New Theory of the Leisure Class*, New York: Shocken Books.

O'Connell Davidson, J. (1996) 'Sex Tourism in Cuba', *Race and Class*, 38 (July/September): 39–48.

Padilla, M. B. (2007a) 'The Embodiment of Tourism among Bisexually-behaving Dominican Male Sex Workers', *Archives of Sexual Behavior*, 37 (5), 783–93.

Padilla, M. B. (2007b) ' "Western Union Daddies" and their Quest for Authenticity: An Ethnographic Study of the Dominican Gay Sex Tourism Industry', *Journal of Homosexuality*, 53 (1–2): 241–75.

Padilla, M. B. (2007c) *Caribbean Pleasure Industry: Tourism, Sexuality, and AIDS in the Dominican Republic*, Chicago: University of Chicago Press.

Parker, R. (1999) *Beneath the Equator: Cultures of Desire, Male Homosexuality, and Emerging Gay Communities in Brazil*, New York: Routledge.

Paz, O. (1985) *The Labyrinth of Solitude* (trans. L. Kemp, Y. Milos and R. Phillips), Belash, NY: Grove Press.

Prieur, A. (1998). *Mema's House, Mexico City: On Transvestites, Queens, and Machos*, Chicago: University of Chicago Press.

Scheper-Hughes, N. (1993) 'Embodied Knowledge: Thinking with the Body in Critical Medical Anthropology', in Borofsky, R. (ed.) *Assessing Cultural Anthropology*, New York: McGraw-Hill.

Scheper-Hughes, N. and Lock, M. M. (1987) 'The Mindful Body: A Prolegomenon to Future Work in Medical Anthropology', *Medical Anthropology Quarterly*, 1 (1): 6–41.

28 Dancing with daemons

Desire and the improvisation of pleasure

Gary W. Dowsett

In this chapter, I want to present two scenarios of bodies-in-sex, which each reveal something about how we do sex, how we understand it and how we are changing it.[1] 'Bodies-in-sex' is a term I coined years ago to capture the contribution of embodied (physical, emotional) *experience* in the social character of sexuality. It aims to register distance from both the empirical cul de sac of essentialism (nature, the natural, instinct, drive) and the discursive perils of social constructionism that simply read the social on the body but could not entertain the body's presence in sexuality (Dowsett 1996).

The first scenario comes from a public domain website devoted to 'Yaoi', originally a Japanese publishing genre, also known as 'Boys' Love', which includes novels, fantasy, short stories and illustrations produced mostly by young women for their peers (McClelland 2000). Yaoi focuses on romantic, emotional and sexual relationships between young men but is marketed primarily to women. The second scenario comes from a second public domain website I am calling MyCam4U, which specialises in real time online chat and webcam video exchange that primarily concerns sexual activity and display:

Yaoi and sexual imaginary

'Please', Narsus breathed as his bones turned to liquid fire and he melted into that kiss. Then, those strong, callused fingers brushed over one nipple the same moment Darun's lips dipped to lap at his neck, and Narsus' faint surprise that Darun was the sexual aggressor disintegrated as his desire rose to new levels ... The warm candlelight besides Narsus' bed brought the slender, yet well-muscled figure of his love into sharp relief. Goddess, he was so beautiful, but ... The trousers Narsus still wore marred the sleek lines of his body, and suddenly Darun wanted, needed, to see more. He drew Narsus close once more, found then loosened the drawstring of the offending garment. As the pants slid down and pooled at Narsus' feet, Darun's breath caught.

'So beautiful ...' He trailed off, awed, excited beyond reason by the unmistakable evidence of Narsus' desire. His lover's penis was fully erect, was long, slender, just as elegant as the rest of him, and was lovelier than anything Darun had ever seen. Irresistibly drawn, Darun reached out to touch, then hesitated just before he made contact ... Narsus opened Darun's belt by touch, then quickly unfastened his lover's trousers. He knelt, following the motion of his hands as he slid the pants down over Darun's slim hips. Finally freed from the restricting cloth, Darun's erection bobbed gently in time to his lover's gasping breaths, so tantalisingly close to his mouth.[2]

Spanking the monkey

'Showerboi' takes his time. They are patient, almost reverential, and will come with him at his pace. He stands in the centre of the bathroom clothed in tight jeans and a crisp, white T-shirt. Slowly, he gets everything ready: the soap, face cloth, back brush, shampoo, clean towel, returning to stand for a minute or two in the centre of the room, the centre of the frame, to entice and attract more before starting this Saturday morning ritual, and then stops to re-arrange the camera at a slightly lower angle.

CAPS start to scream off the screen at him – 'YEH BABY', 'THAT'S HOT', 'GO 4 IT Showerboi'. He returns to the centre of the room, the centre of the frame. The tight T-shirt reveals his gym-toned chest really well. His pecs preen and his biceps bulge under the short sleeves. He turns to adjust the towel on the rail, showing off his back and butt to advantage. The screen screams again: 'Sweet man, take it off', 'Let me massage those delts', 'Lose the T, Showerboi – NOW'. He returns to the centre of the room, the centre of the frame. He undoes his jeans fly buttons and opens the V-shaped space to reveal pristine white Y-fronts with a '2$^{(x)}$ist' waist band, with just a hint of a 'treasure trail'. It's a nice shot; he can see that in his monitor.

The chat is coming fast, maybe thirty punters on board now. 'Showerboi' removes the T-shirt and lowers the Y-fronts in one carefully rehearsed move, but turns his back on the camera at the same time – just to tease a little more – to turn on the shower, moving the clear glass screen and making sure that not too much steam will frost the glass. Turning to his waiting fans, he stands naked, looking gorgeous, he knows, and watches the gasps, smileys and other emoticons and terms he could not repeat to his grandmother surge up the screen, with phone numbers, email addresses, Yahoo IM handles. And then he smiles at himself in the mirror, pleased with the response again, a moment of pleasure-taking unseen by the audience for the frame stops at his chin.

He enters the shower and for the next 15 minutes 'Showerboi' slowly and gently washes every part of his body for them all to see. The chat is frenzied; they plead with him; they 'SCREAM' at each other; they string statements of desire; they signal ecstasy and orgasm. He starts to masturbate but is in no rush. He knows he has the chat room to himself; the others with cam shows have moved to other rooms and left 'Showerboi' to his climax – and he does, ejaculating on the shower screen for the panting fans.

Choreographing computers

It is hard to imagine these two scenarios without the technology that supports them. The Yaoi narrative may not seem very different from the kind of tales found in the heterosexually focused 'bodice rippers' that make millions of dollars for their authors and publishers (such as Mills and Boon) from women readers worldwide. Yet, even if these Yaoi websites have their forebears in print, these electronic sites now allow a rapid sharing of stories and pictures, and inter alia interactive storytelling with each contributor adding to the tale in turn, weaving fantasy and favourite characters between contributors' imaginations and desires. Yaoi and its sexual imaginary are truly breathtaking in its emotional depth, its beauty and its erotic range. While 'bodice ripper' stories elaborate the sexual desires and fantasies, and maybe real experiences, of the women who read and write them, those in Yaoi reside in the imagination and desires of young women who have not experienced such sex acts. Few, I suspect, have even witnessed sex between men. Maybe some have seen versions available in pornography or oblique enactments in films like *Brokeback Mountain*; but really feeling what men have in wonderful, close, sexy and fulfilling encounters – no! Yet, these young women do know something about how the bodies of young men engage each other. After all, erections may not be all that unfamiliar. Kissing is kissing after all. (Is it?) Maybe some of these women have experienced anal penetration so it might not be unknown either (if without the uniquely male sensation of the overstimulated prostate). But an arousal experience at the hands of another man, with all that this entails physically, emotionally, culturally and symbolically – it is textural and textual – no! For these young women, this can only be imagined.

On MyCam4U, we see something equally originative. With the arrival of webcam technology and its widespread use on such sites, the previous anonymity of internet chat is no longer inevitable. Before webcams, chat users could be anyone they wanted to be and respondents might never really know who was chatting with them. Male? Female? Or even transgender? Gay? Straight? Bisexual? How old? What race or ethnicity? Part of the beauty of this moment in cyberspace was (and still is for those who do not use webcams themselves) that users actually do not know the attributes of the persons with whom they are chatting. Indeed, the 'real' identity of chat users can actually be unknowable; the very impossibility of knowing whom users are engaging with and what their real sexual interests are remains part of the allure in chat rooms and cybersex. Straight women can be men and seduce other women (who might also be men); gay men can be women and explore that all time sexual fantasy that no man is really straight after all – and succeed. Everyone can be young and beautiful. In the privacy of one's own room, one can be seduced, masturbate with a complete stranger doing the same somewhere else, sequenced via keyboard text, and still never be certain who or what anyone is. More importantly, one might not want to know – the very characteristics that we sex researchers think choreograph sex are significant in their absence. In a sense, these social categories and conventions serve no purpose and our 'independent variables' are rendered nonsense.

This is not just a cyber-variety of that well-documented identity/practice dissonance evident in the majority of recent behavioural studies of sex the world over, largely generated by the HIV pandemic. Cybersex challenges the very divisibility of identity and practice that sex research has relied on to explain its paradoxical behavioural findings. The internet destabilises the very concept of identity as we have come to utilise it in relation to sexuality, as a category of certainty and difference. The sexual choreography available to users in cyberspace suggests that in the absence of verifiable bodies, identity is only useful in sexuality as an act of endless creation, as performance. As a relatively recent construct in understanding sexuality, identity may become redundant faster than we think.

This scene from MyCam4U exemplifies another more recent shift in the choreography of sex. At the moment of Showerboi's performance, there were over 2500 people chatting in over 25 chat rooms, which operate 24 hours a day, seven days a week. There were 173 live webcams showing at that moment, with a handful of women but mostly men, often stripping or naked, some displaying erections, many masturbating before their cameras and for the audiences they were pulling in the chat room. There was the odd sex toy employed here and there, some cross-dressing, the occasional couple (both same and opposite sex), and now and then people having sex, full intercourse both anal and vaginal. There were some real 'personalities', such as 'TigerWoodie' who auto-fellated his nine-inch penis, and a few who were exercising or cleaning their houses nude – it was not all riveting and arousing. The chat was racy but was not only about sex. However, there was, apparently, a lot of ejaculating occurring. If this indicates anything about how often men 'cum' then, thinking on a global scale at any given moment … ah, I'll let you do the sums.

I have no detailed knowledge on how MyCam4U works technically, but there are also voice chat rooms, email options, preview possibilities and so on. Neither do I know who owns it, how it came into being or how long it has been going. I have no idea how unique it is or how ubiquitous such web sites have become. A 'Google' search on 'live webcams' at the moment of writing revealed thousands of similar sites. They seemed mostly commercial sites. Many were not sex related, but frequent pop-ups and banners revealed the extent to which things sexual dominate the domain. There is, however, very little commercial marketing on MyCam4U. This site is clearly for amateurs, and Showerboi is just another guy, albeit a good-looking one, doing his thing. He is not a sex industry entertainer, stripper, pole dancer or sex worker as we might usually classify these; he showers and ejaculates for his own audience once a week, a part of his own pleasure and for theirs. That is his gift, his thrill, his desire, offered to others for free in ritual orgasm.

The sexed body is less ambiguous here. There is something incontrovertibly male about Showerboi. The camera cannot lie, at least not easily. Neither Showerboi nor TigerWoodie for that matter confuses. They are men. They reveal men's bodies. They display unambiguous erections. They ejaculate. Similarly, the women offer breasts and/or labia to view. The few transgender folk declare it, from what I could tell. Distinction here on gender lines requires little help – nudity is a great clarifier. Sexual 'orientation', however, is another issue. Distinctions *are* made primarily (but not only) between gay and straight. It seems to be a 'boy thing' too. The women rarely bother with such declarations; maybe they have little need of them and that in itself is interesting. Most straight men add 'str8' as a caption; some gay men add 'gay'. There is clearly a 'gay' chat room, understood to be so by everyone, and it is also the busiest. But other rooms are not so clearly non-gay either. There is a considerable degree of banter between gay and non-gay people. Gay men like to play with the 'str8' men, sometimes pretending to be women, enticing them to do more, show more; sometimes they get found out. The straight men know it, or some do, and enjoy the game; some get cross and occasionally there is explicit homophobia. Often the women conspire to get men to reveal more information or flesh if they are hesitant. It is a different game these women play: wily, yet explicitly self-pleasuring in their voyeurism and as ambitious in exercising influence.

There is also considerable boundary crossing: straight men praised by gay men for their bodies, humour, erections or ejaculations often say 'thank you'. There is some cachet for straight men here, some recognition of being a passive yet phallic object of an erotic gaze from both women and men. There is recognition shared with other men, gay and straight, of the obvious pleasure in masculine arousal – a kind of a 'polity of the penis'. Indeed, Showerboi never declares himself one thing or another and enjoys everyone's attention. The blurring of boundaries certainly occurs with declaredly bisexual men or within that rapidly enlarging sexual category 'bi-curious', but that is not adequate as an underlying explanation. An incident with TigerWoodie serves to show how these distinctions are made and tested, and what purpose they serve. After a self-fellation session, TigerWoodie, who acknowledged warmly the men who watch him while declaring himself definitively straight, was asked if he had sucked any other penises. He answered, 'No, only my own because I'm not gay'.

Even with gender distinctions clearly marked by visible bodies, and sexual arousal and satisfaction so clearly linked to men's ejaculation (the women declare they enjoy this too), the boundaries between heterosexual and homosexual are hard to maintain. They have to be worked at constantly or they collapse. An erect, ejaculating penis has no sexual orientation in this domain; sexual action cannot rely on definitive object choice for definition, or as control; pleasures offered by MyCam4U must recognise and accept many sexual interests. Any assertion of sexual orientation dissolves in the act of granting the machine the distribution of attraction and satisfaction.

On the Yaoi sites and in MyCam4U and its like, the process of self-definition, the construction of identity, practice, meaning and experience is amplified, indeed generated, by using multiplying computer categories, and this reveals much about sexual cultures in transition. On the Yaoi sites, the young women are exploring sex through improvisation on their own shared fantasies, for the bodies of the young men they write about (and as illustrated Yaoi stories testify) are highly romanticised and feminised – they are beautiful, lithe young men, even pretty. Yet, these young men's bodies experience desire strongly and with determination. There is always a dominant one and anal penetration is always ecstatic and wildly ejaculatory. His receptive partner succumbs/surrenders to sex; virginity is lost/given to the other. As these young women write and improvise on each other's contributions, they raise the sexual stakes, moving beyond salacity to art, mapping their own sexual desires and envisaging futures beyond the accepted boundaries of their own lives. For in Yaoi desire cannot shame, in part because these stories are written anonymously, in a sense hidden from the other young women and behind their characters, but also because these adventures cannot be completely owned. They remain vicarious, and that is its own pleasure.

For MyCam4U users, the site not only offers the speed of instant communication available on Yaoi, but also the possibility of a definitive presence. Where anonymity might once have provided camouflage and facilitated fantasy in pre-cam chat, now identification and exposure has increasingly become the etiquette. Indeed, the machine itself fosters and encourages a new sexual adventure, one lived within the lives of others, one where shamelessness is foregrounded and the sexual is valued and validated. The choices offered by the machines and their sites, as they become more sophisticated and complex, inspire adventure. A good example is the not-so-old dichotomy between 'top' and 'bottom' in gay parlance: top being the penetrative partner and bottom being the penetrated. These terms top and bottom derive from SM, but have become more common in the last 20 years than their antecedents pitcher/catcher, active/passive, butch/bitch. Given the dominance of heteronormative notions of sex as penetration, and of sex 'roles' as clearly demarked by gender as penetrator (male) and penetrated (female), this current usage is not surprising. However, those endless HIV behavioural surveys of gay men in many countries have revealed that this hard and fast division is not so hard or fast in practice, and the category 'versatile' has been added to gay men's taxonomy to allow for those who enjoy both modes in sexual intercourse. This is a great help in choreographing threesomes.

However, on websites such as MyCam4U and similar chat sites, this modal preference has been enlarged to five categories recently to accommodate more specificity *and* variability in men's interests: there is now 'bottom', 'versatile bottom', 'versatile', 'versatile top' and 'top'. Recently, 'fully top' has been added to the list for added certainty. Faced with these choices, one is encouraged not to limit one's sexual potential. Other such possibilities have multiplied on these sites as well. The sites offer possibilities of defining and refining the sexual self in ways previously unavailable. In the binary code that underpins computing, one is or one is not. Click on a pull-down menu and choose: male, female, transgender, transsexual, transvestite, intersex. Identify as gay, str8, bisexual, bi-curious, queer, questioning. Offer oral sex, kissing, anal sex, toys, SM, watersports. Seek like interests in underwear, Speedos, uniforms, rubber, leather, lycra. Mark the choices as 'like', 'don't like', 'undecided', 'want to try'. Choose a handle (site nickname) that indicates preferences: dirtybttmboi, satin_doll, evil_angel. Post a picture clothed, naked, from the neck down, profiling erections or orifices opened to view. Add a short video intro: strip, dance, sing, ejaculate, penetrate. It is not just the presence of the camera that has smashed through the wall of shame that surrounds desire. Now one can perform, entice, embody desire and claim it as one's own: put one's whole body, face and all, there declaring oneself phallic, desiring, desirable to whoever wants to watch, and do so unashamedly.

The ever increasing specification of categories of desire or pleasure, and the computation of them to find an audience or sex partners (on- or offline) or enhance one's singular pleasures, constitute a remarkable shift in *inciting* desire rather than merely *representing* it. As one is invited to improvise, sexuality's traditional binary categories begin to dissolve in the face of the democracy of a machine that is without prejudice or conscience. There is a fragmenting of hetero/homo 'orientation' into more specified, yet fluid categories of desire, more defined choreographies, declared exclusivities and finer gradings that are potentially less firmly 'fixed'. Rather than new forms of 'sexual identity' tied to old cartographies of desire, these shifts might best be framed as an emerging cultures or as a performative ethics of sex. They represent something new, something shifting within sexuality. Foucault captured this years ago when he wrote:

> Sexuality is something we ourselves create – it's our own creation, and much more than the discovery of a secret side of our desire. We have to understand that with our desires, through our desires, go new forms of relationships, new forms of love, new forms of creation. Sex is not fatality [i.e. not inevitable]; it's a new possibility for creative life.
>
> (Foucault 1998: 138)

The internet as we now know it was not available when Foucault said this, but he does get it right; the only things missing from his formulation are the machines with their programmers and their software. More than ever, it is these that increasingly choreograph the 'deployment of sexuality' and invite improvisation in our pleasuring; they are the daemons with which we increasingly dance.

Notes

1 Thanks to Duane Duncan, Australian Research Centre in Sex, Health and Society, La Trobe University, Melbourne, for research assistance.
2 The site from which this extract was drawn originally seems to have disappeared, so cannot be referenced here. But there are many similar sites: just Google 'Yaoi'.

References

Dowsett, G. W. (1996) *Practicing Desire: Homosexual Sex in the Era of AIDS*, Stanford, CA: Stanford University Press.
Foucault, M. (1998) *Essential Work of Foucault, Volume 1* (trans. R. Hurley), in Heiner, B. T. (2003) 'The Passions of Michel Foucault', *Differences: A Journal of Feminist Cultural Studies*, 14 (1): 42–3.
McClelland, M. (2000) 'No Climax, No Point, No Meaning? Japanese Women's Boy-love Sites on the Internet', *Journal of Communication Inquiry*, 24 (3): 274–91.

29 Sex in motion

Notes on urban Brazilian sexual scenes

Veriano Terto Junior and Fernando Seffner

Abstinence is a good thing, as long as we practice it in a moderate way.

(Anonymous)

The events and descriptions in this chapter highlight the connection between sex and pleasure. They emphasise vividly how erotic sexual encounters can cross boundaries of class, race, gender, sexual orientation and generation. Each of the scenes described was extracted from field research that we have been conducting over the last few years. The names of the places mentioned are real, but the anonymity of the individuals involved has been preserved.

Redenção Park, Porto Alegre, January 2008

Redenção Park is located in a region near downtown Porto Alegre in Brazil. It is bounded by three major avenues, on one of which young male sex workers work at night, catering to men who drive up and down the avenue looking to buy sex. During the day, the park is a recreational setting for local residents: elderly people walking individually or in groups; people walking their dogs; students dating or just enjoying the park; and maids taking small children out for a walk. Service sector workers walk through the park on their way to work or sit on benches to go through documents and call colleagues. Maintenance and cleaning staff keep things tidy, and people hand out pamphlets advertising products for sale.

In the late afternoon, before the sun goes down, there is a higher concentration of people in the park, especially those jogging and exercising. Movement decreases substantially with the arrival of dusk, accompanied by a change in the type of person who goes there. Between early evening and midnight, the park is a popular location for men seeking sexual contact with other men. Between late afternoon and around nine o'clock, these tend to be men returning home from work. Some take short cuts through the park and stay there for an hour or so. About nine o'clock, things change, a different kind of man arrives who stays there longer, usually until after midnight. These men circle around or sit for a time near the pathways, sometimes chatting with friends, sometimes alone, watching what is happening or finding other men with whom to have sex. After midnight, the park begins to empty and stays that way until the early hours of the morning, when the pattern repeats itself. In the early morning, however, some men pass through the park again on their way to work. For a few, there is just enough time to find someone with whom to have sex.

The time of the following scene is around 10 p.m., it is a pleasant and warm evening, with just a few people walking around. The atmosphere is quiet, but the silence is broken by conversation between a group of four gay men, aged between 20 and 35. They chat merrily, all seated on a bench of the park, underneath a lamp post. Their conversation is quite loud, there is laughter and stories are being told. They are friends, and get together here in the park every once in a while. Are all white, dressed in T-shirts, shorts and trainers. A homeless man, not exactly a beggar, already well known in the park where he often spends the summer nights sleeping in some sheltered corner, approaches the group. He is a mulatto, young, aged around 30, but with the appearance of being younger. He carries two backpacks and a bag containing his belongings. He stops in front of the group of gay men. They do not seem to be friends, but certainly know each other. The group acknowledges him and he acknowledges the group.

He says good evening and asks in a loud voice, 'I want a *chupisco* (blowjob). Anyone want to give me a *chupisco*'. The young gay men laugh, a few talk with him making jokes, but he insists: 'I've had a wash in the lake, I'm clean, look my hair is wet'. The young homeless man is in fact good looking and has a captivating smile. Again he says 'I want a *chupisco*'. The gay men know the homeless man which explains the dialogue between such different people, and the request being made in so direct a way. Perhaps a similar scene has happened before. One of the gay men then decides to give the homeless man a *chupisco*. He responds, saying 'Come here, I'll give you a *chupisco*, let's go over there'. The joy of the homeless man is almost touching. He leaves his things next to the bench, backpacks and bags, and then goes into a wooded corner with the gay guy. There they are, hidden by the vegetation, at a distance not more than 20 paces from the whole group, but enough to be in the dark surrounded by vegetation. In the five minutes that follow, some of the younger men shout things to the two hidden in the bushes, encouraging them, and some indicating that they too will soon be there giving *chupiscos*.

Nothing is heard from the bushes, and about five minutes later the two return, the young homeless man expressing his satisfaction, the gay boy emphasising that the homeless man was really excited – that he was 'overdue' and 'needed' to have sex. Hearing this, the young homeless man smiles, and before picking up his things asks the others whether they too don't want to give him a *chupisco*. The group respond saying he has already had too much and to get a move on, but all is said in a tone of joking. It is remarkable how the homeless man expresses himself in a clear, direct, way without any shame either about the request made or the situation. Similarly, the four gay men talk about the matter in a straightforward way, kidding about, accepting the request, responding to desire. All is expressed in clear Portuguese, full of expressions drawn from the world of *bichice* (gay slang).

Seeing that he is not going to receive any more 'sexual favours', the young homeless man thanks them. He takes his belongings and begins to leave, but repeats once again that he will be around sleeping near the lake in case anyone changes their minds and wants to go with him. With that the scene ends. The four men return to their talk and laughter. The young homeless man moves on, walking toward the lake until he is lost from sight. Everything happens in a very 'civilised' way, the whole conversation takes place as if between equals, nothing revealing the enormous social distance between a black homeless man and four white lower middle-class young gay men.

The Astor Cinema, Salvador, April 2008

Since the early afternoon, the movement of men in and out of both the male and female toilets on the mezzanine level of the cinema has been intense. Despite the clear distinction of gender in bright lights above the doors, the two bathrooms serve the same purpose: they are places where visitors can fulfil their physiological needs, but can also flirt, talk and have sex. The men's room, in addition to the cubicles, has sinks and urinals where there is space for up to four men to urinate or display their erections to each other. The women's bathroom has just three cubicles and washbasins. It seems just a bit cleaner than its male counterpart. The cubicles of both bathrooms are occupied by pairs of men seeking to have sex in a more 'private' way than in the cinema itself, or by sex workers serving a customer who pays for sex with penetration or any other activity they do not want to do in the dark of the audience.

The privacy offered by the toilet cubicles is relative, because the doors are small, and it is possible for those who are outside, to see the heads and feet of those who are standing inside. It is quite possible to see when there are two men in the booth and a taller person just has to lean over and he can see what the couple is doing inside the cabin. The walls that divide the stalls are also relatively low, perhaps not two metres in height, which makes it easy for a man in the next booth to stand on the toilet seat and look over to see what his neighbours are doing. Throughout the afternoon, the cubicles are busy in both the men's room and the women's room and are occupied both by heterosexual couples (most usually sex workers and their clients) and by men. Contact between men and negotiation with sex workers happens in the audience, and couples then go to the toilets to do what they cannot do in the shadows of the cinema itself.

There are also those who come alone to an empty stall to climb on a toilet seat and watch what the neighbours are doing, and others who seek to look over and under the doors. These practices of voyeurism do not seem to bother the couples who are having sex without seeming to mind the fact that they are being observed. Outside the cubicles, flirting and kidding around continues among men revealing even more the mixing of heterosexual and homosexual practices. The one seems to reinforce the other: men who seek to observe the couples having sex in the cubicles may touch others next in the queue. Similarly, in the men's room those excited by seeing scenes of heterosexual couples may end up revealing themselves to other men at the urinal, or will look for sex outside with one of the sex workers or any other interested partner in the audience.

The Astor is an old cinema, certainly more than 40 years old, but in good condition for this type of old movie theatre dedicated to showing pornographic films. The films, shown on a single large screen, only portray heterosexual sex. They are projected by DVD projectors and not on film as are the movies shown in non-pornographic movie theatres. Admission is cheap, compared with the non-pornographic cinemas. The Astor, unlike most cinemas in Brazil, which tend to be in large modern shopping malls, is located on one of the most busy streets of downtown Salvador, accessible by the pavement of the street it is on, and near to a number of other shops, bars and offices.

As for those who go there, these are mostly black and mulatto men, together with a few sex workers and *travestis*, who work there during the afternoons every day.

Many of those who go come from the downtown working class. By the same token, it is impossible not to note the presence of many young people wearing shorts and thongs (flip-flops) who are not working, while others carry folders, uniforms and briefcases, demonstrating they have been working or studying in the area. Just a few patrons are middle class or lower middle class judged by the type of clothing they wear: well-ironed shirts, shoes in good condition, etc. The few women and *travestis* observed that afternoon, seemed to dress in a certain careless way, shorts not matching tight tops and tight blouses, an image further damaged by hair or wigs in disarray and nails poorly taken care of, with little or no makeup.

Not all visitors of course are in search of sex, and a considerable part of the public even seem interested in enjoying the movies or maybe masturbate themselves while seated in the audience and the lower mezzanine floor, these both accessible by two stairways, one on each side of the room. Another part of the audience walks around the cinema looking for partners seated in chairs or standing in the entryway of the darkened room, while a few, perhaps the older ones, find friends and acquaintances to chat with while roaming around the cinema. The cinema is often full on weekdays, during working hours, but this is characteristic of this type of movie theatre in other cities of Brazil.

Windsor Cinema, São Paulo, May 2008

In contrast to the quantity of visitors on weekdays, the movement of men in search of sex in the movie theatre seemed very low late afternoon that Saturday afternoon. The small number of people in the audience reflects the quiet and the empty streets and avenues of downtown São Paulo, the largest city in Brazil. The large size of this cinema, almost empty, reinforced the impression of the end of a party in which the people who are left have low expectations of finding someone to have sex with. A few people are still arriving at the cinema, but the numbers of those leaving, as minutes go by, grows. At a particular moment, however, a heterosexual couple arrives, the only one in a cinema normally occupied only by men looking for other men. The two, hand in hand, walk down to the seats at the front of the cinema, closer to the screen. Despite the low number of visitors, there in that part of the cinema some men are having oral sex or masturbating, and others are watching the movie. The couple sit in seats overlooking one of the aisles.

As expected of a dating couple, they embrace for a time, but soon the woman starts to perform oral sex on her partner. The men seated in the same section of the theatre and those who are wandering around seem to realise what is happening and approach the couple. One person seated close by advances then approaches even closer, sitting next to the couple. He begins to masturbate and rub his body gently against the body of the woman next to him. In the aisle, a group of men is standing near the couple and observes the scene. Almost all are already masturbating, some less than a few metres away from the couple. Some of the men masturbating while standing touch each other and reach out to masturbate each other. A circle slowly forms around the couple who continue to watch the movie or look around at those assembled, the woman once in a while continues giving her partner a blowjob. None of the men standing actually touches the couple, only the third party seated next to the woman. Not all cinema viewers go to see what is happening. Some remain where they are just watching the film, flirting or wandering around. However, the circle with the couple in the middle continues to be reinforced, not so much by the number of participants, but because many are touching each other, some ejaculate, while pairs of men a bit further away also begin to have sex, which intensifies an impression of profligacy.

The Windsor Cinema is part of a network of old movie theatres in downtown São Paulo. With the decline of the neighbourhood and loss of prestige, these have since the 1970s been occupied by men in search of homosexual sex. The Windsor is an old movie theatre, possibly more than 50 years old, large, as movie theatres used to be in the middle of the twentieth century. It does not appear in modern gay guides of the city, which demonstrates its low status among places preferred by the current gay population of São Paulo such as saunas, nightclubs and bars located in the middle-class neighbourhoods. Ticket prices are also inexpensive compared to the new sites listed, and the fact that heterosexual pornographic movies are shown enhances the difference from gay settings that exhibit exclusively homosexual movies. Like other old cinemas downtown, the quality of projection is bad, there is a smell of mould and stale cigarettes and the worn-out seats show some sense of abandon and neglect. Men of various kinds go there, most are masculine, many come from the working class, many are married (their wedding rings are visible). In the darkness, men of different ethnicities (whites, blacks, orientals, mulattos, etc.), both old or young, meet in moments such as that just described, and have diverse forms of sex both in public and in toilets, with an intensity that contrasts sharply with the almost funereal-like atmosphere of the aging theatre.

In February 2009, we received news that the Windsor Cinema had closed its doors, possibly due to a ban by São Paulo city council. Other downtown cinemas showing pornography had earlier been closed in 2008, having been refused renewal of their operating licenses.

So what does all this mean?

The scenes described here took place in three major Brazilian cities, in the south (Porto Alegre), in the northeast (Salvador) and in the southeast (São Paulo) of the country. However, similar events take place elsewhere in major metropolises such as Rio de Janeiro and Fortaleza (Terto 1989). The movie theatres described here have in common the fact that they are located downtown, in busy, often slightly run-down areas, in which there is a lot of population movement. Similarly, Redenção Park is located in an area near downtown, and is seen as a place of fun and entertainment for a significant portion of the inhabitants. Despite these common features, each of these settings deserves further study to understand its history, and its specific place in the sexual cultures of each of the urban areas in which our observations were carried out. Significantly, the two types of place here described (cinemas and parks) do not appear in the modern gay guides distributed in these cities. When they are mentioned, they are accompanied by a series of warnings about the risk of robbery and violence, which reinforces their position of marginality and low value on the gay scene.

Compared to those frequenting gay bars, clubs and saunas, men in the chosen settings show remarkable diversity in terms of class, age, occupation, race, preference for paid or unpaid sex, marital status and so on. Activities in Redenção Park show dramatic change throughout the course of day. For some men, the park is a place to go to after work and before going back home, just like a bar may be for other men. Activity varies too with the day of the week. For example, on Saturday nights the park is frequented much more by 'out' gay men, making it a place of sociability and cruising between gays. Married men prefer to visit cinemas between Monday and Friday during working hours rather than at weekends when busy-ness seems to decrease, as does the number of sex workers who are more common during the week. In some cinemas, 'out' gay men are more numerous at weekends.

The scenes also reveal something of the harmonious coexistence between two distinct sexual preferences, heterosexual and homosexual, which rarely coexist outside of these spaces, occupying singular and differentiated territories. In the cinema and in the park, less of a clear boundary is drawn between identities. That does not mean that antagonism and estrangement between heterosexual and homosexual men do not happen in the cinema or in the park, but that such responses appear rare in an atmosphere of overall 'understanding'.

This understanding allows same-sex and heterosexual practices to take place at the same time and paid and unpaid sex to coexist in close proximity, implying quite different uses of the movie theatres and the park. Some go to the cinema to simply watch a movie and some walk through the park and do not want to be bothered by others. Others wander around searching for casual sex or even prostituting themselves. The use of the park by men for homoerotic encounters is shared with *travesti* prostitution, heterosexual couples looking for a free-of-charge motel, drug users, people walking their dogs and those simply exercising their curiosity. In modern-day Brazil, it is hard to imagine two men kissing in a fashionable nightclub for young heterosexuals. In the cinemas and in the park, however, such sexual differences seem to be welcome; instead of being excluded they are integrated without either being denied. If in some social spaces, sexual differences become a reason for conflict and barriers to harmonious coexistence, in other settings such boundaries seem less rigid and exclusionary.

Such diversity of relationships does not occur by chance or by accident. Married men and other men who do not accept themselves as homosexual go to parks and porn movie theatres mainly because they know there are other men there wanting to have sex. Dim light, little need for talk, body-to-body contact and impersonality not only reinforce sexual availability, but also provide protection and anonymity for those who do not wish to show their sexual desires publicly. In a social world increasingly segmented into specialised niches and sexual communities, it is important to draw attention to the survival of these spaces and the investment of men and some women in sexual possibilities less marked by boundaries of identity, class or generation.

Finally, a methodological comment. What are the limits to observational research in settings such as these? We have no answer, but want to stress the tension that exists between that of participant and that of researcher. Even notions of 'participatory research' say little about what is likely to be experienced by researchers in contexts similar to those which we have investigated. Suppose we had not initially gone into these settings with the intention of experiencing these situations, and only later analysing and reflecting on them? Would our analysis and understanding of them have been different if we had initially observed with no intention of collecting data for scientific investigation? The scenes observed, and our interpretations of them, call attention to a researcher's reflexive position – and to the importance of paying attention to reflexivity (which is too often forgotten) in research on sexuality.

Conclusions

Sexuality is a complex plot made up of differences, identities, rights, biomedical discourse on reproduction and health, moral discourses on religion, political positions and many other factors. But it is also, very powerfully, the experience of having sex. The strong meaning of the word 'sex' seems sometimes to be pushed into the background nowadays. On the one hand, there is discourse on gender and power relations defining what the 'free' expression of sexuality, its rights and guaranteed visibility might be. On the other hand, the scenes described here of sexual performance reveal important ways of being, including ways of delineating identities and negotiating their boundary relationships with other forms of self understanding.

Both as social researchers and as activists, we value the emergence of the interdisciplinary field of sexuality studies and sexual rights. But we have worries about some of the demands made by what might be described as the sexual identity and LGBTQ movements. We also question whether some of their achievements do not normalise sex by focusing too much on the 'aseptic' practices that visibility allows. Visibility and rights come with changes in ways of being sexual. These changes often make the pursuit of sex more 'committed', more palatable and more decent, complying to the standards of visibility for all society.

In this chapter, we have focused on areas of sexual practices that do not claim visibility and which lie apart from most discourses of sexual rights. They reveal a less aseptic form of sex, maybe 'nastier', but not necessarily better or worse than that performed by those who opt for greater visibility. Here we may see more of what Foucault (1978) termed an erotic art which values performance and the experience it provides, rather than sexual science focused on knowing our desires and why we like this or that. Visibility implies a confession of practices, while anonymity is often about practices that do not want to show themselves. To convince others of the power and legitimacy of anonymous practice is very different from the ways in which many gay men live their lives and make claims about their legitimacy nowadays.

In the scenes we have studied, sexual practices do not exist independently from other social determinants such as gender, class, race and sexual orientation. If in many places there is antagonistic coexistence of different sexual orientations, in our chosen scenes there is what we might call an antagonism in coexisting. The antagonism is there, but it 'loosens' for a moment of pleasure. As we have indicated earlier, the coexistence of differences in public space is forced by sexual pursuit itself. This is not to suggest that there are social class, sexual orientation and age differences in the cinemas or in the park, but to stress that the sex scene and the performance of those involved involve people of different social classes, ages and sexual orientations. They are not only in the same space, they actively participate in the same scene. And their presence enhances the scene, including individual or group enjoyment and ecstasy.

Finally, we would like to emphasise the significance of regimes of 'darkness' in a similar way to those of visibility. Our focus here has been on areas of practice that might be called 'marginal', not wishing visibility, and which exist in systems of anonymity, silence, darkness and low exposure. We have undertaken silent observation in these places, respecting the privacy of those involved. Despite the diversity, there is the potential for convergence. In other words, the underpinning logic is not one of the different coexisting side by side but of the different in a project of common pleasure. These scenes represent a coming together and a confluence of desires. These are moments of drifting. Individuals are there with no track of time. Within each scene it is always twilight, either the natural twilight of the park or the artificial night of the darkened cinema. In each, there are always shadows helping time to come to a halt, which favour wandering, walking and the quest for leisure. How then can we bring together such regimes of darkness and the more visible discourses of sexual and human rights?

References

Foucault, M. (1978) *The History of Sexuality, Volume 1: An Introduction*, New York: Random House.
Terto Jr., V. (1989) 'No Escurinho do Cinema: Socialidade Orgiástica nas Tardes Cariocas', master's thesis in psychology, Catholic University of Rio de Janeiro (PUC/RJ), Brazil.

Part VI
The darker side of sex

30 Sexual and intimate partner violence

The global picture

Claudia Garcia-Moreno

Introduction

Sexual relationships are considered to be the ultimate expression of intimacy, partnership, love. Yet, far too often, violence and abuse are also part of them. Whether in long-term relationships, dating violence, the first sexual experience, during childhood, for women and children who have been trafficked, in situations of conflict and displacement, this experience has both immediate and long-term impacts on an individual's health and wellbeing. Sexual violence is used as a form of punishment; a tactic of control; to assert masculinity and men's right to sexual pleasure, and often society condones this violence, whether by silence and shame or impunity. Victims rather than perpetrators carry the stigma of their experience.

Gender inequality and other forms of power inequality underlie much of this violence. Although not specific to them, women and girls comprise the majority of victims, and men are the majority of perpetrators. Because of this, this chapter is focused on sexual violence against women, while also referring to sexual violence against men and children. It uses data from a World Health Organisation (WHO) multi-country study on women's health and domestic violence, which provides an overview of women's experience of different forms of violence, to illustrate global prevalence. The study involved population-based face-to-face surveys in over 24,000 randomly selected women aged 15–49 years in 15 sites (both urban and rural) in 11 countries.[1]

The World Report on Violence and Health defines sexual violence as: 'any sexual act, attempt to obtain a sexual act, unwanted sexual comments or advances, or acts to traffic, or otherwise directed against a person's sexuality, using coercion, by any person, regardless of relationship to the victim, in any setting, including but not limited to home and work' (Jewkes *et al.* 2002a: 149). Coercion can here include the use of physical force, psychological intimidation or threats to harm – including losing a job or failing an exam. It can also occur when a person is unable to give consent, either because of mental problems or the use of alcohol or drugs (Jewkes *et al.* 2002a). It includes rape – usually defined legally to refer to forced penetration of vulva or anus, using a penis, other body parts or an object, and attempts to rape. It can happen within intimate partnerships (marriage or cohabitation) or by acquaintances or strangers, and it can happen to children (child sexual abuse), adolescents and adults of any age. Other forms include harmful practices related to sexual control of women such as female genital mutilation; child marriage or virginity tests; forced prostitution and trafficking for the purposes of sexual exploitation.

Prevalence

Child sexual abuse

Child sexual abuse includes any activity by adults or significantly older children on children, for sexual gratification. Most common is the sexual abuse of children by family members (incest) and by other known people who are not family members. It can be non-contact (including indecent exposure or unwanted and inappropriate sexual solicitation), contact (such as sexualised kissing, touching or fondling but not involving penetration) or penetrative (including oral, anal or vaginal intercourse or attempted intercourse (WHO 2002). Using the age of 18 years as a cut-off and based on a meta-analysis of studies of child sexual abuse worldwide (93 for boys and 143 for girls), Andrews and colleagues came up with the following global estimates of childhood sexual abuse victimisation prevalence:

- non-contact sexual abuse (3.1 per cent boys, 6.8 per cent girls)
- contact sexual abuse (3.7 per cent boys, 13.2 per cent girls)
- penetrative sexual abuse (1.9 per cent boys, 5.3 per cent girls)
- any sexual abuse (8.7 per cent boys, 25.3 per cent girls).

The WHO multicountry study on women's health and domestic violence asked women about sexual abuse before the age of 15 years. The prevalence of sexual abuse before age 15 years (child sexual abuse) varied from 1 per cent in Bangladesh to 21 per cent in Namibia. In most cases, only one perpetrator was mentioned, most usually a family member (Garcia-Moreno *et al.* 2005). These rates are higher than often assumed and are likely affected by recall bias and thus likely to be underestimates. Much of the violence happens in the home, but also by neighbours, teachers, priests and other, usually men, in positions of power and trust. In some settings, schools are also places where girls (and boys) can be at risk of sexual abuse, whether sexual harassment or rape by teachers or peers. For example, one study in South Africa identified teachers as responsible for 32 per cent of disclosed child rapes (Jewkes *et al.* 2002b).

Forced first sex

For many girls, the first sexual experience is forced or unwanted. Studies in, for example, Ghana and Zimbabwe found 25 per cent of females aged 15–24 reported that their first sexual intercourse was forced (Glover 2003; Phiri and Erulkar 2000). In Rakai district in Uganda, 14 per cent of young girls reported that heir sexual initiation had been coerced or forced (Koenig 2004). In the WHO multicountry study, between 3 per cent and 24 per cent of women reported that their first sexual experience was forced (Garcia-Moreno *et al.* 2005). In 10 of the 15 settings investigated, over 5 per cent of women reported their first sexual experience was forced, with more than 14 per cent reporting forced first sex in Bangladesh, Ethiopia, Peru province and Tanzania. In contrast, less than 1 per cent of women in Japan and Serbia described their first sexual experience as being forced. In all sites, except Ethiopia, the younger a woman's age at first sex, the greater the likelihood that her sexual initiation was forced (Garcia-Moreno *et al.* 2005).

Rape and sexual assault

A growing number of studies of intimate partner violence document physical, sexual and, to a lesser degree, emotional violence and controlling behaviours, but few population studies have looked at rape and sexual assault outside of intimate partner abuse. While there is no universally agreed definition for emotional abuse and coercive control, it is worth noting that several of the items often considered in the measurement of coercive control (e.g. insists on knowing where you are at all times, gets angry if you speak to another man, is often suspicious that you are unfaithful) are related to the control of women's sexuality.

Studies worldwide find that between 6 per cent and 47 per cent of women report attempted or completed forced sex by an intimate partner in their lifetime (Heise *et al.* 1999). The findings of the WHO Violence against Women Study were consistent with this: between 6 per cent and 59 per cent of women reported ever having experienced sexual violence by an intimate partner, with most sites falling between 10 per cent and 51 per cent and between 3 per cent and 24 per cent for sexual violence during the past 12 months (Garcia-Moreno *et al.* 2006). Sexual violence was usually accompanied by physical violence by an intimate partner.

The range of lifetime prevalence of physical or sexual violence, or both, by an intimate partner was between 15 per cent and 71 per cent (Garcia-Moreno *et al.* 2006). Women also reported sexual violence by non-partners, but with much lower rates (not including child sexual abuse). Between 0.3 per cent and 12 per cent of respondents reported being forced to have sex or perform sexual acts that they did not want to by non-partners since the age of 15 years. The highest levels (between 10 per cent and 12 per cent) were reported in Peru, Samoa and Tanzania. Generally the most frequently mentioned perpetrators were acquaintances (boyfriends) and strangers, but in Japan 16 per cent of women reported 'someone at work' as the main perpetrator (Garcia-Moreno *et al.* 2005). Teachers accounted for between 15 per cent and 56 per cent of reported perpetration of physical violence, but not sexual violence by non-partners since the age of 15 years. In the USA, one in six women has experienced an attempted or completed rape in their lifetime (Centers for Disease Control and Prevention 2006). Of all women surveyed, 18 per cent reported having suffered rape or attempted rape, of whom 22 per cent were younger than 12 years and 32 per cent were between 12 and 17 years when first raped (Centers for Disease Control and Prevention 2006).

Boys and men are also victims of sexual assault, but less is known about this, as few studies exist, and it tends to be an unrecognised problem. Like sexual violence against women it tends also to be underreported due in part to the shame and stigma attached to it, but men may be even more reluctant than women to report it. A population-based study conducted recently on 705 adult men in Virginia, USA, found a lifetime prevalence of 12.9 per cent among men (including child sexual abuse), with 94 per cent assaulted for the first time before the age of 18 (Masho and Anderson 2009). Similar to women, only a small percentage had sought counselling in spite of experiencing mental health problems. Men are also the most frequent perpetrators. While women may coerce young men into sex, qualitative research shows that the experience of being coerced by a woman is quite different to that of being abused by a man (Sikweyiya and Jewkes 2009). Most often it is older men who abuse other young men – whether in the context of child sexual abuse, sexual initiation or rape (Jewkes *et al.* 2002a). In conflict settings, rape of men can also form part of the tactics of war (Burnett and Peel 2001).

Violence against gay, trans- or same-sex attracted men is also much reported, and rates of intimate partner violence in same-sex relationships appear to be similar to rates in heterosexual relationships, although research on this remains limited (Shipway 2004). A study reporting on interviews with 19 gay and bisexual men identified different patterns of forced, coerced or unwanted sex: use of physical force; intoxication affecting men's ability to refuse sex; coercion or pressure by older men (Braun *et al.* 2009). The driving factors behind the abuse were more often linked to notions of masculinity, whereas some of the factors increasing vulnerability were related to the organisation of gay life and its social marginalisation in many communities (Braun *et al.* 2009). Similar to what women experience, barriers to reporting sexual assault, power dynamics in intergenerational sex and the difficulty of refusing unwanted sex, play a role. Stigma affects both women and men, with many remaining silent about their experience for years.

Sexual violence in conflict

In situations of conflict, rape and other forms of sexual violence are often widespread (MSF 2009). They have often been seen as an inevitable part of the collateral damage of war. However, this violence can be used also as a deliberate strategy to humiliate, punish, control, injure, inflict fear and destroy communities, as was seen during the 1994 genocide in Rwanda, the war in Bosnia-Herzegovina, Liberia and many other recent conflicts. While women and girls are the most likely to experience sexual violence, men and boys can also be affected, particularly during conflict. In disaster situations, refugees and internally displaced persons can also face an increased risk of violence, including being forced to exchange sex for food or other commodities. Basic survival tasks like gathering firewood and water place women and girls at particular risk. Impunity becomes an even greater issue in conflict settings where legal and judicial systems can be practically non-existent. There has been some recent progress in this respect with the United Nations Security Council (SCR) resolution 1820 which recognised rape during war as a crime against humanity and a threat to global security (United Nations Security Council Resolution 1820, 2008).

Trafficking

Human trafficking is defined in the *United Nations Protocol to Prevent, Suppress, and Punish Trafficking in Persons, especially Women and Children* as:

> [T]he recruitment, transportation, transfer, harbouring or receipt of persons, by means of the threat or use of force or other forms of coercion, of abduction, of fraud, of deception, of the abuse of power or of a position of vulnerability or of the giving or receiving of payments or benefits to achieve the consent of a person having control over another person, for the purpose of exploitation. Exploitation shall include, at a minimum, the exploitation of the prostitution of others or other forms of sexual exploitation, forced labour or services, slavery or practices similar to slavery, servitude or the removal of organs.
>
> (United Nations 2000: Article 3: 3)

Trafficking occurs in most parts of the world, across international borders and also internally within countries. Although human trafficking is recognised as a global phenomenon, there are no reliable statistics on how many people are trafficked. It is clear, however, that this is a global crime that is not abating – both because it is profitable and because it is difficult to detect. Key features of the crime include movement or confinement of an individual, accompanied by coercion and exploitation, usually for financial profit (IOM 2009). It takes many forms, including for labour exploitation, but the most frequently reported form of trafficking has been the trafficking of women and girls for sexual exploitation.

Harmful practices

Harmful traditional practices against women and children are common in many countries and are often linked to issues of sexuality. They include early and forced marriage, which in turn is associated with early pregnancy and can lead to higher mortality; widow cleansing, which mandates that a woman have sex with the brother or other male relative of her deceased husband; and female genital mutilation, among others.

Female genital mutilation (FGM) refers to all procedures involving the partial or total removal of the external female genitalia or other injury to the female genital organs for non-medical reasons (WHO, UNICEF, UNFPA 1997). Between 100 and 140 million girls and women in the world are estimated to have undergone procedures involving partial or total removal of the female external genitalia or other injury to the female genital organs for non-medical reasons, including in some countries, severe forms that involve stitching together the labia (WHO 2008). For African countries from which there are data, it has been estimated that 92.5 million girls and women above the age of 10 are living with the consequences of FGM, and, of these, 12.5 million are girls between the ages of 10 and 14 (DHS 2004). FGM of the more serious type is associated with serious maternal and neonatal health complications (WHO Study Group on Female Genital Mutilation and Obstetric Outcome 2006). Less is known about its psychosocial consequences.

Causes and consequences of sexual violence

Sexual violence has serious consequences for people's health and wellbeing, both in the short and in the long term. It can lead to unwanted pregnancy and unsafe abortion; sexually transmitted infections, including HIV; fistulae and other genital injuries; as well as pelvic inflammatory disease and sexual difficulties. It also can lead to a wide range of psychosocial and mental health consequences. These include symptoms of shock, fear and anxiety in the initial stages, followed by depression and post-traumatic stress disorder. Women who have experienced sexual violence, compared with women who have not report poorer self-rated health and increased self-harming behaviours, including alcohol and substance abuse and suicidal thoughts (Resick 1993). Women who have been raped have also been found to have more chronic pain symptoms and higher use of medical services compared to non abused controls, even years after the event (Hillel *et al.* 2000; Kernic *et al.* 2000).

Child sexual abuse has been linked to repeat victimisation (sexual assault, intimate partner violence) and to a range of negative health outcomes and behaviours that translate, among other things, into increased sexual risk taking (including early sex, use of drugs and alcohol and not using contraception) by girls during adolescence (Fleming *et al.* 1999; Stock *et al.* 1997). A national study on violence against women in the USA found that women who were raped before 18 years were twice as likely to be raped as adults, compared with those who were not raped as children or adolescents (18.3 per cent and 8.7 per cent respectively) (Tjaden and Thoennes 2000). Less is known about the impact of sexual violence on boys. However, perpetration of sexual abuse is associated with having been sexually abused as a child. A survey of sexual offenders conducted retrospectively in the UK found that 32 per cent of those with paedophilic behaviour had a history of childhood sexual abuse (Balasundaram *et al.* 2009). Mental disorder was observed in 7.69 per cent and 14.1 per cent had significant personality factors (Balasundaram *et al.* 2009). It is estimated that, across the world, child sexual abuse accounts for 7–8 per cent of disability-adjusted life years[2] in females for each of depression, alcohol abuse/dependence and drug abuse/dependence; 13 per cent for panic disorder; 33 per cent for posttraumatic stress disorder; and 11 per cent for suicide attempts (Andrews *et al.* 2004), although some of this effect may also be mediated by other victimisations including intimate partner violence.

Gender inequality and homophobia – key manifestations of underlying social inequalities embedded in a patriarchal ideology and closely linked to notions of sexuality and what constitutes 'good sexual behaviour' – often lie at the root of sexual violence. While these sexual norms may be changing among young people, in many societies, violence against women and children is still condoned socially, and in some countries even legally sanctioned as a means of 'discipline' or punishment. In some countries, murders are carried out – usually by male partners or other male family members – in the name of protecting family honour (Nasrullah *et al.* 2009). In others, girls may be married off to their rapists in order to erase the shame on the family or so-called 'passion crimes' may receive lighter punishments. Many countries still do not recognise that rape is possible within marriage, as sex is seen as part of the obligations incurred with marriage. All these forms of violence constitute violations of international human rights law, which clearly establishes the right of all individuals to be 'free from torture and degrading or humiliating treatment', to 'bodily integrity' and 'to the highest attainable standard of health' (WHO 2007).

Violence, including sexual violence, is associated with patriarchal notions of manhood, male means of asserting control and right to pleasure. Men are expected to be sexually active and even aggressive, while women are generally expected to be sexually passive, remain faithful and not initiate sexual activity. Thus rape and sexual violence may be seen as an acceptable common event, as evidenced by the low conviction rates, even where it is well recognised as a crime (Home Office 2002).

In many societies 'rape myths' abound and tend to blame the victim. Examples of this are that: only certain kinds of women get raped (or 'she was asking for it'), when women say 'no' they really mean 'yes', sex is the primary motivation for rape (rather than power and control), rape always involves physical force and leaves injury, a husband cannot rape his wife, sex workers cannot be raped (WHO 2003). These myths lead to stigma and also impact on the response that women receive when they report or disclose rape, both from society and from service providers.

The lack of empathetic and supportive responses can exacerbate some of the negative psychological consequences of rape and impact on women's willingness to access and use services, even whey they need them. A literature review commissioned by the WHO and the Sexual Violence Research Initiative (SVRI) found that stigma and victim blaming of rape survivors is widespread, including among service providers, and that these negative social reactions are associated with more psychological symptoms and poorer self-rated recovery among survivors (Wang and Rowley 2008). These perceptions are frequently also internalised by victims, and influence their own perception and understanding of their victimisation experience, as well as their coping responses. Victims may recur to avoidance, justification and substance and alcohol abuse as strategies to deal with the experience. The ability to disclose and have access to social networks may act to ameliorate some of the mental health consequences, however, many if not most victims do not disclose immediately and often do not seek medical or other care.

Implications for research and policy

Sexual violence is a widespread, and yet unrecognised, occurrence affecting primarily women and children. Men are also victims of sexual violence, particularly in conflict settings. Gay and same-sex attracted men and women can also be victims of homophobic violence. As a crime and a public health problem sexual violence is still seriously underreported and the majority of research is from high-income countries.

There is a need for further research on the extent of the problem of non-consensual sex (rape, forced and coerced sex and other forms of sexual violence), including among children and young people, as well as its consequences on people's health and wellbeing – including psychological and mental health effects – both short and long term, and on subsequent sexual behaviour. Other gaps in knowledge include a clear identification of victims' needs, and how the responses that they get from the various individuals and systems they come into contact with (health, legal, psychosocial) can help or hinder their recovery. There is a need to develop primary prevention programmes as well as responses that are appropriate to low- and middle-income countries, and to assess the impact of services, traditional healing practices and other interventions on the recovery of victims.

In spite of the growing recognition of sexual and intimate partner violence, in terms of primary prevention few interventions have been subjected to scientific evaluation and the field is still in its early stages. Furthermore, the research that does exist is primarily from high-income countries. Among those interventions found to be successful in reducing sexual and partner violence are: *IMAGE* – an intervention that combines microfinance for women with an education intervention on gender, violence and HIV – and was shown to reduce intimate partner violence by 50 per cent (Kim *et al.* 2007); and *Safe Date*, a school-based 'dating violence' prevention programmes, which has been shown to be successful in reducing both perpetration and experience of sexual violence (Foshee *et al.* 2000; Foshee *et al.* 2008). Community-based interventions to challenge gender norms and raise awareness about sexual violence and its consequences have to date not been very well evaluated. A promising one is *Stepping Stones*, a participatory training programme to improve communication and relationship skills in communities originally developed for HIV prevention but now addressing violence against women and other social problems. An evaluation of Stepping Stones in South Africa indicated that men who had participated in the programme were less likely to commit physical or sexual intimate partner violence in the two years after the programme, compared with the men in a control group (Jewkes *et al.* 2008).

In terms of responding to victims, the health system should be equipped to provide the necessary medical care and treatment needed in the acute phase following rape, including: emergency contraception and safe abortion, prophylaxis for HIV and other STIs as appropriate, full documentation of injuries and first-level psychological care. The role of a comprehensive forensic medical examination will vary depending on the situation, but is of critical importance to build an effective prosecution in court. However, victims should be provided full medical and psychosocial care whether they wish to go to court or not (WHO 2003). A multisector response, involving other systems – legal, social, welfare and education – is needed as well.

The establishment of specialised institutions such as rape crisis centres or programmes can be useful in providing immediate post-rape care, but their functioning depends on good coordination across settings, particularly health, police and judicial systems. These centres, however, are difficult to sustain and may only be available in a few urban areas, so integrating the care of victims of violence into existing health programmes is likely to be more sustainable. Supportive counselling has been shown to be effective in reducing some mental health symptoms, together with efforts to reintegrate victims into their social network. This requires providing skills and training – which is currently not available in many settings – as well as addressing provider attitudes that can revictimise or harm victims further. The same is true for the interaction with the criminal justice system where victims may often face disbelief, denial, blame and other unhelpful responses that can cause further damage.

In many countries, legal reform as well as reform of the judicial system is necessary to be able to deal appropriately with domestic violence, including marital rape, and sexual violence crimes such as honour killings. Models for both primary prevention and multisectoral responses that are effective but also affordable and sustainable in resource-poor settings are badly needed. Efforts must be made to recognise the needs of, and reach out to, men who have been sexually assaulted with information and support services. Most importantly, services need to be responsive to the victims and their needs and ensure that no further damage is inflicted.

Notes

1 Countries include Bangladesh, Brazil, Ethiopia, Japan, Namibia, Peru, Samoa, Serbia, Thailand and the United Republic of Tanzania. The study has now been replicated in Kiribati, the Maldives, New Zealand and the Solomon Islands, and the WHO questionnaire adapted and used in many other settings.
2 The disability-adjusted life year (DALY) extends the concept of potential years of life lost due to premature death to include equivalent years of 'healthy' life lost by virtue of being in states of poor health or disability. One DALY can be thought of as one lost year of 'healthy' life, and the burden of disease can be thought of as a measurement of the gap between current health status and an ideal situation where everyone lives into old age, free of disease and disability.

References

Andrews, G., Corry, J., Slade, T., Issakidis, C. and Swanston, H. (2004) 'Child Sexual Abuse', in Ezzati, M., *Comparative Quantification of Health Risks: Global and Regional Burden of Disease attributable to selected major Risk Factors*, Geneva: World Health Organisation.

Balasundaram, B., Frazer, J. B. and Wood, P. J. (2009) 'Who are Sexual Offenders? A Survey of Pre-trial Psychiatric Reports', *Medicine, Science and the Law*, 49 (1): 33–40.

Braun, V., Schmidt, J., Gavey, N. and Fenaughty, J. (2009) 'Sexual Coercion among Gay and Bisexual Men in Aotearoa/New Zealand', *Journal of Homosexuality*, 56 (3): 336–60.

Burnett, A. and Peel, M. (2001) 'Asylum Seekers and Refugees in Britain: The Health of Survivors of Torture and Organized Violence', *British Medical Journal*, 322: 606–9.

Center for Disease Control and Prevention (CDC) (2006) *Extent, Nature and Consequences of Rape Victimization: Findings from the National Violence against Women Survey*, Washington, DC: US Department of Justice, National Institute of Justice.

DHS (2004) *Female Genital Cutting in the Demographic and Health Surveys: A Critical and Comparative Analysis*, Washington, DC: MACRO International. (Comparative Reports No. 7)

Fleming, J., Mullen, P. E., Sibthorpe, B. and Bammer, G. (1999) 'The Long-term Impact of Childhood Sexual Abuse in Australian Women', *Child Abuse and Neglect*, 23: 142–59

Foshee, V. A., Bauman, K. E., Ennett, S. T., Linder, G. F., Benefield, T. and Suchindran, C. (2008) 'Assessing the Long-term Effects of the Safe Dates Program and a Booster Effect in Preventing and Reducing Adolescent Dating Violence Victimization and Perpetration', *American Journal of Public Health*, 9419–624.

Foshee, V. A., Bauman, K. E., Greene, W. F., Koch, G. G., Linder, G. F. and MacDougall, J. E. (2000) 'The Safe Dates Program: 1-year Follow-up Results', *American Journal of Public Health*, 90 (10): 1619–22.

Garcia-Moreno, C., Jansen, H. A. F. M., Ellsberg, M., Heise, L. and Watts, C. (2005) *WHO Multi-country Study on Women's Health and Domestic Violence against Women. Initial Results on Prevalence, Health Outcomes and Women's Responses*, Geneva: World Health Organisation.

Garcia-Moreno, C., Jansen, H. A. F. M., Ellsberg, M., Heise, L. and Watts, C. H. (2006) 'Prevalence of Intimate Partner Violence: Findings from the WHO Multi-country Study on Women's Health and Domestic Violence', *Lancet*, 368: 1260–69.

Glover, E. K. (2003) 'Sexual Health Experiences of Adolescents in three Ghanaian Towns', *International Family Planning Perspectives*, 29: 32–40.

Heise, L., Ellsberg, M. and Gottemuller, M. (1999) *Ending Violence against Women*, Baltimore, MD: Johns Hopkins University School of Public Health, Population Information Program.

Hillel, M. F., Stenn, P., Davies, F., Stalker, C., Fry, R. and Koumanis, J. (2000) 'Chronic Pain and Healthcare Utilization in Women with a History of Childhood Sexual Abuse', *Child Abuse and Neglect*, 24: 547–56.

Home Office (2002) *Action Plan to Implement the Recommendations of the HMCPSI/HMIC Joint Inspection into the Investigation and Prosecution of Cases involving Allegations of Rape*, London: Home Office, Court Service, CPS; available at http://police.homeoffice.gov.uk/publications/operational-policing/rape-action-plan.pdf?view=Binary (accessed 9 April 2009).

International Organization for Migration (IOM) (2009) *Caring for Trafficked Persons. Guidance for Health Providers*, Geneva: International Office of Migration.

Jewkes, R., Levin, J., Bradshwa, D. and Mbananga, N. (2002b) 'Rape of Girls in South Africa', *Lancet*, 359: 319–20.

Jewkes, R., Nduna, M., Levin, J., Jama, N., Dunkle, K., Puren, A. *et al.* (2008) 'Impact of Stepping Stones on Incidence of HIV and HSV-2 and Sexual Behaviour in Rural South Africa: Cluster Randomised Controlled Trial', *British Medical Journal*, 337: a506; available at www.bmj.com/cgi/content/abstract/337/aug07_1/a506 (accessed 9 April 2009).

Jewkes, R., Sen, P. and Garcia-Moreno, C. (2002a) 'Sexual Violence', in Kruge, E., Dahlberg, L., Mercy, J., Zwi, A. and Lozano, R. (eds) *World Report on Violence and Health*, Geneva: World Health Organisation.

Kernic, M. A., Wolf, M. E. and Holt, V. (2000) 'Rates and Relative Risk of Hospital Admission Among Women in Violent Intimate Partner Relationships', *American Journal of Public Health*, 90: 1416–20.

Kim, J., Watts, C., Hargreaves, J. R., Ndhlovu, L. X., Phetla, G., Morison, L. A. *et al.* (2007) 'Understanding the Impact of a Microfinance-based Intervention on Women's Empowerment and the Reduction of Intimate Partner Violence in South Africa', *American Journal of Public Health*, 97 (10): 1794–802.

Koenig, M. A. (2004) 'Coerced First Intercourse and Reproductive Health in Rakai, Uganda', *International Family Planning Perspectives*, 30: 156–63.

Masho, S. W. and Anderson, L. (2009) 'Sexual Assault in Men: A Population-based Study of Virginia', *Violence Victims*, 24 (1): 98–110.

Médecins sans Frontières (2009) *Shattered Lives. Immediate Medical Care Vital for Sexual Violence Victims*, Brussels: Médecins sans Frontiers.

Nasrullah, M., Haqqi, S. and Cummings, K. J. (2009) 'The Epidemiological Patterns of Honour Killing of Women in Pakistan', *European Journal of Public Health*, 19 (2): 193–7.

Phiri, A. and Erulkar, A. (2000) 'Experiences of Youth in Urban Zimbabwe', Harare: National Family Planning Council.

Resick, P. A. (1993) 'The Psychological Impact of Rape', *Journal of Interpersonal Violence*, 8: 223–55.

Shipway, L. (2004) *Domestic Violence. A Handbook for Health Professionals*, London: Routledge.

Sikweyiya, Y. and Jewkes, R. (2009) 'Force and Temptation: Contrasting South Africa Men's Accounts of Coercion into Sex by Men and Women', *Culture, Health and Sexuality*, 11: 529–41.

Stock, J. L., Bell, M. A., Boyer, D. K. and Connell, F. A. (1997) 'Adolescent Pregnancy and Sexual Risk-taking among Sexually Abused Girls', *Family Planning Perspectives*, 29: 200–3.

Tjaden, P. and Thoennes, N. (2000) 'Full Report of the prevalence, Incidence and Consequences of Violence against Women: Findings from the National Violence Against Women Survey', Washington, DC: National Institute of Justice, Office of Justice Programs, United States Department of Justice and Centers for Disease Control and Prevention.

United Nations (2000) *United Nations Protocol to Prevent, Suppress, and Punish Trafficking in persons, especially Women and Children*. New York: United Nations; available at www.uncjin.org/Documents/Conventions/dcatoc/final_documents_2/convention_%20traff_eng.pdf (accessed on 9 April, 2009).

United Nations Security Council (2008) *Secruity Council Resolution 1820. Women, peace and security. SC/Res1820 (2008)*, New York: United Nations Security Council; available at http://daccessdds.un.org/doc/UNDOC/GEN/N08/391/44/PDF/N0839144.pdf?OpenElement (accessed 9 April 2009).

Wang, S. and Rowley, E. (for the Sexual Violence Research Initiative) (2008) *Rape: How Women, the Community and the Health Sector respond*, Geneva: World Health Organisation.

WHO, UNICEF, UNFPA (1997) *Female Genital Mutilation. A Joint WHO/UNICEF/UNFPA Statement*, Geneva: World Health Organisation.

World Health Organisation (2002) *The World Health Report 2002. Reducing Risks: Promoting Healthy Life*, Geneva: World Health Organisation.

World Health Organisation (2003) *Guidelines for Medico-legal Care for Victims of Sexual Violence*, Geneva: World Health Organisation.

World Health Organisation (2007) *Women's Health and Human Rights: Monitoring the Implementation of CEDAW*, Geneva: World Health Organisation.

World Health Organisation (2008) *Eliminating Female Genital Mutilation: An Interagency Statement*, Geneva: World Health Organisation; available at www.who.int/reproductive-health/fgm/ (accessed on 9 April 2009).

World Health Organisation Study Group on Female Genital Mutilation and Obstetric Outcome (2006) 'Female Genital Mutilation and Obstetric Outcome: WHO Collaborative Prospective Study in six African Countries', *Lancet*, 367: 1835–41.

31 The social production of men's extramarital sexual practices

Jennifer S. Hirsch

For a growing number of women in rural Mexico – and around the world – marital sex represents their single greatest risk for HIV infection (UNAIDS 2004). These women are infected by the very people with whom they are supposed to be having sex – indeed, according to social convention in many countries, the *only* people with whom they are *ever* supposed to have sex. The situation challenges existing approaches to HIV prevention: abstinence is impossible, unilateral monogamy is ineffective and marital condom use is complicated by women's deep, culturally supported commitment to the fiction of fidelity.

This chapter presents the findings from one of the sites involved in a five-site comparative, ethnographic investigation funded by the National Institute of Child Health and Human Development that explored the social organisation of married women's HIV-related risk (Hirsch *et al.* 2007; Parikh 2007; Smith 2007; Wardlow 2007; Phinney 2008; Hirsch *et al.* 2010).[1] The goal was to assess how men contribute to women's risk of acquiring HIV, going beyond the focus on ideological aspects of masculinity that characterises current programmatic approaches to improving women's reproductive health by shifting norms of ideal masculinity (Pulerwitz and Barker 2008; Barker and Ricardo 2005). This work draws on Connell's idea of gender regimes as composed of the intersecting micro- and macro-level domains of labour (who does what work, both domestically and in societies), power (micro-level decision making as well as social, political and military deployment of authority) and affect (socially constructed desires and the emotions that surround those desires) (Connell 1987, 1995; Hirsch *et al.* 2010).

The aim is to extend previous work, which focused primarily on women's perspectives, to explore how social, cultural and economic factors intertwine to shape married women's risk of HIV infection. This chapter also describes the intersection of culturally constructed notions of reputation with structurally patterned sociosexual geographies. Overall, the point is that extramarital sex, although typically portrayed (in Mexico and elsewhere) as a breach of social norms, is a fundamental if tacit dimension of gendered social organisation rather than the product of individual moral failings or a breakdown in social rules. This chapter also presents the concept of *extramarital opportunity structures*,[2] which calls attention to how extramarital sex is produced and facilitated by social, cultural and economic forces (Sobo 1995; Hirsch *et al.* 2002).

Ethnographic context

The present study was conducted in Degollado, a town of approximately 15,000 residents (although the actual population ebbs and flows with the patterns of seasonal migration between Mexico and the USA) situated in the semi-rural western Mexican state of Jalisco. Degollado's main sources of income have traditionally been agriculture and migrant remittances; however, the 2000 census indicates that the balance has tipped decisively away from agriculture, with only 30 per cent of residents reporting agriculture as their main source of support, down from more than 90 per cent in 1960 (Hirsch 2003). The area's distorted age structure reflects the institutionalisation of labour migration: 2000 census data showed that there were 702 men for every 1000 women in the 20- to 29-year age group, traditionally the peak age range for labour migration. The county seat, Degollado also has two banks, a number of schools including a high school, many small grocery stores, a central market and two modern supermarkets, as well as a small private hospital, several internet cafés and a number of other local businesses.

Mexico's HIV epidemic is concentrated, with HIV prevalence rates of 0.3 per cent in the general population and up to 15 per cent among most at risk groups such as men who have sex with other men and sex workers (Instituto Nacional de Estadísticas 1960, 2006b). Of the approximately 160,000 adults with HIV at the end of 2003, two-thirds were men believed to have been infected while having sex with another man (Magis-Rodriguez *et al.* 2003); consequently, the more recent 'heterosexualisation' of the epidemic is thought to be attributable to women becoming infected during sex with male partners who have sex with men (Instituto Nacional de Estadísticas 2006a).

Rural Mexico, where gender ratios among those living with AIDS are lower than ratios in urban areas, is at the forefront of this heterosexualisation, with rural women thought to be at particularly high risk of marital transmission because of the high rates of labour migration from rural areas to the USA and the way in which migration presents a risk factor for HIV infection (Hirsch *et al.* 2002; Fátima Estrada Márquez 2006; Magis-Rodriguez *et al.* 2003; Sobo 1995; Magis-Rodriguez *et al.* 2004; Sanchez 2004). One recent report put the percentage of migrants who are infected with HIV at 1 per cent, three times higher than the percentage among the general population (Magis-Rodriguez *et al.* 2004; Sanchez 2004; Hirsch *et al.* 2002). As reported in 2004 the two states with the highest rates of migration-related HIV infection (above 20 per cent) were Michoacan and Jalisco (Martinez 2005). Degollado sits on the border between these two states. Jalisco also has the third highest number of AIDS cases of any Mexican state.

Data collection approach relied on participant observation, marital case studies, key informant interviews and archival research, with each method contributing distinctly to the triangulation that is so critical to ethnographic reliability (Sanchez 2004). Our final sample included marital case study interviews from 17 couples (with each member interviewed individually) and five additional individuals in which the spouse was either unavailable or unwilling to participate; key informant interviews with two priests, three health professionals, two lesbians, 15 adolescent girls, six feminine-appearing men who have sex with men and nine women with local reputations for 'sexual misbehaviour'; and six months of participant observation. The social ties and understanding of local culture developed through 15 months of fieldwork on an earlier project conducted in this community allowed for much more rapid start-up than would normally be the case for community-based ethnographic research (Bernard 1994).

Men's marital ideals

Previous research, conducted primarily with women, has described an increasingly widespread, companionate marital ideal in which intimacy, communication and sexual pleasure figure prominently as measures of a successful relationship. This companionate ideal frames women's commitment to the appearance of fidelity and the denial of marital risk within the broader goal of building a publicly successful relationship. However, the focus on women in this earlier work has left unanswered the questions of the extent to which men share this commitment to marital companionship and fidelity and, if they do, whether that has any influence on their extramarital sexual behaviour.

In the interviews and case studies conducted in the spring of 2004, we found that young men across social classes share with their wives a marital ideal characterised by emotional intimacy, sexual pleasure, trust and warmth, whereas men of older generations focus more on respect and fulfilment of gendered obligations. Emotional compatibility figured prominently in young men's words both as a reason to get married and as a characteristic of a successful marriage. As in the similar generational shift observed previously with women, the growing prominence of a companionate marital ideal among men does not mean that younger men love their wives more than their fathers did. Rather, the shift is more in the way that emotional intimacy, sexual pleasure and personal satisfaction have gained prominence as goals in and of themselves as opposed to being by-products of a life well lived.

Men's feelings for their wives, although not the sole determinants of their extramarital sexual behaviour, shape the cultural context of marital HIV risk in complex ways (Hirsch *et al.* 2002; Hirsch and Wardlow 2006). For some, the love they have for their wives means that they would not be able to face them if they were unfaithful; for others, it merely means greater discretion so that their extramarital activities do not infringe on the companionate intimacy they are building with their wives.[3] Ironically, this loving attention to appearances may actually increase married women's risk of HIV infection.

Cultural construction of risk: reputation and public sexual selves

One of our major findings was the importance of reputation, rather than object choice (i.e. heterosexual, homosexual), as a locally meaningful axis of sexual identity. People in Degollado almost invariably talked about their own or others' social and sexual identities by using reputational categories. Men, for example, would refer to themselves as *serio* (serious), *calmado* (calm) or similar adjectives or as *sinvergüenza* (lacking in shame) or *descarados* (faceless), and women would talk about themselves as *recogida* (under control) or *volada* (out of control) (see Hirsch 2003: 95–111). When men resist the temptations of extramarital sex, they often talk about preserving their local reputations. One of our participants reported that he had never gone beyond flirting with the attractive young secretaries in his family business:

> [O]ut of fear that someone would say 'that guy is really looking for sex'; it would drag me into a really big problem – [someone would say] 'hey, your husband is coming on to me'. More than anything, I avoid it so I don't get burned. I definitely notice other women, but *'pueblo chico, chisme grande'* [small town, big gossip].
>
> (Hirsch 2003: 100)

This concern with reputation was expressed by manual labourers as well as the business owners for whom they worked and members of the town's professional class.

Reputation is also considered a family characteristic, so that women worry when their daughters marry the sons of notorious adulterers. A woman's adultery constrains the marriageability of her children and shows profound disrespect for her husband. Men have a particularly complex task in regard to these sexual selves; men build relationships with other men by demonstrating an assertive, competent and sexually independent masculinity, but they also demonstrate their respect (and sometimes their love) for their wives through carefully maintaining the appearance of fidelity.[4] There is a type of built-in symbolic tension for men in which succeeding too well at either extreme inherently means failing at the other. This overriding concern with reputation as an axis of sexual identity is reflected in the study area's local sexual geography – which is, in turn, a key element intersecting with the cultural construction of risk intersects to shape patterns of extramarital sexual practices.

Extramarital opportunity structures

Our participant observations, key informant interviews and marital case studies all supported the fact that men quite commonly engage in extramarital sex with partners ranging from scarcely known women or men with whom they have casual sex for money to male friends and acquaintances and the wives of neighbours. We describe here how three elements of extramarital opportunity structures – gendered sexual geography, local forms of kinship and compulsory heterosexuality – facilitate men's participation in extramarital sex.

Men and women in rural Mexico preserve public face by navigating strategically through two parallel dimensions of the local sexual geography. Public, heterosocial spaces such as the central plaza and Sunday market form a sort of stage for the 'performance' of men's and women's respectability.[5] In contrast, in the semi-private spaces in which men drink together, including cantinas, pool halls, table dance bars and liquor stores, men engage in a variety of sexual behaviours, secure in the knowledge that the town's gossip networks do not extend back to their wives. Although not exclusively male, these spaces are known as places 'where women do not go' – that is, where *decent* women do not go (see Hirsch 2003: 95–102). When married men spend the evening visiting a brothel or a table dance bar, they rely on the unspoken agreement that they will cover for one another. One man, remembering how his girlfriend would meet him at a local cantina, noted, 'I would tell her to come meet me, but no one saw us, only the people in the cantina'. (There are no parallel spaces in which women can develop extramarital relationships with the full knowledge of their female friends.)

Men's patterns of movement – and therefore their access to risky spaces – differ quite sharply from women's. These gendered patterns of mobility reflect the gendered organisation of labour, which reflects, in turn, how these very concerns about sexual reputation have traditionally limited women's physical mobility. Men's greater physical mobility resulting from their jobs – manifested locally through their disproportionate access to horses, bicycles, cars and other means of transport and internationally through their participation in labour migration – simultaneously justifies their journeys out of town and gives them money for extramarital sex while they are away. This culturally meaningful gendered physical landscape, intricately intertwined with economic organisation, is one example of what we mean by extramarital opportunity structures.

The conceptual division of social space into a female *casa* (house) and a male *calle* (street) is a cultural reflection of men's historically greater access to economic opportunities; this access to disposable income (whether men spend it on commercial sex or on gifts for a girlfriend) combines with men's physical mobility to create gender differences in opportunities for extramarital sex (Thompson 2005). Interviews and everyday conversations provided countless stories of men who took advantage of this mobility to seek extramarital sex, including a man who drove a highway delivery truck for his family's business and reportedly knew every brothel along the way and a group of prominent businessmen from town who went together to Cuba on what was widely known to be a sex tour. International labour migration provides the most extreme illustration of how the gendered organisation of labour intertwines with these concerns about reputation, with men's long absences lowering the reputational risk of infidelity by ensuring that it occurs far away.[6]

Despite increasingly widespread access to conveniences such as blenders and store-bought tortillas, women face an intensely demanding regimen of chores, and live under constant surveillance that evaluates their performance as producers of clean children with well-combed hair and neatly ironed clothes. (Even the author quickly learned not to leave the house without making sure that her children's hair was combed and slicked back with gel.) The gendered division of domestic labour directs married women's attention and energy toward their children, so that the very organisation of marriage creates opportunities for a man to have one woman to raise his children and provide him with hot food and clean clothes and another (or several others) to provide pleasure and diversion. The gendered reward structure and the immediacy of children's needs clearly push women to excel as mothers rather than lovers. Although women are increasingly employed in the formal labour market after marriage – most commonly in local commerce, as schoolteachers, or (more rarely) as professionals – parenting is still the central means through which women in rural Mexico gain social advancement and prestige and secure family relationships. The frequency with which men spoke of feeling neglected by their wives, of wanting to be 'chiqueado' (coddled) by their wives, reflects tensions between the all consuming maternal career and emerging ideals of marital companionship.

The centrality of marriage as a form of domestic organisation also contributes to the pervasiveness of men's extramarital sex. Ideologically, marriage is increasingly positioned as a structure for intimacy and self-realisation; in actuality, however, many of the couples in this study had remained married despite the affective quality of their relationship rather than because of it. Many unhappy marriages endure, sustained not by love but by social convention, gendered economic opportunities and gendered patterns of social reproduction; men and women may not necessarily like one another, but they need one another.

Compulsory heterosexuality also structures men's engagement in extramarital sex. Marriage is a required step in the journey to being an adult, as well as a means through which men ensure their biological and social reproduction. In rural Mexico, marriage is a requirement and not a choice, so compulsory heterosexuality forces men who experience same-sex desires to marry and seek extramarital pleasure rather than assuming a public gay identity (Rich 1986).[7] Gendered social organisation and traditional sexual cultures in rural Mexico intertwine to produce, simultaneously, great stress on compliance with gendered norms of self-presentation along with a certain degree of flexibility with regard to sexual object choice. As Carrier, Carrillo and others have described (Carrier 1985, 1989, 1995; Carrillo 1999, 2002; González-López 2005) and as was supported by many conversations during our participant observations and interviews with key informants, traditional Mexican constructions of sexual and gender identity divide men who have sex with men into two categories: masculine-appearing *activo* (active 'normal men') or feminine-appearing *pasivo* (literally 'passive' but figuratively 'receptive' or 'insertive').

In Degollado, we became acquainted with a number of feminine-appearing men who had a great number of sexual partners locally, many of them married men, some of whom paid them, some of whom they paid and others with whom they had sex in a context of short-lived romantic affectivity. We also observed masculine-appearing men in pursuit of these feminine-appearing men or, when drunk, in pursuit of each other. This sex between men represented *socially safe sex*: a man could easily slip off to the cantina bathroom for casual sex, cruise the gay disco in neighbouring La Piedad or invite a male sex worker strolling in the plaza to take a late-night ride in his chrome-laden pickup, secure in the knowledge that this was a 'low-risk' activity (socially speaking). Neither man would fall in love (supposedly), neither could get pregnant and another man could certainly be trusted not to tell the other's wife. Both masculine- and feminine-appearing men who enjoy sex with other men almost always marry, both for 'cover' and for convenience. Social modifies the notion of risk in an important way: by using the word risk to describe practices without saying anything about what is being risked, public health practitioners and epidemiologists imply that health is the most salient form of risk to consider. Social risk reminds us that other concerns – preservation of reputation, creation of relationships – may trump health in shaping behaviour.

Social safety and physical risk

We saw in our participant observation how couples collude in maintaining appearances around men's sexual behaviour: women tell men not to be unfaithful or they tell them that if they must be unfaithful, then do it in a way that will not humiliate them; men routinely deny their infidelities, regardless of their actual behaviour, as part of being a good husband, and men seek out sex that is socially safe, rather than necessarily physically safe. Given the importance of public sexual selves, a major element shaping extramarital sex is the ease with which it can be hidden. Most of the men included in our marital case studies talked about deliberately seeking out women who did not pose a risk of emotional or economic entanglement so that there would be no leakage of this semiprivate behaviour onto the public stage of reputation. A majority of rural Mexican men who engage in extramarital sex take great care to practise 'safe sex', not in terms of using a condom but in terms of being discreet: for them, the most visible risk is a contaminated reputation rather than a viral infection.

Commercial sex is the central means through which men seek socially safe sex. Their view is that, despite the fact that commercial sex workers are people's daughters, wives and mothers, their reputation has already been ruined, and they can have sex with these women without running the risk of incurring the moral debt produced by having sex with a 'nice girl'. However, men overwhelmingly perceived STI risks as limited to women who charge for sex acts, and thus some did adopt a strategy for physically 'safe sex', limiting extramarital sex to women with whom they shared an affective tie.

The affective qualities of a marriage were one element that influenced the extent to which widely shared fears of STIs shaped actual sexual behaviour. Men who expressed affection for their wives and who shared pleasurable companionship with them were much more likely to engage in extramarital sex with a commercial sex worker than with a girlfriend, whereas men with less emotionally and physically satisfying marriages were more likely to establish a long-term affective relationship with another woman. Ironically, then, men's commitment to ideologies of modern love may increase marital HIV risk: men who love their wives protect their feelings (although perhaps not their health) by choosing commercial sex. Given the overwhelming ways in which social, cultural and economic factors intertwine to shape men's access to extramarital sex, love alone is not quite enough to ensure fidelity. It does, however, shape how men respond to these extramarital opportunity structures.

Implications for prevention

The reputational dimension of sexual identity has implications both for HIV prevention locally and for the framing of prevention programmes more broadly. Given the ways in which men are expected to manage their extra-domestic sexuality, a man who infects his wife is likely to be the subject of scorn. It might seem that a solution would be to frame HIV-prevention messages around men's responsibility to protect their wives. Public silence, however, has been a crucial strategy through which men protect their wives from the *social* risks of infidelity, and so creating effective community-based dialogues about marital HIV risk faces the formidable challenge of how to raise the issue, as it were, without breaking the silence.

Second, we must take social risk seriously, remembering that the maximisation of their individual health is not necessarily the highest priority of those whose health we seek to promote. The intersection of sexual geography and reputation means that a husband's love for his wife may increase her risk by leading him to seek out relatively higher risk partners. Love, and a shared desire to keep up appearances, shapes both partners' commitment to denying that risk. Third, this notion of sexual geography holds promise for community-based HIV prevention programmes; it is time to go beyond an individual-level emphasis on preventing risky acts and consider the utility of working in risky spaces. Using the idea of sexual geography would mean constructing – in collaboration with affected communities – contextually specific maps of risky spaces and developing spatially specific interventions to modify risks.

Fourth, the concept of externalities – a cost of the production process for which neither the consumer nor the producer pays – helps us link our own patterns of consumption, the global reliance on migrant labour and marital HIV risk. Both this chapter and others from the same comparative study (Wardlow 2007; Smith 2007; Parikh 2007; Phinney 2008) highlight labour migration as a critical element of extramarital opportunity structures; marital HIV risk is an externality of the use of migrant labour, just as surely as carbon dioxide is an externality not yet accounted for by the low cost of incandescent bulbs. The burrito served by Mexican hands in New York and adorned by lettuce, chicken and tomatoes produced by Mexican migrant labour in California and Florida increases the risk for women in rural Puebla or Michoacán. The borders that separate those who benefit from these unmeasured costs and those who bear their burden makes it challenging to conceive of how to ameliorate this situation – but consumers should at least know that their burrito comes with a side of HIV risk.

Fifth, and finally, the structural nature of men's extramarital sex makes clear the inadequacy of strategies that focus on changing individual behaviours and promoting marital fidelity. It may be possible to achieve reductions in the number or frequency of men's extramarital partnerships; however, given the complex and intertwined types of support for such behaviour, merely telling men to decrease their extramarital sexual activities is unlikely to be successful. Instead, our findings argue for taking a 'harm reduction' approach to extramarital sex. Rather than funding interventions that satisfy our own delicate moral sensibilities, we should consider structural interventions to reduce the likelihood that existing patterns of behaviour will serve as the conduits through which the HIV epidemic will continue to grow.

Notes

1 This research was supported by National Institute of Child Health and Human Development, R01 HD041724. The contributions of Sergio Meneses, Brenda Thompson, Estela Mata and Alan Lujambio to the fieldwork discussed here are also gratefully acknowledged.

2 We credit Constance Nathanson for coining this phrase.

3 Many factors other than marital affect that shape men's participation in extramarital sex. Among the couples included in the marital case studies, for example, there were some older men who expressed little warmth and intimacy toward their wives but who nonetheless denied having had extramarital sex; these men refrained from extramarital sex out of a desire to demonstrate public respectability and restraint. Don Carlos (names are pseudonyms), for example, beat his wife Doña Esperanza quite severely in the early years of their marriage – at one point, she recounted that he might have killed her had her brother not intervened – but he also vigorously asserted that to have been unfaithful would have been to be no better than an animal.

4 This same emphasis on the importance of sexual reputation, rather than behaviour, is also seen in terms of public perceptions of adolescent sexual behaviour.

5 The comment 'small town, big gossip' refers to a telenovela, *Pueblo Chico, Infierno Grande* (small town, big hell), that focused on the scandals and suffering simmering just below the surface in small-town Mexico.

6 International labour migration poses challenges to fidelity even for those who remain behind; that is, the distorted population structure creates an intense local competition for men, leading to many marriages of desperation among young women in their late twenties and creating a semi-permanent pool of available young women, some of whom are all too willing to flirt with a married man in the hopes of stealing another woman's husband (such women are typically referred to as 'leftover women'). These marriages of desperation can be in and of themselves reasons that men end up seeking out extramarital sex: they are not always founded on deep emotional intimacy, but men can find this intimacy elsewhere through extramarital relationships.

7 Residents of large urban centres such as Mexico City and Guadalajara can join growing communities of gay-identified men (and women), but these identities and communities barely exist at the local level. In fact, the level of discrimination against men who are perceived to be homosexual in rural areas and provincial cities has been recognised and is being addressed through a national HIV-prevention programme that frames gay rights as a critical element of effective HIV prevention. More information on the Mexican programme on HIV and Human Rights, including the media spots used in the campaign, is available on HIV-related page of the website of the Mexican Commission on Human Rights, www. cndh.org.mx/progate/vihsida/vihsid2.htm (accessed 12 March 2007).

References

'La Preferencia por Frutas y Hortalizas de USA y Chile en México esta Afectando a los Productores Mexicanos', *Mural*, B: 5 (14 June 2004).

'El Frijol Procedente de EU y Canada Inunda el Mercado Mexicano, a Pesar de que aún no se Autorizan Cupos de Importación', *Mural*, B: 6 (15 March 2004).

'Impactan Reglas de EU a Productos Nacionales: Hubo un Incremento de Importaciones de Maíz, Trigo, Frijoles, y Carne de Cerdo y Ave', *Mural*, 7: A (10 May 2004).

Barker, G. and Ricardo, C. (2005) 'Young Men and the Construction of Masculinity in Sub-Saharan Africa: Implications for HIV/AIDS, Conflict, and Violence', in Bank, T. W. (ed.) *Social Development Papers, Conflict Prevention and Reconstruction*, Washington, DC: World Bank.

Bernard, H. R. (1994) *Research Methods in Anthropology: Qualitative and Quantitative Approaches*, Thousand Oaks, CA: Sage.

Carrier, J. M. (1985) 'Mexican Male Bisexuality', in *Bisexualities: Theory and Research*, New York: Haworth Press.

Carrier, J. M. (1989) 'Sexual Behavior and Spread of AIDS in Mexico', *Medical Anthropology*, 10: 129–42.

Carrier, J. M. (1995) *De Los Otros: Intimacy and Homosexuality among Mexican Men*, New York: Columbia University Press.

Carrillo, H. C. (1999) 'Cultural Change, Hybridity, and Male Homosexuality in Mexico', *Culture, Health, & Sexuality*, 1: 223–38.

Carrillo, H. C. (2002) *The Night is Young: Sexuality in Mexico in the Time of AIDS*, Chicago: University of Chicago Press.

Connell, R. W. (1987) *Gender and Power: Society, the Person, and Sexual Politics*, Stanford: Stanford University Press.

Connell, R. W. (1995) *Masculinities*, Berkeley: University of California Press.

Fátima Estrada Márquez, C. M. R. and Bravo Garcia, E. (2006) 'Estigma y Discriminación en Hombres que Tienen Sexo con Hombres', in Carlos Magis Rodríguez, H. B. B. and Bertozzi Kenefick, S. M. (eds) *Sida: Aspectos de Salud Pública*, Mexico City: INSP and Censida.

González-López, G. (2005) *Erotic Journeys: Mexican Immigrants and Their Sex Lives*, Berkeley: University of California Press.

Hirsch, J. S. (2003) *A Courtship after Marriage: Sexuality and Love in Mexican Transnational Families*, Berkeley: University of California Press.

Hirsch, J. S. and Wardlow, H. (eds) (2006) *Modern Loves: The Anthropology of Romantic Love and Companionate Marriage*, Ann Arbor: University of Michigan Press.

Hirsch, J. S., Higgins, J., Bentley, M. E. and Nathanson, C. A. (2002) 'The Social Constructions of Sexuality: Marital Infidelity and Sexually Transmitted Disease – HIV Risk in a Mexican Migrant Community', *American Journal of Public Health*, 92: 1227–37.

Hirsch, J. S., Meneses, S., Thompson, B., Negroni, M., Pelcastre, B. and Del Rio, C. (2007) 'The Inevitability of Infidelity: Sexual Reputation, Social Geographies, and Marital HIV Risk in Rural Mexico', *American Journal of Public Health*, 97: 986–96.

Hirsch, J. S., Smith, D. J., Wardlow, H., Parikh, S., Phinney, H. and Nathanson, C. A. (2010) *The Secret: Love, Marriage, and HIV*, Nashville, TN: Vanderbilt University Press.

Instituto Nacional De Estadísticas (1960) *VII Censo General de Población, 1960, Estado de Michoacan 1*, Mexico City: Instituto Nacional De Estadísticas.

Instituto Nacional De Estadísticas (2006a) *Total Population by Country, Sex and Five Year Age Group*, Mexico City: Instituto Nacional De Estadísticas; available at www.inegi.org.mx/est/contenidos/espanol/rutinas/ept.asp?t=mpob02&c=3179 (accessed 13 February 2006).

Instituto Nacional De Estadísticas (2006b) *Working Population by Country, Sex and Primary Occupation*, Mexico City: Instituto Nacional De Estadísticas; available at http://dgcnesyp.inegi.org.mx/cgi-win/bdiecoy.exe/603?c=13032 (accessed 13 February 2006).

Magis-Rodriguez, C., Bravo-Garcia, E. and Uribe-Zuniga, P. (2003) *Dos decadas de la epidemia del SIDA en Mexico*, Mexico City: Central Nacional de la Prevencion y Control del SIDA.

Magis-Rodriguez, C., Gayet, C., Negroni, M., Leyva, R., Bravo-Garcia, E., Uribe, P. *et al.* (2004) 'Migration and AIDS in Mexico – An Overview based on Recent Evidence', *Journal of Acquired Immune Deficiency Syndromes*, 37: S215–S226.

Martinez, A. (2005) 'Tienen VIH 1 por Ciento de Migrantes: Censida', *La Jornada*.

Parikh, S. (2007) 'The Political Economy of Marriage and HIV: The ABC Approach, "Safe Infidelity", and Managing Moral Risk in Uganda', *American Journal of Public Health*, 97: 1198–208.

Phinney, H. M. (2008) ' "Rice is Essential but Tiresome; You Should get Some Moodles": Doi Moi and the Political Economy of Men's Extramarital Sexual Relations and Marital HIV Risk in Hanoi, Vietnam', *American Journal of Public Health*, 98: 650–60.

Pulerwitz, J. and Barker, G. (2008) 'Measuring Attitudes toward Gender Norms among Young Men in Brazil: Development and Psychometric Evaluation of the GEM Scale', *Men and Masculinities*, 10 (3): 322–8.

Rich, A. (1986) *Compulsory Heterosexuality and Lesbian Existence. In Blood, Bread, and Poetry: Selected Prose 1979–1985*, New York: Norton.

Sanchez, M. A. (2004) 'The Epidemiology of HIV Among Mexican Migrants and Recent Immigrants in California and Mexico', *Journal of Acquired Immune Deficiency Syndromes*, 4: S204–S214.

Smith, D. J. (2007) 'Modern Marriage, Extramarital Sex, and HIV Risk in Southeastern Nigeria', *American Journal of Public Health*, 97: 997–1005.

Sobo, E. J. (1995) *Choosing Unsafe Sex: AIDS-risk Denial among Disadvantaged Women*, Philadelphia: University of Pennsylvania Press.

Thompson, B. (2005) *Protecting your Image: An Ethnographic Look at Courtship and Sexuality from the Perspective of Muchachas in a Mexican Migrant-sending Town*, Atlanta, GA: Emory University, Rollins School of Public Health.

UNAIDS (2004) *Women and HIV/AIDS: Confronting the Crisis*, New York: Joint United Nations Programme on HIV/AIDS, United Nations Population Fund, and United Nations Development Fund for Women.

Wardlow, H. (2007) 'Men's Extramarital Sexuality in Rural Papua New Guinea', *American Journal of Public Health*, 97: 1006–14.

32 Innocence and scandal

Sexuality and the mass media

Lenore Manderson

Contemporary social science understands the body as both biological and social, with each facet shaping and shaped by the other. How these properties or sets of properties interact and interrelate, changing the character of each, continues to be elaborated. Bodily actions carry social and cultural meanings at individual and societal levels, with stigma and other marginalising techniques operating to monitor and constrain actions that are seen to challenge the body politic. Sexuality is especially subject to surveillance, formally through institutions and the laws that govern them, and informally via norms and values. Such norms and values are reiterated through public discourse, and the media plays a particular role in this regard.

The mass media, their technologies and multiple functions, contribute to co-constructions of physical and social bodies, to relations between political bodies, and to values attached to individual bodies, gender and sexuality. Ideas of gender and sexuality are 'mediated' by both the old (conventional) and 'new' media. While the media today still includes newspapers, journals and other print media and radio and television broadcasting, there is greater interactivity and greater opportunities for the expression of diverse opinion: via talk-back and call-in programmes, through the mobile phone and the transmission of text (SMS) and multimedia messages (MMS), and via internet chat rooms, discussion boards, blogs, list serves and social networking sites.

Over the past quarter of a century, bodies have been differentiated theoretically in terms of time, space and function, and in relation to reproduction, regulation, discipline and desire. There are medical bodies and global bodies, social bodies, the political body and bodies (that is, population groups), of consumers, for instance, voters and workers. The media span the interests of all of these dimensions. The interest in individual bodies and their uses – in crime, sport, sex and science – is what sells papers and cranks up ratings. Understanding of how individuals and societies are constructed, and how physical, social and political bodies are characterised and used, helps us unpack sex in the mass media in relation to individual bodies whose activities are monitored and reported 'in the public interest'.

Sex scandals of men in high office

Sex scandals in the mass media are often analysed for the moral lessons they impart, with emphasis given to the listening and/or reading public of the importance of sustaining normative sexuality and other behaviours. But arguably not all sex scandals have moral lessons, and even if they do, sex scandals differ in content, form and direction according to the gender, age and status of the individual, of the presumed audience and the cultural context in which events take place.

In comparing the encounters of three men with prostitutes – televangelist Jimmy Swaggart, actor Hugh Grant and presidential advisor Dick Morris – Gamson (2001) illustrates how each 'story' produces a different moral lesson as a consequence of the office of the man involved. So Swaggart is revealed, through the inconsistency of his preaching and personal action, to be a hypocrite; Grant – consistent with his cultivated public persona and typecast characters – emerges simply as reckless; Morris – because he is a politician – is shown to be amoral and disloyal. The institutional context, and the moral constructs that inform them, shape the telling of the scandal and the lesson to be learnt.

Because of their public access to wealth, and their exercise of power and privilege over other humans and other resources, senior politicians (including heads of state) surrender much privacy and control over their bodies. They are always under surveillance in open state systems because the rest of us are subject to them (they make and/or exercise the laws) and at the same time, we support them electorally and/or fiscally. Out of office, they reclaim privacy and so their individual bodies and their uses. Salacity sells only when there are political reasons for and advantages in gossip and scandal. Recent media scandals provide examples of this.

Sexual scandals are not new, of course. Many scandals of the past 50 years or so have still to sediment as mere footnotes of twentieth-century history, not because of the details of the sex, but because they provided leverage for political action and sometimes constitutional crisis. Before The Second World War, the most obvious UK example is the abdication of King Edward VII to marry twice-divorced American Wallis Simpson. The UK also provides the best example of sex scandal from the Cold War, when tensions between 'the west' and the Soviet Union were at a height. In this case, the Secretary of State for War, John Profumo, had a brief affair with showgirl Christine Keeler. She had also, it transpired, had an affair with a senior naval attaché at the Soviet Embassy, and while the tabloid press made much of the sex and her personal style, the central issues were lies, state secrets and political vulnerability. US President Bill Clinton's famous statements that he did not have 'sexual relations' with Monica Lewinsky, at a White House Press Conference and in his deposition in Paula Jones' civil lawsuit against him (for sexual harassment), echoed earlier reactions by politicians when exposed for impropriety by the media. Although the tawdry details of the Clinton–Lewinsky affair are still part of public memory as well as wiki commentary and archived court files, in the end the media reports faded out. There were many reasons for this, not necessarily because of the actions themselves, but because of general embarrassment of the mundane details, and the fact that, in describing such acts, the corporeal and sexualised body of the man dominated and so undermined the office. More recent examples of scandal do not simply reiterate the ways in which sex is used to destabilise political power. Rather, they test the boundaries of social justice, sexism and heterosexism. To illustrate this, in this chapter I discuss two cases, both from the global south – namely those of Anwar Ibrahim in Malaysia and Jacob Zuma in South Africa. In both cases, sex is the entry point to questions of power and its misuse.

Anwar Ibrahim and the sodomy accusations

From 1968 to 1971, and in the early 1980s, Anwar Ibrahim had been involved in student politics and Islamic student activism, and as a result, under the provisions of the Internal Security Act, spent 20 months under detention without trial. His strong pro-Malay stances were, however, in harmony with those of Mahathir Mohamad, who became Prime Minister in 1981. In 1991 Anwar was appointed Minister of Finance, and in 1993, when he won the position of deputy president of UMNO (United Malays National Organisation), he became Deputy Prime Minister.

Anwar's relationship with Mahathir soured in the mid-1990s, however, when he criticised his colleagues of nepotism, and curdled in 1997 when, as acting Prime Minister, he took steps to implement fiscal policy that countered Mahathir's economic philosophy and policies. In September 1998, after his continued reported public criticism of Mahathir, and allegations of corruption and mismanagement of government, Anwar was fired from Cabinet. The next day he was expelled from UMNO, reportedly because he was being investigated for sodomy and corruption in relation to the arrest of Khalid Jafri. Khalid was the author of *50 Dalil Kenapa Anwar Tidak Boleh Jadi PM* (50 Reasons why Anwar cannot become PM), in which the first allegations in print appeared – that Anwar was 'homosexual and a serial sodomite'. Anwar was tried, condemned and sentenced to six years in prison for corruption in 1999. A year later, he was sentenced to a further nine years for non-consensual homosexual acts. In 2004 the Federal Court reversed the conviction of sodomy, and he was released. In July 2008 he was again arrested over allegations of sodomy. A month later, as leader of the Malaysian opposition, he was re-elected to his old Parliamentary seat, one held by his wife while he was in prison.

In this case as with Clinton and Profumo, among others, the media played a major role. With Profumo, the tabloid press and the then new medium of television sustained reportage. The Clinton story first appeared on the internet, then travelled to a television talk show and then to print media, with debates then played out in the new media. television chat shows, call-in radio, internet columnists and tabloid journalism, Owen (2000) argues, that mirrored soap opera in style and presentation as the scandalous details unfolded, but by virtue of their framing as soap opera or sensationalist tabloid journalism, the office of the president, in the end, remained protected.

In the UK and US sex scandals, the men involved were unsettled politically by lying, not by sex. In Malaysia, it was the sex that mattered, and by association, Anwar's degeneracy, apostasy and political unworthiness. Under Section 377B of the Malaysian Penal Code, even if consensual, sodomy is punishable by whipping and up to 20 years' imprisonment; while this is artefact of colonial law, it is consistent with conservative Islamic precepts. Hence, for legal reasons, there was no space to challenge the fundamentals of the accusation (that homosexuality was criminal). Opposition in private circles, in the streets and on internet, too, focused on political and criminal issues, and while picking up on evidence fixing, evaded questions of sexuality (Nair 2007).

The charges of sodomy, and the evidence presented by the prosecution, pandered to prurient interest and captured front page headlines as in other sex scandals. Among those arrested in Anwar's case under suspicion of engaging in 'unnatural sex' with him were his former speechwriter, his adoptive brother, two of his secretaries and his wife's chauffeur (echoing homosexuality) the transgressions of inequality that also characterised Clinton's various (alleged) liaisons (among other political sex scandals).

And as with Clinton, there was bodily evidence. In Anwar's trial, a mattress, purportedly stained with and identified positively by DNA tests as Anwar's semen, was brought in and out of court more than 20 times. The defence team maintained that while unconscious, Anwar was stimulated anally to ejaculate, evidence of sexual abuse by the police to obtain false (and inaccurately recent) forensic evidence. While the case was being heard, and so *sub judicae*, Prime Minister Mahathir made a number of statements to the press insisting on Anwar's guilt of sodomy and homosexuality. The saga has continued, with new accusations, arguments about a new trial, forced evidence, reports of tampering with evidence, murder and corruption, and more salacious detail, including whether or not Anwar's 'private parts' and circumcision scar were measured at the time of his arrest.

In all this sex and scandal, and protestations of innocence and evidence fixing, there was, as noted, little opportunity to contest the illegality of sodomy. The debate about the law against sodomy therefore was largely on internet list serves and blogs. This provided anonymity and space for those who instead of refuting accusations of Anwar's homosexuality, wanted to take advantage of the moment and advocate decriminalisation. But even in this safer space, debate about the law was muted. Anwar's defence relied on denial of homosexual affinity or acts, and at no time were Muslim laws related to same sex questioned. Others who might find this pertinent knew too that to 'out' Anwar was to feed into the hands of the government. The risk was that media exposure would increase the vulnerability of sexual minorities and increase the risk of police surveillance and harassment.

Although the accusations of sodomy broke in the old (conventional) media, Anwar's example highlights the importance of new media – the use of internet to discuss questions that cannot be aired in a highly charged political forum. Like Anwar's, Jacob Zuma's case, which follows, is about corruption and sexual scandal. The example here highlights the way in which critical commentary was played out, with Zuma emerging as the winner at least in the short term.

Jacob Zuma and the rape of justice

Jacob Gedlehihlekisa Zuma is President of the African National Congress (ANC), the governing political party, which was re-elected on 22 April 2009. Zuma, a polygamist with a very public history of sexual relationships, is now the President of South Africa. On 2 November 2005 he was accused of rape by a relatively young family friend, known by Zuma to be HIV positive. The case opened in the Johannesburg High Court on 6 December, at which his defence team maintained that consensual sex had taken place and that his accuser had a history of false rape claims. Zuma, formerly head of South Africa's National AIDS Council, in response to questions about unprotected sex, maintained that he had taken a shower after sex because this 'would minimise the risk of contracting the disease [HIV]'. The political cartoonist Zapiro (Jonathan Shapiro) lampooned this statement, and depicted Zuma with a shower rose on his head; he and other cartoonists still use this image. Others within civil society were less amused, arguing that Zuma had undermined years of

HIV-prevention education in a country battling with continued high transmission of HIV and significant resistance to preventive action.

Zuma's defence, his use of the woman's past history and his views on HIV were repeatedly discussed in both the conventional and new media. Commentaries via SMS (read out on radio and TV talk-back and magazine programmes), for example, online letters to the editor and independent blog sites and discussion boards maintained on internet by the print media, provided venues for people to express their frustration about the case, protest against the victimisation of the woman and express frustration regarding Zuma's apparent poor knowledge of HIV prevention (Robins 2008).

The rape trial concluded after six months in favour of Zuma, but debate about his suitability as president continued. Then in June 2006 Zuma was dismissed as Deputy President of South Africa, not in relation to the rape charges, but for alleged corruption in an arms deal in 1999. The trial was to be held in Durban in July 2006, and the media, including editorials and guest op-ed pieces, as well as letters to the editor, SMS messages to radio and TV programmes and so on, now dwelt on this to question Zuma's suitability as next president. But, despite media characterisations of Zuma as a buffoon and/or a thug and accusations of corruption, Zuma retained the support of the ANC Youth League and Communist Party Youth League, and remained (as he does at time of writing) head of the ANC.

The corruption trial resumed in Durban in September 2008. There were simmering concerns – as in Malaysia with Anwar – of cronyism and corruption to ensure that the judgement was in his favour, since if convicted, Zuma would not be able to stand for presidential election, which he could be expected to win. But the controversy that exploded related not to the case, but to Zapiro's continued cartoon editorials. The trigger was a cartoon by Zapiro, published in the *Mail & Guardian* on 7 September 2008 and reprinted in the *Sunday Times*, of Zuma, shower rose on his head, unzipping and preparing to rape a woman ('Justice') as she is held down by four of Zuma's 'cronies' – leaders of the ANC, the South African Communist Party (SACP), the ANC Youth League and the Congress of South African Trade Unions (COSATU). While debates about corruption and the constitutional implications of a guilty verdict continued, in the short term the debate focused on the cartoon. Zuma was unhappy; various spokespeople of the organisations implicated in the cartoon described it as racist, disgusting, in extremely bad taste and a direct attack on the ANC, alliance membership and leadership. A further cartoon on 12 September in the *Mail & Guardian* helped sustain the debate: in this, Zuma is shown to reassure the supine woman: 'I just want to say how much we respect you'. The *Sunday Times* and Shapiro, unapologetic in face of further outrage, maintained that interpreting the cartoon as depicting Zuma as a rapist was shallow, and that it was designed to highlight the potential frightening risk to democracy by supporting Zuma. In one op-ed piece in the *Mail & Guardian*, this reading was extended; Charlene Smith (2008) argued that Zapiro's characterisation of Zuma raping the justice system was an apt one given his record of convictions and appeals. So the original cartoon, and those that followed, were not about sex and its violent misuse. But of course, they were. Zuma – posture, gesture, text and shower rose – all reminded readers not of metaphoric rape, but of a real rape case in a country with perhaps the highest rate of sexual violence in the world and one of the highest HIV infection rates. Shapiro justified the depiction of the rape of Justice as a centuries' old allegoric tradition, and remarked that '(t)he fact that Jacob Zuma has this personal history is his problem' (Zapiro 2008). But online blogs, letters to the editor, TV and radio commentary – always alive and vociferous in South Africa – dealt as much with Zuma's sexuality and abuse of personal power, as with corruption, court procedures and his appropriateness to be president.

In the process, the debate elicited comments about and alluded to African sexual prowess, male heteronormativity and Zulu identity. It suggested too parallels elsewhere of the seductiveness of power, as debated in the context of Clinton and Lewinsky (a young White House intern), to various other sex scandals in the USA, and indeed, regarding Anwar (via accusations from his aide and other subordinate staff).

Whose strategies?

These examples of politics, sex and power, and allegories of domestic and civil decay, were scandals because of how they were played out – the nature of the reportage, the precipitation of action and the direction of opinion in editorials and related commentaries. Whether the sex acts of senior politicians, in the main examples, were illegal, foolish, embarrassing or imprudent, the differences in reporting and commentary were the result of a mix of historic moment, cultural setting and technologies of the time. Political actions necessarily use and are confined by available technology, and so there has been extraordinary change with the rapid spread of new media (Pertierra *et al.* 2002). I have illustrated how the media are used to present instances of alleged impropriety to draw attention to underlying political problems. Many of these improprieties suggest poor judgement or bad luck, rather than serious misdemeanour (rape is the exception here). The primary aim of the journalist or commentator, in most cases, would appear to be embarrassment; the lying that follows perhaps demonstrates the success of this strategy.

But as noted, stories of sex and scandal need always to be contextualised. The scandals relating to Anwar and Zuma, for instance, occurred when there was considerable uneasiness in both states regarding the integrity of the regime, succession of leadership and confidence in government. Debates about leadership capacity were framed by alleged moral transgression and duplicity or sexual violence, greed and stupidity. But how the debates are handled in the press and broadcast media give some insight into the political economy of the media and its role in opinion making.

While the new media have allowed considerable democratisation, ownership of the printing and broadcast media is still concentrated. Journalists and their editors making the everyday decisions about stories, but their reportage is shaped by the media owners, whose interests are commercial first, then in relation to government since the former depends on the stability of the latter. Questions that affect civil society and individuals, including sexual rights and protection, are of little interest. In order to achieve their own goals, the key players (men such as Rupert Murdoch) exercise considerable authority in shaping news presentation, instituting sensationalist news formulas as appropriate (Arsenault and Castells 2008) and running editorial lines that ensure outcomes that protect rather than challenge social order.

But these scandals are never frequent enough and extreme enough to continue to sell subscriptions and advertising space. Other scandals appear with far great regularity and perhaps are a better litmus test of public anxieties and their variation across time and space. In mainland southeast Asia at time of writing, for instance, the 'ordinary' sex scandals are stories of rescue and recovery – trucks of women and children intercepted at national borders, brothel raids of illegal immigrants held in sexual slavery and so on. These stories highlight some of the real risks of poor and vulnerable people, while drawing public attention to the boundaries of acceptable behaviour, sexual and commercial. While stories of lack of agency, poverty, marginalisation and risk, they provide arguments that would strengthen state intervention and control but not necessarily protect individuals.

In the UK and Europe, with local variation, the sex scandals of ordinary folks are superficially about unimaginable breakdowns in the social order – extended incest, imprisonment, torture and sadism, often by kin (as famously in the case of Josef Fritzl). Here again, there is a conservative warning, related to the importance of surveillance, the risk posed to society at large and to individuals of liberalism, loosened surveillance and, perhaps, of urbanism and mass society. These accounts of degradation at a household and familial level support the more conservative interpretations of social capital. State surveillance of immigrant families suspected of have the potential to abuse their children for assumed cultural reasons – taking young girls to country of origin for genital cutting, for instance – are reinforced by occasional media accounts that are sufficiently salacious and shocking to legitimise further state action.

Media access as power

I remarked earlier that, to a degree, the soft peddling of accusations of rape against Zuma reflected heteronormativity. Women – including the woman at the centre of the case – are represented as temptresses, with continued tolerance among men of possible ambiguities in gender interactions, sexualised or not. This is consistent with other media representations related to women, although there is diversity in the kinds of scandal, sexism and intrusion and comment on women's private lives, in different cultural settings (Toffoletti 2007). In Australia, for instance, there has been no negative public reaction to lesbians in public office, and no scandals about them. Instead, the print media, including weekend magazines and women's monthly magazines, have featured these women and their partners, very much like high-profile heterosexual couples, in their domestic environments.

The scandals too, as illustrated, suggest considerable shifts in values and response. We have scandal without innocence (Edward VII), with asserted and contested innocence (Profumo and Clinton), with the manipulation of evidence to disprove asserted innocence (Anwar), scandal and its dismissal (Zuma) and the muddying of the territory of sex and power at both textual and subtextual levels where the human body and the body of office are one and the same.

Concurrently, the media provides contexts and spaces for civil engagement and enabling debate. Where apparent public value systems are not enforced through law – as in most cases – the debates appear to work in favour of liberalism. People's understanding of the issues in the Clinton/Lewinsky affair shifted as they reflected on their own vulnerability. To some extent the uneasiness relating to moral judgement has shaped the responses to all such cases – including the silences around the sex at the heart of Anwar's trial.

Internet sites have sustained people's ability to communicate and criticise, arguably enhancing their engagement in civil society and providing growing space for marginal communities beyond the surveillance of the state and conservative civil forces. While some new media (YouTube, for instance, or cam-chat rooms) can be interpreted as a means of empowerment and self-promotion for individuals, groups have particularly taken advantage of digital technology and electronic media to establish virtual communities to sustain dialogue while largely avoiding public surveillance and scandal. The media offer a vehicle of resistance, providing diverse groups of people with new anonymous ways to engage in civil society and political acts.

The debates around sex and sexuality that emerge through the media highlight also the inequalities that prevail – in relation to sexual minorities, certainly, and in relation to gender and sexual violence. The new media may work as infotainment (and sometimes only entertainment), but even so, they allow multiple voices in various registers. This in turn has the potential for community building, as occurs through various websites for sexual minorities. It enables advocacy and political protest, as illustrated by the 2009 example in India when a website was established to campaign against violence against women and to support women's access to public space.[1] The media can victimise and humiliate, but it can also work to reduce stigma, protect individual safety and support dignity and citizenship.

Note

1 I refer here to the web-based Pink Chaddi Campaign, which was launched in Bangalore, India, in February 2009, after women were physically assaulted by a conservative group of older men for drinking in a bar. The assault, and continued organised violence against women, was orchestrated on the pretext of protecting the Indian way of life, cultural identity and female chastity. *Chaddi* is the Hindi word for women's undergarments.

References

Arsenault, A. and Castells, M. (2008) 'Switching Power: Rupert Murdoch and the Global Business of Media Politics: A Sociological Analysis', *International Sociology*, 23 (4): 488–513.

Gamson, J. (2001) 'Normal Sins: Sex Scandal Narrative as Institutional Morality Tales', *Social Problems*, 48 (2): 185–205.

Nair, S. (2007) 'The Limits of Protest and Prospects for Political Reform in Malaysia', *Critical Asian Studies*, 39 (3): 339–68.

Owen, D. (2000) 'Popular Politics and the Clinton/Lewinsky Affair: The Implications for Leadership', *Political Psychology*, 21 (1): 161–77.

Pertierra, R., Ugarte, E., Pingol, A., Hernandez, J. and Dacanay, N. (2002) *Texting Selves: Cellphones and Philippine Modernity*, Metro Manila: De La Salle University Press.

Robins, S. (2008) 'Sexual Politics and the Zuma Rape Trial', *Journal of Southern African Studies*, 34 (2): 411–27.

Smith, C. (2008) 'Zapiro is on the Spot with his Zuma cartoon, thought Leader', *Mail & Guardian Online*, 11 September; available at www.thoughtleader.co.za/charlene-smith/2008/09/11/zapiro-is-on-the-spot-with-his-zuma-cartoon (accessed 20 March 2009).

Toffoletti, K. (2007) 'How is Gender-based Violence covered in the Sporting News? An Account of the Australian Football League Sex Scandal', *Womens Studies International Forum*, 30 (5): 427–38.

Zapiro (Jonathan Shapiro) (2008) 'Zapiro defends Zuma Cartoon', Creamer Media, 9 September; available at www.polity.org.za/article/zapiro-defends-zuma-cartoon-2008-09-09 (accessed 20 March 2009).

33 Engaged research on incest in Mexico

Gloria González-López

By the time my first book was published in 2005, I had been conducting qualitative sexuality research with Mexican immigrant women and men for about eight years. During the formal review process in my third year as an Assistant Professor of Sociology, I revisited this work and the other publications that had resulted from the rich in-depth interviews conducted with many generous informants in the late 1990s. As part of the review process, my academic mentors were urging me to generate a proposal for my second major research project. Considering the question of my next project became a process of unexpected reflection and self-inquiry. In reviewing my previous work and thinking about what I would like to explore next as a feminist sociologist with a special interest in conducting sexuality research with populations of Mexican origin, I was reminded of my unfulfilled desire to create bridges between my professional career, my personal growth and my spiritual life. I kept wondering how these bridges are created. Where and how do I begin?

Activist scholarship wherein researchers explore ways of becoming engaged with the communities they are studying has always been an inspiration for me. I had been exposed to several significant models of this approach through my own mentors and in the feminist sociological literature (e.g. Hondagneu-Sotelo 1993), but tensions regarding whether I had a future in academic life and, later, concerns about what kind of work counts in the tenure process prevented me from successfully incorporating a community-based paradigm into my initial sexuality research with Mexican immigrant populations. Despite my hesitations in this first project, my aspiration was to conduct sexuality research that was more deeply engaged with and beneficial to the informants and communities represented in my projects. I also suspected that this engagement would not only benefit the individuals and communities I was studying, but that it might help me become more whole as a human being. In this chapter, I describe how concepts such as 'activist research' and 'spiritual activism' have given me both the inspiration and the tools to practise these professional and personal goals in my most recent sexuality research.

Activist research and going back home

According to Francesca M. Cancian, activist research refers to a 'research that is "for" relatively powerless groups, and it often involves close social ties and cooperation with these groups' (1993: 92; cf. Naples 2003). For AnaLouise Keating, spiritual activism is a process that 'begins with the personal yet moves outward acknowledging our radical interconnectedness. This spirituality for social change, spirituality that recognises the many differences among us yet insists on our commonalities as catalysts for transformation' (2002: 18). In my own professional development, a driving question has been *how* to successfully incorporate these inspirational paradigms into my research. After surviving the tenure process – which required writing and publishing 'for' colleagues – I experienced more freedom in thinking about ways to do research that could be beneficial to both academic circles and the communities represented in my work. I now feel deeply privileged by my academic institutional status and location, but my recognition of this privilege has prompted me to think even more about ways to generate knowledge that extends beyond these academic expectations to the communities in which I conduct my research. Revisiting the research experience that led to my first book reminded me of many unanswered questions and concerns; issues that I had not been able to address at that stage of my professional development. This awareness of paths not taken enhanced my clarity and motivation to chart this terrain in my subsequent intellectual journey.

In my first study, I was deeply touched by my informants' stories of sexual experiences within the context of family life, especially those that involved coercion and related expressions of violence. Moved by these narratives, I initially considered doing research on incest with Mexican immigrants. However, I did some preliminary research and noticed immediately the invisibility of sociological research on incest in Mexico. This information corresponded with my desire to become a more engaged researcher and led me to consider how a second project might emerge more directly from the actual communities affected by the experiences of sexualised pain. Inspired by feminist models of activist scholarship and spiritual activism, I went back to Mexico – the country in which I was born, raised and educated – for the first extended period since migrating to the USA in 1986. There, I approached activists and mental health professionals advocating for women's rights in Ciudad Juárez and asked them what they considered to be 'urgent' and highly needed areas of research in the field of sexuality studies. My relationship with some of these professionals had been established five years earlier when I had become a sort of long-distance volunteer who visited Ciudad Juárez periodically to offer my sociological and clinical expertise through workshops on gender inequality and sexual violence at two community-based organisations in the city.

When I returned to Ciudad Juárez and asked these activists and clinicians to help me identify pressing research issues in sexuality studies, they confirmed my own instincts: research on incest with Mexican populations was both much needed and a way to be of help to those working so diligently and for so long in the community-based trenches. In these conversations, I learned that while sexual violence against women of all ages had reached perversely high statistical levels in the city, research on incest remained an invisible topic. In the social sciences generally, and even in the areas of sexuality, inequality and social justice, incest was a closeted subject.

The invisibility of incest in Mexican research

The relationship between incest and the social, economic and cultural forces that make some individuals vulnerable to these relationships, remains largely unexamined in Mexican sociological research. Across disciplines, the studies that deal with these relationships are few, and most of them are either historical analyses and descriptive statistical examinations (Castañeda 1989; Vidrio 1991), legal and judicial publications that examine social and cultural forces responsible for incest from a theoretical perspective (Guridi Sánchez 1961; Falconi Alegría 1961; Floris Margadant 1999) or artistic representations that have given a voice to the victims through the production of novels and critical essays in the humanities (see *La Delgadina* in Pérez 1993; Foladori 2005). In short, although incest has been examined in classical western sociology (i.e. Durkheim 1963; Parsons 1974), sociological research about incest in Mexican society is non-existent.

Why is sociological research on incest in Mexico so invisible? Similar to other western and westernised countries and cultures, incest is a taboo in Mexican society. But incest and related topics (both consensual and non-consensual intra-familial sex) are not only matters of silence within and across the families witnessing these sexualised exchanges, sexuality research in the social sciences has not yet examined this sensitive topic. Although emerging empirical research studies in sexuality have paved the road with groundbreaking studies across disciplines and on a wide diversity of themes exploring sexuality, inequality and social justice in Mexican society, the subject of incest remains unexplored. At the same time, passionate activists and other scholars concerned about issues involving violence against children and women have become increasingly invested and committed in the communities struggling for the establishment of prevention and healing projects, clinical training programmes, legal and social reform and the most basic human rights related to these sensitive areas.

The dynamics of invisibility might be the case in any society. However, they have special implications in Mexico. Generally defined, incest involves sexual activity between individuals belonging to the same immediate or extended family. Thus, talking about incest involves not only talking about sexuality, but also talking about sexual activity within the family. Sexuality research with Mexican populations consistently identifies Mexico as a society characterised as especially silent with regard to issues related to sexuality, a dynamic identified with the concept of 'sexual silence' (Alonso and Koreck 1993; Marín and Gómez 1997; Díaz 1998; Carrillo 2002). This pattern is not unique to Mexico. Deeply rooted in colonial society, a family ethic of honour and respect forces children and youth to be silent with regard to their sex lives or to avoid discussing any sexuality-related question they may have as a way to show respect to their parents and other authority figures within the immediate and extended family.

I was aware of this pattern from my upbringing in Mexican society and it was confirmed for me in my initial sexuality research with Mexican immigrants (see González-López 2005). In this research, I learned about and explored these dynamics. For instance, among the 60 adult immigrants (40 women, 20 men) living in Los Angeles who participated in this study, 12 of the women and one of the men reported being exposed to some type of sexual violence, including coercive sexual contact by brothers, uncles, fathers and cousins. All of them reported that they had rarely talked to their parents about the abuse because of this family ethos. Thus, in Mexico, sexual silence *and* family dynamics may be central factors that prevent children and adult survivors of incest from talking to others and making legal reports of the abuse about this painful experience. Recently, as their understanding of incest and other forms of sexual violence has become more articulated, community-based agencies offering psychotherapy and legal services to incest survivors have begun to acknowledge this pattern of silence (E. Chávez Cano, personal communication 2005).

With these reflections in mind and heeding the desire to be of help as a researcher, I secured funding and immersed myself in the field to conduct in-depth tape-recorded individual interviews with a total of 60 adult women and men with histories of incestuous relationships and 35 professionals (therapists, attorneys, priests, activists, among others) working with these populations. The research took place at four of the largest urban areas in Mexico (Ciudad Juárez, Guadalajara, Mexico City and Monterrey) during 2005 and 2006. I identified these informants through community-based organisations and advocacy groups that included women's rights organisations as well as other grassroots and professional networks. My professional and personal relationships within these community-based institutions evolved through my keen desire to learn how to engage and be of help beyond simply gathering information. This motivation was a key factor in the responsiveness of the agencies I worked with and I am profoundly grateful for the generosity of their support.

Impressions from the field

The benefits of engaged research became particularly apparent in the unexpected and surprising information I gained. I had expected the stories of incest to be raw and traumatic but the conversations with informants resulted in several findings that will not only shape my analysis in new ways but may also have useful implications across disciplines (i.e. clinical mental health). For instance, I was unprepared for the fact that in many cases their sharing with me was the first time several inform-ants had revealed their incest experiences. In this way, the interview became an occasion in which I served not only as researcher but also as a significant witness to their testimony. My initial understanding of incest was also challenged when I learned that some relationships between family members are consensual, especially if they involve individuals of similar age and a romantic context. Another extension of the concept involves sexual abuse by priests, which is an activity that some survi-vors identified as incestuous given their perceptions of a priest as *el padre* and the church as *la madre iglesia.*

One particularly revealing moment occurred when talking with an informant who had experienced extreme physical and sexual violence from her father but who nonetheless reported very little trauma and was in a healthy adult relationship herself. When I asked her for her insights on why some adult survivors of incest appeared unaffected by the experience while others remained locked in perpetual trauma she stated without hesitation: '[B]ecause my mother believed me and took action'. I later heard similar stories that suggest the significance of validation from a trusted adult in recovery and healing. When I asked 'is it possible to heal from this ordeal?', I was repeatedly moved by the processes leading to forgiveness among some survivors and intrigued by those whose own healing was tied to a belief that life would extract an equal measure of justice from their tormentors.

From professionals, I learned how significant the gap is between the high preva-lence of incest and the legal avenues available for seeking justice. For instance, most state criminal codes in Mexico define incest as a crime against the family such that, semantically, the legal concern is for the institution of family rather than individual children. It is also difficult to get accurate incident statistics because reports of incest are conflated with and get lost within the general domestic and sexual violence categories. Many times a person may indentify domestic violence or rape as a reason for seeking therapy but a history of incest may emerge during treatment, however, this is never documented in the statistical records.

Conducting fieldwork on incest has also revealed to me the reasons why there is no empirical research on incestuous relationships, especially with women and men who have experienced them within contexts of extreme pain and abuse. Inviting informants to open up their wounds so I could immerse myself in their stories was an unexpected ethnographic adventure. My attempts to engage them in ways that were gentle and compassionate were emotionally exhausting as well as intellectually stimulating. In addition, identifying potential informants involved methodological considerations that I had not anticipated when I started the research. In attempts to identify individuals who qualified for the study, I met with professionals at community-based agencies who would refer potential informants to me, for example, people who had gone to their organisations seeking legal advice. In these meetings, I found myself being interviewed by highly curious potential informants who had an endless list of questions about the project. I was asked about my age, my professional training, my credentials and cultural competency, the rationale for my study, and my level of personal and professional comfort with regard to pain and other intense emotions. Many times, I was asked if I had a personal history of incestuous relationships or abuse as a child. In these inquisitions, which at times took more than an hour, I was being evaluated on my ability to explore a sensitive topic.

During the interviews, many informants asked for my opinion about some of their unresolved issues and concerns. For example, more than one informant asked my opinion about relationships, HIV and AIDS, sex education for children, among other topics. At all times I avoided giving a personal opinion or professional advice during my interviews. Instead, I referred interviewees to a professional clinician or a professional organisation where he or she could receive help in exploring these concerns. Although none of this was new to me, and while I was following the same protocol as in the previous project, I was beginning to discover something unexpected: the interview process was having a transformative effect on me.

These interviews became life-transforming dialogues for me. In these conversations I experienced a multidimensional state of consciousness that I had not experienced in my previous project or in my training as a psychotherapist. At the core of these conversations, I was beginning to identify a new state of consciousness as a sexuality researcher. Conducting the interviews required me to engage in a multilayered process of inquiry that involved intellectual, emotional and spiritual levels. Intellectually, I followed my endless curiosity as I explored the many complex social, family and cultural processes and dynamics responsible for my informants' fascinating sex stories. Spiritually, I learned to remain present, non-judgmental, peaceful, respectful and compassionate as I participated in an exquisite process of human connection I have no words for. And emotionally, I used my psychological *self* while immersing *myself* inside the sexualised wounds that my informants so unconditionally and generously opened up and exposed to me (see also González-López 2006).

As I finished my very last interview in Mexico City, and was unplugging my tape-recorder, organising my handwritten notes and getting ready to say goodbye, my informant, a kind married woman, inquired, 'May I ask you a personal question?' 'How do you take care of yourself? How do you handle all these intense emotions?' She asked me while crying and thanking me for taking the risk of immersing myself in her story. She asked me if she could give me a big hug as I cried and realised that all the effort was not only becoming part of my professional development but also an unexpected, unfolding spiritual and personal journey.

Doing research on incest hurts more than what I expected – now I know – but it would hurt even more not to do it, especially now that I know the sociological relevance of these narratives of humanity and sexuality. Intellectually, spiritually and emotionally, I became vulnerable to my informants during the data collection but the vulnerability did not stop there. My views of incestuous relationships have evolved continuously throughout the research. I have learned that each story is unique, nuanced and not necessarily surrounded by intense trauma.

The process of revisiting these powerful stories for the purposes of the analysis and organisation is also taking longer than expected. The rich and multilayered nature of the data requires both intellectual and emotional labour. Meditation, exercise, a good cry, restful sleep and the support of people who love me deeply, including my 'thera-friends' who specialise in sexual abuse and who have offered me their support for cathartic purposes, have been an integral aspect of this journey from the beginning. Priceless memories of the many expressions of gratitude that my informants so kindly offered to me have also given me strength while validating the importance of doing work on these issues beyond the challenges and exhaustion this may represent.

The idea of spiritual activism keeps coming to my mind now as I revisit and read the still unfinished transcriptions of my interviews with those who have experienced incest and the professionals who work with them. These professionals in particular – highly committed activists and agents of change – have taught me so much while conducting this research. Through continued reflective, active engagement I hope to be a bridge between them and my mentors and colleagues within academe who believe in scholarship for social change. I dedicate this modest critical essay to all of you – *con amor.*

References

Alonso, A. M. and Koreck, M. T. (1993) 'Silences: "Hispanics", AIDS, and Sexual Practices', in Abelove, H., Barale, M. A. and Halperin, D. M. (eds) *The Lesbian and Gay Studies Reader,* New York: Routledge.

Cancian, F. (1993) 'Conflicts Between Activist Research and Academic Success: Participatory Research and Alternative Strategies', *The American Sociologist,* 24 (1): 92–106.

Carrillo, H. (2002) *The Night is Young: Sexuality in Mexico in the Time of AIDS,* Chicago: University of Chicago Press.

Castañeda, C. (1989) *Violación, Estupro y Sexualidad: Nueva Galicia 1790–1821,* Guadalajara: Editorial Hexágono.

Díaz, R. M. (1998) *Latino Gay Men and HIV: Culture, Sexuality, and Risk Behavior,* New York: Routledge.

Durkheim, E. (1963) *Incest: The Nature and Origin of the Taboo,* New York: L. Stuart.

Falconi Alegría, F. (1961) *El Delito de Incesto: Estudio Dogmático,* Mexico City: Universidad Nacional Autónoma de México, Facultad de Derecho.

Floris Margadant, G. (1999) *La Sexofobia del Clero,* Mexico City: Miguel Angel Porrúa.

Foladori, R. (2005) *El Tabú del Incesto: Su Representación en La Mujer del Puerto;* available at www.cem.itesm.mx/dacs/publicaciones/logos/anteriores/n46/rfoladori.html (accessed 24 October 2008).

González-López, G. (2005) *Erotic Journeys: Mexican Immigrants and Their Sex Lives*, Berkeley: University of California Press.

González-López, G. (2006) 'Epistemologies of the Wound: Anzalduan Theories and Sociological Research on Incest in Mexican Society', *Human Architecture: Journal of Sociology of Self-Knowledge*, IV: 17–24.

Guridi Sánchez, J. (1961). *Ensayo sobre Dogmatica del Delito de Incesto en el Derecho Penal Mexicano*, Mexico City: UNAM.

Hondagneu-Sotelo, P. (1993) 'Why Advocacy Research? Reflections on Research and Activism with Immigrant Women', *The American Sociologist*, 24 (1): 56–68.

Keating, A. (2002) 'Charting Pathways, making Thresholds … a Warning, an Introduction', in Anzaldúa, G. E. and Keating, A. (eds) *This Bridge We Call Home*, New York: Routledge.

Marín, B. V. and Gómez, C. A. (1997) 'Latino Culture and Sex: Implications for HIV Prevention', in García, J. G. and Zea, M. C. (eds) *Psychological Interventions and Research with Latino Populations*, Boston: Allyn & Bacon.

Naples, N. A (2003) *Feminism and Method: Ethnography, Discourse Analysis, and Activist Research*, New York: Routledge.

Parsons, T. (1974) 'The Incest Taboo in Relation to Social Structure', in Coser, R. L. (ed.) *The Family: Its Structures and Functions*, 2nd edn, New York: St. Martin's.

Pérez, E. (1993) 'Speaking from the Margin: Uninvited Discourse on Sexuality and Power', in de la Torre, A. and Pesquera, B. M. (eds) *Building with Our Hands: New Directions in Chicana Studies*, Berkeley: University of California Press.

Vidrio, M. (1991) *Estudio Descriptivo del Abuso Sexual en Guadalajara: Violación, Incesto, Atentado al Pudor y Estupro*, Guadalajara: Editorial Universidad de Guadalajara.

34 Brutal logic[1]

Violence, sexuality and macho myth in South African men's prisons[2] and beyond

Sasha Gear

Researchers working in South African men's prisons have observed the readiness of the perpetrators of male, same-sex rape behind bars to report this violence as compared to the bashfulness of victims (Woodin 2002; Gear 2007a). While providing a jolt to assumptions, this situation is well explained by the social place of sexual violence in prison. Here, the meanings with which inmate culture imbues violence and the gender identities that violence is perceived to bring about, lead victims to go unrecognised or to receive only stigmatised and humiliating attention. Perpetrators, by way of contrast, go unchallenged and/or are valorised.

Potent ideas of masculinity and sexuality coming out of South Africa's history have often been intertwined with violence – connected, for example, to numerous young men's fights for or against apartheid. Today powerful notions of manhood remain ensnared by violence as men negotiate their identities in a 'new' South Africa characterised both by humane and peaceful ambitions (in strong contrast to the country's past) and by exceptionally high levels of interpersonal violence.

With the dramatic increases in incarceration that democracy has paradoxically ushered in, growing numbers of young men especially, are experiencing the socialising force of the prison (Gear 2007b). Drawing on research with (ex) prisoners and analyses from a project focused on sexual violence in prison, this chapter examines the ways in which prison experiences legitimate and add momentum to brutal notions of masculinity and sexuality. These notions make no space for vulnerability in 'manhood', non-violent 'men' or same-sex desire. And while they do not go unopposed, emerging well-intentioned contestations that seek to address the damage, have apparently left sinister elements of the supporting discourses intact.

Making women, taking wives

The ways in which sexual violence in men's prisons is understood and lived is largely framed by dominant inmate culture – the behaviours and understandings considered 'normal' in that context, upheld by those wielding most power. While inmate culture's hierarchies and practices are interwoven with sexual violence, its discourses simultaneously make it invisible. That male victims of prison sexual violence are no longer even acknowledged as men, but are commonly believed to have been turned into 'women' provides striking example. One young prisoner explained:

If … sex [is done to you] … you are now a woman … There is nothing we can do … and we don't care … When [you] walk past people want to touch [you] or threaten to rape [you].

It is predominantly through rape and coercion that a portion of the male prison population is positioned within the inmate world as 'women' to be regarded as sex objects and domestic servants. They are regularly taken as 'wives' or *wyfies* in long-term coerced relationships known as 'marriages' (reportedly the most common site of sexual interaction in prison) by other inmates identified as 'men'.

'Marriages' and these gendered relations are entrenched in the workings of prison gangs and inmate culture generally.[3] Gangs, for example, have masculine and feminine rankings and new members are often classified as either 'men' or 'women'. Classification seems to boil down to whether the recruit has displayed traits that are perceived as feminine (and that also predict vulnerability to sexual violence) or not. Newcomers especially are vulnerable because their unfamiliarity with the unwritten rules of prison sees them easily tricked and manipulated by other inmates. To be naive and needy are seen as signals of *woman*-ness and the risks increase for the poor, physically weak, 'pretty', prisoners linked to 'sissy' crimes and identifying as gay or transsexual. While ultimately no one is immune from danger, inmates' responses to violence are perhaps most fundamental: those showing fear and unwillingness to use violence are likely targets.

Violence reconstituting heterosexuality

Forced sexual penetration is understood to cast on victims a detested feminised identity while endorsing the masculinity of the perpetrator. In this social system, where gender is conflated with a strictly delineated sex role, rape performs the social function of reconstituting heterosexual relations within the all-male prison environment (Gear 2005).

The conflation of gender with a fixed sex role corresponds with Butler's (1990) analysis of dominant gender constructions. These constructions insist on fixed genders that adhere to fixed sexualities and specifically hetero ones. The genders are also defined in opposition to each other. In men's prisons where all inmates are male, the requirement for opposite, fixed sexes is translated into that for oppositional sex roles – 'men' being exclusively penetrators and 'women' exclusively receivers. And the powers that be do not take kindly to deviations.

One such deviation is the (largely) consensual practice of *ushintsha ipondo*. Because in this, participants take turns to sexually penetrate and receive, the practice upsets the equation of gender with a fixed sex role. Inmate power structures relatedly view it as 'homosexuality', regard it as a threat and treat it as a punishable offence. Even so *ushintsha ipondo* is reportedly the next most common site of sexual interaction following the forced 'marriage' situation.

Importantly, other configurations challenging dominant norms also emerge. Moreover as time passes, the dynamics of relationships may shift, and even in those relationships that seemingly occur along the rigid lines of forced marriage, individuals may negotiate different ways of relating under this guise (Gear 2005). This said, existing research points to the power of the dominant, coercive patterns and interviewees maintain that sexual and gendered relations play out largely in conformity with them.

Vanishing violence

Various legitimating discourses support dominant abusive relations. Like female rape victims outside, inmate victims are blamed for what has happened to them. Here, it is for supposedly not having been man enough to prevent it, or for 'asking for it' by being fearful, gullible or effeminate so building the perception that rape is the victim's fault and the perpetrator has done nothing wrong. 'You can never allow another man to come on top of you if you do not like it', said one young prisoner.

That much sexual violence is contained within prison marriages, which in turn mimic dominant heterosexuality, also serves a justificatory function. Inmates often draw on outside relations to describe prison relations, saying things like 'prison wives are treated just like women outside' or 'you can't rape your wife'.[4] Conceptually, prison 'marriages' smooth over the anxiety-provoking issue of violence by disappearing its protagonists: they turn victims into wives and perpetrators into men.

Manhood: brutal by definition

Deeply implicated in the violence are notions of prison manhood constructed as the vastly superior opposite of the despised state of womanhood imposed on rape victims. In addition to self-sufficiency and manipulation skills, a capacity to use and withstand violence is considered integral to masculinity (Gear and Ngubeni 2002; Steinberg 2004) – so much so that 'women' seeking promotion out of humiliation are usually required to perform violence to prove worthiness of 'manhood'. 'Manhood' is further endorsed by having a 'woman' or 'wife':

> [He's saying] … 'This one is my wife' … boasting, boasting … He get[s] proud of himself – that he's a man [among] those gangsters.
>
> (Young inmate)

Antony Whitehead's (2005) conceptualisation of male violence is pertinent to the gendering nature of prison sexual violence. He considers ways in which violence can function in men's interactions with each other, particularly in contexts of 'masculine anxiety', these being situations where men fear for their manhood. Such anxiety is certainly fuelled in identity-robbing, single-sex prisons that offer few opportunities for self-expression. The fear, Whitehead argues, comes from the romanticised ideal that manhood exists in 'transcendental courage' which in reality, can only be intermittently achieved (Hearn and Whitehead 2006). Violence, however, may be utilised to assert it. Sometimes this masculinity-asserting violence is understood to involve victims who are 'manly' themselves and therefore 'worthy rival[s]'. But other times, which often entail sexual humiliation, violence may function to 'exclude the victim from the category "man" as unworthy of belonging there', positioning him as a non-man while affirming the perpetrator's manhood. Whitehead terms this 'exclusive violence' (Whitehead 2005: 416–17).

Male rape clearly constitutes a form of exclusive violence: it is viewed as demolishing the victim's manhood for failure to meet the requirements of idealised manhood. The notion that real men succeed in fighting off attackers and therefore cannot be raped is widespread in society generally, and the stigma of demasculation keeps many victims enduring shame in silence (Rumney and Morgan-Taylor 2004; Singh 2005).

The potent gendered identities then, that prison violence generates, shed light on the relative willingness of perpetrators to share their perpetration compared to the reticence of victims. Other discursive processes that also coalesce in constructions of gender and sexuality further contribute to this situation. Among them is a tendency to muddle definitions of homosexuality and violence.

Anxious muddlings of sex and violence

In South Africa, opportunities for much needed engagement with issues of sexual violence, inmates' health and rights have tended to get besieged by outcry that instead fuels and expresses destructive myths. Specifically, two of society's most profound taboos – homosexuality and male rape – are stirred up and confused: sexuality and violence are conflated. The result is that same-sex desire gets demonised and male rape victims go unacknowledged.

Television depictions of same-sex male prison rape, for example, have been interpreted as homosexuality, generating uproar in which it is difficult to tell whether there is more distress about the screening of 'homosexuality' or of male rape. In a similar vein, the term homosexuality is often used to refer to all sexual encounters in prison, with inmates and staff referring to 'victims' of homosexuality and newcomers being 'afraid of homosexuality' when, in fact, they are scared of being forced to have sex. References to the 'problem of sodomy' and so-and-so being 'sodomised' often also fail to distinguish coercive from consensual practices. Although in South Africa 'sodomy' now refers to anal penetration and is not an offence, misperceptions likely come from criminalisation of male same-sex penetration prior to 1998. Even more recently – and until the end of 2007 – South African legislation failed to acknowledge that men *do* get raped.

The Department of Correctional Services' procedures are along the same discriminatory lines. Quite literally, for example, rape is absent in prison records of violence because no category catering for it exists. And in the absence of policy on sexual matters, there is much disagreement among both staff and inmates about what is allowed and what is not. These situations contribute to the confusion which in turn perpetuates criminalised notions of same-sex desire, and obscures violence by conflating coercion with homosexuality. One manifestation of this is that coercive sex is regularly mistaken for and dismissed as consensual.

Attempting to explain the muddle

That these muddlings have been felt in other countries too (Scarce 1997; Wooden and Parker 1982) points to links between South Africa's specific evolving legal and moral terrain with wider processes. So what is behind the tendency to blur sexuality and violation that sees society treating male victims of rape as existent only as 'nonmen' and homosexuals as criminals, both being regarded with similar disgust?

One explanation lies in dominant constructions of masculinity, which, as we have outlined already, insist first that having manhood means being a heterosexual male while a woman is a heterosexual female, and, second, that manhood relies on its opposition to womanhood. The status quo therefore depends on heterosexuality, and other forms of male sexuality constitute a fundamental threat to masculinity (Connolly 1991). While homosexuality threatens masculinity, femininity represents its opposite 'other'. And as Weeks (1985: 190) noted, hegemonic masculinity is only 'precariously' achieved by consistently repelling its primary threats: femininity and homosexuality.

Male rape evokes notions of both femininity and homosexuality. Because dominant notions of gender make vulnerability a defining feature of femininity, and sexual contact with another man (even unwanted) is allied to homosexuality, same-sex male rape becomes connected to both of masculinity's defining threats: femininity through vulnerability, and homosexuality through same-sex contact.

The taboos of male rape and homosexuality are then linked by the threat they pose to hegemonic masculinity. Consequently, homophobia is generated and male victims of prison rape are alternately 'disappeared' from sight or brought into sight only as stigmatised non-men.

Stuck in the manhood = violence paradigm

Thanks to a scattering of activists, however, discourses seeking to remedy the invisible nature of male rape victims have begun to emerge. Unfortunately, however, some of these well-intentioned discourses inadvertently cause harm. In attempts to get prison victims recognised and paid the attention they deserve, many writers and activists have pointed to the potential for victims to engage in violent compensatory behaviour – usually rape (Donaldson 1993; Harvey 2002; Singh 2005; PMG 2004).

In essence, the emerging activist discourse argues that we should give male victims attention to avert the threat of them becoming future perpetrators. While this approach draws much needed attention to rape victims, a damaging by-product is that it feeds a situation whereby we are only prepared to recognise that men can be victims if we are afraid of them. We thereby risk unintentionally stigmatising men further – as future rapists – by refusing to recognise that they are more than just possible perpetrators. This is because we are inadvertently demanding violence and the commanding of fear from victims in exchange for acknowledging their experiences. Ultimately, we thereby echo the tyrannical requirements of dominant masculinity and the inmate culture it shapes.

Certainly, linkages between 'manhood' and violence make future abuse plausible outcomes of prison rape. But while these at least sometimes will be perpetrated by victims, aggression and violence are not necessary responses to victimisation, and the potential connections require further investigation. Furthermore, these progressively intentioned discourses single out victims as future perpetrators while overlooking the aggressors and coercers (the 'men'). It is likely however, that prison experiences entrench in those identified as prison 'men' abusive notions of masculinity, and that many of them will presumably slot relatively smoothly back into harmful gendered relations in broader society. In overlooking 'men's' potential future violence this discourse abides by the prison discourses that define perpetrators not as perpetrators but as 'men' in 'marriage' and therefore draw attention away from their violence.

No doubt a general inquiry into how prison rape may produce future violence (as opposed to efforts specifically to get victims recognised) may more readily consider prison perpetrators. Nevertheless, an unintended effect of the current approach in relation to both victims and perpetrators is that it supports a normalisation of men's violence. Thus, attempts to build a discourse of male vulnerability again entwine men with violence, so sustaining the very ideas that need to be debunked.

Socialising homophobia

From this exploration of dominant masculinity in South African men's prisons it is already clear that understandings of homosexuality get very short shrift. The compromised place of homosexuality in prison warrants consideration in other respects as well. Inmates' experiences of prison sexual relations also contribute to conflations of homosexuality with violence. Paradoxically, here it is exposure to the types of relationship that homophobic prison culture considers heterosexual – 'marriages' that fuel the linkage. Witnessing or experiencing prison sex and sexual violence is some prisoners' first exposure to male-on-male sex (Gear and Ngubeni 2002). For some inmates, abusive prison relations are their only benchmark for understanding sexual interactions occurring between men. It follows, in this context, that notions of coercion may get confused with homosexuality. Prison experiences are likely to impact on understandings of sexuality even if not constituting inmates' first such encounters (Gear 2007b). 'Gays' are people with whom 'you have to sleep' when you do not know what is going on, said one young offender. Prison experiences, then, can for many[5] inmates, be considered a socialisation into homophobia.

Conclusion

In prison, potent and destructive notions of what it means to be a man gain ascendancy. Related to this, it is difficult to ignore that homophobia and misogyny are alive, well and bred in prison. If prevailing inmate structures had their way, no sex would be happening other than in power-defined interactions between 'men' and 'women'. Relatedly, prisons are environments in which it is acceptable – admired even – for an inmate to be a perpetrator of sexual violence while victims are marked by stigma usually suffering in isolated shame. This is the outcome of the repressive grip of constructions of masculinity and sexuality that are enmeshed with violence – the sexual forms of which are legitimised by being obscured from sight.

Tempting it may be to see this set of relations as an obvious consequence of housing together society's most 'deviant' members. Indeed, in South Africa, where violence and fear feature big on the post-apartheid landscape, questions of inmate wellbeing are often drowned in public animosity. And prisoners, as the most visible face of violence, attract angry public attention and are regularly dismissed as entirely 'other' to the rest of us, morally devoid and deserving of pain.

On the contrary, however, scrutiny of prison relations underscores their connections to wider societal processes. Simultaneously, they underscore the constructed nature of gender. Inmates are not in the business of creating from scratch a whole new society but rather adapting identities and ways of relating that they bring from the outside. In turn, these will be fed to the outside when inmates are released. Prison manifestations of these identities and modes of interaction may be exaggerated along particularly tyrannical lines, but they are also the logical outcome of an unforgiving construction of masculinity that has a clutch on society more generally.

Patterns of interaction resonate strongly with many people's treatment of each other outside and inmates highlight these connections with statements like '[*wyfies*] are treated just like women outside'. Locally and across continents this masculinity is felt in official procedures, recent legislative history (which in some places remains current) and in fervent responses to the issues that conflate violence and homosexuality. These conflations feed the denial of male rape while stigmatising same-sex desire.

Oppositional discourses that have emerged to show up the plight of male rape victims, while sorely needed, have neither adequately deconstructed damaging ideas of 'manhood' nor succeeded in making vulnerability a legitimate facet of masculinity. Inadvertently, they predicate acknowledgement of men on the same fear-demanding basis as the brutal definitions of masculinity and the inmate culture they feed.

Notes

1 This research on which this chapter is based was conducted under the Criminal Justice Programme of the Centre for the Study of Violence and Reconciliation, Johannesburg. Thanks to Amanda Dissel and Kindiza Ngubeni for their work in the Sexual Violence in Prison Project and to the Heinrich Böll Stiftung and Ireland Aid for their generous support. Thanks too to all our interviewees who were willing to share their stories.
2 This chapter draws substantially on arguments first published (and presented in greater detail) in Gear, S. (2007) 'Behind the Bars of Masculinity: Male Rape and Homophobia in and about South African Men's Prisons', *Sexualities*, 10: 209–27.
3 While gangs are custodians of these relations, there is nevertheless some contestation among members on issues of sex (Gear and Ngubeni 2002).
4 South Africa made marital rape a crime in 1993.
5 See Gear and Ngubeni 2002, where, in contrast to other interviewees, one ex-prisoner described leaving prison with greater understanding of and tolerance for homosexuality than when he had arrived.

References

Butler, J. (1990) *Gender Trouble*, London: Routledge.
Connolly, W. E. (1991) *Identity/Difference*, Ithaca, NY: Cornell University Press.
Donaldson, S. (1993) 'The Rape Crisis Behind Bars', *New York Times*, 29 December; available at www.spr.org/docs/nyt.html (accessed 10 January 2000); now available at www.nospank.net/rape2.html
Harvey, E. (2002) 'Rape in Prison: An Intervention by Rape Crisis at Pollsmoor Prison', *Track Two*, 11 (2): 44–51.
Hearn, J. and Whitehead, A. (2006) 'Collateral Damage: Men's "Domestic" Violence to Women Seen Through Men's Relations With Men', *Probation Journal*, 53: 55–74.
Gear, S. (2005) 'Rules of Engagement: Structuring Sex and Damage in Men's Prisons and beyond', *Culture, Health and Sexuality*, 7 (3): 195–208.
Gear, S. (2007a) *Fear, Violence and Sexual Violence in a Gauteng Juvenile Correctional Centre for Males*. Briefing Report No. 02, Johannesburg: CSVR.
Gear, S. (2007b) *Doing Time in a Gauteng Juvenile Correctional Centre for Males*, Briefing Report No. 01, Johannesburg: CSVR.
Gear, S. and Ngubeni, K. (2002) *Daai Ding: Sex, Sexual Violence and Coercion in Men's Prisons*, Johannesburg: CSVR.
PMG (2004) 'Minutes of the Correctional Services Portfolio Committee Meeting "Friends Against Sexual Abuse": Briefing', 13 October; available at www.pmg.org.za/viewminute.php?Id=4690 (accessed 3 November 2004).

Rumney, P. N. S. and Morgan-Taylor, M. (2004) 'The Construction of Sexual Consent in Male Rape and Sexual Assault', in Cowling, M. and Reynolds, P. (eds) *Making Sense of Sexual Consent*, Farnham: Ashgate.

Scarce, M. (1997) *Male on Male Rape*, Cambridge, MA: Perseus Publishing.

Singh, D. (2005) 'Women and Men as Vulnerable Victims', in Davis, L. and Snyman, R. (eds) *Victimology in South Africa*, Pretoria: Van Schaik.

Steinberg, J. (2004) *Nongoloza's Children*, Johannesburg: CSVR.

Weeks, J. (1985) *Sexuality and its Discontents*, London: Routledge & Kegan Paul.

Whitehead, A. (2005) 'Man to Man Violence', *Howard Journal*, 44 (4): 411–22.

Wooden, S. and Parker, J. (1982) *Men Behind Bars*, New York: Plenum Press.

Woodin, N. (2002) 'Charting Domains of Silence: A Process of Feminist Training Addressing the Rape of Men in Prison', dissertation for master of arts, clinical psychology, University of Cape Town.

35 Beyond pseudo-homosexuality

Corrective rape, transactional sex and the undoing of lesbian identities in Namibia

Robert Lorway

In 2001, I began ethnographic research with a community of young people engaging with queer rights discourses emanating from the Namibian sexual minority rights NGO known as the Rainbow Project (TRP).[1] From 1995 until 2005, when President Sam Nujoma finally stepped down from office, numerous government officials from the ruling party, the South West African People's Organisation (SWAPO), vilified gays and lesbians, likening them to infectious diseases, genetic mutation, anti-nationalism, neocolonialism, corruption and globalisation. My original concern was how this intensely homophobic climate and the resultant public health silences shaped the HIV vulnerability of young people living in the impoverished township of Katutura.

I also grew fascinated with some young people's vivid displays of gender sexual non-conformity, which appeared remarkable at a time when ruling government officials were deploying virulent anti-homosexual rhetoric. However, multiple overlapping forms of violence periodically interrupted their gender-dissident performances, as the following description excerpted from my field notes for May 2003 illustrates:

> After many long hours, our HIV/AIDS awareness committee finished painting the walls of TRP in preparation for a safer-sex poster exhibition. As some of us began crumpling up the newspapers that served as a drop cloth, from the corner of my eye I watched a heated argument spark between Hanna, a self-identified 'butch lesbian', and Melvin, who often dressed in partial feminine drag. Hanna accused Melvin of sexually coercing a young, gay friend of hers at a 'safer sex' educational weekend organised by the Rainbow Project (TRP) a few weeks previously. Melvin adamantly denied it.
>
> Despite our best attempts to settle the argument it continued to escalate, especially when Melvin placed his hands on Hanna's shoulders. We all knew that this physical contact would further 'set off' Hanna who had endured intense physical and sexual abuse at the hands of men since she was a child. As more members of the working group became drawn into the dispute, a barrage of insults flew, such as: 'at least *my* mother didn't die of AIDS', 'Your aunt is a prostitute and has a sugar daddy', 'You only have Standard 6 [education level]', 'Ovambos are dirty' and 'Damaras don't have real culture'. Such deeply cutting insults culminated into physical violence between six of the members. The eventual casualties included a bloodied lip, a broken tooth, a slashed-open knee and other bodily bruises.
>
> Beyond the physical injuries, what unsettled me most was the gendered form that the violence took during the episode. The previously proud composure of

the butch lesbians noticeably drew downward while the posture of the three 'feminine' males inflated. Earlier that day I witnessed these same feminine males request 'the men' (Hanna and some of the other butch lesbians) to move the furniture in preparation for the painting, gesturing that they were physically too delicate to accomplish the task themselves; and Hanna and her butch friends were more than happy to demonstrate their strength. Now, the vibrant physical presence of these women diminished. They appeared vulnerable and tentative, similar to when other young women in Katutura encountered violence from men. As for the dainty, feminine-acting males, they appeared to drop all traces of effeminacy before my eyes, transforming into violent and aggressive men.

The episode reached an abrupt denouement when Hanna noticed two 'non-members' lurking about outside the office. She insisted that both young men, *botsosos* [criminals] she called them, wanted to rob TRP. One of them asked if he could enter the centre, even though it was well after hours. Hanna instantly shouted '*Nie* [no] man ... you can't come in' and then bent down and began to draw an imaginary outline around the front of the office door with her hand while repeating, 'This is LGBT safe space. You are not allowed in here'. One of the men began ridiculing Hanna and the other butch lesbians saying 'why are *you* dressing like men?' He then called us all 'moffies', with great distain, and proceeded to hurl a large, empty beer bottle at one of the newly painted walls inside the centre, sending fragments flying, just missing a few of us. In the midst of this commotion, Hanna, with almost manic devotion, repeated her mantra: 'This is LGBT safe space'.

When 'butch bodies' draw downward and become vulnerable during such violent episodes, what does this suggest about the pursuit of lesbian modes of self-determination in Namibia? How does the idealistic notion of safe space, as iterated by Hanna, and other queer rights discourses of bodily integrity shape sexual self understandings in their continual collision with gender-based violence, and its refraction – homophobia?

This chapter specifically examines moments in which female gender-sexual reversals appear to unravel as they get caught in the complex web of power relations between deeply entrenched gender-sexual inequality and the transnational ensemble of human rights interventions designed to improve the wellbeing of Namibian sexual minorities. I place *less* emphasis here than elsewhere (Lorway 2008) on how these young women achieve and sustain their enactments of butch defiance. Rather, I choose to focus on the underside of such identity formation, highlighting moments of insecurity, anxiety and uncertainty surrounding the pursuit of a lesbian identification in Namibia. From this perspective, we may better understand how multiple and sometimes contradictory subjectivities emerge along a winding trajectory. This perspective coincides with contemporary approaches within gender and sexuality studies that have increasingly moved away from the concept of sexual identity in favour of sexual subjectivity (Boellstorff 2005), which I loosely define as the way individuals understand and experience gender and sexuality within shifting relational fields of power. Furthermore, this conceptualisation avoids the idea of a singular sexual identity that stands whole prior to social inequality. Instead, I recognise the ways sexual self-understandings register in subjectivity *as* social inequalities unfold and iterate in people's lives.[2]

Three hegemonic discourses have come to characterise a particular set of truths about the sexual experience of African lesbians with men – pseudo-homosexuality, corrective rape and survival sex – and currently disseminate through TRP's human rights development projects, feeding out from and into larger public debates in southern Africa (particularly South Africa). Read together, these discourses provide fertile terrain for public commentators to explain the prevalence of heterosexual behaviour among Namibians who self-identify as lesbians. Furthermore, these discourses allow African lesbians themselves to construct narratives of authenticity to achieve a sense of belonging within the larger transnational LGBT rights networks that connect through TRP. However, by semantically cementing their sexual relationships with men to trauma, abuse and exploitation, the pervasiveness of these discourses raise a significant question: Is oppression the only lens through which to interpret the sexual relationships that form between African lesbians and men?[3]

In the next section, I sketch out the broader discursive terrain that articulates the experience of being a lesbian in southern Africa and I provide some interrogation. Drawing on recent fieldwork conducted in the Coastal Namibian town of Walvis Bay, I then illustrate how local versions of these discourses surface, in conflicting ways, within the subjectivities of young women who have begun to pursue sexuality training programmes offered by TRP in 2007.

Reigning discourses

Pseudo-homosexuality

On 14 July 2007, a white South African Pastor and educational consultant from Inclusive and Affirming Ministry held a public talk at TRP's head office in Windhoek entitled 'My Child is Gay – What Now?' This well-attended presentation was offered to help parents 'cope' with the 'loss' of discovering that their child is gay. 'Such loss includes', the pastor emphasised, 'the loss of the dream of grandchildren'.

This presentation followed on a series of training workshops that taught spiritual (Christian-based) counselling techniques to young TRP members. Drawing on O'Neill and Ritters' (1992) eight phases of 'spiritual awakening for lesbians and gay men', the lesbian pastor, with her usual rousing tone, insisted that parents and youth could 'transform loss into a liberation. The journey doesn't have to end in victimisation. There can be freedom at the end!'

Of all TRP-sponsored presentations and workshops I attended over the years, Christian, religiously oriented workshops always drew the largest crowd from TRP youth and the wider public. During interviews with young people, it also became evident that it was tremendously important for them to reconcile being gay and being a Christian. Although TRP workshops generally set forth delineations between lesbian-gay-bisexual-transgender identities, the religious workshops, by contrast, *rarely* referenced bisexuality.

From my ethnographic work, I knew that many of the lesbian women sitting in the audience practised bisexual behaviour and had children, so I posed the following question to the pastor during the discussion period: 'How would O'Neill's stages work for parents who discover that their child is *bisexual?*' Some of the women nodded in agreement with my question, a few also grinned at me slightly. The pastor paused looking mildly perplexed and began muttering for a few moments. Then, with a tone of conviction she cited the term 'pseudo-homosexuality' stating: 'Some people are not true homosexuals ... for example, if a woman is sexually abused she may think that she is a lesbian. But she is not a true lesbian and she must therefore seek counselling'. A few of the women squirmed in their seats, others crinkled their faces. However, the usually vocal TRP members remained respectfully silent.

The issue of sexual abuse and lesbian authenticity resurfaced in 2008 during TRP's public forum held in conjunction with the Media Institute of Southern Africa as part of their new gay–straight alliance initiative entitled Straight Talk with Straight Friends. The forum began with a presentation by a prominent young, black lesbian activist who rose to define a range of sexual identity terms: anatomical sex, gender, sexual identity, bisexuality, transgenderism, transvestitisms, intersexuality, etc. Then, during the question period, a male audience member asked 'can a woman become a lesbian if she is raped by a man?' This question captured the audience's interest as a lively debate on the subject ensued. Attempting to settle the debate authoritatively a German psychotherapist, who worked at a local violence and trauma counselling NGO, known as PEACE, responded firmly: 'Yes, it is possible for a woman who has become sexually abused by a man to believe that she is a lesbian'.

Corrective rape

The term corrective rape recently came to the fore in the international press when the South African Human Rights Commission released a report on 12 March 2008, stating that: 'There is a growing phenomenon of corrective rape ... where a male learner rapes a lesbian female learner in the belief that after such a sexual attack the learner will no longer be lesbian' (McGreal 2008). However, this disturbing phenomenon made its strongest appearance in 2003 when 33 South African lesbians publicly released their stories of sexual abuse:

> Lesbians are being raped, assaulted and victimised every day in the townships, in an attempt to force a change in their sexual orientation. Since January this year, 33 black lesbians have come forward with their stories of rape, assault, sexual assault and verbal abuse to organisations fighting hate crimes in Johannesburg townships. Zanele Muholi, a reporter for the lesbian and gay publication *Behind the Mask*, has documented 12 rapes, four attempted rapes, six verbal abuse cases, three assaults with a deadly weapon and two abductions. She said:
>
> > Since we started on this project [The Rose has Thorns] we've realised that this kind of thing happens every day, everywhere ... The age group of the victims ranges from 16 to 35 years, and two of the rape survivors are teenagers ... 24 of the 33 women who were subjected to hate crimes were 'butch' women who had been victimised ... Kekeletso Khena fled from Soweto after being raped three times before she turned 19 ... It's a practice called corrective rape, where men try to turn you into a real African woman. I was raped because I was a butch child. I was 13 years old the first time it happened.
>
> (Mufweba 2003)

Currently, notions of corrective rape has become a hallmark for representing the human rights struggles of Namibian lesbians in local forums. For example, the rape of lesbians feature prominently in a new video documentary sponsored by TRP entitled, 'Forgotten Survivors'. In 2007 and 2008, TRP screened this film before LGBT youth throughout Namibia as well as at the national film festival held in the capital city. It has also won a few awards in southern Africa. In one poignant scene, two butch lesbians in their early twenties sit together outside a shack in a small southern Namibian township as one begins to recount the following story:

> My friend's name is Barbara and she was raped in 2003. This was done by a guy who was HIV positive. We were together in the afternoon. She went into town to drink. While on her way back, the guy followed and raped her … The guy was not found guilty. She passed away. We were very scared afterwards. The same guy also threatened to kill us.

During interviews I conducted in the township of Katutura, lesbians' stories commonly carried accounts of rape and attempted rape, often committed by men known to their family. For instance, during my first interview with 21-year-old Monica, she stated:

> When I was 11, if a man tried to touch me, I always had a fist for him. If a woman did, well that was a different thing. A friend of my family, he came and told me I must do it [have sex] … I was 15. I didn't want to. He forced me and that day I was pregnant. That was the only time I had sex with a man. That day I also became HIV positive.

As I came to Monica over the coming years, I learned that she did have sexual relationships with other men, on occasion, for money. 'I just don't make enough selling fish, you know; I have to pay school fees for [my child] and my younger brother and sister. I am the oldest daughter'.

Transactional sex

How African women become vulnerable to HIV infection through 'transactional sex' has received significant attention from academics and policymakers. By 2004 local multimedia campaigns in Namibia began to portray the danger of sugar daddy relationships on billboards, posters and small television spots. Today, sugar daddy relationships are commonly referred to in daily discussions of sexual politics in the townships. But it is only recently that these relationships have become associated with African lesbians in the emerging HIV prevention discourse on WSW or women who have sex with women. In 2007 the Dutch humanitarian foundation, Schorer, expanded its global health development programme known as the Prevention Initiative for Sexual Minorities (PRISM) to include Botswana, Zimbabwe, Namibia and South Africa. I was involved in the development of the community-based methodology for Namibia's needs assessment sponsored by Schorer. At a planning workshop, lesbians and WSW, defined as 'closeted women in heterosexual settings', were identified as a vulnerable group that needed to be targeted for the needs assessment. Representatives from the Netherlands and various African sexual minority rights organisations concluded that because of economic dependence and stigma, WSW frequently came to be in unwanted heterosexual relationships.

In my research, the narrative of survival sex was also invoked by participants with respect to motherhood:

> I mean I am proud to say I am a lesbian but then people say 'but you have children?' That is the one thing that was hurting me the most … We all have a pressure to belong, because of the society, the pressure out there. Somehow there were pressures from my family to have children. There was a reason why I had to go out and sometimes [have sex with men]. I don't reject my children; they are a blessing in my life. But just the fact of how they came made me unhappy …
>
> It was not because I really wanted [sex with men] but because of circumstances. Sometimes I had nowhere to sleep. I even never wanted to drink or smoke, but having to be with men when I didn't want to … it dragged me into that! … That is how I got my first child. His father took advantage of my weaknesses and the circumstances I was in and I had no choice and I needed a place to sleep, and something to eat … [T]hat is how it happened and with my second and third child as well. Until I realised that this is not getting me anywhere, this is just hurting me more.
>
> (Audrey, aged 26)

These discursive formations variously figure the sexual lives of African lesbians in terms of oppression. However, they pivot on a similar bounded notion of sexual identity that maintains a hetero-homo binary. Part of what is understood to constitute the traumatic character of sexual abuse and exploitation is the deformation, dissolution or crossing of this boundary of authenticity.

The discourse of pseudo-homosexuality proffers a degenerative narrative whereby sexual abuse damages the integrity of heterosexual identity – posited, tacitly, as an original and impressionable surface – corrupting its 'natural' separation from homosexuality. This implies a psycho-pathological state in which the sexually abused individual falsely recognises herself as a homosexual to escape from the anxieties surrounding the sexual abuse event(s). Employing this logic, the lesbian pastor not only positions heterosexuality as the normative, healthy default sexuality, but she casts African female bisexuality as a conflicted sexual subject position: where heterosexual remnants continually return to resist the foreclosure of a 'false' lesbian identity enforced by traumatic memories. In other words, the pastor's deployment here calls into question the authenticity of the lesbian identification taken up by many of the women in her audience, thus inadvertently undermining their space of political belonging. Although these women hold a firm connection to global lesbian activism in their personal and collective pursuits of sexual self-determination, many have shared (and continue to share) sexual intimacies with men and have encountered various forms of sexual-gender violence over their lifetime. But what I find salient in the discourse of pseudo-homosexuality pertains not only to concerns over authenticity and belonging, per se. I am particularly troubled by how its deployment seals over potentially wider political resonances between these women's struggles and other non-lesbian identifying women.

In the case of corrective rape, it is held out in the media as a particularly heinous form of rape – a homophobic hate crime – that is distinguishable from heterosexual rape, which is widespread and frequent in southern Africa. This distinction prompts us to accept that the experience of lesbian corrective rape is innately different from heterosexual rape, even though, by definition, both forms are committed against unwilling individuals. Does this distinction suggest that the spectrum of heterosexual rape encompasses a possible grey zone shaded by sexual desire, where heterosexual desire itself becomes exploited? And are we to only understand the experience of lesbian rape contrastively: as strictly devoid of this zone of (different sex) sexual desire? What is clear about the discourse of corrective rape is that it takes as given, and therefore reifies, the boundaries of sexual difference assumed to exist between lesbians and heterosexual women.

Although social scientists recognise that 'women approach transactional [sexual] relations not as passive victims, but in order to access power and resources in ways that can both challenge and reproduce patriarchal structures' (Hunter 2002: 101), do deeply embedded structural inequalities and the local fields of economic strategy they bring into play occlude all possibilities of affection forming between men and women in these relationships? In the emergent public health discourse on WSW, lesbians involved in transactional sex are made to exemplify 'true' sexual exploitation and 'survival sex', for it is based on the notion that a lesbian could never truly experience pleasure or affection in her sexual relationships with men. Similar to the discourse of corrective rape, the distinction made between 'lesbians' and 'heterosexual women' in the discourse of transactional sex upholds the division and opposition between homosexual and heterosexual desires.

In the next section, I demonstrate how the narratives of young, lesbian-identifying women living in Walvis Bay in many ways coincide with these discursive formations. However, the extended time spent inhabiting the ordinary social spaces where young people regularly socialise allows me to present a more nuanced picture of the sexual intimacies that form between lesbian-identifying women and men.

Some lived realities

I first met Loran during a TRP sexuality training workshop at Walvis Bay in August 2007. She sat around the workshop table wearing long baggy shorts with her legs sprawled widely apart and her arms folded in a masculine way much like her three butch friends who sat near to her. It was their first time attendance at this kind of workshop, although Loran informed me that she had already learned about 'LGBT' identities from her butch friends in Windhoek. During the first interview, 22-year-old Loran identified her gender and sexual identity:

> I describe myself as a lesbian, but not a man, but as a woman. In my community we didn't use it [the term 'lesbian'] in the beginning; we were called tomboys. When I heard the word 'lesbian' for the first time, it felt so much better to use the word 'lesbian' than the word 'tomboy'.

A month later I met Loran at TRP's head office in Windhoek for a training workshop on community-based research, which I was asked to lead. TRP's health officer and I had decided to train unemployed youth as the researchers from three high-HIV prevalence zones in Namibia (Oshakati, Walvis Bay and Windhoek). Loran was selected for the community research training because she was very intelligent, well-known and well-respected among her peers in Walvis Bay.

At the conclusion of the training, we all headed to the Angolan dance club, Chez Ntemba. However, while we waited in the queue, Loran, who entered ahead of us, quickly exited the club. Looking very upset, she pulled me aside to explain why she was refused entry. During the regular weapons check, the female security guard told her that pregnant women were not allowed in the club in case a fight broke out. On the verge of tears, and somewhat intoxicated, she said: 'Please just tell the group that I have to go back to my room because I forgot my money or some-thing. I am really embarrassed, I don't want them to know that I am pregnant or they will wonder "how is this lesbian pregnant? She cannot be a real lesbian."' Ironi-cally, many of the other lesbians waiting in the line had given birth to children already.

I saw Loran again in January 2008 when I returned to Walvis Bay to conduct inter-views with LGBT youth. She invited me to her home to meet her family and see her new baby girl who had been born prematurely and extremely underweight. Her mother beamed with pride when she showed me the sleeping baby. Loran just rolled her eyes and then quickly whisked me away to meet her butch friends who lived nearby.

Over the next two months, I came to spend a great deal of time with Loran's mostly unemployed friends at places where they regularly hung out: at Independ-ence Beach, the soccer fields, the nearby *cuca* shops (pubs) and a few *shebeens* (small drinking establishments). Over the Easter long weekend, I witnessed numerous drinking binges that lasted from Friday afternoon until Sunday evening. The cost of alcohol was much less than escalating food prices, and it was especially cheap in the township where beer could be bought almost at cost. That weekend, Loran's mother threatened to take the baby away shouting: 'you are not looking after the baby prop-erly. You are running off with your friends drinking when you should be saving money for your baby's milk!'

Eventually Loran explained why she felt some resentment toward her baby:

> I was turning 17 – my first time with a man. There is pressure from the com-munity to be straight. Mostly I got from people 'how could you be with a woman? Why don't you take a man?' It felt very offensive to me.
>
> From my side of view, I have a baby and [hesitates] ... basically there wasn't the bonding of love or anything when I had sex with the father; it was the alcohol while I was drinking. I don't want to blame it on the alcohol, but it was all done while I was under the influence of alcohol.

In clubs, *sheebeens* and *cuca* shops, I watched as the butch lesbians tried and usually succeeded in 'hooking up with the ladies', many of whom were sex workers. I also witnessed many flirtations between the butch women and men as more alcohol was consumed. Late one evening Loran and one of her butch friends grew excited when one guy dressed all in white, dressed like R&B artist Art Kelley, approached. 'He is looking so fly!' 'He is very sexy', they commented.

Learning that I was intrigued by how lesbian women came to have sexual rela-tionships with men, Loran stated during an interview:

> Lots of my friends are having sex with men. I mean I feel that women who are identifying as lesbians who are having sex with men ... I don't think there is

anything wrong with that. I guess some of the butches may feel ashamed to talk about it openly because they are suppose to be men, and they are afraid of what other people will say.

During the daytime, Loran regularly took me along to visit with her friends like 25-year-old Linda, who also had a young baby. After we had been introduced, Linda said how difficult she was finding it to get any work other than washing the neighbours' clothing. 'This didn't pay much money', she explained.

After attending TRP workshops, Linda began to reflect on her struggles with men, linking them to the discrimination faced by the LGBT community in Walvis:

> I started dressing like a man since I was 14 years of age, but I only heard of lesbians when the president was saying bad things about them ... in the 90s. I learned about what a lesbian was only recently at TRP, their workshops, you know. I only attended two workshops so far. After that I am feeling now that we lesbians must protect ourselves from people. Maybe I am in a club for example and they are saying like 'you moffie' and wondering if I want a drink and then later on they want sex in payment ... well this one guy after we had sex, it was for money, he beat me and didn't pay me. Lesbians are experiencing it a lot here from men.
>
> (Linda, aged 25)

People living in Kuisebmund commonly supplemented their household income with selling drugs: *dagga* (marijuana) and *rocks* (crack). When I was introduced to Loran's friend Kenya, I was asked to first wait by the gate until her family could hide some of the drugs they were organising for sale.

Kenya and I sat outside in the backyard discussing her life story and how she came to understand her gender and sexuality after taking TRP's sexuality training:

> I feel I am a lesbian and a man. Well I guess I am transgender then [pauses to reflect]. I very much liked the workshops because I learned more about who I am and about how to protect myself from HIV.
>
> (Kenya, aged 23)

When we came to the subject of sexual violence between lesbians and men, Kenya said:

> There are these boys ... Oh! They beat this one lesbian. They also beat me last weekend [shows stitches on her scalp] ... they said 'oh you moffie! You see, I am going to bring you down. I am going to make you straight again'.

'What did they beat you with?' I asked. She responded:

> I was beat like this with a bottle. I didn't even say any word. I didn't even swear at them. They just came up and beat me and took my cell phone. They call us and they said I want you to be my girlfriend ... but they know [we are lesbians].

I was surprised when 23-year-old Kenya showed up at a beach party with her two young boys. By this time she had grown comfortable with me and she said: 'These are my children. I was much younger when I had them, I thought I liked men then, I was drinking a lot then'.

Kenya and Loran insisted that I meet another lesbian, 'Boy', who had also suffered an attack. Boy's mother led us to the back of her cinder-block house to a smaller, makeshift shack. 'This is Boy's place', she said with a slight grin. Twenty-year-old Boy greeted us at the door with a wide smile and invited us in so we could be properly introduced.

Boy was anxious to tell me his harrowing tale of violence. 'It is important for you to know the problems facing my community'. His intense political sensibility was cultivated in Windhoek while receiving human rights training:

> I am a lesbian ... a man. The first time I heard it was from a friend, a member of TRP because I asked her about it. I was 13 when I knew what I was, although I didn't know the word 'lesbian'. I told my parents at 15, they are OK with it ... I am 'out of the closet'. I told my mum that I am feeling more comfortable with women and I don't want to be with men. They fully accept me now.

When we came to the subject of violence, Boy recounted his recent assault:

> [We] were drinking and this guy started asking questions. He approached me saying 'I want to date you' and I said 'no I am not into men I am a lesbian'. And then he said 'you lesbian people, you are illegal here in Namibia' and he slapped me in the face and I slapped him back and ran, and he hit me on the head with a broken bottle and cut it open ... see here [shows stitched-up wound].

Boy stated that it would be good for my research to interview his girlfriend, Kathe, who was a 'real lady'. Because Kathe had not attended a workshop yet she was somewhat tentative in her discussion of her sexual identity:

> I see myself as a lady, not a lesbian. Although I am not really sure what a lesbian is. I do not define myself as a lesbian. I mean I have a girlfriend but I am bisexual. When my boyfriend found out about her he tried to kill me, to strangle me [laughs]. This is my first relationship with a woman. It's only 2 months. It is better than being with a man ... when my boyfriend is working at the sea and coming back he is drinking with his friends, he is partying till late.
>
> (Kathe, aged 19)

The theme of absent male partners arose during interviews with several of Loran's young friends, including Naomi:

> I never went off with guys really but, but one guy he came and decided to give me a child and then ran away. He is working as a fisherman down the coast at Lüderitz, and he just left me pregnant and that is why I decided to become a lesbian.
>
> (Naomi, aged 21)

Among the 20 women I interviewed, fear of HIV infection was the most common theme used to explain how they came to engage in same-sex sexual practices:

Before I started to date women, I was going out with boys. I am a bisexual. My parents say 'what is the problem?' now that I start to date women. I said because of AIDS I see too many of my friends dying of AIDS, and that is why I've turned my life to women, because of safety. My mum and my grandmum reacted negatively because they say a woman is supposed to take a man so they can produce children. They said: 'How will you get children if you are with another woman?'

Conclusion

The lived realities of participants point to a set of interrelated axes around which sexual subjectivities emerge: the HIV epidemic, gender inequality, poverty and the identity politics disseminating from TRP programmes. But it is important to look beyond the three reigning discourses, their confining politics of truth/authenticity and the pathologising framing they impose. Determining whether or not the participants in this study are in fact 'true lesbians', is less fruitful for considering possibilities for emancipation than, I propose, acquiring an *appreciation* for the complex quality of their engagement: how these women cross numerous borders, establishing connections between domains cordoned off in human rights and development discourses. Recognising their continual crossing not only calls the realness of these borders into question but brings the participants' struggles into a wider focus and resonance. Indeed, their struggles for sexual self-determination do not exist outside the political economy of sexuality that configures gender inequities for other women in their community. An appreciation for how these women make political connections as they cross between the multiple borders of nationhood, class, gender and identity opens up an avenue to explore greater possibilities for alliance between the advancement of sexual minority rights and global health and development projects concerned with furthering gender rights.

Notes

1 Many thanks are due to the members and staff of the Rainbow Project in Windhoek and Walvis Bay. Gratitude is also owed to the Wenner-Gren Foundation, which generously supported the most recent phase of this research.
2 My thinking here borrows insight both from Monique Wittig's (1980) thesis (how the 'straight mind' is produced by gender inequality) and from Diana Fuss' (1989) interrogation of Wittig's thesis (41–5).
3 Sexual abuse and rape committed against African lesbians is also emphasised in life stories discussed in Morgan and Wieringa (2005: 317).

References

Boellstorff, T. (2005) *The Gay Archipelago: Sexuality and Nation in Indonesia*, Princeton: Princeton University Press.
Fuss, D. (1989) *Essentially Speaking: Feminism Nature and Difference*, New York: Routledge.
Hunter, M. (2002) 'The Materiality of Everyday Sex: Thinking beyond "Prostitution"', *African Studies*, 61 (1): 99–120.
Lorway, R. (2008) 'Defiant Desire in Namibia: Female Sexual-gender Transgression and the Making of Political Being', *American Ethnologist*, 35 (1): 20–33.
McGreal, C. (2008) 'Traumatised South African Children play "Rape Me" Games', *Guardian*,

13 March; available at www.guardian.co.uk/world/2008/mar/13/southafrica.internation-alcrime (accessed 30 July 2008).

Morgan, R. and Wieringa, S. (2005) *Tommy Boys, Lesbian Men and Ancestral Wives: Female Same Sex Practices in Africa*, Johannesburg: Jacana Media.

Mufweba, Y. (2003) 'Corrective Lesbian Rape makes You an African Woman', *Saturday Star* (South Africa), 18 November; available at www.globalgayz.com/RSA-news03-04. html#article14 (accessed 4 April 2005).

O'Neill, C. and Ritter, K. (1992) *Coming Out Within: Stages of Spiritual Awakening for Lesbians and Gay Men*, New York: HarperCollins.

Wittig, M. (1980) 'The Straight Mind', *Feminist Issues*, 1 (1): 103–11.

Part VII

From sexual health to sexual rights

36 Sexuality education, US federal abstinence policies and young people's right to health information

John S. Santelli, Rebecca Schleifer and Andrea J. Melnikas

Human rights principles have not played a prominent role in discussions of health in the USA. Human rights discussions in the context of medicine or public health have usually been limited to patients' rights and notions of informed consent. Little attention has been paid to broader human rights obligations that are critical to ensuring fundamental human rights to health, such as rights to information or non-discrimination based on gender or sexual orientation. In this chapter, we will examine US Federal government promotion of abstinence using a human rights perspective that builds on international documents such as the United Nations Convention on the Rights of the Child. A critical focus here is on the 'right to information' – as articulated in multiple of these international accords.

This chapter focuses in particular on the rights issues raised by US government promotion of 'abstinence until marriage' or 'abstinence only'. First, we examine public health critiques of abstinence-only policies and programmes, as these perspectives are important in grounding a human rights analysis in public health realities. Then we review the human rights of adolescents and young people as related to health and government responsibilities to promote the information needed to protect young people's lives and health. We conclude that recent US government efforts to promote abstinence-only education are inconsistent with the internationally accepted right to health information. Based on this analysis, we suggest that US government policy should embrace a vision for sexuality education grounded in access to complete and accurate sexual health information, articulated as a basic human right and recognised as essential to realising the human right to the highest attainable standard of health.

Public health and abstinence-only and abstinence-until-marriage policies

Timing of first sex and its importance to health

First sexual intercourse is an important developmental milestone from both social and public health perspectives. Sexual intercourse is a normal and natural part of human development and is essential for human reproduction. However, sexually active young people face considerable risk for unplanned pregnancy and sexually transmitted infection (Weinstock *et al.* 2004; Finer and Henshaw 2006). The median age at first intercourse in the USA is 17 years (Abma *et al.* 2004), which is similar to other developed countries. Teenagers in the USA have much higher birth and pregnancy rates compared with many of their European counterparts, primarily because of lower contraceptive use (Godeau *et al.* 2008; Santelli *et al.* 2008). The US Public Health Service has identified delay in initiation as a public health goal (US Department of Health and Human Services 2000) in addition to a variety of goals related to risk reduction. Abstinence-only proponents have identified delay until marriage as the sole goal that is acceptable to them.

Although some abstinence proponents have claimed that initiation of sex outside marriage or during adolescence is likely to lead to mental health problems (Rector *et al.* 2003), research does not support these assertions (Santelli *et al.* 2006). While the initiation of sexual intercourse between the ages of 12–14 years has been associated with mental health problems, early initiation is also associated with poverty, family instability and physical and sexual abuse – all of which may give rise to mental health problems (Sandfort *et al.* 2008).

Sexual health, sexuality education and abstinence programmes

Sexual health has been defined as:

> [A] state of physical, emotional, mental and social well-being in relation to sexuality; it is not merely the absence of disease, dysfunction or infirmity. Sexual health requires a positive and respectful approach to sexuality and sexual relationships, as well as the possibility of having pleasurable and safe sexual experiences, free of coercion, discrimination and violence. For sexual health to be attained and maintained, the sexual rights of all persons must be respected, protected and fulfilled.
>
> (World Health Organisation 2006: 5)

Knowledge of sexuality and one's body is essential to protecting oneself from STIs and unplanned pregnancy. Professional health groups, which see the results of sexual ignorance first hand, have strongly supported sexuality education (Society for Adolescent Medicine 2006; American College of Obstetricians and Gynecologists 2003; American Public Health Association 2005; American Academy of Pediatrics 2001). There is also broad public and parent support in the USA for comprehensive sexuality education in schools and for abstinence as part of that education (Albert 2004). Few parents support education that focuses exclusively on abstinence.

The impact of comprehensive sexuality education programmes which also promote abstinence and abstinence-only programmes is available from several recent systematic reviews (Underhill *et al.* 2007a; Underhill *et al.* 2007b; Kirby 2008). These reviews examined studies that were peer reviewed and included several well-designed evaluations of abstinence-only programmes. Criteria used to select studies included the use of experimental or quasi-experimental research designs and measurement of behaviours and not just behavioural intentions. These reviews concluded that many comprehensive sexuality education programmes demonstrate efficacy in delaying initiation of intercourse and in promoting other protective behaviours such as condom use. In contrast, these reviews found no strong scientific evidence that abstinence-only programmes demonstrate efficacy in delaying initiation of sexual intercourse.

Observation studies have also examined the impact of 'virginity pledges' – components of many abstinence-only programmes in the USA and elsewhere – on sexual behaviour. Pledging is a marker for both abstinence intentions and exposure to abstinence-only educational programmes. Virginity pledges are associated with delay in sexual initiation in some but not all studies (Bruckner and Bearman 2005; Rosenbaum 2008). When pledgers do initiate intercourse, they may be more likely to engage in risk behaviours such as unprotected vaginal, anal and oral sex – than non-pledgers.

History of abstinence education in the USA

While the Federal government began supporting abstinence promotion programmes in 1981 via the Adolescent Family Life Act (AFLA), since 1996 there have been major expansions in Federal support for abstinence programming. Additionally, there has been a shift to funding programmes that teach abstinence exclusively and restrict information about condoms and other methods of contraception (Dailard 2002). Federal programmes prohibit disseminating information on contraceptive services, sexual orientation and gender identity and other aspects of human sexuality. Section 510 provides an eight-point definition of abstinence-only education (see Box 36.1) and specifies that programmes must have as their 'exclusive purpose' the promotion of abstinence outside marriage and may not in any way advocate contraceptive use or discuss contraceptive methods except to emphasise their failure rates (Dailard 2002).

Box 36.1

Under Section 510, abstinence education is defined as an educational or motivational program which:

A   has as its exclusive purpose, teaching the social, psychological and health gains to be realised by abstaining from sexual activity;

B   teaches abstinence from sexual activity outside marriage as the expected standard for all school age children;

C   teaches that abstinence from sexual activity is the only certain way to avoid out-of-wedlock pregnancy, sexually transmitted diseases and other associated health problems;

D   teaches that a mutually faithful monogamous relationship in the context of marriage is the expected standard of human sexual activity;

E   teaches that sexual activity outside of the context of marriage is likely to have harmful psychological and physical effects;

F   teaches that bearing children out-of-wedlock is likely to have harmful consequences for the child, the child's parents and society;

G   teaches young people how to reject sexual advances and how alcohol and drug use increases vulnerability to sexual advances; and

H   teaches the importance of attaining self-sufficiency before engaging in sexual activity.

In 2006 the US federal government issued new rules that more clearly defined abstinence but also more clearly prohibited dissemination of any positive information about contraception or condoms (Administration for Children and Families 2006). For example, grantees must not 'promote or encourage the use of any type of contraceptives outside of marriage or refer to abstinence as a form of contraception', and must teach that 'contraception may fail to prevent teen pregnancy and that sexually active teens using contraception may become pregnant' (Dailard 2006: 19). Such language reveals an overt bias against condoms and contraception. Such bias reflects the moral beliefs of many in the abstinence movement and directly conflicts with the human right to information.

Medical accuracy of abstinence-only curricula

Assuring the medical accuracy of health education curricula is essential in guaranteeing the human right to information (Santelli 2008). A 2004 review of abstinence-only curricula from the Committee on Government Reform of the US House of Representatives found that 11 of the 13 curricula commonly used in federally supported programmes contained false, misleading or distorted information about reproductive health including inaccurate information about condom and other contraceptive effectiveness, the risks of sexual activity and the risks of abortion, as well as other scientific errors (United States House of Representatives 2004). The Committee also found that some of these curricula promoted gender stereotypes as scientific fact and blurred religious and scientific viewpoints.

We recently examined the accuracy of condom information in three abstinence-only curricula still used by federally grantees (Lin and Santelli 2008). We found that these curricula explicitly and implicitly convey the message that condoms fail to provide protection against HIV, cite out-of-date references, misrepresent cited research, use faulty reasoning to explain infection risk and promote misinformation about condoms (such as pores in latex) that has been repudiated by scientific consensus. We concluded that these curricula do not provide complete, current or accurate medical knowledge about condoms in preventing infection.

Impact of abstinence-only policies on public health programmes

Abstinence-only goals have permeated domestic public health programmes and US foreign aid programmes. Abstinence-only education has replaced more comprehensive forms of sexuality education in many parts of the USA. For example, in 2004 the Texas Board of Education decided to remove most information about contraception from new health education textbooks and today Texas provides almost exclusively abstinence education in its classrooms (Wiley *et al.* 2009). Human rights organisations and popular media have described censure of teachers and students who respond to questions or discuss sexuality topics that are not approved by the school administrators (National Coalition against Censorship 2002) as well as restrictions on access of HIV and AIDS experts to classrooms (Human Rights Watch 2004).

At a national level, surveys on health educational practice provide quantitative evidence of an erosion of comprehensive sexuality education, coincident with the rising emphasis on abstinence education. Between 1988 and 1999, sharp declines occurred in the percentage of teachers who supported teaching and actually taught about birth control, abortion and sexual orientation; in 1999 one-quarter of sex education teachers reported that they were prohibited from teaching about contraception (Darroch *et al.* 2000). Between 1995 and 2002 a declining percentage of young people reported receiving formal education (primarily from schools) about birth control methods while most (>85 per cent) reported receiving abstinence education in both years (Lindberg *et al.* 2006).

An emphasis on abstinence has also influenced other critical public health programmes that serve young people, including US family planning and HIV prevention programmes (Santelli *et al.* 2006; Dailard 2003). Human rights groups have criticised US government policy as a source for misinformation and censorship in countries receiving US foreign aid (Human Rights Watch 2004). Likewise, an emphasis on abstinence appears to have reduced condom availability and access to accurate information on HIV and AIDS in some countries (Human Rights Watch 2004). The President's Emergency Plan for AIDS Relief (PEPFAR), enacted in 2003, required grantees to devote at least 33 per cent of HIV prevention spending to abstinence-until-marriage programmes. These spending requirements – according to the US Government Accountability Office can limit 'efforts to design prevention programmes that are integrated and responsive to local prevention needs' (Government Accountability Office 2006: 2). The US Congress, which in 2008 reauthorised PEPFAR, has continued to impose arbitrary funding directives to encourage abstinence-only-until-marriage programmes, findings by expert agencies regarding their harm notwithstanding (US Agency for International Development 2008).

Implications of abstinence-only education for sexually active youth and gay, lesbian, bisexual, transgender and questioning youth

Abstinence programmes that are geared to young people who have not yet engaged in coitus and who are presumed to be heterosexual systematically ignore the sexual and reproductive health needs of sexually experienced adolescents and gay, lesbian, bisexual, transgender and questioning (GLBTQ) youth. These young people need access to complete and accurate information about contraception and risk reduction, their legal rights to healthcare and ways to access sexual and reproductive health services, none of which is provided in abstinence-only programmes. Abstinence-only programmes largely ignore homosexuality (except when discussing transmission of HIV) or stigmatise homosexuality as deviant and unnatural behaviour (Kempner 2001). Homophobia in schools and communities contributes to health problems such as suicide, feelings of isolation and loneliness, substance abuse, HIV infection and violence among GLBTQ youth (Garofalo and Katz 2001). US federal law and most state laws limit marriage to heterosexual couples. Thus, lifelong abstinence is the implied goal for GLBTQ youth, an unrealistic standard markedly different from that expected of their heterosexual peers.

Ethical and human rights perspectives

The perspectives of both human rights and medical ethics are helpful in analyzing abstinence-only policies and their relationship to adolescent health.

Young people and human rights

Government obligations to protect the human rights of young people are set out in a number of international treaties, including the 1966 International Covenant on Civil and Political Rights (ICCPR), the 1966 International Covenant on Economic,

Social, and Cultural Rights (ICESCR) and the 1989 Convention on the Rights of the Child (CRC). The CRC specifically protects the rights of children up to age 18, and is interpreted and updated by the Committee on the Rights of the Child (Committee on the Rights of the Child, 2003a). Young people of this age are 'active rights holders' i.e. persons with their own rights. The Convention recognises that adolescents demonstrate emerging capacity for independent decisions about health but at the same time deserve continuing special protections, given their unique vulnerabilities. Likewise, parents have responsibilities, legal rights and duties to provide direction and guidance to children and adolescents. Parents' rights and responsibilities should take into account the child's age and maturity while providing a safe and supportive environment. The right to health is recognised in numerous international agreements including Article 25.1 of the Universal Declaration of Human Rights (United Nations 1948), the International Covenant on Economic, Social, and Cultural Rights (1966), the Convention on the Rights of the Child (1989) and the Programme of Action of the International Conference on Population and Development – Cairo 1994 (United Nations 1994).

The specific rights of young people related to health include the right to non-discrimination, the right to express views freely, the right to legal protections about healthcare, the right to information, the right to privacy and confidentiality and right to protection from abuse, neglect, violence and exploitation (Committee on the Rights of the Child 2003b). The right to non-discrimination is inclusive with regard to race, colour, sex, language, religion, political opinion, disability, sexual orientation and health status (including infection with HIV) and national, ethnic or social origin.

The human right to health information

The CRC and the ICCPR both provide that all people have the right to 'seek, receive, and impart information and ideas of all kinds', including information about their health. The Children's Rights Committee and the Committee on Economic, Social and Cultural Rights (the expert body that monitors implementation of the ICESCR) have also emphasised the importance of protecting the right to complete and accurate HIV/AIDS and sexual health information as critical to protecting the right to the highest attainable standard of health (Committee on the Rights of the Child 2003b; Committee on Economic, Social and Cultural Rights 2000). Access to complete and accurate HIV/AIDS and sexual health information has also been recognised as a basic human right and essential to realising the human right to the highest attainable standard of health (Freedman 1995). International treaties and human rights statements support the rights of all people – including young people – to seek and receive information vital to their health:

> All couples and individuals have the basic right to decide freely and responsibly the number and spacing of their children and to have the information, education and means to do so.
>
> (United Nations 1994: Principle 8)

The following statement further emphasises the importance of access to health information as a human right:

Information, education and counseling for responsible sexual behaviour and effective prevention of sexually transmitted diseases and HIV should become integral components of all reproductive and sexual health services.

(United Nations 1994: para. 7.32)

Furthermore, special attention is paid to the importance of meeting the educational and service needs of young people:

As part of their commitment, full attention should be given to the promotion of mutually respectful and equitable gender relations and particularly to meeting the educational and service needs of adolescents to enable them to deal in a positive and responsible way with their sexuality.

(United Nations 1994: para. 7.3)

The UN Committee on the Rights of the Child emphasised in 2003 that:

Consistent with the obligations of States parties in relation to health and information (parts. 24, 13 and 17), children should have the right to access adequate information related to HIV/AIDS prevention and care, through formal channels (e.g. through educational opportunities and child-targeted media) as well as informal channels (e.g. those targeting street children, institutionalised children, or children living in difficult circumstances).

(Committee on the Rights of the Child 2003a: para. 16)

The following is also stated in the same section of the document:

The Committee wishes to emphasise that effective HIV/AIDS prevention requires States to refrain from censoring, withholding, or intentionally misrepresenting health-related information, including sexual education and information ... State parties must ensure that children have the ability to acquire the knowledge and skills to protect themselves and others as they begin to express their sexuality.

(Committee on the Rights of the Child 2003a: para. 16)

These treaties and human rights statements strongly assert that governments have an obligation to provide accurate information to their citizens in government-funded health education.

Medical ethics and health information

Perhaps a more common language than a human rights framework to health workers in the USA is the principles of medical ethics. However, both human rights and medical ethics share common themes that are useful in discussions of young people and adolescents, abstinence policies and the right to information.

The current US approach emphasising abstinence challenges a key ethical principle of medical research and practice known as 'respect for persons' which was central in the developed research ethics in the 1970s and published in the Belmont Report (1979) also called 'respect for autonomy' (Beauchamp and Childress 2001):

> [T]his principle requires respectful treatment in disclosing information and fostering autonomous decision-making ... Respect for autonomy obligates professionals in healthcare and research involving human subjects to disclose information, to probe for and ensure understanding and voluntariness, and to foster adequate decision-making.
>
> (Beauchamp and Childress 2001: 64)

Respect for persons is the ethical principle that underlies the concept of informed consent. Informed consent requires that persons receive accurate and complete information, that information is provided in a way that people can understand the information and that the person is allowed to make a free choice and is not coerced to choose any particular option (National Commission for the Protection of Human Subjects of Biomedical and Behavioral Research 1979). Informed consent is not limited to adults.

Children and adolescents are provided informed consent under the notion of assent which requires that information be presented that is sensitive to a young person's social and cognitive developmental. Adolescents from about age 12 or 14 exhibit many of the cognitive qualities of adults in providing informed consent (Weithorn and Campbell 1982). While assent with minor adolescents is often supplemented by the permission of a parent, this practice never envisions that misinformation be provided to children.

A second principle – the notion of beneficence (i.e. do good and avoid harm) – can also be invoked in considering health education. Health education, whether provided in clinics or classrooms, is designed to do good, that is, to promote health. Health information allows a person to protect his or her health. Accurate health information is necessary – if not always sufficient – to improve or safeguard health. Likewise, complete and accurate health information on sexual and reproductive health is essential to protection against unintended pregnancy and STIs, including HIV. Providing health education might not beneficial if sexuality health education *increased* risk behaviour (e.g. led to earlier sexual initiation) leading to adverse reproductive health outcomes. Considerable scientific evidence finds that access to information through sexuality education *does not* increase risk behaviour (Kirby 2008). Rather the weight of scientific evidence finds that comprehensive sexuality education decreases sexual risk behaviours.

In discussions of abstinence-only education, we have frequently invoked an example from medical ethics. We have described a hypothetical oncologist who presented only the benefits or only the risks of cancer therapy – or who only provided information about the specific treatments but not others that might also be beneficial. The oncologist would be widely denounced as failing in his or her obligations to the patient. Similarly, it is unethical to provide misinformation or withhold information from young people about sexual health, including ways for sexually active young people to protect themselves from STIs and pregnancy. Withholding information on contraception to induce young people to be abstinent is inherently coercive. It violates the principle of beneficence (i.e. do good and avoid harm) as it may cause the individual to use ineffective (or no) protection against pregnancy and STIs.

Summary

US government policies focusing on abstinence-only education or abstinence-until-marriage have multiple problems, including serious ethical and human rights concerns. Programmes are required to withhold information on contraception and to promote scientifically questionable positions. Programmes provide misinformation by overemphasising or mis-stating the risks of contraception. They fail to require the use of scientifically accurate information. Such programmes are inherently coercive – attempting to change young people's behaviour (i.e. promote abstinence) by withholding health information (about contraception). By limiting discussion in the classroom and the clinic, health educators and other public health professionals are placed in a terrible ethical quandary, forcing them to choose to between withholding potentially lifesaving information and breaching US federal government guidelines.

The tide appears to be turning however on support for abstinence-only education. Health professional associations and human rights groups have identified the health and human rights problems with this approach. Concerns about the efficacy and the scientific accuracy of abstinence-only curricula have been raised by researchers and health practitioners. By the end of August 2008 25 US states had rejected federal funding for these programmes (Sexuality Information and Education Council of the United States 2008).

Looking to the future, it is possible to see how human rights perspectives can guide the development of new approaches to sexuality education in the USA and elsewhere. International treaties and human rights documents support the rights of all people, including adolescents, to seek and receive information vital to their health. As such, governments have an obligation to provide accurate information to their citizens in government-funded health education and healthcare services for youth. Likewise, patients and students have rights to accurate and complete information; healthcare providers and health educators have ethical obligations to provide this health information. US government policy can and should embrace a vision for sexuality education grounded in human rights – one that recognises that access to complete and accurate sexual health information is essential if young people are to realise their right to the highest attainable standard of health.

References

Abma, J. C., Martinez, G. M., Mosher, W. E. and Dawson, B. S. (2004) 'Teenagers in the United States: Sexual Activity, Contraceptive Use and Childbearing', *Vital Health Statistics*, 23: 1–87.

Administration for Children and Families (2006) Funding Opportunity No. HHS-2006-ACF-ACYF-AE-0099, 'Community-Based Abstinence Education', Washington, DC: US Department of Health and Human Services.

Albert, B. (2004) *American Opinion on Teen Pregnancy and Related Issues 2003*, Washington, DC: National Campaign to Prevent Teen Pregnancy.

American Academy of Pediatrics (2001) 'Sexuality Education for Children and Adolescents', *Pediatrics*, 108: 498–502.

American College of Obstetricians and Gynecologists (2003) *Sexuality Education. Appendix B: Healthcare for Adolescents*, Washington, DC: ACOG.

American Public Health Association (2005) *Sexuality Education as Part of a Comprehensive Health Education Program in K-12 Schools*, Washington, DC: APHA.

Beauchamp, T. L. and Childress, J. F. (2001) *Principles of Biomedical Ethics*, New York: Oxford University Press.

Bruckner, H. and Bearman, P. (2005) 'After the Promise: The STD Consequences of Adolescent Virginity Pledges', *Journal of Adolescent Health*, 36: 271–8.

Committee on Economic, Social and Cultural Rights (2000) General Comment No. 14: The Right to the Highest Attainable Standard of Health, UN Doc. E/C.12/2000/4; available at www.unhchr.ch/tbs/doc.nsf/(Symbol)/40d009901358b0e2c1256915005090be?Opendocument (accessed 5 April 2009).

Committee on the Rights of the Child (2003a) General Comment 3: HIV/AIDS and the Rights of the Child, UN Doc. CRC/GC/2003/3; available at www.unhchr.ch/tbs/doc.nsf/(symbol)/CRC.GC.2003.3.En?OpenDocument (accessed 3 April 2009).

Committee on the Rights of the Child (2003b) General Comment 4: Adolescent Health and Development in the Context of the Convention on the Rights of the Child, UN Doc. CRC/GC/2003/4; available at www.unhchr.ch/tbs/doc.nsf/(symbol)/CRC.GC.2003.4.En?OpenDocument (accessed 3 April 2009).

Dailard, C. (2002) 'Abstinence Promotion and Teen Family Planning: The Misguided Drive for Equal Funding', *The Guttmacher Report on Public Policy*, 5: 1–3.

Dailard, C. (2003) 'Understanding "Abstinence": Implications for Individuals, Programs and Policies', *The Guttmacher Report on Public Policy*, 6: 4–6.

Dailard, C. (2006) 'The Other Shoe Drops: Federal Abstinence Education Program becomes more Restrictive', *The Guttmacher Policy Review*, 6: 19–20.

Darroch, J. E., Landry, D. J. and Singh, S. (2000) 'Changing Emphases in Sexuality Education in US Public Secondary Schools, 1988–1999', *Family Planning Perspectives*, 32: 204–65.

Finer, L. B. and Henshaw, S. K. (2006) 'Disparities in Rates of Unintended Pregnancy in the United States, 1994 and 2001', *Perspectives on Sexual and Reproductive Health*, 38: 90–6.

Freedman, L. P. (1995) 'Censorship and Manipulation of Reproductive Health Information', in Coliver, S. (ed.) *The Right to Know: Human Rights and Access to Reproductive Health Information*, Philadelphia: University of Pennsylvania Press.

Garofalo, R. and Katz, E. (2001) 'Healthcare Issues of Gay and Lesbian Youth', *Current Opinion in Pediatrics*, 13: 298–302.

Godeau, E., Gabhainn, S. N., Vignes, C., Ross, J., Boyce, W. and Todd, J. (2008) 'Contraceptive Use by 15 year-old Students at their Last Sexual Intercourse – Results from 24 Countries', *Archives of Pediatrics & Adolescent Medicine*, 162: 66–73.

Government Accountability Office (2006) Global Health Spending Requirements Presents Challenges for Allocating Prevention Funding under the President's Emergency Plan for AIDS Relief, GAO-06-395; available at www.gao.gov/new.items/d061089t.pdf (accessed 3 April 2009).

Human Rights Watch (2004) *Access to Condoms and HIV/AIDS Information: A Global Health and Human Rights Concern*, New York: Human Rights Watch.

Kempner, M. (2001) *Toward a Sexually Healthy American: Abstinence-Only-Until-Marriage Programs that Try to Keep Our Youth 'Scared Chaste'*, New York: NY: Sexuality Information and Education Council of the United States.

Kirby, D. (2008) 'The Impact of Abstinence-only and Comprehensive Sex and STD/HIV Education Programs on Adolescent Sexual Behavior', *Sexuality Research and Social Policy*, 5: 18–27.

Lin, A. J. and Santelli, J. S. (2008) 'The Accuracy of Condom Information in three Selected Abstinence-only Education Curricula', *Sexuality Research and Social Policy*, 5: 56–70.

Lindberg, L. D., Santelli, J. S. and Singh, S. (2006) 'Changes in Formal Sex Education: 1995–2002', *Perspectives on Sexual and Reproductive Health*, 38: 182–90.

National Coalition against Censorship (2002) *Abstinence Only Education? A Joint Statement*, New York: National Coalition against Censorship.

National Commission for the Protection of Human Subjects of Biomedical and Behavioral

Research (1979) *The Belmont Report: Ethical Principles and Guidelines for the Protection of Human Subjects of Research*, Washington, DC: US Department of Health and Human Services.

Rector, R. E., Johnson, K. A. and Noyes, L. R. (2003) 'Sexually Active Teenagers Are More Likely to Be Depressed and to Attempt Suicide', Report of the Heritage Center for Data Analysis, CDA03–04.

Rosenbaum, J. E. (2008) 'Patient Teenagers? A Comparison of the Sexual Behavior of Virginity Pledgers and Matched Nonpledgers', *Pediatrics*, 123: e110-e120.

Sandfort, T., Orr, M., Hirsch, J. S. and Santelli, J. (2008) 'Long-term Health Correlates of Timing of Sexual Debut: Results from a National US Study', *American Journal of Public Health*, 98: 155–61.

Santelli, J. (2008) 'Medical Accuracy in Sexuality Education: Ideology and the Scientific Process', *American Journal of Public Health*, 98: 1786–92.

Santelli, J., Ott, M. A., Lyon, M., Rogers, J., Summers, D. and Schleifer, R. (2006) 'Abstinence and Abstinence-only Education: A Review of US Policies and Programs', *Journal of Adolescent Health*, 38: 72–81.

Santelli, J., Sandfort, T. and Orr, M. (2008) 'Transnational Comparisons of Adolescent Contraceptive Use: What can we Learn from these Comparisons?',*Archives of Pediatrics and Adolescent Medicine*, 162: 92–4.

Sexuality Information and Education Council of the United States (2008) 'Sexuality Education and Abstinence-Only-Until-Marriage Programs in the States'; available at www.siecus. org/index.cfm?fuseaction=Page.viewPage&pageId=668&grandparentID=478&parentI D=487 (accessed 6 April 2009).

Society for Adolescent Medicine (2006) 'Abstinence-only Education Policies and Programs: A Position Paper of the Society for Adolescent Medicine' (prepared by Santelli, J., Ott, M. A., Lyon, M., Rogers, J. and Summers, D.), *Journal of Adolescent Health*, 38: 83–7.

US Agency for International Development (2008) *Tom Lantos and Henry J. Hyde United States Global Leadership Against HIV/AIDS, Tuberculosis, and Malaria Reauthorization Act of 2008*, Washington, DC: US Department of Health and Human Services.

US Department of Health and Human Services (2000) *Healthy People 2010: Understanding and Improving Health*, Washington, DC: US Government Printing Office.

Underhill, K., Montgomery, P. and Operario, D. (2007a) 'Sexual Abstinence-only Programmes to Prevent HIV Infection in High-income Countries: Systematic Review', *British Medical Journal*, 335: 248.

Underhill, K., Operario, D. and Montgomery, P. (2007b) 'Systematic Review of Abstinence-plus HIV Prevention Programs in High-income Countries', *PLoS Med*, 4: e275.

United Nations (1948) 'International Bill of Human Rights: A Universal Declaration of Human Rights'; available at www.un.org/en/documents/udhr/ (accessed 12 March 2009).

United Nations (1966) 'International Covenant on Economic, Social and Cultural Rights'; available at www.unhchr.ch/html/menu3/b/a_cescr.htm (accessed 12 March 2009).

United Nations (1989) 'Convention on the Rights of the Child'; available at www.unhchr.ch/ html/menu3/b/k2crc.htm (accessed 12 March 2009).

United Nations (1994) *Report of the International Conference on Population and Development*, New York: United Nations; available at www.un.org/popin/icpd/conference/offeng/poa.html (accessed 3 April 2009).

United States House of Representatives (2004) 'Committee on Government Reform – Minority Staff. The Content of Federally Funded Abstinence-only Education Programs'; available at http://oversight.house.gov/documents/20041201102153-50247.pdf (accessed by 3 April 2009).

Weinstock, H., Berman, S. and Cates, W. (2004) 'Sexually Transmitted Diseases among American Youth: Incidence and Prevalence Estimates, 2000', *Perspectives on Sexual and Reproductive Health*, 36: 610.

Weithorn, L. A. and Campbell, S. B. (1982) 'The Competency of Children and Adolescents to make Informed Treatment Decisions', *Child Development*, 53: 1589–98.

Wiley, D., Wilson, K. and Valentine, R. (2009) *Just Say Don't Know: Sexuality Education in Texas Public Schools*, Austin, TX: Texas Freedom Network Education Fund.

World Health Organisation (2006) 'Defining Sexual Health: Report of a Technical Consultation on Sexual Health', 28–31 January 2002, Geneva; available at www.who.int/reproductive-health/publications/sexualhealth/index.html (accessed 3 April 2009).

37 Bodies and beyond

Where sexual health meets sexual rights

Radhika Chandiramani

Sexual health is both a state of wellbeing as well as an approach to working on issues of sexuality. While one cannot quarrel with the notion of sexual health as a health goal to be attained, as an approach to working on sexuality more generally it has perhaps got some limitations. What, then, is lacking in a sexual health framework? Put in a nutshell, while claiming that sexual health is not just the absence of disease, sexual health work still limits sexuality to bodies and essentialises sexuality as a biological construct. Because of its focus on health, it does not give sufficient weight to non-biological or non-physical expressions and aspects of sexuality such as desires, fantasies and cravings, as well as the gender and power relations that govern gender and sexual expressions.

In the few cases when sexual health extends its ambit to the provision of education, such as in the form of sexuality education and sex and relationships programmes, the perspective is once again often one of prevention – of HIV, STIs, unplanned pregnancy, sexual abuse, all very worthy causes, deserving of attention. But insufficient attention is often given to more positive goals such as the pursuit of happiness, pleasure or of achieving one's full (sexual) potential. Because of their normative focus, notions of sexual health also run the risk of setting up standards of what is to be considered 'sexually healthy', which can become a trap in itself. For instance, monogamy may be promoted as a standard HIV prevention message. But what if Partying Penis and Vagrant Vulva, users of lubricants and condoms, want to have a good time with as many people as they possibly can? Or, what if someone wants to do something that may not be considered 'good' for them, such as participation in sadomasochism or watersports?

These problems and others call for a more expansive framework that recognises that people have different sexual desires, that sex manifests itself and is understood differently in different places and across time (Weeks 1986) and that sexual categories that exist today, such as 'homosexuality' were invented in relatively recent times (Katz 1990). As contributions elsewhere in this volume highlight, there is a growing awareness that gender is also not quite as fixed a category as it was thought to be, and the possibility of authentic expression for gender non-conforming people traverses a range of landscapes, from the beautifully vibrant to the agonisingly bleak.

Crucially, sexual health is not about making lifestyle choices. The woman who lives in poverty and does not use contraception is doing so not because she has made a choice. She may do so in order to protect herself from violence from a husband who beats her up if she suggests the use of condoms. She could use a government-supported injectable contraceptive, you might say, to take care of her contraception-related sexual health. Yes, she could, provided it were proved to be safe, which it is not yet, and she was aware of all the risks. The woman who lives in a mansion and is forced to have yet another abortion because the foetus is female, is doing so not because she has made a choice. It is because her husband and her in-laws with whom she lives are forcing her to do so in a society that values sons over daughters. These are real-life examples from our work on the TARSHI sexuality helpline in New Delhi, India.[1]

For people to achieve sexual health, the material, economic and social conditions affecting their lives need to change. For example, a woman who needs to insert a diaphragm as a method of contraception must have access to clean water in order to wash her hands; an anaemic pregnant woman needs nutritious food; a gender-non-conforming person must be able to find a job and just wages. Callers on the TARSHI helpline reveal their inability to engage in more pleasurable or more frequent sex because of the lack of privacy that results from living in cramped accommodations in which children sleep with their parents. The lack of information in a society where sex is not considered an appropriate topic of education, let alone conversation, and where marriage is arranged for many people, leads to questions on the helpline as well as in sexuality advice columns in newspapers, such as:

> I am going to be married soon, to someone my parents have chosen for me. I am 28 years old, a quiet and shy kind of guy. I barely know the woman who will be my wife. She also seems to be quite shy. Must we have sex on the first night itself? What should I do? How do I go about it?
>
> (Chandiramani 2008: 153)

To achieve sexual health, people must also be able to exercise control over their own sexual lives. Sex as practice is relational, even if there is no other person physically present. Even if there are no bodies in contact with each other, as may be in the case of phone sex or cybersex, there are still two or more imaginations at play, each exerting its power over the other. When it comes to actual bodies in contact, power – and the exchange or assertion of it – becomes more readily apparent, whether it be a consensual or non-consensual sexual encounter. To what degrees are people able to make decisions that empower them to exercise control over their own sexual lives? Who gets to make these decisions and who does not? And, why?

For different groups of people, in various parts of the world, the answers will be different. In some places, it will be the case that young girls have no say in having their clitoris removed or their vagina sewn up; in other contexts, rape is used as a weapon of war on both women and men; in some places, sex between consenting heterosexual adults outside marriage is punished while in others it is variously tolerated, expected and approved of. The list goes on. The factors that govern societal responses to these actions have to do with tradition, laws, religious beliefs, commerce and many other influences that have very little to do with health, sexual or otherwise. We need to go beyond notions of health alone in order to address injustices.

Sexual rights offer such a framework. Sexual rights are based on the core ethical principles of bodily integrity, autonomy, equity and non-discrimination (Corrêa and Petchesky 1994). Sexual rights approach sexuality positively, as a part of life that has the potential to offer excitement, pleasure, comfort, intimacy and all the other joys that sexuality can offer. But sexuality has a dark side as well, and sexual rights seek to prevent and address violence and discrimination that are the reality of many people's sexual lives, for example people who do not conform to gender and sexual norms, rape survivors, sex workers and many other people. If indeed sexuality is integral to and of value to people's lives, this aspect of life is also worthy of human rights protections. Just as women's rights are human rights and reproductive rights are part of human rights, so also sexual rights must be claimed as human rights.

Historically, and as Jane Cottingham's chapter in this volume explains, reproductive rights predate sexual rights in terms of their formal articulation. However, as a notion, sexual rights subsume many reproductive rights. With the advent of new technologies such as assisted reproductive technologies as well as the increasing popularity of adoption, there are also areas where the two sets of rights, reproductive and sexual, do not meet, because now reproduction is not necessarily dependent on sex. As conditions of life change, so also do the demands for rights.

Corrêa and Petchesky (1994) offer a framework of the evolving articulation of sexual rights that includes: the right to be free from discrimination, coercion and violence and rights based on positive ethical principles such as those of bodily integrity (my body is mine), personhood (right to make one's own choices), equality (between and among men, women and transgender people) and respect for diversity (in the context of culture, provided the first three principles are not violated).

It is important to note that the articulation of sexual rights is evolving and is a site of contestation among both its detractors as well as its promoters. As in all sites of political struggle, there are opposing camps, as well as factions within camps. Sexual orientation has been a matter of much debate at the international level of the United Nations (Saiz 2004) since at least 1994. It continues to be. On 18 December 2008 Argentina read a statement supported by 66 states that condemned violations based on sexual orientation and gender identity and endorsed a Declaration on Human Rights, Sexual Orientation and Gender Identity at the UN General Assembly (IGLHRC Press Release, 19 December 2008). In response, 57 other states signed an alternative text read by the delegate from Syria and promoted by the Organisation of the Islamic Conference. According to this counter-statement, notions of sexual orientation and gender identity have no legal foundation and should not be linked to international human rights documents (UN Webcast, 18 December 2008).

The struggle for sexual equality and rights continues at local levels as well and is not limited to matters of sexual orientation. One example is provided by the events around Valentine's Day in India, every year over the last decade, with various right-wing groups threatening and beating up romancing heterosexual couples and the counter-protests by students' unions and civil society groups claiming the 'right to live and love in freedom' (Sharma 2009).

So, how do sexual rights work? Or rather, how might we put them to work? Sexual rights use the principle of consent rather than that of procreation or marriage or the gender of partner to determine what is acceptable sexual behaviour. Consent, in simple terms, means that a person has willingly, of their own free choice, agreed to participate in an activity, with adequate knowledge of its possible consequences. Sexual rights recognise that people bring their own meanings to different sexual acts – that is to say what for one may be highly erotic, for another might be unacceptable (Rubin 1984). This means that a judgmental attitude towards people's gender and sexual expressions (that are practised consensually) is also a form of violence in and of itself. Because this approach privileges the consent and choice of *all* people and not just a few, it encourages work with people who have traditionally been neglected (Miller 2000).

For example, once we acknowledge that people with disabilities have sexual feelings, we will include them in sexuality education programmes and reproductive and sexual health and rights interventions. Ann Finger (1992) points to how the sexuality of people with disabilities is ignored, even within the disability rights movement:

> Sexuality is often the source of our deepest oppression; it is also often the source of our deepest pain. It's easier for us to talk about – and formulate strategies for changing – discrimination in employment, education, and housing than to talk about our exclusion from sexuality and reproduction.
>
> (Finger 1992: www.newint.org/issue233/fruit.htm)

We will also recognise that different groups of people negotiate differently for sexual rights. Take the sexual right to decide if, when and how many children to have, as an example. The struggles in most parts of the world have been and continue to be around women's right to seek an abortion. However, when it comes to women living with a disability or women living with HIV, the struggle is to avoid being coerced into having an abortion, and preceding that, also the struggle to be able to assert their right to engage in sexual activities of their choice. Again, in societies where son-preference exists, the issue is not one of the right to seek an abortion, but of not being forced to abort a female foetus (Visaria 2007).

Similarly, if we are able to discern the differences between sex work and trafficking for sexual exploitation and believe that sex work is best understood as work, and is not always 'exploitation', we will not expend our energies in trying to 'rescue' sex workers and 'rehabilitate' them in meaningless and frequently demeaning ways, but will instead work towards claiming sex workers' rights. This is what one sex worker has to say about her being 'rehabilitated':

> I was also a subject of rehabilitation. They gave me a buffalo. Well, I had this small room [in a house] which I now found myself sharing with the buffalo. You see the buffalo eats a lot, and as I was expected to stop sex work after rehabilitation, there was not much money. I didn't mind for myself, but I couldn't bear to see the buffalo wasting before my eyes. So soon I found myself doing twice the sex work to feed the buffalo and me. Well, now the buffalo was in heat, and I had to get her 'crossed'. I was told that it would cost 100 rupees per attempt. So there I was now being forced to do sex work to pay for the buffalo to have sex! That was enough. I decided I had enough with rehabilitation.
>
> (Revathi 2002: 7)

Sexual rights also push us to look at the question: 'What is our standard of sexual legitimacy?' If we make consent rather than gender our bench mark for acceptability, it allows us to work with and for the rights of same-sex desiring people. For instance, in Colombia, because of the work of the LGBT rights group Colombia Diversa, the human rights group Dejusticia and the Group for Public Interest Rights from the Universidad de los Andes, the Colombian Constitutional Court ruled on

28 January 2009 that same-sex couples must be granted the same rights as those in heterosexual common law marriages. The decree (No. 029 of 2009) grants sweeping civil, political, social, economic, immigration and criminal rights to gay and lesbian couples. Until now, these rights had only been reserved for non-married heterosexual couples (Colombia Diversa 2009).

In India, the Supreme Court is expected to pass a judgement on Section 377 of the Indian Penal Code that criminalises 'carnal intercourse against the order of nature' and is used by the police to harass and extort money from *hijras* and men who have sex with men and, in some instances, also beat and torture them. The arguments to remove Section 377 from the statute book are based on consent, privacy, equality, dignity and the right to health. The last argument is made because Section 377 is also used to harass HIV prevention outreach workers who work in areas where men cruise for sex with other men.

Section 377 presents a case of consensual sexual behaviour being penalised, simply because it is interpreted on the basis of gender even though the wording of the law is gender neutral and in its interpretation could be applied also to heterosexual couples who engage 'in carnal intercourse against the order of nature', simply by using contraception. Strangely, in the same country, non-consensual sexual behaviour in heterosexual marriage is not penalised. Based on consent as a standard, heterosexual married women who face marital rape should be able to take it on as an issue.

Variables such as gender expression, marital status, sexual preference, age, socio-economic status, race, ethnicity, poverty, caste and religion are some of the axes of privilege or discrimination that intersect not only with one another but also with matters of sexuality. An affirming approach to sexuality must necessarily take into account the fact that people live in multiple dimensions and while they might experience privilege in one of these, they might be disadvantaged in another, or that they might be multiply disadvantaged. For example, a young lesbian from a minority ethnic group may be disadvantaged because of her age, sexual preference, gender, marital status and her ethnicity and may therefore not have the same access to sexual health services that a married woman from a dominant ethnicity may have.

By acknowledging that sexual and gender expression take many different forms, sexual rights offer the possibility of being inclusive of *all* people. All over the world, there are vibrant and various ways in which people express their gender and sexual identities – ways that defy simple categorisation of people into man–woman or heterosexual–homosexual. For instance, think of the *travestis* in Latin America, the *warias* in Indonesia or the *hijras* in India. Let us look at age as another example. Sexual rights apply to young and old, not just to people who are in the reproductive age range. Given this, sexual health and sex and relationships education programmes need to go beyond the 15–45 age range.

In the area of policy as well, sexual rights can be used towards ensuring there are policies that uphold and do not violate people's rights. For example, same-sex sexual relations between men are prohibited in more than 80 countries in the world, and in more than half of them this remains as a colonial legacy under which same-sex desiring people are harassed and oppressed (Human Rights Watch 2008). Sexual rights are not just about gay rights or the right to have sex. They engage with people's fundamental rights to equality and privacy. For example, the Basic Law in Hong Kong states that all residents of Hong Kong shall be treated equally before the law and are entitled to protection under the law without any discrimination. In 2005 a young gay man in Hong Kong, William Leung, then 20 years old, mounted a challenge to the laws which criminalise consensual sex between men aged over 16 years but under 21 years while allowing sex between consenting heterosexuals aged 16 and over. This led to an amendment to the law lowering the age of consent for sex for homosexuals in Hong Kong in August 2006.

Sexual rights also require us to analyse the underlying motives with which funding support is given. The US President's Emergency Plan for AIDS Relief (PEPFAR) has until recently endorsed the ABC approach (Abstain, Be faithful, use Condoms) and mandated that 33 per cent of the HIV prevention funds be used for abstinence-until-marriage programmes. This was changed in 2008 to requiring organisations that spent less than 50 per cent of their funds on abstinence-only programmes to explain why they did so (obviously pressurising them to spend more) (PlusNews, 21 January 2009). Given the circumstances and realities of many people's lives, this is an entirely inappropriate proposition. For instance, how many women, especially in regions like Asia and Africa, have the power to insist on their male partners being 'faithful', let alone use condoms or be abstinent? Joke van Kampen from Malawi offers a searing critique of how the ABC approach is leading to a D – D for disaster – in Africa. Her arguments are valid in other parts of the world as well, as she notes how unrealistic the approach is and points out the gender double standards that it perpetuates as well as the inaccurate connections that it creates. She says:

> In a sort of strange side effect of the abstinence mantra, manuals on sex education linger on virginity for pages. While virginity might seem a desirable state of being to some people, it is as useful in HIV/AIDS prevention as advising people to stay inside in order to reduce traffic accidents. Full blown double standards go unchallenged in the virginity discourse, since virgins are, we all know this, female.
>
> The same double standards are resulting in hilarious communication hazards. One of the many NGOs here that were circulating messages on the occasion of World AIDS Day published two posters here: one portraying women in a village, pouring maize, the other portraying men drinking beer and playing trick track (ok, let's not split hairs here). The theme of World AIDS Day being Keeping the Promise, the women on the poster say: 'I promise to be mutually faithful', the men promise 'to reduce the number of my sexual partners'. Apart from the fact that it is hard to imagine how an individual can promise to be mutual, note that these promises, when kept, will lead to infection indeed.
>
> (Kampen 2006: www.comminit.com/drum_beat_345.html)

In addition to this disastrous intervention, recent US law has also required organisations receiving US global HIV/AIDS and anti-trafficking funds to adopt the anti-prostitution oath. This means that organisations cannot in any way be seen to support prostitution. Therefore, organisations that work to support sex workers' rights to health, clean water, food, health services, education for their children and other meaningful forms of employment are thwarted in their aims, and are also not able to use the skills that sex workers have to train others including rural youth on safer sex practices. PEPFAR Watch has evidence that these restrictions are already undermining promising interventions. As Meena Seshu, who works with people in prostitution, says:

> Many of the women I work with are what are known as *devadasis*, called temple prostitutes in some parts of India. For them, prostitution is a way of life. The fact is some of the women are strong fighters, who negotiate with the police, who negotiate with health systems and doctors all the time, and come out with flying colors. And they're the best educators of their male clients I have seen. These women are able to talk to them straight. All of the truths we'd assumed were challenged by them. There are women here. They're saying something. Isn't it right that we listen?
>
> (Kaplan 2006: www.alternet.org/rights/33284?page=2)

And, of course, as Françoise Girard has pointed out:

> These are only some of the sexuality-related policies of the Bush Administration. They nevertheless give an idea of the Administration and their allies in Congress in their drive to remake America and the world in line with their moral and religious values. Sexuality is not an afterthought, but a center piece of their thinking. Large sums of money are being spent to make this vision of a mythical, heterosexual, conjugal sexual past, a reality.
>
> (Girard 2004: 30)

Fortunately, with a recent change of administration in the USA there are some signs of improvement. It has been announced, for example, that the 'Mexico City Policy' has been revoked (ABC News, 23 January, 2009). This regulation, also called the 'global gag rule' by abortion rights activists, prohibited the use of Federal funds by international family planning groups to promote or perform abortions, even if the funding for these activities came from other sources. This resulted in a lack of sexual and reproductive health services for countless women and was a serious violation of their sexual and reproductive rights.

That is why we need to get beyond bodies and health to see how we can build on and promote sexual rights for all – for young people who may be vulnerable and marginalised, for lesbians and gays and other same-sex desiring people who may not yet have a name for themselves, for indigenous as well as rural women, for people with disabilities and also for heterosexuals who, because of their very 'ordinariness', may be neglected, apart from being 'targeted' by HIV prevention interventions that do not take pleasurable sexuality into account. Sexual rights are for all, not just the chosen few.

Note

1 The TARSHI helpline has been operating for 13 years and has responded to more than 60,000 calls from people between the ages of 10 and 70+ years. For more information, see www.tarshi.net

References

ABC News (2009) 'Obama Overturns "Mexico City Policy" implemented by Reagan'; available at http://abcnews.go.com/Politics/International/story?id=6716958&page=1 (accessed 26 February 2009).

Chandiramani, R. (2008) *Good Times for Everyone: Sexuality Questions, Feminist Answers*, New Delhi: Women Unlimited.

Colombia Diversa (2009) 'Colombia's Constitutional Court Rules for Equality – Same Sex Couples', SOGI online posting; available email: Sogi@list.arc-international.net (accessed 31 January 2009).

Corrêa, S. and Petchesky, R. (1994) 'Reproductive and Sexual Rights: A Feminist Perspective', in Sen, G., Germain, A. and Chen, L. C. (eds) *Population Policies Reconsidered: Health, Empowerment and Rights*, Boston, MA: Harvard University Press.

Finger, A. (1992) 'Forbidden Fruit', *New Internationalist*, 233; available at www.newint.org/issue233/fruit.htm (accessed 16 February 2009).

Girard, F. (2004) 'Global Implications of US Domestic and International Policies on Sexuality', International Working Group on Sexuality and Social Policy, Mailman School of Public Health, Columbia University. (Working Paper No. 1)

Human Rights Watch (2008) 'This Alien Legacy: The Origins of "Sodomy" Laws in British Colonialism'; available at www.hrw.org/en/node/77014/section/2 (accessed 15 February 2009).

IGLHRC Press Release (2008) 'United Nations: General Assembly Statement Affirms Rights for All', 19 December; available at www.iglhrc.org/cgi-bin/iowa/article/pressroom/pressrelease/826.html (accessed 16 February 2009).

Kaplan, E. (2006) 'Pledges and Punishment', in *AlterNet*; available at www.alternet.org/rights/33284?page=2 (accessed 15 March 2006).

Katz, J. (1990) 'The Invention of Heterosexuality', *Socialist Review*, 20 (1): 7–34.

Miller, A. (2000) 'Sexual but not Reproductive: Exploring the Junction and Disjunction of Sexual and Reproductive Rights', *Health and Human Rights*, 4 (2): 69–109.

PEPFAR Watch; available at www.pepfarwatch.org/index.php?option=com_content&task=view&id=23&Itemid=37 (accessed 20 January 2009).

PlusNews (2009) 'A New and Improved PEPFAR under Obama?'; available at www.plusnews.org/Report.aspx?ReportId=82494 (accessed 3 February 2009).

Revathi (2002) 'Buffalo Blues', *Of Veshyas, Vamps, Whores and Women*, (1) 2: 7.

Rubin, G. (1984) 'Thinking Sex: Notes for a Radical Theory of the Politics of Sexuality', in Vance, C. S. (ed.) *Pleasure and Danger: Exploring Female Sexuality*, Boston, MA: Routledge & Kegan Paul.

Saiz, I. (2004) 'Bracketing Sexuality: Human Rights and Sexual Orientation – A Decade of Development and Denial at the UN', *Health and Human Rights*, 7 (2): 48–81.

Sharma, P. (2009) 'Delhi Celebrates "the Right to Live and Love in Freedom"', *The Hindu*, 15 February; available at www.hindu.com/2009/02/15/stories/2009021557130100.htm (accessed 15 February 2009).

UN Webcast (2008) available at www.un.org/webcast/ga.html.

van Kampen, J. (2006) 'The ABC Disaster', *The Drum Beat*, 345; available at www.comminit.com/drum_beat_345.html (accessed 16 February 2009).

Visaria, L. (2007) 'Sex-selective Abortion in Gujarat and Haryana: Some Empirical Evidence', in Visaria, L. and Ramachandran, V. (eds) *Abortion in India: Ground Realities*, New Delhi: Routledge/Taylor & Francis Group.

Weeks, J. (1986) *Sexuality*, London: Tavistock.

38 Political agents or vulnerable victims?

Framing sexual rights as sexual health in Argentina

Mario Pecheny

In 1998 I wrote a paper with the title 'Sexual Orientation, AIDS, and Human Rights in Argentina: The Paradox of Social Advance Amidst Health Crisis' (Pecheny 2003). In this optimistic text, I described how the HIV epidemic helped redefine the status of homosexuality and contributed to the promotion of gay rights. That process was not exceptional. Since the 1980s, HIV and AIDS have been a window of opportunity to render homosexuals visible, foster social movements and NGOs and advance the recognition of gay rights almost everywhere (Altman 1994; Roberts 1995).

Concurrently, advocacy for reproductive health has helped the advance of women's status. Human rights, population and women's issues came together in the promotion of women's empowerment and autonomy (Marques-Pereira 1995; Pecheny 2002). International United Nations Conferences in Vienna (1993), Cairo (1994) and Beijing (1995), and subsequent national and regional conferences have provided transnational public spheres in which women – and men – can discuss the relationship between health, rights, gender and sexuality, contributing to political action and networking at local, national and global levels (Petchesky 2003; Corrêa *et al.* 2008).

In Latin America, such events coincided with the transition from authoritarian regimes to formal democracies. Since the 1980s the rule of law, liberal rights, free elections and legitimate social mobilisations have become defining features of the political landscape in countries such as Argentina.

Considering these global processes of sexual and gender advance – in addition to political democratisation – why not be optimistic? Why not recognise the value of recent struggles and the advance of political and sexual rights? Intelligent pessimism, as Gramsci (1977: 19) put it, invites us to rethink some of the tensions inherent to these processes. In this chapter, I want to examine if and how the short-term politicisation of sexuality through health exists in tension with a broader and longer term process of the depoliticisation of sexuality and gender relations. According to my hypothesis, if HIV and reproductive health have contributed to the greater recognition of reproductive and sexual rights, they have done so in ways that need to be critically analysed: through allied processes of victimisation (or victimism), medicalisation and judicialisation.

In sexual and reproductive health, as well as in the first wave of sexual rights, subjects were framed as victims: victims of unwanted pregnancies, violence, HIV or social and gender inequalities. Little room was left for political agency, collective projects and historical and structural thinking. We witness now a gradual movement from sexual health to sexual rights. This process opens the door to repoliticise sexuality.

However, the original framing has installed the idea that powerful, publicly speaking up and acting subjects – that is, *political* subjects – are suspect.

We can witness here a particular dynamic: the more sexual an issue or a subject appears to be, the more 'political' it is. Yet such actions are political in a specific and stigmatised way: considered as particular, interest based and conflictive. Inversely, the more desexualised an issue or a subject appears to be, the more apolitical it is: considered as impersonal, value or interest free and in harmony with the social order. The challenge, therefore, lies in how to sexualise and politicise issues and subjects in a democratic way, and in the direction of erotic justice.

If we rethink sexuality and politics dialectically, it is possible to identify three key moments in recent Latin American history. First, the widespread use of health discourse as a vehicle for the promotion of sexual rights. Second, the recognition of health discourse as an obstacle to the evolution of sexual rights. Third, the questioning of both health and rights languages as forms of depoliticisation of sexuality practices, parallel to the recognition of sexuality practices as inherently conflictive, and as impossible to reduce to the rational, the public and the normative.[1]

In this chapter, I discuss these issues using the experience of Argentina and other Latin American countries as a case study. I draw examples from the fields of reproductive health, abortion, feminist politics and women's rights, HIV and AIDS, sexual liberation politics and lesbian, gay, bisexual and transgender (LGBT) rights, in order to ask to what extent the language of health and rights is hindering the constitution of sexual subjects and the idea and practice of erotic justice.

Victims or subjects: the depoliticisation of sexual issues

In Latin America, sexual rights have advanced thanks to the incorporation of health issues, in particular reproductive health and HIV, in the public agenda. However, both conceptually and in practice, these advances increasingly reveal the existence of limitations, tensions and contradictions. In other words, the language of health obliterates the advance, diversification and deepening of sexual rights. We might as well ask to what extent the language of gender (in its equating of gender with women and in its desexualised versions) and the language of rights itself have lost their potential for social transformation.

In the policy domain, sexuality issues have been rendered as amenable to political decision making and policy intervention. In the domain of rights, similar processes of framing have also led to forms of depoliticisation. As a result, sexuality remains hidden behind languages that inherently violate its logic: the languages of health policies as well as the language of formal, positive and enforceable rights. These liberal languages suppose identifiable and stable subjects, and the possibility of ownership of one's body, in contradiction with alternative practices that are more substantive, fluid and blurred.

Latin American societies have developed a sexual rights agenda and sexuality-related policies since the last wave of democratisation, in the 1980s and 1990s. Advances have been recorded in fields such as civil rights equity for women and men; access to contraception and sex education; freedom of sexual expression and diversity; access to abortion (in a few cases); redress for sexual and gender violence; HIV/AIDS; sex work; and transgender rights. There are key pending issues, but a long road has been travelled, which provides a degree of optimism (Cabal *et al.*

2001; Pecheny 2003; Amuchástegui and Rivas 2004; Vianna and Lacerda 2004; Amuchástegui and Aggleton 2007; Petracci and Pecheny 2007; Dides *et al.* 2008).

However, this agenda often presupposes the notion of sexual victims rather than sexual subjects (Raupp Rios 2004). In sexual and reproductive health, as well as in reproductive and sexual rights, subjects were originally framed as victims. For example, abortion is often more visible as a maternal mortality issue than as a woman's right to choose her own sexuality and reproduction; and abortion is framed as an individual moral decision or as an involuntary individual fate, rather than the product of gender and class structural relations of inequality and oppression. Social movements often reinforce these ideas and crystallise social interactions based on a logic of the competition among victims, within each social movement and between social movements (Pecheny 2004; Kapur 2005; Polletta 2006). This hegemonic 'victimist' framing makes powerful, publicly speaking up and acting political subjects less entitled to rights than to reparations or privileges.

By depoliticisation, I mean the ideological eradication of structural conflicts. After long periods of dictatorship and violent struggle, political conflicts are conceived of today as susceptible of being resolved. The new democratic regimes have framed political conflict as clashes of opinions, rather than the results of social contradictions that may not be amenable to consensus or even compromise. Institutional politics, by definition, institutionalises social conflicts. The possibility of institutionalisation separates 'civilised' from 'barbaric', Hobbesian social interactions (Benasayag and del Rey 2007). Institutional democracies tolerate conflicts and conflictive actors only when they are able to fit within the norms of this institutionalisation.

How then can societies coexist with their oppressed, inadmissible conflicts? In political theory, the paradigmatic case is the problematic coexistence of capitalism and democracy (Przeworski 1986), but gender relations and particularly sexualised relations or sexuality practices are also at the root of conflicts hard to institutionalise through normal politics. Normal politics implies the construction of conflicts as decidable issues within the political agenda and as the potential objects of public policy. Conflicts framed as clashes of opinions rely on the liberal assumption that all individuals have an equally valuable point of view. The idea that opinions are organically linked to structural and radical conflicts contradicts the vision of an ultimately harmonic order that lies at the base of formal democracy. Political order only institutionalises conflicts that do not question its own foundations.

In addition, governments implement policies on legitimate issues. According to its own validity claim, democratic legitimacy depends on formal procedures such as the majority rule, in a context of fairness. Even within this idealised state, the scope of government tasks means that there is no rational argument for accepting majority rule if this will lead to decisions on topics that ought to remain free from government interference and/or which are beyond politics. Sexuality practices constitute one such area in which government intervention is problematic. It is the self-image of democratic legitimacy that fosters this paradox: the more sexual an issue or a subject appears to be, the more it is considered as personal, conflictive – in other words, beyond democratic legitimacy and government's legitimate interference.

In this context, how should the sexual nature of some issues and subjects be taken into account in the pursuit of erotic justice? As Sonia Corrêa (2007: 12) has put it:

A challenge sexuality and development thinkers must tackle is to consolidate sexual rights as a foundation of erotic justice. Erotic justice endorses principles of pleasure, fulfilment and delight in sexuality, consent in sexual practices between partners, and a public climate that restricts violence, stigma and discrimination. This concept is inspired by Gayle Rubin (1984). Erotic justice should have the same policy legitimacy as the long-standing and widely accepted principle of social justice and the more recently recognised premise of gender justice.

Erotic justice provides a potent political discourse for actors making claims within the public sphere, but it is less useful as a guide for institutional politics and public policies. Translating principles of erotic justice into laws and policies is more difficult than the cases of social and gender justice. What should be the role of the state in respecting, fulfilling and promoting erotic justice (García and Parker 2006)? What measures and policies can social movements claim? Who are accountable, and what are they accountable for? What is the connection between social justice and erotic justice?

Since the 1980s and the new wave of democratisation, an evolution of sexual rights and a transition from gender- and sex-based inequalities to more equal relations or patterns have been recorded in most Latin American countries. In spite of some pending issues – such as the decriminalisation of abortion – the process of evolution has been so rapid that it may be perceived as the manifestation of linear progress. Nevertheless, there are critical contradictions within sexual democratisation, as well as serious tensions in the political democratisation processes throughout the region.

The consolidation of formal democracies, together with the rule of law, political liberalisation and processes of citizenship (i.e. processes that encourage individuals to consider themselves the subjects of rights (Amuchástegui Herrera and Rivas 2004; Paiva 2003, 2006)), are crucial for political democratisation. By political democratisation, I mean that the scope of rights recognition, as well as that of citizenship, increasingly extends to reach a larger number of subjects and a wider range of matters. New categories of subjects have access to acknowledged rights; societies and legal systems acknowledge new rights; rights contents expand; and the field of application of rights broadens (Lefort 1981, 1986; Jelín 1996; Pecheny 2002).

As a dynamic process, political democratisation implies reflecting on the politicisation of relations and matters framed as necessary, natural and/or private. Ideologically, structural social relations have been constructed as though they are necessary, essential or unavoidable (i.e. they could not be otherwise), as private (i.e. in opposition to the political and the public domains); and as natural (i.e. not social and cultural). A process of politicisation implies shedding light on the fact that social relations are contingent (i.e. are not inevitably so), that they are not (purely) private and that they do not derive from a natural order (Pecheny 2002). This alternative political framing authorises social actors to act politically in a transformative direction.

Sexual democratisation refers to patterns of greater equity in personal relations and the contestation of the frontiers between legitimate sexual practices, identities and relations, as illustrated by Gayle Rubin's (1984) well-known binary oppositions between good, natural and blessed sex and bad, unnatural and sinful sex. In a narrow sense, sexual democratisation means the recognition, protection and promotion by the state of rights related to sexuality. Let us consider here the politicisation of sexuality in a context of democratisation through neoliberal and neopopulist forms. For the purpose of this chapter, I do not consider these forms as exclusive, but as a continuum; since the 1990s, Latin American neoliberalism has been compatible with historically populist parties, discourses, identities and folklore.

Particularly since the International Conferences on Human Rights (Vienna 1993), Population (Cairo 1994) and Women (Beijing 1995) and in the context of recurrent structural adjustment and neoconservative reduction of political demands, one of the most common strategies for advancing claims for sexual rights has been to frame them as public health needs (Pecheny 2003; Parker *et al.* 2004). Simultaneously, advances in health have permitted the promotion of sexual rights, because even in contexts of privatisation and neoliberal reform, health is still recognised as a universal good. A Latin American colleague once said, quite ironically: 'Because in my country we do not have high rates of maternal deaths related to abortion, it is more difficult to demand the decriminalisation of abortion'. Her comment illustrates a common feeling among activists. In the region, many feminists find that public health's need to reduce maternal deaths is a more effective argument for the decriminalisation of abortion than is a demand for women's sexual rights.

To what extent is health discourse a useful strategy or an ideological perspective? To what extent have the gains been obtained at the price of their depoliticisation? Politicisation, which involves both argument and struggle, is a process through which social relations are resignified as contingent, as political and public, as well as socially, culturally and historically constructed. This process presupposes the recognition of conflicts inherent to a particular historical moment and social structure. In addition, politicisation is a process by which individual, isolated experiences are inscribed within a broader collective experience, in the sense that 'I am not the only one'. Take, for example, the experience of assuming one's HIV seropositivity. For many years, most individuals who received an HIV diagnosis experienced this moment alone, isolated from others (Terto 2000; Pecheny and Manzelli 2008). A politicisation of seropositivity occurred when individuals were able to make sense of their own personal experiences within a community of peers (Pecheny 2002; Paiva 2003).

Other subjects face similar situations of isolation: a young person who realises s/he has desires for a person of the same sex; a rape victim; a girl or a woman with amenorrhoea who faces the possibility of terminating a pregnancy; and a victim of sexual violence. In all of these cases, politicisation means the inscription of individual experiences within a larger whole. Something that 'does not happen to me as a woman', but happens to us 'as women', provides a way of politicising an individual experience. Such a process allows for the possibility of recognising sexual questions not (only) as individual destinies, but as framed by conflicts intrinsic to a structure of unjust and/or unequal social relationships at a particular historical moment.

In contrast, depoliticisation processes entail concealing or sequestering the historical, structural and political character of specific practices and relations. Depoliticisation can take different forms. Victimisation (or victimism) assumes that individuals or groups deserve to be listened to in their claims only as the victims of injustices, and not as the full subjects of rights. Medicalisation supposes that social problems can be framed and solved objectively by the intervention of doctors and the medical system. Judicialisation refers to the notion that claims should be brought before judges in individual cases, and that injustices should be resolved in terms of individual reparations.

In Latin America, these three mechanisms have allowed for advances in sexual rights, provided individual reparations and improved the relative position of subaltern groups, but at the price of fragmentation and competence between groups. They have stimulated between 'victims', a perverse competition whose characteristics are consistent with current processes of social disarticulation and with neoliberal political dynamics (Pecheny 2004).

Throughout the region, procreation, abortion, HIV and AIDS, gender, sexual education, gay and lesbian rights, transgender identity, sex work, etc. are usually framed as public health, human rights and/or population issues or policies, rather than as issues of sexuality. The sexual dimensions of an issue (practice, problem) are usually silenced, by policy- and decision-makers but also by activists and social movements. Depoliticisation is thus intimately linked to desexualisation.

Victimisation is the process through which situations of misfortune or injustice (Shklar 1990) are signified from the perspective of victims who need or ask for reparation – 'I can speak because of what happened, it happened to me; what happened to me gives me the authority, the dignity, to be listened to and get a response'. Victimisation confers moral virtues and personal dignity on individuals or groups (Polletta 2006). Sometimes it may be necessary to add a redundant adjective before the term victim as in 'innocent' victims, as if 'guilty' victims might deserve less.

As a way of obtaining a response, strategies of victimisation have provided benefits to different individuals and groups. However, victimisation reaffirms individual stigma and disempowers the collective. When a rape victim appears as a sexed, sexual and desiring subject, her claim for reparations from the act of sexual violence becomes suspect. It seems as if a pure victim, incapable of acting and devoid of desire and reasoning, better deserves her rights than a full person who is the subject of her own body, actions and reason.[2] In the long term, victimisation contributes to depoliticising conflicts and to the incapacity of acting politically. It hinders the constitution of subjects as political subjects and as collective ones and hinders the possibility of framing social claims as universal. Consequently, victimisation strategies tend to social fragmentation and reducing structural conditions to individual situations.

Victimhood's temporality is also problematic: is one a victim at the very moment of the victimising acts or does one remain a victim 'forever'? Given that being a victim is a short-term state and/or it refers to the past, victimism impedes structural and strategic thought. Although it works, it responds to a model of individual amends and avoids a commitment to a more universalising model of rights. This phenomenon happens at national and global levels. By supporting 'those who suffer the most', well-intentioned, patronising international donors, non-governmental organisations and government agencies encourage this way of acting.

Moreover, victimism renders political representation logically impossible, as in claims such as 'You're not HIV positive, so you have no say in this' or 'There are no lesbians on the panel!' Only authentic victims can speak in the name of other victims, and ultimately only a victim can speak for herself. When it comes to sexual issues, it is common to find this pre-modern idea of representation, which defines it as physical representation, rather than a more modern notion of representation, which is an abstract one. Should the represented subject always be physically 'there'? Should everybody be mentioned on a panel or in a committee, paper, law or policy, in order to 'be represented'? This kind of physical representation becomes a key aspect of the competition among victims: to be visible, named, mentioned, specified, and not be subsumed into any form of abstract or universal category.

Victimisation obliterates and impedes the possibility of acting responsibly and speaking of plurality, which, according to Arendt (1992), are the human condition of politics. As agency and expression imply suspicion, the rights of the victim remain linked to silence and helplessness. It is possible to think, as Bruckner (1995) has pointed out, that victimisation is but a fake version of privilege. We are no longer in the field of universal rights here, but in the field of privileges derived from suffering.

Radical victimisation raises aspects that are more controversial. The idea of the absolute victim justifies, in a Hobbesian dynamic, any measure of her part. If my own being is at risk, everything is justified. The victim is sacralised, in a religious sense.

If we agree that victims do not speak nor act, then the dead, the disappeared, embryos, foetuses (Boltanski 2004), the dying or animals, are victims par excellence. All these are absolute innocents, and so they are right a priori. This a priori rightness is non-political and, to some extent, non-human. By definition, pure victims do not speak out. There is a large gap between silence and political discourses. Is silence a political discourse without the context of a hermeneutic process of signification of that silence as political? The political performance of different discourses is critical. In this sense, how performatively powerful are silence, complaints, ironies and protests?

An individual complaint is a discourse that returns to itself, powerless, with no consequences. This typically 'feminine' discourse remains at the private level (Amorós-Puente 1990). At the private level too, we also find the irony, a discourse that allows an individual to look, in perspective, at themselves in his or her own situation. This is the gay or Jewish discourse (Kaplan 1997): not powerless, yet not powerful either, because subjects need to introduce their political claims into the public sphere. In public, they become the contentious discourses of protest, of political confrontation in a conflictive situation. As such, the contradiction between speaking subjects and speechless victims becomes clear.

Victimisation is particularly harmful for the politicisation of sexuality. Pro-choice and anti-abortion sides each identify their own victims. Debate becomes impossible at this point. The embryo, the 'unborn child', incapable of agency, is an absolute victim, while women are also reduced to non-subjects. Victims are transparent, while subjects are contradictory. The subjective experience of abortion is not coherent, neither is public opinion, while the absolute victim always displays coherence. The unborn child has the right to life from the time of conception, and this is coherent with how this figure has been constructed (Bajos and Ferrand 2006). Arendt (1997) warned, too, against coherent political discourse deductive principles of action, potentially leading to totalitarianism.

My argument here against victimisation does not deny the existence of persons who are victims of something or someone (Cole 2007). Critics of victimisation do not deny the atrocities or inequalities that have caused victims to suffer. The main problem lies in the construction of victims as subjectivities devoid of the potential for becoming political subjects. To accompany someone, to join someone in his or her tragedy, is not the same as to join a collective fight for the future, in positive or utopian terms. In other words, this form of depoliticisation also renders compromises and alliances among different social actors impossible.

Concluding remarks

Recent Latin American history shows a political evolution in sexual matters. However, the politicisation and depoliticisation of sexuality through processes of victimisation, medicalisation and judicialisation invites us to rethink the link between sexuality and politics. These phenomena are, of course, part of broader processes of depoliticisation and objectivation of social practices. Practices and claims are legitimate only when they appear to be impersonal or neutral. In capitalist societies, the logics of social action are ideologically homogenised, as in the case of capitalists and workers (Offe 1985). Different degrees of interest are determined by structural differences of class position, and available political forms of liberal democracy provide the members of different classes with unequal chances of articulating their interests (Offe and Wiesenthal 1985). Critics of political democracies have shown that structural class inequalities are critical to determining the social conditions of formal equality and, inversely, how formal political equality has contributed to the reproduction of class inequalities. In a similar sense, concepts such as sexual citizenship and/or intimate citizenship have recovered this kind of approach to examine political equality in relation to structural differences based on gender and sexuality (Plummer 2003; Cáceres *et al.* 2004; Corrêa *et al.* 2008). In other words, these concepts may help us understand how inequalities based on gender and sexuality determine the social conditions of political equality and, inversely, how formal political equality has contributed to the reproduction of gender and sexuality-related inequalities.

Contemporary Latin American societies tend to repress both class and gender/sexuality structural and historical conflicts. If politics is a way of transforming unequal and unjust social relations, processes of depoliticisation should be analysed critically. Processes of depoliticisation conceal the political nature of sexuality practices, which parallels the ideological process of the concealment of sexualised political dimensions in social relationships. Both politicisation and sexualisation make conflicts visible and mobilise passions. In contrast, depoliticisation and desexualisation objectify sexuality and other social practices. They make social practices impersonal and consistent with the rational-bureaucratic legitimacy of health policies.

Objectivation takes place through the language of public health, but also in the language of gender (most usually in non-relational versions of gender as women) and the language of rights (premised on coherently identifiable sexed/gendered subjects). All these processes and languages related to policy legitimacy reify and homogenise the diversity of projects of happiness, including those related to sex, eroticism and loving relationships.

When we rethink sexuality and politics dialectically, three key moments in recent Latin American history can be identified: health discourse as a vector of sexual rights; health discourse as an obstacle to the evolution of sexual rights; and both health and rights as veiled forms of the depoliticisation of sexuality practices. My analysis of these processes shows the limits policies have when dealing with sexuality, and the value of politics considered as inherently conflictual.

According to Honnig (1993: 15):

> To affirm the perpetuity of the contest is not to celebrate a world without points of stabilisation; it is to affirm the reality of perpetual contest, even within an ordered setting, and to identify the affirmative dimension of contestation.

At the same time, this analysis invites us to think about more strategic, contextual, long-term policies, geared towards creating more favourable environments for local, subaltern political struggles, as well as more favourable environments for sexual and erotic practices.

Notes

1 I use here the expression 'sexuality practices' to emphasise that I am talking of social practices, experiences and actions rather than of an epistemic field.
2 Interestingly, the Penal Code in Argentina allows abortion only in the case of danger to the life or health of the pregnant woman; and when the pregnancy results from a rape committed to a woman legally declared insane or mentally retarded.

References

Altman, D. (1994) *Power and Community. Organizational and Cultural Responses to AIDS*, London: Taylor & Francis.

Amorós-Puente, C. (1990) *Mujer: Participación, Cultura Política y Estado*, Buenos Aires: de la Flor.

Amuchástegui Herrera, A. and Rivas Zivy, M. (2004) 'Los Procesos de Apropiación subjetiva de los Derechos Sexuales: Notas para la Discusión', *Estudios Demográficos y Urbanos*, 19 (3): 543–97.

Amuchástegui, A. and Aggleton, P. (2007) '"I had a Guilty Conscience because I wasn't Going to Marry Her": Ethical Dilemmas for Mexican Men in their Sexual Relationships with Women', *Sexualities*, 10 (1): 61–81.

Arendt, H. (1992) *Condition de l'Homme Moderne*, Paris: Agora.

Arendt, H. (1997) *L'Impérialisme*, Paris: Seuil.

Ayres, J. R. (2002) 'Conceptos y Prácticas en Salud Pública: Algunas Reflexiones', *Revista Facultad Nacional de Salud Pública* (Colombia), 20 (2): 67–82.

Bajos, N. and Ferrand, M. (2006) 'La Condition fœtale n'est pas la Condition humaine', *Travail, Genre et Sociétés*, 15: 176–82.

Benasayag, M. and del Rey, A. (2007) *Éloge du Conflit*, Paris: La Découverte.

Boltanski, L. (2004) *La Condition fœtale. Une Sociologie de l'Engendrement et de l'Avortement*, Paris: Gallimard.

Bruckner, P. (1995) *La Tentation de l'Innocence*, Paris: Grasset.

Cabal, L., Roa, M. and Lemaitre, J. (eds) (2001) *Cuerpo y Derecho. Legislación y Jurisprudencia en América latina*, Bogota: Termis.

Cáceres, C., Frasca, T., Pecheny, M. and Terto Jr., V. (eds) (2004) *Ciudadanía Sexual en América Latina: Abriendo el Debate*, Lima: Universidad Peruana Cayetano Heredia.

Cole, A. M. (2007) *The Cult of True Victimhood: From the War on Welfare to the War on Terror*, Stanford: Stanford University Press.

Corrêa, S. (2007) 'Realising Sexual Rights', available at www.ids.ac.uk/ids/bookshop/outputs/RealisingSRids.pdf (accessed 12 December 2008).

Corrêa, S., Petchesky, R. and Parker, R. (2008) *Sexuality, Health and Human Rights*, London and New York: Routledge.

Dides, C., Marques, A., Guajardo, A. and Casas, L. (2008) *Chile: Panorama de Sexualidad y Derechos humanos*, Santiago: FLACSO/CLAM.

García, J. and Parker, R. (2006) 'From Global Discourse to Local Action: The Making of a Sexual Rights Movement?', *Horizontes Antropológicos*, 12 (26): 13–41.

Gramsci, A. (1977) *Pasado y Presente*, Buenos Aires: Granica.

Honnig, B. (1993) *Political Theory and the Displacement of Politics*, Ithaca, NY: Cornell University Press.

Jelín, E. (1996) 'Human Rights and the Construction of Democracy', in Jelin, E. and Hershberg, E. (eds) *Constructing Democracy: Human Rights, Citizenship, and Society in Latin America*, Boulder, CO: Westview Press.

Kaplan, M. B. (1997) *Sexual Justice: Democratic Citizenship and the Politics of Desire*, New York and London: Routledge.

Kapur, R. (2005) 'The Tragedy of Victimisation Rhetoric: Resurrecting the "Native" Subject in International/Postcolonial Feminist Legal Politics'. in *Erotic Justice: Law and the New Politics of Postcolonialism*, London: Routledge.

Lefort, C. (1981) 'Droits de l'homme et politique', in *L'Invention démocratique*, Paris: Fayard.

Lefort, C. (1986) 'La Question de la Démocratie', in *Essais sur le politique*, Paris: Seuil.

Marques-Pereira, B. (1995) 'Les Droits reproductifs comme Droits de Citoyenneté', in Marques-Pereira, B. and Bizberg, I. (eds) *La Citoyenneté sociale en Amérique Latine*, Bruxelles and Paris: L'Harmattan.

Offe, C. (1985) 'Introduction', in *Disorganized Capitalism*, Cambridge: Polity Press.

Offe, C. and Wiesenthal, H. (1985) 'Two Logics of Collective Action', in Offe, C. *Disorganized Capitalism*, Cambridge: Polity Press.

Paiva, V. (2003) 'Sem Mágicas Soluções: A Prevenção do HIV e da AIDS como um Processo de Emancipação Psicossocial', *Divulgação em Saúde para Debate*, 27: 58–69.

Paiva, V. (2006) 'Analisando Cenas e Sexualidades: A Promocao da Saúde na Perspectiva dos Direitos Humanos', in Cáceres, C., Careaga, G., Frasca, T. and Pecheny, M. (eds) *Sexualidad, Estigma y Derechos humanos: Desafíos para el Acesso a la Salud en América Latina*, Lima: FASPA/UPCH.

Parker, R., di Mauro, D., Filiano, B., García, J., Muñoz-Laboy, M. and Sember, R. (2004) 'Global Transformations and Intimate Relations in the 21st Century: Social Science Research on Sexuality and the Emergence of Sexual Health and Sexual Rights Frameworks', *Annual Review of Sex Research*, 15: 362–98.

Pecheny, M. (2002) *La Construction de l'Avortement et du Sida en tant que Questions politiques: Le Cas de l'Argentine*, Lille: Presses Universitaires du Septentrion.

Pecheny, M. (2003) 'Sexual Orientation, AIDS and Human Rights in Argentina', in Eckstein, S. and Wickham-Crowley, T. (eds) *Struggles for Social Rights in Latin America*, New York and London: Routledge.

Pecheny, M. (2004) 'Lógicas de Acción Colectiva de los Movimientos por los Derechos Sexuales: Un Análisis con Aires abstractos de Experiencias bien concretas', in Cáceres, C., Frasca, T., Pecheny, M. and Terto Jr., V. (eds) *Ciudadanía Sexual en América Latina: Abriendo el Debate*, Lima: Universidad Peruana Cayetano Heredia.

Pecheny, M. and Manzelli, H. (eds) (2008) *Estudio Nacional sobre la Situación Social de las Personas Viviendo con VIH en la Argentina*, Buenos Aires: UBATEC.

Petchesky, R. (2003) *Global Prescriptions: Gendering Health and Human Rights*, London: Zed Books.

Petracci, M. and Pecheny, M. (2007) *Argentina: Derechos humanos y Sexualidad*, Buenos Aires: CEDES-CLAM.

Plummer, K. (2003) *Intimate Citizenship: Private Decisions and Public Dialogues*, Seattle: University of Washington Press.

Polletta, F. (2006) 'Ways of Knowing Stories Worth Telling: Why Casting Oneself as a Victim Sometimes Hurts the Cause', in *It was like a Fever. Storytelling in Protest and Politics*, Chicago and London: University of Chicago Press.

Przeworski, A. (1986) *Capitalism and Social Democracy (Studies in Marxism and Social Theory)*, Cambridge: Cambridge University Press.

Raupp Rios, R. (2004) 'Apuntes para un Derecho Democrático de la Dexualidad', in Cáceres, C., Frasca, T., Pecheny, M. and Terto Jr., V. (eds) *Ciudadanía Sexual en América Latina: Abriendo el Debate,* Lima: Universidad Peruana Cayetano Heredia.

Roberts, M. W. (1995) 'Emergence of Gay Identity and Gay Social Movements in Developing Countries: The AIDS Crisis as Catalyst', *Alternatives*, 20 (2): 243–64.

Rubin, G. (1984) 'Thinking Sex: Notes for a Radical Theory of the Politics of Sexuality', in Vance, C. (ed.) *Pleasure and Danger: Exploring Female Sexuality*, London: Routledge & Kegan Paul.

Shklar, J. (1990) *The Faces of Injustice*, New Haven, CT: Yale University Press.

Terto Jr., V. (2000) 'Male Homosexuality and Seropositivity: The Construction of Social Identities in Brazil', in Parker, R., Barbosa, R. and Aggleton, P. (eds) *Framing the Sexual Subject. The Politics of Gender, Sexuality and Power*, Berkeley: University of California Press.

Vianna, A. and Lacerda, P. (2004) *Direitos e Políticas Sexuais no Brasil – O Panorama atual*, Rio de Janeiro: CEPESC.

39 Sexuality, identity and citizenship in contemporary Mexico

Ana Amuchástegui and Rodrigo Parrini

Eleven men sue the Mexican government for dismissing them from the army on the grounds of having HIV (Suprema Corte de Justicia de la Nación 2007), while 302 same-sex couples sign civil partnership agreements in Mexico City (Comisión de Derechos Humanos del Distrito Federal 2008). More than 10,000 women have legal abortions for the first time in history in the capital city's public hospitals (Grupo de Información sobre Reproducción Elegida 2009), while a group of gay men become an important pressure group for political candidates in municipal and state elections in the southern city of Tenosique. Between 2006 and 2008 Mexico witnessed unprecedented change in legal political activity related to sexuality. Each of these groups, however, approached the process of advocating for their rights from a very different perspective, working to secure these rights by assuming different 'identities.'

Internationally over the last two decades, the concept of sexual rights has been promoted by two rather different social movements, but both of them have made identity the basis of their claims. Women have been constructed as the subjects of sexual rights within the long-term struggle for women's rights in general (Petchesky 2000), while movements for lesbian and gay rights have made sexual identity the foundation of their political claims.[1] Connections between identity, sexuality and rights seem to be the expression of an ongoing process of radicalisation of the meanings of democracy that struggles to broaden subjects' rights beyond the civil and the political.

The emergence of these 'new political subjects' has made possible the politicisation of a new series of social relations, among them those anchored in sexuality, eroticism and desire (Parker 1994; Terto 2000; Weeks 1991, 1993; Amuchástegui and Rivas 2008). This has caused a radical transformation of the political, in that 'we are confronted with the emergence of a *plurality of subjects*, whose forms of constitution and diversity it is only possible to think if we relinquish the category of "subject" as a unified and unifying essence' (Laclau and Mouffe 2001: 181).

The construction of sexuality as a field of rights is closely linked to western understandings of democracy and citizenship (Bell and Binnie 2000). It has implied both the historical deployment of sexuality as an object of experience and identity, and the emergence of a series of discursive 'subject positions'[2] that have claimed related rights. The relatively recent character of identities pertaining to sexual rights – especially gay identities – suggests that these are discursive practices possible only within particular historical conditions. Identities are thus constructed through identification processes that, although part of an individual narrative project (Weeks 1999), can only exist at certain historical and subjective conjunctures.

For example, while in the countries of the north, 'the deployment of sexuality' (Foucault 1978: 24) has made sexual self-definition a central marker of identity, in the south the concept of sexuality per se has not penetrated as deeply or as extensively. Such is the case in Mexico, where research has shown that men's sexual practices (with other men) do not necessarily link to particular sexual identities (Carrillo 2005; Parrini 2007; Nuñez 2007; Prieur 1998). How then does the relationship between sexuality, identity and rights play out in different settings and situations?

In this chapter, we will address this question by analysing field data produced in the context of a series of major changes to Mexican law regarding sexuality. In order to better understand the subjective processes associated with these changes, we developed a series of case studies to shed light on the issues involved (Stake 1994: 237). By analysing observational records, autobiographical narrative interviews (Lindón 1999) and conversations, we were able to look at the subjective processes and discursive construction of identities involved in different groups' appropriation of rights.

The case studies

Soldiers dismissed as a result of HIV

In 2005 the Mexican Ministry of Defence publically accepted that 110 soldiers had been summarily dismissed for having HIV (Medellín 2003). By 2007, many of the men concerned had sued the government, and 11 of their appeals had reached the Supreme Court. Through their legal counsel, we were able to interview four men under the condition that we kept their personal details confidential. While some men came from poor rural and minority ethnic communities, others from a better socioeconomic position had received better educational opportunities.

The men were of different ranks. One of them had won and another had lost his case shortly before the interview. The appeals of the remaining two were being discussed in court at the moment. Their dismissal would deprive them of their livelihood, housing and, more importantly, of health services and access to antiretroviral treatment. This is why one of the interviewees spoke of his dismissal as a 'death sentence.' For him, the alleged offence that had triggered this sentence was the army's presupposition of his homosexuality. However, it was not sexuality that was seen as the area of violation, but men's right to work, to health services and to be free of discrimination on the basis of health status.

Women who received legal abortions in Mexico City

Following the decriminalisation of abortion by Mexico City's Legislative Assembly in April 2007, local hospitals were required to provide the necessary services. During 2007 and 2008 we conducted a study of the consequences of this in one public hospital, interviewing doctors, nurses, social workers and 12 women who came to receive the procedure. Half of the women concerned were married or in a long-term relationship; the rest were single. Four of them did not have children, most had secondary education. They all came to the hospital because they could not afford and did not trust private abortion services, since most of them were self-employed or housewives without an income of their own. Relations of subordination were vividly described in the interviews, so much so that for some women the interruption of pregnancy was described as the first truly autonomous decision they had made.

The Club Gay Amazonas in Tenosique

The Club Gay Amazonas was established in 1996 by a group of gay men and *travestis* in Tenosique, southern Mexico. Besides being a social and psychological support group where gay men from Tenosique can socialise, the club organises services such as hairdressing, party decoration and *quinceañeras* (sweet 16) ceremonies in the local community.

The Club is also a political group that has established a dialogue with local authorities in their struggle for the promotion and protection of human rights of gay people and people living with HIV, as a way of responding to the HIV epidemic, which, by the beginning of the 1990s, had begun to affect the residents of this city of ranchers, peasants and migrant workers. The group also conducts HIV prevention work among gay people, sex workers and the population in general.

Fieldwork at the Club began in 2007. Since then, more than 30 interviews have been conducted with club members, government officials, politicians and other relevant social actors, trying to understand the space that the Club had won in a strongly homophobic context.

Men and women in sociedades de convivencia (civil partnerships) in Mexico City

It took five years of intense activism for the law on civil partnerships to be approved by Mexico City's Legislative Assembly in 2006 (Cuenca 2006). Although its passing was taken as a victory by the gay rights movement, paradoxically the law makes no specific mention of sexuality. In this case study, we wanted to understand the experience of those involved in exercising the right to establish a civil partnership, so we interviewed eight couples jointly – four of them men and four of them women. In most cases, one of the members of the partnership was or had been a gay rights activist.

Identity, sexuality and rights: subject positions and subjective processes

The subject positions displayed in each of these groups' discourses present differences and all are marked by different structural conditions hindering the exercise of rights related to sexuality (Parker and Aggleton 2002). Because of fear, lack of information, isolation, poverty, gender inequality or homophobia, all individuals concerned had travelled a long road in their struggle to have their rights respected. Consequently, there was no *one* subject position that underpinned all these processes. Instead, subject positionality was over-determined by a range of different social factors such as class and gender.

In one sense then, our analysis does not intend to explain exhaustively the complexity and fluidity of the political action displayed by these groups, since politicisation is strictly a historical outcome; that is achievable but not inevitable. Critically, this process needs to be anchored by specific subjective and biographical coordinates such that while certain historical conditions may be present, they will only become factors for the transformation of social relations if they can be identified, read off and actively used by subjects themselves.

The analysis of the subject positions produced by different social actors in each of the events just described reveals how they are part of a struggle to expand a narrow of definition of citizenship beyond individuals' legal status, by formulating and claiming new rights. Following Isin and Wood (1999), rather than seeing citizenship and identity as antinomic principles, we view the rise of new identities and claims for collective group rights as a challenge to *modern* interpretations of the notion of universal citizenship.

Although in legal terms all rights related to sexuality are individual rights, in these interviews individualities emerge as multiple and belonging to different collectives. Sometimes these subject positions relate to the political action of groups such as the Mexican gay and lesbian movement, civil society struggle against AIDS and the feminist and women's movements. Importantly, the subject positions taken up by men and women in the case studies do not have their foundation in an abstract individual subject, but in the relationship of this subject to a collective identity linked variously to citizenship, desire, reproduction and/or gender. In a sense then, subject positions are articulated as a collective and unstable product, crystallising in the actions of particular individuals expanding their rights as provided by law.

At first glance, all the cases mentioned could be described as examples of the defence of sexual rights. However, such an assertion is problematic in two ways. First, in Mexican law there is no formal specification of 'sexual rights' and therefore no possibility of their legal protection (Morales 2008). Consequently, the frequent use of the term by Mexican activists and NGOs has resulted much too often in a confusion between its political dimension and its legal operation, bringing discredit to the notion of sexual rights itself.

Second, sexuality was not the foundation for *all* the subject positions sustaining these claims. Among interviewees for this project, only those who had signed civil partnership agreements and a few members of the Club Gay placed sexuality at the centre of their identity, making it a focus for political action. Soldiers and women receiving legal abortions did not. Thus, the place of sexuality in these legal processes was different as was the relationship between sexuality, identity and rights.

Sexuality at the intersection of identity and rights

The nature of the collectivities constructed in the interviews we conducted was not homogeneous. When the members of the Club Gay Amazonas spoke of 'we', they were talking about a specific group of people who knew and worked with one another, while those men and women who had signed civil partnerships constructed an imaginary community of 'gay people' to which they belonged. In both of these cases, it was desire and sexuality that sustained political action and rights claims, albeit in different ways. Individuals in civil partnerships seemed to adhere strongly to a globalised 'gay' identity in that the way they use the term 'suggests not just a sexual but also an emotional definition' (c.f. Altman 1996) in which same-sex relationships mark the creation of a specific sexual identity. As one of the men interviewed said: 'Signing a cohabitation society is a social recognition that helps to shape your personal identity.'

For their part, the men from the Club Gay defined their 'gayness' in their own terms; besides their desire and sexual practices, they spoke of themselves as a group that shared a common space with a similar biographical destiny. Identity, and specifically sexual identity, provided the space within which rights were founded, and demands were made for recognition and respect by society and the law:

> Being 'gay' allows for a transformation of capital importance in the subjective and collective trajectories of the subjects that we are looking at. It allows people to move from traditional, fundamentally derogatory and exclusionary identities, to others that have better connotations, with elements of pride and self-affirmation and not only abjection. This is the step from 'faggot' to 'gay', from heteronomy and hetero-denomination, and to a certain autonomy and self-denomination.
>
> (Parrini and Amuchástegui 2008: 185)[3]

Such actions reveal a process of politicisation of social relations and symbolic constructions involved in naming (in the case of the Club) and forms of alliance and marriage (in civil partnerships). Both members of civil partnerships and of the gay Club insist on bending symbolic intelligibility in order to be included and recognised for their own specificity within conditions of equality (Butler 2004). Based on the performative practices of bodies and social relations, their discourse carves space within naturalised notions of gender and heteronormativity.

Sexuality as irrelevant for the intersection of identity and rights

Women who had legal abortions, by way of contrast, spoke of 'we women' as a clearly defined collective subject that served as a platform for the subjective appropriation of rights. This imagined collectivity had its foundations in bodily events which only women could experience – namely, pregnancy and abortion. Here, the 'we' was not founded in performativity but was marked by the reproductive body in all its materiality. This 'we' is a naturalised construction, not so much of the body as of biology and the common experience of the body.

In interviews, abortion was always described as a woman's individual and private decision, not so much as a right. Women spoke, rather, of *legal* abortion as a sort of concession by 'the government'. However, the fact that abortion became a right served as an authorisation of such decision with important subjective consequences. Since women's lives are marked by structural conditions of poverty, dependency and subordination, abortion was often experienced as a constitutive practice of autonomy whose repercussions went beyond the reproductive event itself and produced a subjective effect of citizenship. In this case – in contrast to the two mentioned earlier – the subject position of 'women' as the bearers of rights came *after* rather than before the law.

Why then did women not construct their sexuality as the matter of their rights? In the context of the social relations of economic dependency and violence in which they lived, the separation of sexuality from reproduction had not become a full reality, so sexuality was less an experience of desire or pleasure than a potential field of damage and subordination. This is particularly true in a culture where mother-hood is considered the landmark of femininity, or even the condition for it, and in which reproduction is not so much a choice but a prescription (Amuchástegui and Rivas 2008). In fact, women in this case study did not speak about a lack of desire to be mothers, but about the impossibility of having *that* particular child in order to be better mothers to their remaining children, for economic reasons, absent fathers, personal projects, etc.

Thus, the subject positions played out in the interviews relied on a previous process enacted by the women's and the feminist movements which, in contrast to the gay communities, did not aim for the recognition of a particular identity – that of women – but for the politicisation of such identity through the demand of recognition of themselves as *subjects* with the right to decide over their own bodies.[4]

If women emphasised the specificity of their bodies and subjectivities as the plat-form for the exercise of the right to abortion, soldiers moved in the opposite direc-tion: by avoiding specification of their sexuality and/or sexual identity. Instead, by affirming their universal identity as *citizens*, they argued that dismissal was a discrimi-natory act based on their health status and a violation to their right to work, health-care and equality, not to their sexual freedom or autonomy. One man, in particular, was very articulate about this:

> In my case they just fired me … and it was an unfair dismissal. Although there is a law that regulates grounds for dismissal, it is a law that clearly violates human beings' most fundamental rights. Among them, we have the right to health, the right to non-discrimination, the right to equality, the right to be heard and defended in trial, the right to due legal process. These are fundamental princi-ples within our Constitution.

Citizenship is here a form of political identity that consists of identifying with the political principles of modern, pluralist democracy, including 'the affirmation of liberty and equality for all' (Mouffe 1999: 120). While it is true that all four groups discussed have struggled to expand restrictive definitions of citizenship, the soldiers paradoxically also use citizenship in its narrow definition of legal status in order to assert their rights.

In fact, their actions were strictly individual in that they filed only their own claims against the army. It is only a posteriori when they talk of their experience in the process – for instance, in the army hospital – that they construct another collec-tivity: namely, that of 'soldiers living with HIV'. However, this was not a subject posi-tion in a strict sense, in that it was not the matter for political activity: the 'we' that soldiers construct eschews any biographical, sexual or bodily particularity. It remains abstract in the form of 'we as citizens' and 'we' as the bearers of inalienable rights.

It is interesting to note that, although never intended as collective action, sol-diers' individual suits made it possible for others in the same situation to benefit from the Supreme Court's ruling[5] and promoted intense social debate regarding citizenship and rights regarding sexuality. Although buried and silenced, the sexual aspects of HIV infection were alluded to again and again during the legal process. In interview, men said that the spectre of homoerotic practices followed HIV infec-tion 'like a shadow', so much so that once their fellow soldiers found out about their diagnosis, accusations and insults relating to homosexuality followed. In a deeply homophobic, violent and discriminatory institution such as the army, it was not only that advancing rights through sexuality claims was not an option for these soldiers – in contrast to the gay groups discussed earlier – but that they did not construct sexuality as the area to be protected. It is not surprising, therefore, that they purged sexuality from their legal claims.

As these analyses have shown, there is no one universal way in which sexuality, identity and rights intersect. Each of these cases reveals how sexuality was differentially included or excluded from political processes and from the exercise of rights. Subjective processes such as recognition or autonomy related to bodies, desires and identities may or may not lead to subject positions in discursive structures linking sexuality and citizenship together. Whether or not sexuality was present depended, among many other factors, on the kind of experience that sexuality entailed for those involved: while for gay men and women it was an anchor to their full social inclusion, for both soldiers and abortion recipients sexuality was the site of subordination and danger. While the former acted politically in order to prevent the damage of sexuality, the latter struggled to repair the damage caused by its consequences.

All three cases involving homosexuality, however – the Club Gay, civil partnerships and the soldiers – highlight a disjunction with gender because of the presence of non-normative desires, and a struggle to denaturalise desire and sexual experience. In contrast, heteronormativity and the naturalisation of gender seem to stand in the way of fully politicising women's experiences, since abortion needed to be explained and/or justified by adverse life circumstances, and not simply the lack of desire to have another child. In any case, taken as a whole, the ideological and political turbulence that these events produced in Mexican society was an important event in the battle for hegemony over the intersections between citizenship and sexuality. A radical conception of citizenship which includes sexuality under its wing:

> [C]an only be adequately formulated within a problematic that conceives of the social agent not as a unitary subject but as the articulation of an ensemble of subject positions, constructed within specific discourses and always precariously and temporarily sutured at the intersection of those subject positions.
>
> (Mouffe 1999: 71)

Although not always intended, the political and subjective processes described in the four case studies here linked different subject positions to one other, triggering unprecedented social debate over what it means to be a citizen. As a historical process, the struggle in Mexico continues.

Notes

1 Much of the mainstream literature on sexual rights and/or citizenship seems to take for granted the affirmation of a particular sexual identity as a condition for the exercise of sexual rights (see Bell and Binnie 2000; Weeks 1999; Evans 1993; Plummer 2003).
2 We here use Laclau and Mouffe's concept of subject position as 'a discursive position, [that] partakes of the open character of every discourse; consequently, various positions cannot be totally fixed in a closed system of differences' (2001: 115).
3 Authors' translation.

4 The Grupo de Información sobre Reproducción Elegida (2008), one of the main driving forces behind this recent legislative change, has declared that legal abortion is the most important legal decision in the history of the recognition of women's rights in Mexico.
5 By August 2007 the Supreme Court had ruled that the claimants – and consequently all those in the same situation – should be reinstated in the army and their withheld income and benefits returned, along with full access to healthcare. However, this was not a total victory because the Court allowed the army to perform frequent health examinations on the soldiers living with HIV so that, were they to develop AIDS before their twentieth year in service, they could be legally dismissed (Pedro Morales, attorney, personal communication 2007).

References

Altman, D. (1996) 'Rupture or Continuity? The Internationalization of Gay Identities', *Social Text*, 14 (3): 77–94.

Amuchástegui, A. (2008) 'Construcción subjetiva de Ciudadanía Sexual en México: Género, Heteronormatividad y Ética', in Szasz, I. and Salas, G. (eds) *Sexualidad, Derechos Humanos y Ciudadanía. Diálogos en Torno a un Proyecto en Construcción*, Mexico City: El Colegio de México.

Bell, D. and Binnie, J. (2000) *The Sexual Citizen. Queer Politics and Beyond*, Cambridge: Polity Press.

Butler, J. (1990) *Gender Trouble: Feminism and the Subversion of Identity*, New York: Routledge.

Butler, J. (2004) *Undoing Gender*, New York: Routledge.

Carrillo, H. (2005) *La Noche es joven. La Sexualidad en México en la Era del Sida*, Mexico City: Océano.

Comisión de Derechos Humanos del Distrito Federal (2008) 'A un Año de la Aplicación de la Ley de Sociedades de Convivencia', press bulletin, 14 March; available at www.cdhdf.org.mx/index.php?id=bol5508 (accessed 10 March 2009).

Cuenca, A. (2006) 'Aprueban en lo General Ley de Sociedades de Convivencia', *El Universal*; available at www.eluniversal.com.mx/notas/386883.html (accessed 9 July 2008).

Evans, D. T. (1993) *Sexual Citizenship. The Material Construction of Sexualities*, London: Routledge.

Foucault, M. (1978) *The History of Sexuality, Volume I: An Introduction*, New York: Pantheon Books.

Grupo de Información sobre Reproducción Elegida (2008) 'La Suprema Corte de Justicia de la Nación declaró constitucional la Despenalización del Aborto', press bulletin; available at www.gire.org.mx/publica2/Boletin_4aSesionDespenalizacionSCJN_280808.pdf (accessed 10 March 2009).

Grupo de Información sobre Reproducción Elegida (2009) 'Cifras sobre Aborto en el DF 2007–2008', available at www.gire.org.mx/contenido.php?informacion=222 (accessed 10 March 2009).

Isin, E. E. and Wood, P. K. (1999) *Citizenship and Identity*, Thousand Oaks, CA: Sage.

Laclau, E. and Mouffe, C. (2001) *Hegemony and Social Strategy. Towards a Radical Democratic Politics*, London: Verso.

Lindón, A. (1999) 'Narrativas Autobiográficas, Memoria y Mitos. Una Aproximación a la Acción Social', *Economía, Sociedad y Territorio*, 11 (6): 295–310.

Medellín, A. J. (2003) 'Crece el SIDA como Problema en Sistema de Salud Castrense, México', *El Universal*, 23 September; available at www2.eluniversal.com.mx/pls/impreso/noticia.html?id_nota=102332&tabla=nac (accessed 10 March 2009).

Morales, P. (2008) 'Los Derechos sexuales desde una Perspectiva Jurídica', in Szasz, I. and Salas, G. (eds) *Sexualidad, Derechos humanos y Ciudadanía. Diálogos sobre un Proyecto en Construcción*, Mexico City: El Colegio de México.

Mouffe, C. (1999) *El Retorno de lo Político. Comunidad, Ciudadanía, Pluralismo, Democracia radical*, Barcelona: Paidós.

Nuñez, G. (2007) *Masculinidad e Intimidad: Identidad, Sexualidad y SIDA*, Porrúa: PUEG/ UNAM, El Colegio de Sonora.

Parker, R. (1994) *A Construção da Solidariedade. AIDS, Sexualidade e Política no Brasil*, Río de Janeiro: ABIA/ IMS/UERJ, Relume Dumará.

Parker, R. and Aggleton, P. (2002) *HIV/AIDS-related Stigma and Discrimination: A Conceptual Framework and an Agenda for Action*, New York: The Population Council.

Parrini, R. (2007) *Panópticos y Laberintos. Subjetivación, Deseo y Corporalidad en una Cárcel de Hombres*, Mexico City: El Colegio de México.

Parrini, R. and Amuchástegui, A. (2008) 'Un Nombre propio, un Lugar común: Subjetividad, Ciudadanía y Sexualidad en México', *Debate Feminista*, 37: 179–96.

Petchesky, R. P. (2000) 'Sexual Rights: Inventing a Concept, mapping an International Practice', in Parker, R., Barbosa, R. and Aggleton, P. (eds) *Framing the Sexual Subject. The Politics of Gender, Sexuality and Power*, Berkeley: University of California Press.

Plummer, K. (2003) *Intimate Citizenship. Private Decisions and Public Dialogues*, Seattle: University of Washington Press.

Prieur, A. (1998) *Mema's House, Mexico City. On Transvestites, Queens and Machos*, Chicago: University of Chicago Press.

Suprema Corte de Justicia de la Nación (2007) Dirección General de Comunicación Social, 'Concluye SCJN discusión de 12 amparos promovidos por militares',; available at www2. scjn.gob.mx/consultas/Comunicados/Comunicado.asp?Pagina=listado.asp&Numero=931 (accessed 10 March 2009).

Stake, R. (1994) 'Case Studies', in Denzin, N. and Lincoln, Y. (eds) *Handbook of Qualitative Research*, Thousand Oaks, CA: Sage.

Terto Jr., V. (2000) 'Male Homosexuality and Seropositivity: The Construction of social Identities in Brazil', in Parker, R., Barbosa, R. and Aggleton, P. (eds) *Framing the Sexual Subject. The Politics of Gender, Sexuality, and Power*, Berkeley: University of California Press.

Weeks, J. (1991) *Against Nature. Essays on History, Sexuality, and Identity*, London: Rivers Oram Press.

Weeks, J. (1993) *El Malestar de la Sexualidad*, Madrid: Talasa.

Weeks, J. (1999) 'The Sexual Citizen', in Featherstone, M. (ed.) *Love and Eroticism*, London: Sage.

40 From reproductive to sexual rights

Carmen Barroso

In the mid-1980s, during a discussion on sex education on the periphery of São Paulo, Brazil, I asked a group of young people whether the rights of women were different from the rights of men. I did not expect bona fide feminist answers, but the one I got from a young man recently arrived from a remote rural area of the country caught me by surprise. He confidently asserted that it was right for women to be good wives and for men to be good providers. I soon realised that the concept of human rights was not part of his vocabulary, and this is still the case for millions of human beings centuries after the French Revolution, and many decades after the landmark Universal Declaration of Human Rights of 1948.

If the notion of rights itself is still not universally understood and accepted, reproductive and sexual rights face even greater hurdles. Their history being shorter, their content being more deeply at odds with many traditional practices in many cultures, they are still met with suspicion and resistance in many quarters. This resistance notwithstanding, there is increasing acceptance of reproductive rights, and the rate of dissemination of the concept is so fast that it defies common patterns of cultural change. In the years leading up to the International Conference on Population and Development (ICPD), in the first of a series of meetings of leading foundations and governments interested in population issues, I heard a representative from a European country object to the use of reproductive rights because there was not such a term in his native language. Soon afterwards, this same person played a key role in negotiating the acceptance of reproductive rights as the bedrock of the plan of action adopted from this same meeting in 1994 in Cairo.

The road to Cairo has been analysed from many angles. Most analysts recognise – with praise (Girard 2007) or dismay (McIntosh and Finkle 1995) – the role played by feminists without borders in introducing the concept of reproductive rights and gaining the support from government delegates. They succeeded because of several factors, an important one being that the human rights discourse had gained new political traction the year before with the success of the World Conference on Human Rights held in Vienna. Feminists had moral authority to promote a new paradigm based on human rights because they had gained prominence exactly by criticising population policies for their supposed lack of regard for human rights.

Within the loose networks of feminists, however, there were heated discussions about the reproductive rights strategy. In some quarters, reproductive rights were seen as too vague while in others as too narrow, especially because in the USA reproductive rights seemed to mean only the right to abortion. More basically, however, radical feminists feared the possible co-opting of their agenda by the population establishment, and so-called cultural feminists preferred not to mingle in the world of policy, seen as either hopelessly perverse or utterly irrelevant for the purpose of deep transformation in gender relations.

After Cairo, the implementation of the plan of action proceeded at a different pace in different countries, but a remarkable gradual incorporation of the reproductive health and rights discourse in policymaking circles took place. This change in discourse was accompanied by a number of concrete steps at the policy level in many countries. In Latin America, for instance, governments adopted new policies and worked to improve access to reproductive health services. They started providing free contraceptives in their health facilities, a practice that was virtually non-existent and unthought-of before Cairo. As a result, overall contraceptive use increased steadily in the 1990s, with 64.5 per cent of women aged 15 to 49 now using modern contraceptives in the region (UN 2008). Reproductive rights started to become a reality not only at the theoretical but also at the practical level.

Seven years later, the victory of conservatives in the USA and their sustained fight against rights in general – and reproductive rights in particular – placed new obstacles to the realisation of the Cairo Plan of Action. After its prominent role in drafting the Cairo consensus in 1994, and the support it offered to the plan implementation in the following years, the US government shifted right, adopting a conservative agenda and declaring open war on reproductive rights. In 2001, the newly elected Bush administration reinstated the 'global gag rule', prohibiting organisations that receive US funding from using their own money to carry out legal abortions, provide information or even discuss abortion in public. As a result, non-governmental organisations outside the USA were forced to choose between defending women's health and rights or losing their US funding, which in many cases was vital for their financial survival.

In intergovernmental meetings since 2002 the USA ignored the international consensus of 1994 and systematically opposed reproductive rights language. In meeting after meeting, US delegations questioned the use of the terms 'reproductive health services' and 'reproductive rights', contending that such terms promote abortion and declaring that the USA supports the sanctity of life from the moment of conception to the moment of natural death.

But the USA was not able to get the support needed to impose its agenda and, in many cases, ended up isolated in its crusade against reproductive rights. For example, in the 50th session of the United Nations Commission on the Status of Women (2006) it was the only one of 42 countries to reject a resolution on the release of women and children hostages because it contained language reaffirming the Beijing Platform for Action. In the ICPD+10 meetings held in Asia, Africa and Latin America, the USA pressed other countries to repudiate the ICPD agenda, especially the points related to reproductive health and rights for women and young people, but again failed to gain support. In the Open-ended Meeting of the Presiding Officers of the Economic Commission for Latin America and the Caribbean, held in Santiago de Chile in 2004, the USA was the only one of 38 countries to oppose a declaration supporting the ICPD Plan of Action.

Even if the concerted efforts of US conservatives did not succeed at the intergovernmental arenas, they were quite successful in energising the conservative forces of other countries, which became instrumental in delaying progress towards the consolidation of reproductive rights in many cases, in countries such as Uruguay,[1]

Chile,[2] and Nicaragua,[3] for example. Furthermore, the purse strings controlled by Washington have a powerful effect in intimidating agencies that depend on its largesse. Some of its symptoms include the preference for the term reproductive health instead of sexual and reproductive health and rights. This might appear a mere semantic issue but often ends up influencing the kind of programmes and services that are implemented at local level.

Despite these attacks, reproductive rights are now well accepted by the international community and at the national level in many countries. The most recent victory on the acceptance of reproductive rights took place at the 2005 World Summit. Governments from all over the world committed to 'achieving universal access to reproductive health by 2015 [and to integrate] this goal in strategies to attain the internationally agreed development goals, including those contained in the Millennium Declaration, aimed at reducing maternal mortality, improving maternal health, reducing child mortality, promoting gender equality, combating HIV/AIDS and eradicating poverty' (UN 2005: 16) Sexual rights, however, are not part of the mainstream discourse yet.

Emergence of sexual rights

The International Conference on Population and Development (ICPD) was a watershed event, but it failed to address the issue of sexual rights. It noted for the first time that 'reproductive rights embrace certain human rights that are already recognised in national laws, international human rights documents and other consensus documents' (ICDP 1994), specifically defining reproductive rights and making clear that population issues should be addressed by focusing on the needs of individual men and women rather than on demographic targets.

This leap forward, however, did not happen overnight. A number of smaller steps preceded it. The first of them occurred in 1968, at the First International Conference on Human Rights held in Tehran, when the right of couples to make family planning decisions was established by recognising that parents have a basic human right to determine freely and responsibly the number and spacing of their children. Throughout the following two decades reproductive rights evolved, starting from a so-called negative right to not being coerced by a population control approach to the inclusion of the positive individuals' right to reproductive self-determination and autonomy. At the 1984 International Conference on Population in Mexico City, reproductive rights were redefined to state that all couples and individuals have the basic right to decide freely and responsibly the number and spacing of their children and to have the information, education and means to do so. ICPD built on the women's rights and reproductive decision-making rights established in the previous decades and combined them to elaborate a new concept of reproductive rights.

Only in 1995, at the Fourth World Conference on Women (FWCW) held in Beijing, were sexual rights mentioned for the first time, even then not explicitly. Paragraph 96 of the Beijing Platform for Action spelled out the main elements that should be included under the sexual rights category: 'The human rights of women include their right to have control over and decide freely and responsibly on matters related to their sexuality, including sexual and reproductive health, free of coercion, discrimination and violence' (FWCW 1995).

Activists who had hoped for a more inclusive and expansive definition were disappointed, especially by the omission of the right to seek pleasure and by the lack of explicit mention of sexual diversity. Nevertheless, the acceptance in this important United Nations document of the autonomy of decision making and the right to freedom from discrimination, coercion and violence was a great step forward and became crucial in energising the sexual rights movement (Girard 2007).

More recently, in 2004, the movement was energised by the landmark report to the UN Commission on Human Rights by Paul Hunt, then the Special Rapporteur on the Human Right to Health. This report concludes that 'the correct understanding of human rights principles, as well as existing human rights norms, leads ineluctably to the recognition of sexual rights as human rights. Sexual rights include the right of all persons to express their sexual orientation, with due regard to the well being and rights of others, without fear of persecution, denial of liberty or social interference' (Hunt 2004: 15).

The sexual rights movement was long in gestation. After all, many of the feminists that re-emerged in the 1970s had claimed sexuality as one of their main battlegrounds. In the USA and Germany, feminists published best sellers with their new approach to sexuality. The book *Our Bodies, Ourselves* (Boston Women's Health Book Collective 1973) had translations all over the world. When feminist researchers from the Carlos Chagas Foundation in Brazil published a booklet on sexuality education in the early 1980s, its title was *Much Pleasure!* and the cover photo was a demonstration of feminists carrying the sign 'The pleasure is ours!' in front of the cathedral in São Paulo. All this, of course, did not happen without resistance from the conservatives, and even from fellow feminists who preferred to stick to less controversial issues such as equal pay for equal work. Particularly in Latin America this resistance was very strong because the feminists were emerging in the opposition milieu dominated by a version of orthodox Marxism that was not sympathetic to the libertarian tradition of Rosa Luxemburg and others.

More recently the sexual rights movement has grown as a result of several factors, among them the interest expressed by respected social scientists on the topics of sex and sexuality and the impossibility of hiding the central role of sex in the HIV pandemic. Public discussion about AIDS broke taboos in every country, the gay and lesbian movements were strengthened, and they in turn put sexual rights high on their agenda. Long-time victims of egregious violations of many of their human rights, gays, lesbians – and more recently transgender people – have become outspoken defenders of sexual rights, especially after the HIV epidemic made clear the threats to their right to life. Given the centrality of sexual rights for sexual orientation and gender identity, and given the relative lack of enthusiasm for sexual rights both among many advocates for women's rights and among many activists for reproductive rights, sexual rights became synonymous with rights of sexual minorities in the minds of many.

This started to change when a broader array of sexual rights issues became the object of controversy and many in the human rights movement developed a deeper understanding of the concept of indivisibility of rights. This concept re-emerged strongly at the Vienna Conference on Human Rights in 1993. Initially it was applied more to the need to link the widely accepted civil and political rights to the mostly neglected economic, social and cultural rights. Gradually, however, it also led to an understanding that violations of rights of sexual minorities are linked to a lack of respect for the sexual rights of all.

Controversy around a broad set of sexual rights issues was created by the growing political power of conservative religious forces. Through their actions, the US Christian right, the Vatican and radical Islamists have somewhat paradoxically resexualised national and international debates (Corrêa *et al.* 2008). Of particular interest, given the sheer size of the population affected and the breadth and depth of the policy implications, are the sexual rights of young people. The violation of young people's sexual rights, including their right to a comprehensive sexuality education, puts them at serious risk and in a disadvantaged position. Many young people – whose civil, political, economic and social rights also tend to be neglected – have no access to appropriate, accurate and science-based sex education and as a result are especially vulnerable.

In many countries, there is a general agreement that it is necessary to decrease pregnancy and sexually transmitted infections among young people, but when it comes time to find ways to do so, there is no consensus because of general disapproval and denial of young people's sexual lives, their desires, their different sexual orientations and new types of relationship. The difficulties are even more extensive, because the very idea that youth under age 18 have rights – in fact that human rights in general also apply to young people – is relatively new and was only established internationally in 1989, in the Convention on the Rights of the Child, which has now been ratified by 191 countries (the only countries that have not ratified it are the USA and Somalia). This convention added a new concept to international law, one with profound implications: the principle of the evolving capacities of the child.

The evolving capacities of the child include his or her physiological ability to reproduce, his or her psychological ability to make informed decisions about counselling and healthcare and his or her emotional and social ability to engage in sexual behaviours in accordance with the responsibilities and roles that this entails. The convention emphasises development and intellectual maturity, the ability to understand complex concepts, to make informed decisions and to understand the possible consequences of their choices. With regards to sexuality, intellectual maturity is generally considered together with emotional or social maturity. It includes, for example, the formation of identity and the ability to decide responsibly and in an informed manner about sexual relations and behaviours.

A young person as a rights holder is a relatively new concept. By the same token, the vulnerability of children and their need for care, counselling and protection by parents, communities and the state is widely recognised. The doctrine of evolving capacities of the child manages this double identity of the child in a flexible and contextual manner in order to apply legal rights and protections in accordance with the evolving stages of maturity and development. This framework is useful for promoting the sexual and reproductive rights of young men and women and for building a social milieu in which young people are capable of making informed and responsible decisions about their bodies and lives.

Are sexual rights subsumed under reproductive rights or vice versa?

As we have seen, sexual rights were initially not more than an appendix of reproductive rights. Corrêa *et al.* (2008) point out that this implies that sexuality is only heterosexual. In that sense, the growing separation between sexual rights and reproductive rights is a step towards greater clarity of conceptualisation. More work needs to be done, however, in examining the overlapping of the two realms of rights, because they are not totally unrelated. The question of subsuming one under the other is a false one, but greater clarity about their linkages would be useful.

It is possible that different rights might be thought of as reproductive or sexual depending on the circumstances or the rationale. A case in point is the right to abortion. Its most common rationale is the link to the right to decide freely on whether or not to bear children, and it is therefore a reproductive right. When one considers, however, that one of the most frequently used arguments against the right to abortion is its alleged detrimental effect on the attempts to maintain women within the boundaries of accepted sexual behaviour, it clearly becomes a matter of sexual rights. In recent years, when I have been to several Latin American countries promoting the IPPF publication *Death and Denial: Unsafe Abortion and Poverty* (IPPF 2006), I have often faced questions from audiences on radio and television about the danger of promiscuity that would follow legalisation of abortion. If abortion is linked with the right to decide on matters of sexuality, it can be thought as a sexual right.[4]

Both sexual and reproductive rights share a common neglected characteristic: their linkages to gender power dimensions. Until today, much of the discourse on rights is either totally focused on women or entirely gender neutral. Conceptual clarification is needed on the differences and possible tensions between the rights of women and the rights of men.

It is possible that a tension between sexual and reproductive rights will persist for some time. But it is also possible that the recognition of both their distinction and their interdependence might be useful for political negotiations in different arenas. In some forums, reproduction – although still a much contested terrain – might be easier to be elevated to a higher level in the international and national policy agenda, for being seen as a relatively safer ground, as compared with sexuality. Other factors that may enter the equation are that reproduction might be seen as a basic necessity for societies, while sexual pleasure might – very mistakenly – be considered a luxury. In any case, there is no doubt that reproduction is more public and sex is more private.

Rights and responsibilities

As indicated earlier, the debate over rights and responsibilities, specifically those related to sexuality, becomes especially clear when discussing the sexual rights of young people. Adults who are opposed to young people being sexually active tend to talk about responsibility, using this concept in a restrictive way. From this perspective, responsibility means that individual young people must avoid any and all types of risk. This discourse blames the victim, because it places responsibility for the harmful consequences that may occur from exercising their sexuality on the shoulders of individual young people to whom opportunities are not being offered for the development of their capacity to make sound judgments. Contrariwise, because advocates for the rights of youth consider it unfair to blame young people when they have not been given the information and means necessary to make good decisions, they tend to avoid using the word 'responsibility'.

It would be more constructive to begin a discussion to more clearly define the responsibilities not only of young people, but also of fathers and mothers, of other family members, of society and of governments.

Parents, for instance, have the responsibility to provide young people with the support needed to lead healthy and fulfilling lives. They must focus on helping young people avoid unprotected and unwanted sexual behaviours, rather than asking them to abstain from sexual behaviours altogether. They must help young people develop the values, attitudes, maturity and skills needed to become sexually healthy individuals. Also, in those cases where close relationships between parents and children exist, parents need to support their children's decisions regarding their sexual and reproductive lives; but when that is not the case parents need to be respectful of their children's decisions. Finally, parents need to be ready to 'let go': when young people acquire enhanced competencies there is a reduced need for parental guidance and, consequently, a greater capacity for young people to take responsibility for those decisions affecting their lives.

States have the responsibility to provide the means necessary to ensure the fulfilment of young people's sexual rights. They have an obligation to provide accurate and comprehensive information through state-supported sexual and reproductive health education and services. They also have the responsibility to respect young people's rights by supporting their decisions on sexual matters. They must ensure young people's freedom in choosing whether or not to abstain from sexual activity, the type of contraceptives they decide to use, etc. Finally, states have the responsibility to protect young people from exposure to activities or situations likely to cause them harm. For instance, they need to guard young people – through the adoption and enforcement of adequate legislation and policies – from abduction and prostitution, sexual trafficking, female genital mutilation and so on.

Finally, young people have the responsibility to act on the information and services made available to them. The right to information and health services comes with the responsibility to protect themselves and their partners against unintended pregnancies and sexually transmitted infections, including HIV. If they decide to engage in sexual activity and do not want to conceive, young people need to use contraceptives in a consistent and effective manner. And they should develop the skills needed to rank and assess risks, which should be clearly understood and not imposed from the outside.

In an ideal world, this triangular relationship between states, parents and young people would work harmoniously: rights would be universally applied, with no distinctions in terms of gender, age and socioeconomic status; and the ensuing responsibilities would be fully and adequately exercised by each party. As we do not live in an ideal world, pushing for progress should try to achieve a balance among the three actors. Focusing only on the responsibility of young people might result in blaming the victim, who does not receive from parents and states the enabling conditions for developing individual responsibility.

The International Planned Parenthood Federation and sexual rights

The International Planned Parenthood Federation (IPPF) adopted a Charter on Reproductive and Sexual Rights in 1994, which gave new impetus to its promotion of a rights-based approach to the provision of reproductive health services by its 152 member associations throughout the world. Grounded on internationally agreed human rights, the Charter included mention of sexual rights, but the main emphasis was on reproductive rights. In the last few years, some IPPF associations in the western hemisphere started to request a more fully elaborated document on sexual rights to better guide their work, especially with young people and with sexually diverse populations. After an extensive process of consultation with staff and volunteers at all levels, in all regions and guided by a panel of experts that included Paul Hunt, Alice Miller and Hossam Baghat, IPPF adopted a Declaration on Sexual Rights in 2008 (IPPF 2008).

The Declaration, developed with the support of the Ford Foundation, includes 10 basic sexual rights and recognises that 'sexual rights are a component of human rights, which are an evolving set of entitlements related to sexuality that contribute to the freedom, equality and dignity of all people' (IPPF 2008: 1). It stresses the importance of sexual rights for the enjoyment of the highest attainable standard of physical and mental health, highlighting the interrelatedness between sexual rights and the rights to development, freedom, equality and dignity. Furthermore, it includes seven general principles that underlie all sexual rights and that recognise, among other things, that sexuality is an integral part of the personhood of every human being, and that the pleasure deriving from it is a central aspect of being human, whether or not a person chooses to reproduce.

One of IPPF's prime motivations in developing this declaration derived from its work promoting the rights of sexual minorities and youth. The prejudice and silence surrounding sex can have deadly effects, particularly among marginalised groups. Fear of sexuality, for instance, represents a social barrier that prevents many young people from accessing sexual and reproductive health services. Stigma and discrimination prevent individuals from seeking the services that meet their specific needs, increasing their vulnerability to poor health outcomes. It was against this backcloth that IPPF realised that specific interventions to promote the sexual rights of marginalised groups would not be enough to make a difference. *Sexual Rights: An IPPF Declaration* is expected to contribute to streamlining sexual rights into the work carried out throughout the entire federation, not only related to sexually marginalised groups but to all individuals, and also as a powerful tool to advocate at the national and international levels for the full recognition and respect of sexual rights. IPPF thinks it can add its weight to the very valuable work already being done by advocates for sexual rights.

While there was prompt acceptance of the so-called negative rights – freedom from discrimination and from violence and coercion – the positive rights of self-expression and the pursuit of pleasure were the subject of more contentious discussions. Some IPPF member associations found it harder than others, due to more conservative cultural and religious backgrounds, to instantly embrace sexual rights. In the end, the Declaration served as an internal advocacy tool that helped to develop our understanding of the nature of human rights in general and the nature of human rights related to sexuality in particular.

By focusing on guaranteeing sexual rights in the health services it provides, IPPF hopes to create a society in which women will not have to risk their lives with unsafe abortion, young people are not denied lifesaving information and where sexual orientation is not a barrier to full citizenship.

Conclusion

I have no doubt the young man I met in the 1980s today has a much broader view of human rights in general and sexual rights in particular. Every day we have pleasant surprises about how widespread are the changes in attitudes supporting sexual rights. We also are constantly appalled by the backlash that this progress brings from more extreme quarters. Vigilance against the backlash and constant effort to push the agenda forward is needed in order to make this world a happier and more secure place for all.

Notes

1 On 5 May 2004 the Uruguayan Senate rejected, by 17–13, a bill that would have made abortion legal in the first trimester of pregnancy, would have promoted sex education, contraceptive distribution and maternal healthcare services. The bill had already passed Uruguay's House of Representatives. Members of the United States Congress sent letters to Uruguay's senators urging them not to 'legalise the violent murder of unborn children'.
2 In 2008 the Chilean Constitutional Court banned the distribution of emergency contraception in public health centres. The ruling comes after a group of conservative parliamentarians filed a petition to overturn President Michelle Bachelet's decree authorising free distribution of the contraceptive to women, including teenagers.
3 In 2006 the government of Nicaragua passed a total ban on abortion. In this way, Nicaragua became one of the few countries in the world to ban medical abortions, even when a pregnant woman's life is at risk.
4 I am grateful to Sonia Corrêa for this insight.

References

Boston Women's Health Book Collective (1973) *Our Bodies, Ourselves*, New York: Simon & Schuster.

Corrêa, S., Petchesky, R. and Parker, R. (2008) *Sexuality, Health and Human Rights*, London and New York: Routledge.

FWCW (Fourth World Conference on Women) (1995) Platform for Action of the Fourth World Conference on Women; available at www.un.org/womenwatch/daw/beijing/platform/health.htm (accessed 7 January 2009).

Girard, F. (2007) 'Negotiating Sexual Rights and Sexual Orientation at the UN', in Parker, R., Petchesky, R. and Sember, R. (eds) *SexPolitics: Reports from the Frontlines*, Sexuality Policy Watch; available at www.sxpolitics.org/frontlines/home/index.php (accessed 7 January 2009).

Hunt, P. (2004) 'Economic, Social and Cultural Rights: The Right of Everyone to the Enjoyment of the Highest Attainable Standard of Physical and Mental Health', Report of the Special Rapporteur, UN Commission on Human Rights, 60th session, 16 February.

ICPD (International Conference on Population and Development) (1994) 'Programme of Action of the International Conference on Population and Development', article 7.3; available at www.unfpa.org/icpd/icpd-programme.cfm (accessed 8 January 2009).

IPPF (International Planned Parenthood Federation) (2006) *Death and Denial: Unsafe Abortion and Poverty*. London: International Planned Parenthood Federation; available at www.ippfwhr.org/files/Death_Denial_EN.pdf (accessed 8 January 2009).

IPPF (International Planned Parenthood Federation) (2008) *Sexual Rights: An IPPF Declaration*, London: International Planned Parenthood Federation International Planned Parenthood Federation; available at www.ippfwhr.org/files/SexualRightsIPPFdeclaration.pdf (accessed 8 January 2009).

McIntosh, C. A. and Finkle, J. L. (1995) 'The Cairo Conference on Population and Development: A new Paradigm?', *Population and Development Review*, 21 (2): 223–60.

UN (United Nations) (2005) Resolution adopted by the General Assembly 60/1, World Summit Outcome; available at http://daccessdds.un.org/doc/UNDOC/GEN/N05/487/60/PDF/N0548760.pdf?OpenElement (accessed 8 January 2009).

UN (United Nations) (2008) *World Contraceptive Use 2007*. New York: UN Department of Economic and Social Affairs, Population Division.

41 Sexual rights for young women

Lessons from developing countries

Deborah L. Tolman and Sarah H. Costa

Sexual rights for adolescent girls and young women are at a precarious yet also unprecedented historical moment. While the concept of these rights has achieved a potentially powerful public status in many parts of the world, their full articulation and promotion remains fragile. Ironically, this instability is particularly pervasive in the USA, where the politicisation and commodification of young women's sexuality has combined with the practice of keeping education, health and development in 'separate silos', working in a parallel rather than an integrated way. In this chapter, we would like to suggest that this silo effect is brought into relief and alternative approaches become evident in examining effective efforts that support girls' sexual rights in developing countries.

We will begin by briefly reviewing the concept of sexual rights for girls and how they are addressed globally and in the USA. Based on a review of programmes and interventions in the developing world that seem to get it right, we will then identify a menu of components we have distilled that holds the potential to enable girls' sexual rights. Finally, we will argue that what is needed and possible for advancing young women's sexual rights in the USA can be more transformational than a restricted set of implementations or even curricular tweaks. Ultimately, we suggest that these efforts can and must be anchored in a more imaginative 'out of the box' approach that goes far beyond constrained initiatives in overburdened schools: initiating, mobilising and supporting a social movement for girls' sexual rights, led by and with young people, enabled and supported by adults who care about them.

Women's and girls' sexual rights

The Fourth World Conference on Women (Beijing) Platform for Action put forward the groundbreaking concept that the right of women to control their sexuality – the basis for their sexual rights – is an indivisible part of their human rights, and that without it, women cannot fully realise their other human rights. This construction of women's sexual rights as human rights has been reaffirmed at several subsequent international meetings (Molyneux and Razavi 2006).

Sexual rights are often conceptually connected to the right to sexual health for women and girls; sometimes the two are even equated or conflated. Importantly, sexual rights are *necessary but not sufficient* for sexual health (Klugman 2000) that is, women and girls must have their rights to control and define their own sexuality – not only to be free from any coerced sexual behaviour and risks to give consent or not, to express their own sexual wishes not simply do whatever their partners demand, to have pleasurable and meaningful sexual experiences – in order to pursue the taller order of sexual health. This distinction underscores the importance of making explicit and integrating what has been referred to as 'the sexuality connection' (Dixon-Mueller 1993: 269; Higgins and Hirsch 2007: 133) in sexual and reproductive rights and health. Sexual rights for girls and women must also be understood within a recognition that gender inequalities at both the individual and structural levels are produced and perpetuated through patriarchal social systems require a specific claim for them, i.e., a neutral (ungendered) claim for sexual pleasure as a human right does not account for the still pervasive subordination and exploitation of women in service of men's sexual pleasure (Higgins and Hirsch 2007; Oriel 2005; Petchesky 2000b).

Following the Cairo UN Conference on Population in 1994 and the Beijing UN Conference on Women in 1995, sexual health and sexual rights gained greater currency and have since gained some recognition in the services, programmes and legal frameworks in many parts of the developing world (Petchesky 2000a). Most recently, the International Planned Parenthood Federation (IPPF) has put forward a Declaration of Sexual Rights (IPPF 2008). However, even in countries that do embrace the significance of women's and girls' sexual rights, in practice, few countries' laws or policies or everyday cultural practices provide women and especially girls with effective protection from coercion, discrimination and violence or with 'enabling conditions' (Corrêa and Petchesky 1994: 120) for developing and acting on a sense of entitlement and empowerment, one of the key psychological and material roots of sexual rights. Fundamentalist states and movements all over the world consistently target women's sexual and reproductive autonomy. Since 2001 this challenge has been compounded by US policies that compromise women's and girls' (and all young people's) sexual rights, both within and outside the USA.

Young women's and girls' sexual rights in the USA: a 'missing discourse'

In the USA, the development of effective tools for action within legal, education and health arenas has seriously lagged behind progress made in many developing countries, despite what would appear to be insurmountable political and structural challenges in these contexts. Hampered by the conservative and religious forces that have suppressed, resisted and punished dialogue and efforts and even public discourse, the USA is far behind even in acknowledging sexual rights as fundamental for women and girls. Rather, the USA has taken the lead in a newly potent commodification of sex that perverts the notion of girls' and women's sexual rights even before we begin to act on them as conceived on the international stage. At this conjuncture, we have the opportunity to draft a rough map, to act as surveyors for how the USA can and must infuse sexual rights into the current rights discourses for women and especially for adolescent girls.

In recent years in the USA, sexual rights understood as human rights for lesbian, gay, bisexual, transgender, queer (LGBTQ) youth has become part of the larger discourse about human rights, and in a growing number of cases, put into practices due in part to federal mandates for safety in schools (National Safe Schools Partnership 2007). This interpretation of sexual rights has been fundamentally and almost exclusively liberal, that is, compelling access, freedom from harm, discrimination and violence for the expression of diverse sexual orientations. Many important cases have pushed forward this vital agenda for securing equal status for a population that has been victimised and marginalised through discrimination, intolerance, coercion and violence.

For young people themselves, this progress has been instigated and sustained in schools by the work of organisations like the Gay, Lesbian and Straight Education Network (GLSEN), which strives to assure all members of the school community are valued and respected regardless of sexual orientation or gender identity/expression (www.glsen.org). Sexual citizenship, a rights-based status, has been construed largely in terms of the freedoms denied and now due young people with alternative sexualities and genders and their expressions (Fields and Hirschman 2007). While this sexual rights discourse has yielded legal protections for LGBTQ people and diminished intolerance, this conceptualisation of sexual rights has to this point been predicated primarily on sexual orientation (Klugman 2000; see www.hrc.org).

What has remained unsaid in the USA is that there is a palpable need for a public discourse of sexual rights for all women and girls, acknowledging the variability of political, economic, race and class barriers for different populations and communities, as well as the stubbornly entrenched cultural ideologies that serve as barriers to, and sometimes obfuscators of, these rights. As the recent advances in this realisation of rights for the LGBTQ community demonstrate, now is a unique and vital moment for action not only in legal efforts for access and resources, but for multiple efforts to front and forward sexual rights for adolescent girls in the USA. In this chapter, we look outside the legal framework towards civil society actions, programmes and practices already up and running in developing countries that can enable and instantiate these rights for girls.

Supporting girls' and young women's sexual rights in developing countries: 'rough maps' to success

The good news is that we do not have to start from scratch. Non-governmental organisations (NGOs) in developing countries have been engaged in this work for years and thus offer tremendous insights and information about what is necessary to enable and ensure girls' sexual rights. What can a country such as the USA learn from these ongoing efforts in developing countries? To this end, we have reviewed a variety of community-, school- and service-based programmes and interventions in developing countries that are up and running which formally and informally support the realisation of girls' and young women's sexual rights. These programmes have demonstrated results not only in terms of girls' empowerment, ability and motivation to know and act on their sexual rights themselves but also to press their communities for the enabling conditions required for them to do so.

It is possible to identify seven persuasive components or strategies characterising these programmes and using selected examples, we outline them later. While some of these programmes incorporate multiple interlocking elements, which we argue is critical to their success vis-à-vis sexual rights for girls, others exemplify how one of these elements contributes to effectiveness. We suggest that these seven essential elements offer routes towards building an integrated and transformational approach to young women's sexual rights in countries such as the USA, which we begin to map in the conclusion to this chapter.

The first key element is the holistic and integrated approach of these programmes. This quality takes into account the complexities of the social contexts and basic social needs of girls and recognises the centrality of gender and sexuality to all aspects of their physical and social development. These are often broader community efforts, involving less 'surgical' approaches to sexuality education. They offer more than what not to do, and do more than just address problems, elaborating how sexual health and respecting sexual rights benefits young girls' psychosocial development, confidence, sense of entitlement to health – and how these contribute to the *health and progress of the society.* This systemic approach allows more linking activities across different sectors and engages actors from different services and support systems.

In Nigeria, for example, the Girls' Power Initiative (GPI) is addressing the challenges girls face in the society and equipping them with information, skills and opportunities for action to grow and realise their full potential. The initiative serves more than 1500 girls in 28 schools across four states and reaches thousands more through a newsletter and radio programme. This programme is intended not only to enhance sexual health but to empower girls across their roles and experiences in their communities, in fact to be agents of community change that create enabling conditions for women and girls to protect and enjoy their sexual rights (see www.gpnigeria.org).

Another example is the work of Afroreggae with young women and men in the slums of Rio de Janeiro, Brazil. Using art, afro-Brazilian culture and education, the organisation promotes social inclusion, social justice and citizenship. The goal is to build girls' and boys' self-esteem and agency as a strategy to steer them away from the endemic violence of poverty and organised crime. Recognising the very high prevalence of teenage pregnancy and HIV among young people in these communities, peer educators encourage girls and boys to explore their gender, sexuality and sexual rights concerns through music and theatre venues. Afroreggae also works closely with local schools and businesses to maximise young people's access to education and employment opportunities and create alternative routes for personal development (see www.afroreggae.com.br).

A second and related strategy is that many of these programmes do not explicitly focus on or have a stated intention on 'promoting the sexual rights of girls'. Instead, such promotion is often woven into the very fabric of efforts and activities that are charged with intervening at a broader level of young people's lives, including rethinking sexuality and in particular the notion that girls are sexual people with rights to their sexuality and sexual pleasure, as well as boys not having right of access to girls' bodies as potential property. A shared strength of these programmes is that they are built on the premise that adolescents, especially older ones, are sexual beings and are likely to be sexually active. As such, activities are not guided by the notion there is something wrong that needs to be prevented or fixed but instead support and reinforce healthy and less risky sexual choices. This dimension is critical to creating the basic conditions for young women understanding and feeling empowered to claim sexual rights and for young men to be respectful as well.

A third quality is the consistent emphasis programmes place on relational and social contexts for young people's development in general and their sexuality in particular. Not only is a rights-based framework undergirding these efforts, we also discern an ethic of care and connection as a fundamental characteristic for reaching young people (Gilligan 1982; Gilligan *et al.* 1990) which is generally not embraced in rights-based work (R.

Petchesky, personal communication 2008). Effective approaches frequently include mentoring, peer-led education and social networking components.

Straight Talk, a communications youth-centred sexuality and reproductive health initiative launched by the Kenya Association of Professional Counsellors (KAPC), facilitates collaborative partnerships with young people with the aim of developing coping strategies and life skills that will help young people remain in control of their behaviour. At the core of all Straight Talk activities is youth participation. The initiative aims to foster peer-to-peer discussion of sexuality, gender and HIV by encouraging young people to share opinions about and experiences with confronting high-risk situations and by helping them develop behaviour-negotiation skills through role-playing activities. Hosted within schools across the country, Straight Talk Clubs discuss issues raised in the newspaper, hear guest speakers, visit health centres and the disabled and engage in community service projects. Another goal is to increase dialogue between young people and teachers, and between young people and their parents to stimulate cross-generational dialogue and community support systems (see www.comminit.com).

A fourth characteristic is the centrality of acknowledging and challenging gender power arrangements that undermine girls' sexual rights. This takes two forms: a focus on the empowerment of girls, and analysis of and challenge to gender power arrangements (and cultural norms/products) that perpetuate coercion, violence and sexual discrimination. These programmes have in parallel or are partnered with programmes for boys that educate *them* about social norms endorsing violence against girls and women, and encourage them to question such masculinity norms and to imagine new forms of masculinity that embrace emotional, concerned and creative equality of partnerships between women and men.

GPI (referred to earlier) is a model for educating young women about human rights and gender equality. Reaching thousands of girls every year, GPI's comprehensive curriculum is infused with vital information about gender relations and girls' rights and responsibilities, empowering them to take control of their reproductive and sexual lives and realise their full potential as individuals. Their successes include supporting young women to challenge community practices (genital cutting, refusal to sell condoms to girls) and providing them with the information they need to champion their goals, needs and desire (Tolman *et al.* 2005).

The Conscientising Male Adolescents (CMA) programme, also in Nigeria, has worked with adolescent boys and men under 20 to counter the social prejudices against women by instilling in a generation of youth a new set of values, human rights and citizenship, as well as manhood. The programme teaches respect, health and faithfulness – and in the process helps to prevent and protect young women and men from violence, coercion and risky behaviours (see www.iwhc.org).

Similarly, Instituto Promundo is a NGO working in Brazil and other developing countries to promote more equitable power relations between men and women with the goal of changing the prevailing culture of violence. It has demonstrated the importance of addressing gender norms in programmes for young men to prevent HIV/STIs and violence and promote sexual and reproductive health for boys is critical. Through research, workshops and community-based campaigns the organisation's workers have also demonstrated a critical association between higher levels of education and support for more equitable norms and the critical thinking skills necessary for the development for questioning inequitable or more traditional norms reinforcing the need for broader cross-sectoral approaches in this work (see www.promundo.org.br).

A fifth characteristic is being anchored in communities and commitment to community change (specifically around HIV, sexuality and reproductive health). While all the programmes cited earlier illustrate the importance of community intervention, particularly since so many young people in the developing world are not in school, another example is the work of the International Centre for Reproductive and Sexual Rights (INCRESE). Based in central Nigeria, where sharia (Islamic law) has posed a serious threat to girls' and women's rights since 2002, INCRESE is advocating for sexual rights among the country's most disenfranchised groups, including young people, survivors of sexual violence and sex workers. Through its education and community programmes, INCRESE seeks to promote an understanding of sexual rights that is both protective (the right to say no) and affirmative (right to sexual expression), and challenges the culture of silence around sexuality despite fundamentalist religious opposition (see www.increse-increse.org).

A sixth strategy is that programmes often use innovative media and communication tools to educate the public, mobilise support, build knowledge and influence attitudes and knowledge. One powerful example is the programmes being developed by the Centre for Integral Support of the Adolescent (CRIA) in Brazil, which uses theatre, dance and music to raise awareness of the daily issues girls and boys face in relation to their sexuality, reproductive health, HIV infection and physical violence. Working with predominately poor black youth in Bahia in the northeast of Brazil, CRIA trains girls and boys to use dramatic arts to stimulate discussion between teens, as well as within families, classrooms and in the broader community. Through this approach, CRIA has succeeded in building collaborative relationships with education and health officials. They have successfully influenced the curriculum on sex education of local public schools. At the same time, young people build their own self-confidence and communication skills (see www.cria.org.br.).

Last, effective programmes have strong advocacy and alliance building components to push for sexual health and rights reform and policy change. This advocacy experience has contributed to girls' empowerment and strengthened their leadership skills, thus not focused on but still enabling them to critique the undermining of their sexual rights and developing their sense of entitlement to living full lives, including having sexual rights and healthy sexuality.

The Nigerian NGO Action Health Incorporated (AHI) has initiated peer-led 'life planning' clubs in schools to address the growing rates of teenage pregnancy and HIV and other STIs and lack of education about sexuality and reproduction. When the Ministry of Health shut down the clubs in 1992, claiming sexuality would corrupt Nigeria's youth, AHI youth and staff and their allies organised to lift the ban. They carried out an intensive media campaign and the government began to back down. The clubs were reinstated. After that victory, the coalition sought to have a wider policy impact. In 1996, it participated in the development of 'Guidelines for Comprehensive Sexuality Education in Nigeria' and won approval from the National Council on Education to introduce them into all of Nigeria's schools. Today, AHI continues to collaborate with a network of governmental and non-governmental organisations, community leaders, media practitioners, trade unions, parents and young people to share knowledge and resources and expand sexual rights policy within the region (see www.actionhealthinc.org).

Another poignant example is the work of ELIGE, Youth Network for Reproductive and Sexual Rights, in Mexico that empowers young women and men through activism and mobilising. The Network has played a key role in defending girls' and women's sexual and reproductive rights in the region and more recently was very involved in successful advocacy efforts to change the criminal code on abortion in Mexico City (see www.elige.net).

Conclusion

In this chapter, we have argued that the sexual rights of adolescent girls and young women are missing as part of public and private discussions, and public discourse and debates about young people's sexuality and their overall development in the USA, in contrast to many countries in the developing world. To identify 'rough maps' for instigating and mobilising a comparably bold commitment to girls' sexual rights in the USA, we have reviewed a number of programmes and interventions in developing countries to elucidate seven topographic components from efforts targeting the sexual health and/or the overall development of youth that are also enacting a commitment to the sexual rights of girls.

How might we use this information to shape sexuality, sexual rights, and thereby sexual health and education for girls in countries such as the USA, where the infrastructure and enabling conditions are in many ways superior to those in the developing world, yet where the commitment to girls' sexual rights has yet to be made? We return to the urgency and opportunity of this possibly unique historical moment, perhaps a deep but narrow window for the kind of profound change that we believe young people and those who care about them are hungering and ready for.

Surprisingly perhaps, the separation of sexuality from the fabric of society is less marked in many parts of the developing world, which facilitates more holistic and integrative approaches addressing sexuality as a nexus of other aspects of life. It is notable that many of these programmes have developed ways to creatively operate outside the formal education system, allowing them to reach broader cross-sections of young people as well as other relevant actors, such as policymakers and community elders.

A commitment to girls' sexual rights may provide a fulcrum in the USA, a catalyst, for linking the restless rumbling and outright outrage at the spiralling commodification of sexuality to the legacy of fear about – and a vacuum of entitlement to – healthy sexuality and relationships, the detritus left by a decade of abstinence-only sex education and the urgent yet narrow focus on fighting for access to even the most basic information for young people in the USA. This struggle has left many of those who care about young people's sexuality in a rut, which needs to be exited so that we can consider, be open to and imagine other approaches to the enhancement of healthy sexuality and its development. Taking the initiative from the bold and creative, often courageous, work of those in developing countries, we have rough maps for what it will take to inspire, instigate and inform a redirection towards larger social change.

Taken together, these observations force us to recognise and confront a very difficult reality, the growing understanding in such developing countries that girls' (and the women they become) sexual rights are at the heart of social and economic rights and development and transformational change, not an add-on or the elephant in the room to be feared, manipulated or ignored. These programmes *taken together* illuminate the necessity for linkages among the different kinds of institution, space and actor where community-based work is much needed and can thrive. They provide a menu of possible routes for how countries such as the USA can move away from walled-off sex education that has remained so bound by the limits of public discourse and panicked anxiety. These seven components suggest that it is unlikely that a continued, exclusive emphasis on schools will yield the kind of 'education' and social change that a sexual rights agenda requires and inspires. Ironically, adolescent and young people's sexuality may be overly designated to 'safe spaces' such as schools and family planning clinics thus maintaining its atomised status outside the then untouched fabric of society, which is where a sexual rights approach may be ushered in.

From this perspective, there are some untapped leads that become visible for transforming budding boulevards into fast-track highways to enable *us to act quickly and gain more traction* to build momentum for a grassroots' movement for girls' sexual rights. There are efforts dedicated to youth development in the USA that may offer fertile ground for articulating and planting seeds for a social movement for girls' sexual rights, where young people learn through various media for instance to develop critical perspectives and hone their sense of social justice rather than simply commit to preventing bad sexual outcomes. There are other places outside schools where young people and those who care about them gather that may be ready to engage girls' sexual rights, as disparate as progressive churches, mother–daughter workshops, community centres, organisations supporting girls' and young people's overall wellbeing, web-based social networks for girls, innovative interventions using text messages, if girls' sexual rights and the 'rough maps' that developing countries offer us are disseminated through public discourse and new technologies. Linking disparate programmes, interventions and conversations through a shared stated commitment to girls' sexual rights may transform into a less rough map of a social movement for sexual rights of girls that are real, not the airbrushed commodities with which girls more than anybody currently struggle. These programmes, strategies and places offer ramps for initiating such a social movement. What we are suggesting is that an explicit commitment to girls' and young women's sexual rights may offer the impetus for paradigm change that many are seeking in the post-abstinence-only US landscape.

Such a social movement cannot be legislated for, slotted into a curriculum or mandated, although changes in these societal organising tools can and should be critical first steps. A movement for girls' sexual rights will challenge the terms of demands for evidence-based interventions, because *a change in what constitute successful outcomes* will become evident. A movement pushes for change through symbiotic wrangling with the terms of public debate. We believe these lessons offer alternative paths, moving away from an exclusive focus on school-based sex education curricula towards broader community engagement, responsibility and demands for girls' and young women's sexual rights. A sexual rights movement explicitly for girls and young women is necessary as a next step to building an inclusive social movement for changing the way we talk about, understand and experience sexuality in the USA.

Note

1 See Fine (1988).

References

Corrêa, S. and Petchesky, R. (1994) 'Reproductive and Sexual Rights: A Feminist Perspective', in Germain, A. and Chen, L. (eds) *Population Policies Reconsidered,* Cambridge: Harvard University Press.

Dixon-Mueller, R. (1993) 'The Sexuality Connection in Reproductive Health', *Studies in Family Planning,* 24: 269–82.

Fields, J. and Hirschman, C. (2007) 'Citizenship Lessons in Abstinence-only Sexuality Education', *American Journal of Sexuality Education,* 2: 3–28.

Fine, M. (1988) 'Adolescent Females, Sexuality and Schooling: The Missing Discourse of Desire', *Harvard Educational Review,* 58 (1): 29–53.

Gilligan, C. (1982) *In a Different Voice,* Cambridge, MA: Harvard University Press.

Gilligan, C., Rogers, A. and Tolman, D. (1990) *Women, Girls and Psychotherapy: Reframing Resistance,* New York: Harrington Park Press.

Higgins, J. and Hirsch, J. (2007) 'The Pleasure Deficit: Revisiting the "Sexuality Connection"', *International Family Planning Perspectives,* 33: 133–9.

International Planned Parenthood (IPPF) (2008) *Sexual Rights: An IPPF Declaration,* London: IPPF.

Klugman, B. (2000) 'Sexual Rights in South Africa: A Beijing Discourse or a Strategic Necessity?', *Heath and Human Rights,* 4: 144–73.

Molyneux, M. and Razavi, S. (2006) 'Beijing Plus 10: An Ambivalent Record on Gender Justice', Geneva: United Nations Research Institute for Social Development. (Occasional Paper No. 15)

National Safe Schools Partnership (2007) 'Bridging the Gap in Federal Law: Promoting Safe Schools and Improved Student Achievement by Preventing Bullying and Harassment in Our Schools'; available at www.glsen.org/cgi-bin/iowa/all/library/record/2102.html?state=policy&type=policy (accessed 13 May 2009).

Oriel, J. (2005) 'Sexual Pleasure as a Human Right: Harmful or Helpful to Women in the Context of HIV/AIDS?', *Women's Studies International Forum,* 28: 399–404.

Petchesky, R. (2000a) 'Reproductive and Sexual Rights: Charting the Course of Transnational Women's NGOs', Geneva: United Nations Research Institute for Social Development. (Paper No. 8)

Petchesky, R. (2000b) 'Sexual Rights: Inventing a Concept, Mapping an International Practice', in Parker, R., Barbosa, R. and Aggleton, P. (eds) *Framing the Sexual Subject: The Politics of Gender, Sexuality, and Power,* Berkeley: University of California Press.

Tolman, D., Madanagu, B. and Osakawa, G. (2005) 'Supporting Subjectivity: Girls' Power Initiative as Gender Practice', *Feminism & Psychology,* 15: 50–3.

Part VIII
Struggles for erotic justice

42 Reaffirming pleasures in a world of dangers[1]

Rosalind Petchesky, Sonia Corrêa and Richard Parker

Reacting to decades of single-minded attention to abuse, victimisation and torture by feminist and human rights activists, writers on sexual rights since 2000 have shifted the balance towards 'pleasure'. At issue here is the principle that 'positive' or affirmative rights – those that explicitly enhance capabilities, the range of freedoms and the enabling conditions necessary to exercise them – are as important as 'negative' rights – those that prohibit abuses and violence (Petchesky 2000; Garcia and Parker 2006; Corrêa *et al.* 2008). With respect to sexuality, the ICPD Programme of Action (1994) defined sexual health in terms of people being 'able to have a satisfying and safe sex life' aimed at 'the enhancement of life and personal relations, and not merely counselling and care related to reproduction and sexually transmitted diseases' (para. 7.1). A decade later, Paul Hunt, the UN's Special Rapporteur on the Right to Health 2002–8, likewise defined sexual health as 'a state of physical, emotional, mental and social well-being related to sexuality, not merely the absence of disease, dysfunction, or infirmity'. In addition to his inclusion of sexual orientation and gender identity in the list of 'fundamental human rights' related to sexuality, Hunt remarked that 'sexual health requires a positive and respectful approach to sexuality and sexual relationships, as well as the possibility of having pleasurable and safe sexual experiences, free of coercion, discrimination and violence' (Hunt 2004: 14–15).

Implicit in these definitions is an awareness that positive and negative rights are inseparable: 'Not only does a person's right to fully develop and enjoy her body and her erotic and emotional capacities depend on freedom from abuse and violence, and on having the necessary enabling conditions and material resources [to make such enjoyment possible]; it may also be that awareness of affirmative sexual rights comes as a result of experiencing their violation' (Petchesky 2000: 97). Nonetheless, as religious and ideological conservatism have strengthened their hold on policy-making in many national and international arenas, it remains far easier and more acceptable to oppose abuse, discrimination and hate crimes than to assert pleasurable and safe sexual experiences as a positive right – particularly for unmarried women, young people and all varieties of sexual and gender outlaws. This is because of not only external threats (the political risks of being accused, from the left and the right, of 'hedonism', 'narcissism' and 'bourgeois' or 'Satanist' values) but also internal divisions, including the confusions and disagreements among feminist and lesbian, gay, transgender and intersex activists about what positive, collective values for sexual pleasure and wellbeing we actually share. At the same time, restricting advocacy to negative freedoms has unacceptable costs:

The negative, exclusionary approach to rights, sometimes expressed as the right to 'privacy' or to be 'let alone' in one's choices and desires, can never in itself help construct an *alternative vision* or lead to fundamental structural, social, and cultural transformations. Even the feminist slogan 'my body is my own', while rhetorically powerful, may be perfectly compatible with the hegemonic global market, insofar as it demands freedom from abuse but not from the economic conditions that compel a woman to sell her body or its sexual or reproductive capacities [in other words, radical changes in those conditions].

(Petchesky 2000: 91)

Freud's *Civilization and Its Discontents* (1962), often seen as a pessimistic resignation to the irresolvable conflict between Eros and Thanatos in modern societies, may seem an unlikely source to draw on here. But this early-twentieth-century text may also be read as a cautious critique of civilisation's inability to tolerate unfettered love, and an argument on behalf of 'sexuality as a source of pleasure in its own right'. Later Foucault (1978: 157) famously called for a 'counterattack against the deployment of sexuality' as a domain of power and biopolitical regulation, a counterattack that could have as its motto 'bodies and pleasures'. Many researchers on sexuality and advocates of sexual rights across sexual and gender differences have taken up this call, beginning with Rubin's (1984) conceptualisation of erotic justice and injustice and her appeal for 'rich descriptions' that would abandon 'hierarchies of sexual value' and simply document 'bodies and pleasures' in all their enormous variety. This literature reflects an attempt to escape the focus on normalisation, 'sexual scripts' and the techniques of biopolitics – that is, the very view of sexuality as discourse and regulatory power that Foucault exposed – and to focus instead on what Gary Dowsett (2000) has called bodies in desire: what people feel and do in everyday life. As Connell and Dowsett remark, 'social framing theory', more commonly known as social construction, has a 'tendency to lose the body' and intimate relationships in its preoccupation with discourses and techniques (1999: 191).

One example of this recent critical literature is Peter Jackson's detailed ethnographic exploration of the 'explosion of Thai identities' and the ways they 'are simultaneously gendered and sexualised'. Jackson elucidates the 'endless circuit of mutual referencing' between 'the categories of gender and sexuality' as they became manifest in the profusion of popular discourses for expressing different ways of being sexual, having sex and doing gender in mid-twentieth-century Thailand. He challenges the frameworks of theorists such as Foucault and Sedgwick who tend to separate 'sexuality' from gender. Instead, Jackson wants to 'talk of "eroticism" and "discourses of the erotic"' and to frame 'Thai identities as eroticised genders rather than sexualities' (Jackson 2007: 352, 343). In doing so, he implicitly recasts Thai erotic subjectivities as active agents, self-naming and living their desire, rather than as objects of regulatory discipline.

In a different way, Sylvia Tamale (2006) defies stereotypes of African women as always victimised by 'harmful traditional practices', and recovers local forms in which African women may redeploy such practices as vehicles of women's sexual empowerment. In a study of the *ssenga* (female erotic teachers and counsellors) among the Baganda people of Uganda, Tamale finds a complex mix of aims and effects in sexual initiation rituals. Along with messages to young women and girls that convey strict heteronormativity and the need to fulfil wifely duties, she uncovers a strong sense of entitlement to sexual pleasure and wellbeing for women. In addition to messages about the importance of economic independence from husbands and rights to be free from cruelty and abuse, *ssengas* (whose practices have now become commercialised) convey information about aphrodisiacs, lubricants, 'sexual paraphernalia and aids' and a variety of sexually suggestive terms. Tamale even defends the traditional practice of elongating the labia of pre-menarchal girls, condemned by the World Health Organisation as a form of female genital mutilation (FGM), as pleasure enhancing for both women and men. Among the younger generation of *ssenga* trainees, many are rejecting the more traditional gender norms that privilege male sexuality, make motherhood women's ultimate identity and fail to train men in how to please their women partners. These young Baganda women 'regard sex not primarily for procreation but for leisure and pleasure, relocating sex from the medicalised/reproduction plane to the erotic zone' (Tamale 2006: 93).

It may be one of the strange ironies of the HIV pandemic that it has created a space for more open talk about sexuality, sexual behaviour and erotic pleasure. The Pleasure Project (2007) cites evidence that HIV prevention and safer sex programmes incorporating and promoting sexual pleasure can increase the consistent use of condoms and thus improve public health outcomes. The project has identified a wide range of such programmes in countries as diverse as Cambodia, India, Mozambique, Sri Lanka, Zambia and Zimbabwe. Some, focusing on the familiar 'target groups' such as men who have sex with men, sex workers and young people, involve interventions by peers and co-workers; others, focusing on married couples, involve such unlikely participants as 'local Catholic priests and nuns'. The project catalogues a surprising array of techniques for eroticising both the male and female condom and using them to enhance stimulation. It introduces sexy language and tasty lubricants in training people how to use tongues, lips, hands and eyes to make insertion a sensual experience, and it uses media campaigns to convey the general message that safer sex (with condoms) is exciting, 'natural' and fun (Philpott *et al.* 2006; Knerr and Philpott 2006). Reminiscent of decades of feminist campaigns for safe, effective and female-friendly contraceptives, these programmes are committed to a 'power of pleasure' message as well as to the enabling conditions of availability, affordability and good quality. All, they imply, are essential components of sexual rights as human rights.

The 'sexy' marketing of safer sex products may seem like an instrumentalist cooption of 'pleasure in its own right' – pleasure as a means towards prevention. Yet, to the extent that millions of people across the globe – disproportionately young African, South Asian and African-American women – receive knowledge of sexuality filtered through the prism of HIV and AIDS, there is no better site in which to move pleasure to the foreground. This solemn coupling of health crisis and the erotic should remind us that 'the construction of sexual desirability' is 'already social', whatever the context (Connell and Dowsett 1999: 191–2).

HIV and programmes to address it are prominent scenarios for producing gendered and sexual 'scripts' (Paiva 2000; Simon and Gagnon 2007), but they merely illustrate the reality that 'bodies and pleasures' are never unmediated. Alas, Foucault was right; they are always and everywhere produced, shaped and made intelligible through a field of discursive meanings (Butler 1993; Fausto-Sterling 2000). This in turn raises questions about the complex variety of whatever we may mean by 'pleasure' and the uneasy tension between pleasure as an infinitely variable lived experience and the more inflexible categories of 'rights':

> The idea of sexual pleasure, its definitions, its language, its expression, all typically come from below, from the local context where people experience life. These interpretations emerge from cultural systems of meaning and significance that are a mélange of popular culture intersecting with elite culture, mechanically reproduced and ideologically mediated ... The tendency of *categorising* rights does not easily lend itself to the multiple and fluid interpretations of pleasure and desire.
>
> (Garcia and Parker 2006: 24–5)

Lewis and Gordon (2006) make a compelling case for why the call to bring pleasure back into sexual rights may be rhetorically appealing but glosses over the enormous ambiguities and complexities that the idea of sexual pleasure involves. Enumerating dozens of hypothetical contexts in which sexual encounters occur, or reasons why people may engage in sexual acts – along a broad continuum from coercion to lust – they observe, 'the possibility and nature of "pleasure" is utterly different in all these situations'.[2] Not only does 'context [shape] sexualities and sexual encounters'; it also shapes what pleasure feels like (p. 110). A few of their examples illustrate this dramatically:

> If your children or grandparents are starving or ill, if you are unemployed or poor, if you are in a conflict zone far from home, then a paid sexual encounter could be joyful not because of actual physical or emotional satisfaction, but because you are accessing possibilities of affirmation ... If you are far from home in a risky conflict situation, far from the intimacies of family or community, living in discomfort, facing the unknowns of danger, injury or death, under pressure to keep up a 'front' in mostly male company, then the pleasure of sex with a local woman, enabled by financial exchange, may not be just about orgasm, but involve a whole range of reassurances and comfort. If you live in a civil war, with collapsed social infrastructure, widespread abject poverty and minimal family resources and violence in the home, your sexual experience with the older sugar daddy (who is enabling your only possible access to education as a girl) may also be the kindest, most pleasuring relation you have.
>
> (p. 111)

Here, we are reminded of the classic narrative by the nineteenth-century African-American former slave, Harriet Jacobs, when she begs her readers to stretch their moral compass to understand why she, as a 15-year-old enslaved girl, would willingly give herself to an older, unmarried man 'who is not her master': 'There is something akin to freedom in having a lover who has no control over you, except that which he gains by kindness and attachment' (Jacobs 1987 [orig. 1861]: 385). Pleasure comes in many forms and may involve successful trades within conditions of racialised and gendered subordination, or warding off 'the fragile edges of pride, anxiety, humiliation and rejection that haunt traditional masculinities' (Lewis and Gordon 2006: 115).

But this kind of careful attention to the infinite nuances of pleasure and the 'contextual realities of real relations, real bodies in real life situations of survival' seems to require an entirely different vocabulary from that of human rights. Lewis and Gordon ask, 'is the language of "needs to be met" and "rights to be fulfilled" radically off key, dissociating sexual pleasure from social context and insulating it from the tides of ordinary daily lives?' (2006: 113). Here we come up against the limitations of rights as an ethical framework and discourse; the ways in which its tendency to press sexuality into discrete identity categories and to focus on violations fails to capture either the range of erotic experience or 'the sexual diversity within each of us' (Sharma 2006: 55). One way to address this problem is to broaden our understanding of eroticism itself and thus of what a human rights of sexuality might encompass. We need to return to something closer to Audre Lorde's (1984) conception of the uses of the erotic and the ways in which eroticism is about empowering and energising not only my body but also my community. This is similar to what Vera Paiva suggests in proposing a form of public education around HIV/AIDS that would merge a Freirian approach to politicisation as self and community empowerment with a Brazilian cultural affirmation of the erotic potential in all of us. From this perspective, eroticism and public, communal engagement are entirely interdependent: '[E]ncouraging people to be the agents of their whole life – subjects who are capable of choosing and deciding' and 'to look beyond [their] own narcissistic reflection [toward] psycho-social emancipation' is a means for 'creating political agency and stimulating desire at one and the same time' (Paiva 2003: 200–1).

When the National Network of Sex Worker Organisations in Kerala insists on both 'an enabling environment ... in which [sex workers] can live as free citizens' and 'the right to safe and pleasurable sex', its actions reflect a similar understanding (see Corrêa *et al.* 2008: Chapter 9). So does Outsiders, the UK-based organisation for people with various forms of disability, when it holds sex parties for differently abled people of diverse sexual and gender orientations, making recognition of their sexual lives as important as access to physical, public spaces (Ilkkaracan and Jolly 2007). Erotic justice and social justice are not one and the same, but they are deeply tied to one another; and a human rights framework worth fighting for must embrace their deep interconnections.

The appeal to relink bodies with communities, and erotic justice with social justice, brings us back from the nebulae of ethics to the more solid but shifting ground of politics. But what sorts of politics will make these linkages possible in the world as it currently is? Over a quarter of a century ago, Derrida's dream of dancing beyond all the sexual binaries – 'feminine-masculine, ... bi-sexuality, ... homosexuality and heterosexuality' – was a vision of queerness that anticipated the eruption of 'incalculable choreographies' of sexual and gender variance across the globe (Derrida 1982: 76). Today, that vision seems like more than a dream, still much less than a liveable reality free from stigma and harassment, for the millions who attempt to live it. The issue we inevitably come back to is how to transform visions into practical possibilities: what obstacles still exist to bridging theory and practice? What concrete strategies, organisational forms and ways of building viable coalitions are beginning to emerge for sexual rights activism? And, to what extent can that activism overcome some of the troubling limits of human rights as discussed earlier?

An inhospitable global landscape makes these questions all the more daunting. In scornful reaction to the choreographies of pleasure, three powerful forces – rampant militarism, hegemonic capitalism and dogmatic religiosity – continue to produce violent, commodified, covert, apologetic or otherwise distorted forms of sexuality. The institutions of states and intergovernmental organisations, to which previous generations looked for social solidarity and the promise of equality, have become discredited by corruption, privatisation, paralysis and complicity with militarism, global capitalism and radical religion. Meanwhile, religious institutions are themselves caught in scandals of sexual predation (the Catholic Church) and agendas of military aggrandisement (imperial Christianity, radical Islam, Hindutva communalism, militant Zionism). In the interstices of these large-scale forces – at the level of the micro-politics of everyday life – biomedical authorities continue to pathologise, and states to police, criminalise and persecute, sexual deviants of many kinds. New local and transnational actors constantly emerge, but they face, on the one hand, scarce resources and marginalisation within, or on the fringes of, left and feminist movements that have themselves become increasingly fragmented and marginalised; and, on the other hand, the risks of cooption that come from reliance on international development agencies and donor agendas.

Yet, external forces and constraints are only part of the picture. A revitalised language and politics of sexual freedom needs to overcome a number of binary traps – false double binds – that hobble our movements and keep political practice lagging behind recent theoretical advances regarding sexuality and gender. Among these traps, the following are most worrisome.

Culture vs. political economy

A division between erotic justice and social justice (and consequently between movements for sexual rights and those aimed at economic development and ending poverty and war) derives from an epistemological error that extracts intimate and bodily experience from its social matrix. Such a division makes no sense in the context of real people's lives. A sex worker's struggle against poverty, police brutality, HIV and moral stigma is a multipronged struggle for a whole and dignified life. A transgender or intersex person's capacity to be who she/he is, in public without shame, or to access necessary health and prenatal care, is inseparable from her/his ability to find work in an environment free of discrimination and harassment. The exposure of Iraqi women, gay men and transgenders to daily threats of sectarian, sexual and gender-based violence, and their exclusion from the political space, are part and parcel of their collective oppression due to the US-led military invasion and occupation (Susskind 2007).

Treating sexuality as something separate from political economy ignores the fact that healthcare access, affordable housing, adequate nutrition, safe environments and secure livelihoods are indispensable for safe and pleasurable erotic experience to be real. This false dichotomy not only obscures the necessary enabling conditions for sexual rights across lines of gender, class, race, ethnicity and geography. It also disregards the *materiality* of sexual expression and wellbeing, a materiality rooted, not in some essential biological drive or genetic predisposition, but rather in the ways that bodies 'matter' and become materialised through the same regulatory norms and power relations that produce gender, class, race, ethnicity and geography to begin with (Butler 1993; Corrêa *et al.* 2008). If bodies themselves – genes, hormones, sexual and reproductive organs – are always imbued with, and made intelligible through, norms and practices, the cultural and economic/political dimensions of those norms are also closely intertwined. And the *indeterminacy* of these relations (fluid, unpredictable, changing) makes it all the more urgent that advocacy for erotic justice and advocacy for economic justice be similarly bound together.

Secularity vs. religion

As work on our recent book, *Sexuality, Health and Human Rights* (Corrêa *et al.* 2008) came to a close, the US presidential elections crowded the mainstream media with speeches by leading candidates professing 'faith' and belief in the divinity of Jesus Christ. At the same time, militant Islamists in Sudan were calling for the death of a British teacher who allowed her pupils to name a teddy bear Muhammed, and a religious court in Saudi Arabia sentenced a female rape victim to 300 lashes for being seen in a car with men to whom she was not related. In such a climate, many advocates of both erotic justice and economic justice must feel pressed into a staunch defence of secularism – indeed, they must even feel nostalgia for what seemed to be a calmer, more rational era in which secularity governed public space, and religion was a matter of private conviction and ritual. But it is precisely because religion has become so intensely politicised in the post-Cold War world that secularity has taken on an aura of either a lost golden age or the demonic and godless opposite of religious virtue. In other words, we again confront a false dichotomy, a highly rhetorical construction, that evades the complex ways in which 'faith' and 'reason', religion and politics, have always been interpenetrating, overlapping domains, although in different ways and in different historical and local contexts (Asad 2003; Derrida and Vattimo 1998).

In the present geopolitical context – and possibly for the foreseeable future – feminist and sexual rights activists and intellectuals will need to re-engage with religion without 'returning' there. What this means, in terms of political analysis and strategy, is bringing a critical perspective to bear on religion as a continuous but changing aspect of political and social reality, not its 'opposite'. On the one hand, this kind of critical engagement means challenging – loudly and forthrightly – the injustices perpetrated in the name of religion, however and wherever they occur, while also disavowing Islamophobia, anti-Semitism and other forms of religious bigotry sometimes proclaimed in the name of sexual rights. On the other hand, it could also mean opening doors that a dogmatic or defensive secularism leave closed – for example, examining the spiritual, ecstatic and mystical dimensions of sexuality, or forging alliances with religious identified groups where we share common goals and values. Sisters in Islam in Malaysia, the Coalition for Sexual and Bodily Rights in Muslim Societies and Catholics for a Free Choice provide examples of groups that have moved in this direction.

Individual vs. community

Both the Marxist left and the religious right dismiss claims concerning sexual freedom and expression as 'individualist' by definition and therefore 'bad' –

whether because such claims are subordinate to the presumably 'collective' aims of ending poverty, securing universal healthcare, empowering workers and so on, or because they represent 'selfish' and 'hedonistic' moral values. We argue, instead, for a vision that encompasses *both* singularity and interdependence (of bodies, persons, desires). By insisting on the singularity of bodies we point to the indeterminacy and infinite variety of desire, even as bodies and pleasures are always lived within, and dependent on, multiple relationships and social ties. We also remind ourselves that economic and social rights accruing to communities (for safe water, healthcare, livelihoods, etc.) are ultimately about the individual bodies that need these resources to live. Rights are always individual and social at the same time, just as persons are. No one else can get inside 'my' body and experience its particular pain, terror, yearning or ecstasy. But the pain, terror, yearning and ecstasy are the effects of power relations and interdependencies that make us who or what we are, embed us within community and kin networks and simultaneously produce community and kin as social constructs.

Identity vs. humanity

The project of reconceptualising individual claims within matrices of community and kin relationships – a holistic perspective that emphasises the social and relational dimensions of sexual rights – is closely linked to that of rethinking identity politics. Here again we are faced with an array of imagined dichotomies that end up enervating social movements and weakening their capacity for radical transformation. In the realm of sexual and gender politics, there exist tensions between two unsatisfactory tendencies. First, there is the totalising and gratuitously additive character of acronyms (LGBT, LGBTQ, LGBTQI, etc.) that glibly cover over the specifically different situations of each subgroup, as well as the power differentials among them. Second, there is the also troubling prospect, and the reality, of 'splinterings', in which each of the subgroups breaks away into its own identity-based enclave. The contempt that some gay men, lesbians and straight feminists have sometimes shown toward trans men and women who wish to join their gatherings, and the reaction of trans and intersex groups who seek to establish clearly defined communities of their own, reinforce the fragmentation that critics of identity politics have bemoaned for some 15 years. Just as problematic is the reluctance of many HIV and AIDS groups to take on and defend issues of sexual diversity, equality and pleasure, in addition to the safer discourses of public health. All this replays the tensions between commonality and difference (of race, ethnicity, class, region, sexual orientation) that have disturbed feminist politics for decades.

How therefore do we create meaningful and politically viable linkages across a wide range of identity-based groups without erasing the real social differences among them or returning to the empty and historically contaminated (and anthropocentric) abstraction of 'humanity as a whole'? The vision here is one of a politics of the body and its integrity, freedom, social connectedness and pleasures that would form the ground for working coalitions and solidarity across many diverse activist groups – whether feminist, lesbian, gay, transgender, queer, intersex and people living with HIV or groups mobilised against torture, militarism, racism and ethnic violence and those for healthcare, reproductive justice, comprehensive sex education, food security and disability rights. Good models for such work across identity boundaries do exist, but they are still few and far between. At the national level, they include the campaigns in Turkey to reform the civil and penal codes (Ilkkaracan 2007); the human rights response to HIV and AIDS in Brazil (Berkman *et al.* 2005); and the fight to revoke Section 377 in India (Corrêa *et al.* 2008, Rama-subban 2007). At the international level, they include the drafting and adoption of the Yogyakarta Principles (2007) (O'Flaherty and Fisher 2008; Sanders 2008) and the coalitions working to bring awareness of sexual, reproductive and health rights to the UN Human Rights Council.

Here there are lessons to be learned from another, related false dichotomy: that between the local and the global. All the examples of good models cited earlier are ones in which key actors have combined deep knowledge of local conditions, insti-tutions and cultures with awareness of, and experience in, shaping international human rights principles. They exemplify the observation made earlier that the global and the local are intersecting spaces rather than separate spheres, particu-larly in conditions of globalisation and the proliferation of information and com-munication technologies (ICTs) (Tan 2009). Yet tensions between these spaces persist, as illustrated by the Zina cases in Nigeria in which international activists attempted to intervene in complete disregard of the strategies of local sexual rights activists (see Corrêa *et al.* 2008: Chapter 3). Commenting on the resulting discord-ance, Imam remarked:

> To respect the beliefs, tenets, and practices of both local cultures and interna-tional human rights agreements requires a double 'claim and critique' strategy. This consists of claiming ownership of both local cultures and international human rights discourses (including the right to participate in the defining content of each), while privileging neither local nor international as automati-cally superior and thus being able to criticise both.
>
> (Imam 2005: 66)

Imam's caveat reminds us once again that human rights/sexual rights discourse and practice constitute a terrain of political struggle that is constantly shifting. We cannot dispense with the language of human rights, but neither can we accept it as fully adequate or complete. As Jacques Derrida has said, 'we must [*il faut*] more than ever stand on the side of human rights', but they 'are never sufficient' (in Bor-radori 2003: 132). Rather, the political project of human rights and sexual rights is to continually reinvent their meanings so they are social and individual, global and local, theoretical and practical, inclusive and specific, visionary and operational, about the body and about the collective body, all at the same time. The 'beyond' beyond dichotomous thinking is political solidarity.

Notes

1 The text of this chapter was originally published in Sonia Corrêa, Rosalind Petchesky and Richard Parker, *Sexuality, Health and Human Rights* (London and New York: Routledge, 2008), pp. 212–24. It is reprinted here with minor revisions by the authors and with the permission of the publisher.
2 The list includes: 'marital duty or fear of abandonment; ... the need to perform and prove yourself; because you have no choice; business; education funding; fear of violence; self-esteem boosting; boredom; kindness and generosity; pity; fear that the man's balls will

burst or he will go mad; worn down by constant demand; to be allowed to sleep; to have children; to feel powerful; for exercise; self-affirmation; love; … for revenge; because there are electricity cuts at night; … to lose weight; … because you cannot sleep; to reduce tension in the home; to share intimacy … to forward your career; to get good grades' and on and on (Lewis and Gordon 2006: 111).

References

Asad, T. (2003) *Formations of the Secular: Christianity, Islam, Modernity*, Stanford, CA: Stanford University Press.

Berkman, A., Garcia, J., Muñoz-Laboy, M., Paiva, V. and Parker, R. (2005) 'A Critical Analysis of the Brazilian Response to HIV/AIDS: Lessons Learned for Controlling and Mitigating the Epidemic in Developing Countries', *American Journal of Public Health*, 95 (7): 1162–72.

Borradori, G. (2003) *Philosophy in a Time of Terror: Dialogues with Jürgen Habermas and Jacques Derrida*, Chicago: University of Chicago Press.

Butler, J. (1993) *Bodies that Matter: On the Discursive Limits of 'Sex'*, New York and London: Routledge.

Connell, R. W. and Dowsett, G. W. (1999) '"The Unclean Motion of the Generative Parts": Frameworks in western Thought on Sexuality', in Parker R. and Aggleton, P. (eds) *Culture, Society and Sexuality: A Reader*, London: University of London Press.

Corrêa, S., Petchesky, R. and Parker, R. (2008) *Sexuality, Health and Human Rights*, London and New York: Routledge.

Derrida, J. (1982) 'Choreographies', *Diacritics*, 12 (12): 66–76.

Derrida, J. and Vattimo, G. (1998) *Religion*, Stanford, CA: Stanford University Press.

Dowsett, G. (2000) 'Body Play: Corporeality in a Discursive Silence', in Parker, R., Barbosa, R. M. and Aggleton, P. (eds) *Framing The Sexual Subject: The Politics of Gender Sexuality and Power*, Berkeley: University of California Press.

Fausto-Sterling, A. (2000) *Sexing the Body: Gender Politics and the Construction of Sexuality*, New York: Basic Books.

Foucault, M. (1978) *The History of Sexuality, Volume 1: An Introduction*, New York: Pantheon Books.

Freud, S. (1962) *Civilization and Its Discontents*, New York: Norton.

Garcia, J. and Parker, R. (2006) 'From Global Discourse to Local Actions: The Makings of a Sexual Rights Movement', *Horizontes Antroploógicos*, 12 (26): 13–42.

Hunt, P. (2004) 'Economic, Social and Cultural Rights: The Right of Everyone to the Enjoyment of the highest attainable Standard of physical and Mental Health', Report of the Special Rapporteur, UN Commission on Human Rights, 60th Session, 16 February.

ICPD Programme of Action (1994) United Nations International Conference on Population and Development, Cairo; available at: www.un.org/ecosocdev/geninfo/populatin/icpd. htm (accessed 7 September 2007).

Ilkkaracan, P. (2007) 'How Adultery Almost Derailed Turkey's Aspiration to Join the European Union', in Parker, R., Petchesky, R. and Sember, R. (eds) *SexPolitics: Reports from the Frontlines*, Sexuality Policy Watch; available at: www.sxpolitics.org/frontlines/home/index. php> (accessed 22 November 2007).

Ilkkaracan, P. and Jolly, S. (2007) 'Gender and Sexuality: Overview Report', BRIDGE/Development, Institute of Development Studies, Brighton; available at www.bridge.ids.ac.uk/ reports/CEP-Sexuality-OR.pdf (accessed 22 November 2007).

Imam, A. (2005) 'Women's Reproductive and Sexual Rights and the Offence of Zina in Muslim Laws in Nigeria', in Chavkin, W. and Chesler, E. (eds) *Where Human Rights Begin – Health, Sexuality, and Women in the New Millennium*, New Brunswick, NJ: Rutgers University Press.

Jackson, P. (2007) 'An Explosion of Thai Identities: Global Queering and Re-imagining Queer Theory', in Parker, R. and Aggleton, P. (eds) *Culture Society and Sexuality: A Reader*, London: Routledge.

Jacobs, H. (1987) 'Incidents in the Life of a Slave Girl', in Gates Jr., H. L. (ed.) *The Classic Slave Narratives*, New York: New American Library.

Knerr, W. and Philpott, A. (2006) 'Putting the Sexy back into Safer Sex: The Pleasure Project', *IDS Bulletin*, 37 (5): 105–9.

Lewis, J. and Gordon, G. (2006) 'Terms of Contact and Touching Change: Investigating Pleasure in an HIV Epidemic', *Sexuality Matters, IDS Bulletin*, 37 (5): 110–16.

Lorde, A. (1984) *Sister Outsider: Essays and Speeches*, Trumansberg, NY: The Crossing Press.

O'Flaherty, M. and Fisher, J. (2008) 'Sexual Orientation, Gender Identity and International Human Rights Law: Contextualizing the Yogakarta Principles', *Human Rights Law Review*, 8 (2): 207–48.

Paiva, V. (2000) 'Gendered Scripts and the Sexual Scene: Promoting sexual Subjects among Brazilian Teenagers', in Parker, R., Aggleton, P. and Barbosa, R. M. (eds) *Framing the Sexual Subject: The Politics of Gender, Sexuality, and Power*, Berkeley, Los Angeles and London: University of California Press.

Paiva, V. (2003) 'Beyond Magical Solutions: Prevention of HIV and AIDS as a Process of Psychosocial Emancipation', *Divulgação em Saúde para Debate*, 27: 192–203.

Petchesky, R. (2000) 'Sexual Rights: Inventing a Concept, Mapping an International Practice', in Parker, R., Aggleton, P. and Barbosa, R. M. (eds) *Framing the Sexual Subject: The Politics of Gender, Sexuality and Power*, Berkeley, Los Angeles and London: University of California Press.

Philpott, A., Knerr, W. and Boydell, V. (2006) 'Pleasure and Prevention: When Good Sex is Safer Sex', *Reproductive Health Matters*, 14 (28): 23–31.

Pleasure Project (2007) www.thepleasureproject.org (accessed 29 September 2007).

Ramasubban, R. (2007) 'Culture, Politics, and Discourses on Sexuality: A History of Resistance to the Anti-sodomy Law in India', in Parker, R., Petchesky, R. and Sember, R.(eds) *SexPolitics: Reports From the Frontlines*, Sexuality Policy Watch; available at: www.sxpolitics.org/frontlines/home/index.php (accessed 22 November 2007).

Rubin, G. (1984) 'Thinking Sex: Notes for a Radical Theory of the Politics of Sexuality', in Vance, C. (ed.) *Pleasure and Danger: Exploring Female Sexuality*, Boston: Routledge & Kegan Paul.

Sanders, D. (2008) 'The Role of the Yogyakarta Principles'; available at www.sxpolitics.org/wp-content/uploads/2009/03/yogyakarta-principles-2-douglas-sanders.pdf (accessed on 17 June 2009).

Sharma, J. (2006) 'Reflections on the Language of Rights from a Queer Perspective', *IDS Bulletin*, 37 (5): 52–7.

Simon, W. and Gagnon, J. H. (2007) 'Sexual Scripts', in Parker, R. and Aggleton, P. (eds) *Culture, Society and Sexuality: A Reader*, 2nd edn, London and New York: Routledge.

Susskind, Y. (2007) *Promising Democracy, Imposing Theocracy: Gender Based Violence and The US War on Iraq*, New York: MADRE.

Tamale, S. (2006) 'Eroticism, Sensuality and "Women's Secrets" among the Baganda', *IDS Bulletin*, 37 (5): 89–97.

Tan, M. L. (2009) 'Where were You in 1981: Reflections on the Digital Revolution, Gender and Sexuality', paper presented at the Sexuality Policy Watch Asian Dialogue on Sexuality and Geopolitics, 10–12 April, Hanoi, Vietnam; available at: www.sxpolitics.org/wp-content/uploads/2009/05/hanoi-tan-april2009.pdf (accessed 17 June 2009).

Yogyakarta Principles (2007) www.yogyakartaprinciples.org/index.php?item=25 (accessed 9 September 2007).

43 Law, sexual morality and subversion[1]

Urban sex work in Uganda

Sylvia Tamale

What is Love?
Love is something natural
Love is a key to life
Love is education
Love is science
Love is light
Love is a gift of speaking in strange tongues
Love is beyond human control
Love is secret
Love creates hope
Love is history ...
 (graffiti on the wall of a brothel in Kisenyi)

One of the most exciting (and humbling) aspects of doing field research is the surprises it throws up. The last thing I expected to find on the wall of a slum brothel was poetry. The experience of seeing and reading the poem I have reproduced here opened my eyes to the deeper reality of people's lives, beyond the rough of the wall, breathing between the reality of the lives of the people. Those simple lines sent out a powerful message of a voiceless marginalised and subculture community.

Police swoops of prostitutes on Ugandan streets and various brothels are a relatively common occurrence that is often reported in the local media. In spite of being outlawed, this form of subversive sexuality has boldly endured across time and space shaped and reshaped by forces such as colonialism, racial and gender supremacy, capitalism and globalisation. The study described in this chapter sought to explore and analyse the link between sex work, gender and the law, and the nexus between labour, desire and female offending.

Under Ugandan law, prostitution is illegal and has been penalised by the Criminal Law.[2] The legal regime is based on the belief that effective law enforcement and repression can and should reduce prostitution. Section 138 of the Penal Code defines a prostitute and prostitution thus:

> In this code a prostitute means a person who, in public or elsewhere, regularly or habitually holds himself or herself out as available for sexual intercourse or other sexual gratification for monetary or other material gain and 'prostitution' shall be construed accordingly.

This definition limits culpability of the offence to the sellers of sex (the majority of whom being women) and not to the clients (mostly men). What this means is that if a woman is found guilty of 'selling sex', she is liable to a sentence of up to seven years while the client that paid for her service walks away free. Furthermore, the dependants of a sex worker such as her children, elderly parents, etc., may also be sentenced to seven years' imprisonment for living 'wholly or in part on the earnings of prostitution'.

The problem

Prostitution or the exchange of sex for 'monetary gain/material gratification' is as old as humankind. Despite its criminalisation, the trade remains a resilient force that continues to flourish unhindered. Why is this? Does it make sense for there to be a continued criminalisation of prostitution? What substantive harm does sex work pose to society? More particularly, the law on prostitution clearly demonstrates the double standards that are employed in sexuality morals for men and women. What influence does this hybrid social construction of sexuality have on gender relations in Uganda? Whose interests does it serve and to what end? How does the commercialisation and banalisation of sex affect gender/power relations in Uganda? These were some of the questions the present study sought to address.

In Uganda, some of the reasons attributed to women's entry into sex work include poverty, the disintegration of the traditional African family, domestic violence, orphanhood, peer pressure, armed conflict, sexual violence and premarital pregnancies (see Slum Aid Project 2002). In his study on Kampala sex workers, Richard Ssewakiryanga (2002) analyses the various ways in which sex workers construct their identities in relation to societal structures of power and the material contexts. His findings indicate that age, education, space, ethnicity and sex were critical factors in the self-identities and discursive social identities of sex workers. Such constructions were fraught with contradictions and competing desires. For example, he found that while retaining a 'youthful' look was vital for the marketability of sex workers, advanced age becomes a lucrative identity when clients seek 'experienced' women. Education (especially proficient articulation in the English language) allows sex workers to access different kinds of spaces as well as mobilise different identities. Many times, sex workers have to negotiate different identities to fit different contexts.

Methods

Data collection and analysis in this study were primarily guided by feminist methods of research, which foreground the experiences of sex workers, as well as the meanings that they attach to these experiences. Thus, although quantitative methods were employed (e.g. in the gathering of basic demographic data), qualitative research techniques of non-participant observation, informal interviews and focused group discussions were also used. It was particularly important to use methods that examine sociopolitical processes and allow for linkages between women's sexuality, power and control. We took care not to objectify participants and to avoid hierarchical representations of knowledge about their lived experiences.

Data-gathering techniques included a desktop review of existing literature, reports, legislation and so forth. Five focus group discussions were conducted with sex workers in Kampala and Jinja. We also conducted in-depth interviews with at least 30 female sex workers and six male informants who had interacted with and/ or used the services of sex workers. A further 11 interviews were conducted with representatives of non-governmental organisations that deal with women's rights issues and/or managers of and bureaucrats associated with sex work. Informants were primarily identified using snowball sampling.

We also employed the non-participant observation, whereby we spent time at places where sex workers are commonly picked up. This technique enabled us to gain useful insights into the lived experiences of sex workers. During data analysis, interview notes were reviewed and tentative themes highlighted. Recurring concepts that emerged from the data were identified and patterns noted. As analysis and data-collection progressed, questions became more focused, seeking more in-depth understanding of their meanings from participants.

Ethical concerns were integral to this study. As far as possible, participants were furnished with information relating to the objectives and outcomes of the study and their informed consent to participate duly sought. All possible measures were taken to treat participants with utmost respect and total confidentiality. For example, no material from the study is identifiable to participants' true identity. With the exception of a clear indication of real identities (e.g. in the cases of government officials and NGO activists), pseudonyms are used throughout.

Findings

Evolution of sex work in Uganda

Sex work has not always been a criminal offence in Uganda. Customary law, for example, did not penalise sex work. It did, however, cover rape and adultery (Morris and Read 1966: 290–1), but married men were only penalised for adultery when it was committed with a married woman or a betrothed girl. Hence, the exchange of material gain for sexual services was generally tolerated under pre-colonial Uganda. However, with the unprecedented rural–urban migration in the 1910s and 1920s, the growth of Kampala city and the attendant 'social explosion', sex work flourished (Southall and Gutkind 1957; Obbo 1980; Musisi 2001). In a bid to chastise and curb illicit sexual behaviour and commercialised sex, the colonial Penal Code of 1930 criminalised sex work. Henceforth, the cultural landscape that had accorded spaces for non-procreative sexuality was changed by the stroke of the colonial pen.

The colonial law against prostitution was, needless to say, very much modelled on that of England at the time.[3] The dye of Victorian Common Law morality and Judaeo-Christian culture was firmly bound into all the sexual penal offences. All of them imposed female sexual monogamy and chastity. Similarly, in the Buganda kingdom where the capital, Kampala was located, the elite members of the *Lukiiko* (Buganda parliament) with their colonial education and missionary influence felt the need to curb what they perceived as moribund morality. Hence in 1941, the Buganda government enacted a separate legislation to prevent sex work in the royal capital. It criminalised sex work and prohibited 'an unmarried girl under twenty years of age to enter employment or engage in any kind of work which takes her away from the home of her parents or lawful guardians at night'.[4] Many women were rounded up under this law and herded back to rural regions (Gutkind 1963).

In practice, the law is used as a 'scarecrow' by the patriarchal state in order to control women's sexuality. Since it is difficult to pin down a prostitute in 'the legal act' of prostitution, most sex workers are arbitrarily prosecuted for the offences of being 'idle and disorderly' or being 'rogues and vagabonds'.[5] Another common and extraordinary charge levelled against sex workers by local government authorities is that of 'disturbing peace by using violent or scurrilous or abusive term of reproach'.[6] The law has become an instrument of harassment and abuse by the police. Most arrests are not pursued in courts of law. Sex workers are forced to either buy their way out of jails or to succumb to rape by the people that are supposed to enforce the law against them.

The present-day context

The study revealed the existence of three main types of sex work in Uganda. The first one is outdoor sex work, which constitutes street sex work. The second type is indoor sex work, which includes a wide array of sites such as brothels, hotels and lodges, bars and clubs, residential homes and massage parlours. The third type is export sex work whereby Ugandan sex workers ply their services in foreign lands such as China, Dubai, Hong Kong and Kenya. Both the expansion of sex work and state responses to its rapid growth point to the paradoxes and contradictions arising out of Uganda's capitalist economy, its embattled patriarchy, globalisation and HIV/AIDS (White 1988, 1990; Davis 2000; Musisi 2001).

Of malayas *and* malaikas ...

The ancient whore/Madonna paradigm is alive and well in Uganda's patriarchal society. In local parlance, the whore is *malaya* and the Madonna is *malaika*. The livelihood of a sex worker completely goes against the defined notions of femininity and domesticity imposed on Ugandan women by patriarchal society, culture, religion and the law. Patriarchal morality emphasises the need for 'good women' to be chaste, modest and monogamous while secretly desiring 'immoral *malayas*'.

Erotic sexuality is thereby constructed as a 'private/intimate' issue and is shrouded in secrecy and taboos. Hence when it is peddled in the public realm as work, it throws up challenges to the heteronormative notions of sex, gender and sexuality. As one sex worker participant in the present study stated: 'The most critical persons in this work are our clients. During the day they say one thing and at night they come for our services' (Connie, aged 27, Jinja).

In an earlier study of a cultural/sexual initiation institution (the *ssenga*) of the Bagda in Uganda,[7] I reported that the basic message passed on to tutees is: 'Be a nice, humble wife, but turn into a *malaya* (prostitute) in your bedroom!' (Tamale 2005: 27). In other words, the 'performance' of a demure and coy woman must be shed once she steps into the bedroom in order to have a healthy sexual relationship with her partner. In this sense, regular Ugandan women are required to perform a version of femininity that is difficult to reconcile for its sheer perversity. The following observation by a Ugandan feminist interviewed in the course of the research sums the situation up well:

We are all prostitutes! A married woman is not in control of her sexuality ... In order for her to satisfy her man, she must engage in prostitute-like behaviour. Moreover, if she needs a *gomesi* (traditional female outfit) or a car, it's through sexual satisfaction. Isn't that sex in exchange for material gain? Women will remain in a sad marriage for economic gains. So whether you're on the street or in the comfort of your home, we are all prostitutes!

Gender roles and women's impoverishment

Women make up only 35 per cent of the waged employment in Uganda and occupy the least ranking and least paying jobs. Almost 68 per cent of female-headed households are also single-parent homes. Women spend more than nine hours a day (compared to one for men) doing care labour activities. The fact that women are the primary care providers in Ugandan society in the context of gender discrimination in education, diminished employment opportunities in the structurally adjusted economy, widowhood, single motherhood, increased orphaning due to HIV/AIDS and armed conflicts – all drive women into sex work. Most women turn to sex work as the only available means of earning money and many hold very traditional family values, despite the stereotypes that are depicted about them in the media:

> Most of us have a side job to mask our involvement in the sex business ... Many of us are Owino market vendors officially. Others have a stall in a shop on Luwum Street. Some of us are married women.
>
> (Focus group discussion, Kisenyi)

> I am a Muslim and go to the mosque regularly ... But I have to do what I have to do in order to survive. I am the mother and father to my children. I have responsibilities.
>
> (Hadija, aged 21, Kampala)

> I have been able to help my siblings since both my parents passed away and all the property was grabbed by our relatives.
>
> (Samali, aged 29, Kampala)

Sex workers put on a strategic performance, much like stage actresses, to achieve a specific goal. Depending on the time of day, opportunities, demands, resources and challenges that a sex worker encounters, her body moves in and out of the various roles that she fulfils. Indeed, the phenomenon of 'shifting identities' that most women are familiar with (e.g. from mother to wife to career woman) apply to sex workers in similar ways. The boundaries of personal ethics and morality that they draw for themselves constitute their self-actualisation.

Issues of masculinity

We were curious to find out whether the unequal gender relations in wider society were replicated in the sex worker/client relationship. Given the fact that the transactions take place in an underground economy, under conditions of patriarchy, one would expect the scales of power in the sale of sex to tip heavily in favour of the male buyers. Indeed, the fact that it is the male client that decides on whether or not to have sex with the commercial sex worker gives him some degree of power over her. Furthermore, extensive evidence of violence against sex workers is a clear indicator of unequal power relations between clients and their customers.

The relations of power within the Ugandan gender systems are not always adhered to for the entire duration of commercial sex encounters. Power dynamics are somewhat destabilised in the face of a non-passive partner whose profession involves displaying sexual prowess and expertise. The leverage begins to kick in the reverse direction during price negotiations and the actual sex act when the sex worker is likely to set the boundaries of the encounter and even draws the lines in the power game (Izugbara 2005).

Hence, even as the work that women do in the sex industry renders them vulnerable, they also wield some degree of power through their transgressive activities. Indeed, many times, their skills and experience inevitably subvert the dominant sexual male and subordinate sexual female construct. Interview excerpts illustrate these paradoxical power dynamics between Ugandan sex workers and their customers:

> Yes, the fact that I seek out the prostitute and buy her services means that I am in control ... I must say though that contrary to common belief about commodifying the prostitute's body, whenever I am with a Malaya it is me who feels like ... [pause] a commodity, with her telling me what to do and being totally in charge of the whole act ... You literally feel your power over her slipping with every passing minute and you tend to oblige, to kind of resign to fate and ... you know, to pleasure.
>
> (Oola, aged 35, Kampala)

> Most men are emotionally weak and they come to us for TLC [tender loving care]. They can talk, talk and go on about their personal lives, cry like babies ... We offer a listening ear and comfort them then they go back to their bickering wives. So, you can see that we malayas do in fact stabilise marriages [laughter]. That is a service that we offer but society overlooks it.
>
> (Damali, aged 26, Jinja)

The seesaw of power relations during the paid for sex encounter underlies the complexity of gender relations in eroticised situations. As the contours of power are shifted and reconfigured at different points of the encounter, so do the levels of control that participating individuals wield over each other. The encounter deconstructs the radical notion that views sex work as the quintessential practice of female exploitation and inequality.

Victims versus survivors

The ever present threat of violence has led sex workers to hone their survival skills. One of the most effective ways of coping with the difficult conditions under which they work is by distinguishing, both conceptually and practically, the material body from the symbolic social spaces that their bodies occupy when they are working. In this context, women's resistance takes various forms and may include negotiating a way out of a violent situation through feigning total submission and offering free sex to boosting the macho ego through flattery and praises.

Protection may also be achieved by collaborating with lodge security guards, bartenders, local councillors and even street children who 'look out' for them; by working in pairs, requesting the client to pay in advance and ensuring that a partner takes the money; by using sign language to alert one another of impending danger; and by confiscating the property (e.g. watches, shoes, cell phones) of non-paying or violent clients, especially in brothels. Other techniques include weaving the hair in tiny long braids and clumping them together to form a hiding place for their money; using humour to deal with the pain and difficulty associated with their work; and using alcohol and other drugs to 'numb' the pain of humiliation and ostracism.

Contrary to the popular image of sex workers as 'conveyers of disease' (Ministry of Health 2006: 56), most sex workers we talked to in this study were extremely cautious about sexually transmitted diseases, particularly HIV/AIDS. Most insist that their clients use two condoms, one provided by themselves. As one male client recounted:

> One time in the haste to wear a condom, I put it on the wrong way. You know … inside out. I tried to turn it and wear it the correct way but she insisted that I put on another one. Those girls take no chances.
>
> (Phillip, aged 48, Kampala)

Class differences in sex work

Despite the popular belief that all sex workers are needy, vulnerable individuals, there are obvious class-related differentials that exist in the Ugandan sex work industry. This study revealed an extremely variegated world of sex work that ranges from 12-year-olds selling sex on the street to a very sophisticated setup of 'call girls', charging hundreds of dollars. The stereotype that paints the sex worker as a poor, illiterate, non-skilled woman disregards the power and complexities associated with this profession.

While many sex workers that operate from Kampala slums like Kisenyi, Katanga, Kivulu and Bwaise or Jinja slums like Loco or Buwenda are undeniably disadvantaged and undeniably poor, our work encountered many who did not even remotely match that stereotype. 'High-class' women who operate from upscale bars and hotels or from their homes are protected from police harassment, abuse and violence. By the same token, street prostitutes and those working in slum brothels face the wrath of police brutality and the law:

> I really don't care whether prostitution is legalised or not … I do my business without any interference.
>
> (Trish, aged 28, Kampala)

Most sex workers that we talked to did not share the 'class privileges' that Trish enjoys. So just as class mediates and brings meaning to the lives of ordinary women, so too does it underpin sex work.

Increased market opportunities

Globalisation is transforming sex work in unprecedented ways. With easier transcontinental movement and advanced communication systems in a globalised world, come wider markets and opportunities for sex trade. However, African sex workers in foreign lands are vulnerable to gender/racial violence from their male clients and law enforcement officers. Olga operates mostly from Dubai and she related this harrowing story:

> One time I went with a police detective that we all knew very well. He picked me from a bar and after using me he drove me into the desert and ordered me out of his car. He spat on me and told me to return to Africa. He left me in the middle of nowhere ... I was stark naked and it was extremely cold in the sand. I walked for a very long time and when it was almost light I got to a gate of a house ... The Arab lady of the house was very kind. She gave me an old skirt and a cloth to cover myself; she also gave me some money for transport.
>
> (Olga, aged 30, Kampala)

The global web has also engulfed sex work in a different way. Conservative donor agencies, such as USAID, influence sexuality policies in donor-receiving countries such as Uganda. The US government has developed several plans that act as 'blueprints' for African women's sexuality such as the conditionalities attached to the PEPFAR (President's Emergency Plan for AIDS relief) funds, including a pledge by the potential recipient that they do not support the decriminalisation of prostitution (du Bruyn 2005).

The expanding space for the commercial sex trade in Uganda occasioned by increasing tourism, hotel facilities, the entertainment industry, etc., has spurred sex workers to organise themselves to demand for their rights and challenge societal attitudes. In Kampala, the Lady Mermaid Bureau was established in 2002 (note the play on the word 'bureau' here, where the public think that they are dealing in money exchange). In Jinja, the Uganda Association for Prostitution was established in 2003, but later changed its name to the Good Shepherd Touch Organization, and is currently known as the Organization for Good Life of the Marginalized. Most notable about these organisations, however, is the fact that the most vocal and visible managers of both bodies were men who were not sex workers themselves. Obviously, there is need for women sex workers in the bourgeoning movement to take control of their groups through union-style organising in order to legitimise sex work.

Conclusions

The paradoxes highlighted in the paper reveal that prostitution laws and policies are influenced by the patriarchal state, sexism and classism, propped up by religious moralism. The tensions set out in the paper surface the complexities surrounding sex work and explode the common and simplistic assumptions that mainstream society holds about sex workers. Transactional sex work is neither clearly liberating nor oppressive; it simultaneously offers both the opportunities of liberation or oppression, with a whole range of experiences and possibilities in between.

The paradoxes, ambiguities and contradictions discussed here also have important implications for the relationship between sex workers and government, aid agencies as well as NGOs. Most times, these bodies deal with sex workers in oblivion to the complexities inherent in the lives of the last. Their lives are often portrayed against a negative backdrop of immorality, disruption and disease. This partial understanding of the lives of sex workers leads to ineffective policies and rehabilitation programmes.

However, in addition to the western conceptualisation of sex work as one form of work and/or an issue of human rights, sex work in Uganda must also be situated within the broader context of underdeveloped economies in Africa. In the context of few education opportunities for women, staggering rates of unemployment, low incomes for farmers and unskilled workers and the extent of gender discrimination and oppression, many women are left with no 'choice' but to engage in sex work. Despite this, it must be noted that the conditions under which Ugandan women enter the trade are highly variable.

The fact is that for most women in Uganda sex work is neither a criminal nor a morality issue, but an economic one. It is economic survival (and therefore emancipatory) for the women who engage in the profession. Adult sex work is no different in this context. It is a form of work, 'chosen' primarily for economic reasons, not moral ones. It is ultimately the duty of the state to provide safe working conditions, free of violence and abuse, for all types of work – whether it is in the home, factory, office, markets, bars, streets or brothels.

From the analysis of gender and sexuality, particularly commercial sex work, African feminists can draw up a progressive agenda in the short, medium and long term. The movement for the decriminalisation of sex work must be launched within the radical women's movement as a subversive force against patriarchal control and oppression. Organised religion and its hypocritical moral code that is so influential in the lives of the wider population in Uganda must be engaged with. Feminists should organise against the various fundamentalisms and institutionalised hypocrisy with corresponding meticulousness and care.

Notes

1 I wish to acknowledge with gratitude the support extended to me by Baxter Bakibinga and Rita Birungi in collecting data for this study. I also thank J. Oloka-Onyango who read through earlier drafts of this report and provided valuable suggestions and wise counsel.
2 See Section 138 of the Penal Code Act, Chapter 120 of the Laws of Uganda (2000).
3 While the British law focused on the 'public nuisance' aspects, banning solicitation for the purposes of prostitution, in addition, the Ugandan law criminalised the sale of sex for money.
4 Legal Notice No. 101 of 1941, Uganda Laws, pp. 102–3, the Buganda Law for the Prevention of Prostitution.
5 Sections 167 and 168 of the Penal Code Act, Chapter 120 of the Laws of Uganda (2000). Section 167(a) of the Penal Code provides: 'Any person who being a prostitute, behaves in a disorderly or indecent manner in any public place shall be deemed an idle and disorderly person, and is liable on conviction to imprisonment for seven years'.
6 Contrary to Rules 27(c) and 72 of the Urban Authorities Rules, Statutory Instrument 27–19, Kampala Law Report's Local Government Practice Legislation of Uganda (2003).
7 The term *ssenga* literally means paternal aunt. She performs the role of tutor to her nieces on a wide range of sexual matters, including menstrual etiquette, pre-marriage preparation, erotics and reproduction.

References

Davis, P. (2000) 'On the Sexuality of "Town Women" in Kampala', *Africa Today*, 47 (3/4): 29–60.

Du Bruyn, M. (2005) 'Women, Gender and HIV/AIDS: Where are we Now and Where are we Going?' available at www.stopaidsnow.nl/documenten/Hivos%20gender%20paper.pdf (accessed 6 July 2007).

Gutkind, P. (1963) *The Royal Capital of Buganda: A Study of Internal Conflict and External Ambiguity*, The Hague: Mouton & Co.

Izugbara, O. (2005) ' "Ashawo Suppose Shine Her Eyes": Female Sex Workers and Sex Work Risks in Nigeria', *Health, Risk & Society*, 7 (2): 141–59.

Ministry of Health (2006) *Uganda: HIV/AIDS Sero-Behavioural Survey, 2004–2005*, Kampala: Ministry of Health.

Morris, H. F. and Read, J. (1966) *Uganda: The Development of its Laws and Constitution*, London: Stevens & Sons.

Musisi, N. (2001) 'Gender and the Cultural Construction of "Bad Women" in the Development of Kampala-Kibuga, 1900–1962', in Hogson, D. and McCurdy, S. (eds) *Wicked Women and the Reconfiguration of Gender in Africa*, Portsmouth, NH: Heinemann.

Obbo, C. (1980) *African Women: Their Struggle for Economic Independence*, London: Zed Books.

Slum Aid Project (2002) *Manual for Working With Commercial Sex Workers*, Kampala: Slum Aid Project.

Southall, A. and Gutkind, P. (1957) *Townsmen in the Making: Kampala and Its Suburbs*, Kampala: East Africa Institute of Social Research.

Ssewakiryanga, R. (2002) 'Sex Work and the Identity Question: A Study on Sex Work in Kampala City', Kampala: Centre for Basic Research (CBR Working Paper No. 75).

Tamale, S. (2005) 'Eroticism, Sensuality and "Women's Secrets" Among the Baganda: A Critical Analysis', *Feminist Africa*, 5: 9–36.

White, L. (1988) 'Domestic Labour in a Colonial City: Prostitution in Nairobi, 1900–1952', in Stichter, S. and Parpart, J. (eds) *Patriarchy and Class: African Women in the Home and the Workforce*, Boulder, CO: Westview Press.

White, L. (1990) *The Comforts of Home: Prostitution in Colonial Nairobi*, Chicago: University of Chicago Press.

44 Being young and living with HIV

The double neglect of sexual citizenship

Vera Paiva, José Ricardo Ayres and Sofia Gruskin

> It is important for people to know that teenagers with HIV ... date, kiss, go to the movies ... People think to themselves 'she is sick' ... but I do have a life!
>
> (Maria, 14-year-old girl)

Maria was born in 1987 in São Paulo, Brazil. Interviewed in 2002, she shared with us many stories about her daily life as a young woman living with HIV in a foster care home, where she has been since her mother died of AIDS. Paulo, who had been born two years before and found out he was HIV positive when he was aged 15, when asked about plans for his future, said:

> I think I am the first person that just doesn't care ... I will be happy anyway. One day I will be a father, having children is essential!
>
> (Paulo, 17-year-old boy)

For many health professionals, parents and foster parents, these statements do not celebrate the beneficial outcomes of the challenging circumstances facing young people living with HIV. Young people's sexuality is often defined as a problem in the health literature and something to be controlled, changed or postponed (Paiva 2005). The sexuality of people living with HIV has also been approached predominantly as a difficulty, with public health attention being focused on unsafe sex and other issues believed to threaten the control of the epidemic.

Against this background, this chapter discusses the challenges of sexual health and rights promotion among young people living with HIV as an emblematic case relevant to the sexual rights of people living with HIV and of young people more generally.

The growth of a rights perspective in defining sexual health

The last few decades have seen dramatic changes in understandings of human sexuality and sexual conduct, deeply affected by responses to the HIV epidemic and the growth of social constructionism as an approach to understanding sexuality growing out of rights activism and a critique of the 'sexological' approaches hegemonic in the mid-twentieth century (Gagnon and Parker 1995). The International Conference on Population and Development (ICPD) in 1994 was a landmark in mobilisation around human rights concerning sexuality and gender. This meeting focused attention on reproduction free from discrimination, coercion and violence, in line with internationally agreed commitments to the protection of human rights (UNFPA 1994). Yet, sexual health was defined as part of reproductive health as 'the integration of the somatic, emotional, intellectual and social aspects of sexual being in ways that are positively enriching and that enhance personality, communication and love', statements that were drawn from a WHO Technical Report that was almost 20 years old (WHO 1975: 6). Just 1 year later, the 1995 UN World Conference on Women recognised the right of women to control their own sexuality, free from coercion, discrimination or violence, highlighted in Paragraph 96 of its Platform for Action (UN 1995), even as such a right was not recognised for men or for adolescents.

In 2002[1] the World Health Organisation (WHO) organised a Technical Consultation to update its definitions of sexual health. A document emerging from this meeting provides 'working definitions' of sex, sexuality, sexual health and sexual rights (see Box 44.1) with the intent of advancing understanding in the field of sexual health. This same document stresses, however, that these definitions 'do not represent an official position of WHO' (WHO 2006: 4–5).

Box 44.1 Working definitions of sex, sexuality, sexual health, sexual rights*

Sex

Sex refers to the biological characteristics that define humans as female or male. While these sets of biological characteristics are not mutually exclusive, as there are individuals who possess both, they tend to differentiate humans as males and females. In general use in many languages, the term sex is often used to mean 'sexual activity', but for technical purposes in the context of sexuality and sexual health discussions, the above definition is preferred.

Sexuality

Sexuality is a central aspect of being human throughout life and encompasses sex, gender identities and roles, sexual orientation, eroticism, pleasure, intimacy and reproduction. Sexuality is experienced and expressed in thoughts, fantasies, desires, beliefs, attitudes, values, behaviours, practices, roles and relationships. While sexuality can include all of these dimensions, not all of them are always experienced or expressed. Sexuality is influenced by the interaction of biological, psychological, social, economic, political, cultural, ethical, legal, historical, religious and spiritual factors.

Sexual health

Sexual health is a state of physical, emotional, mental and social well-being in relation to sexuality; it is not merely the absence of disease, dysfunction or infirmity. Sexual health requires a positive and respectful approach to sexuality and sexual relationships, as well as the possibility of having pleasurable and safe sexual experiences, free of coercion, discrimination and violence. For sexual health to be attained and maintained, the sexual rights of all persons must be respected, protected and fulfilled.

Sexual rights

Sexual rights embrace human rights that are already recognised in national laws, international human rights documents and other consensus statements. They include the right of all persons, free of coercion, discrimination and violence, to:

- the highest attainable standard of sexual health, including access to sexual and reproductive healthcare services;
- seek, receive and impart information related to sexuality;
- sexuality education;
- respect for bodily integrity;
- choose their partner;
- decide to be sexually active or not;
- consensual sexual relations;
- consensual marriage;
- decide whether or not, and when, to have children;
- pursue a satisfying, safe and pleasurable sexual life.

The responsible exercise of human rights requires that all persons respect the rights of others.

World Health Organisation 2006: 5.

Sexual health and the rights of people living with HIV

A number of initiatives have taken place globally in pursuit of the goal of promoting the sexual health and rights of people living with HIV. However, it was only in 2006 that recommendations to support the sexual and reproductive health and rights of people living with HIV were published in a document issued by UNAIDS (UNAIDS/ Guttmacher Institute 2006). The impact of an HIV diagnosis on affective and sexual life, the fear of disclosing HIV status to partners, the challenge of lifelong adherence to condom use and the desire to have children are not new issues. What is more recent, is the need for, and the existence of, health services dedicated to children who have grown up with HIV and who are entering into young adulthood. Delay in organising a coherent response to the sexual health and human rights of people living with HIV can be seen as a major failure within the context of global efforts to ensure the right to 'the highest attainable standard of sexual health, including access to sexual and reproductive healthcare services' as indicated in Box 44.1. The question needs to be asked, therefore, would people with any other disease, or women and men who want to conceive after the age of 45, face the same neglect of their sexual citizenship?

The rights of people living with HIV in relation to partnership, family, conjugality and parenthood should not only be recognised rhetorically, but operationally by public services around the world. In the meetings that led to publication of these recommendations, participants from all over the world cited examples of people living with HIV wanting to have children, but facing stigma, rejection and discrimination by health services, actions which imply rights violations as well as contribute to new HIV infections. In this and subsequent discussions, the notion of sexual health has been strongly linked to sexual rights (UNAIDS/Guttmacher Institute 2006; Lusti-Narasimhan *et al.* 2007; Gruskin *et al.* 2007).

Human rights were explicitly referred to in the first Global AIDS Strategy (WHO 1987), the first time they had been cited in any high-level public health document endorsed by national governments (Gruskin and Tarantola 2005). Framing the strategy in human rights terms allowed it to be anchored in international law, making governments and intergovernment organisations publicly accountable for their actions (Mann and Tarantola 1998). Delay in responding to the sexual and reproductive health needs of people living with HIV is emblematic of the synergy of stigmas associated with sexuality and HIV that affects the daily lives of HIV seropositive people, their partners and families.

In countries where there is access to HIV treatment, large numbers of children who were infected through parent to child transmission are growing into young adulthood. And for young people infected during adolescence, the fact that they are sexually active suggests a rights and health challenge for long-term high-quality care beyond the offer of good-quality treatment (Frederick *et al.* 2000; Rotheram-Borus *et al.* 2003; Kmita *et al.* 2002, Ayres *et al.* 2006).

The Brazilian response

Since its inception in the 1990s, the Brazilian response to HIV and AIDS has stressed a human rights perspective, in line with principles of universality, comprehensiveness, equality and community participation. These are the principles of what is called the unified health system (Sistema Unico de Sande – SUS), which is dedicated to promoting and protecting health as a right in line with the 1988 Brazilian Constitution (Berkman *et al.* 2005). Developing healthcare in line with SUS principles is understood as contributing to *cidadania* or citizenship – a very special concept in Latin America. *Cidadania* has its origins in the democratic movements replacing the dictatorships that ruled in many Ibero-American countries before the 1980s. It aims to foster both the fulfilment of the human rights for all, and to maintain debate concerning the new rights and the expansion of existing ones – critically, these include sexual rights. This notion of *cidadania* is based on a commitment to openness and emancipation, on the idea of equality with concern for the differences, surpassing people's oppressions and exclusions – based on, for example, race, gender, age, sexual orientation (Santos 2005).

Throughout Brazil, local and national HIV programmes have aimed to integrate prevention and care to ensure access to the quality treatment, condoms and sexuality education, and explicit programming to reduce stigma and discrimination. Concern for social and individual vulnerability and a desire to promote human rights has guided national AIDS programme efforts over the last decade. But what exactly is vulnerability and why is it relevant here?

Vulnerability analysis begins by identifying the physical, mental and/or behavioural factors that predispose people to health problems. The next step involves examining the deeper social dimensions of vulnerability – political, economic, institutional, cultural and moral – so as to identify key contextual factors. Finally, programme analysis examines the way in which particular policies, programmes and services hold the potential to mitigate or increase vulnerability to HIV. A human rights perspective offers a point of departure for vulnerability analysis in that it helps not only to identify situations of social vulnerability – the growth of the epidemic may offers a *proxy* for human rights violations – but also to guide health services and programming towards the broader dimensions of health.

A series of studies conducted in Brazil[2] have examined the concepts of HIV vulnerability and have led to the development of the conceptual framework shown in Figure 44.1. Within this framework, individual level experiences are understood not in sociocognitive terms but in terms of the intersubjectivity of the citizen rights holder and others influencing his or her social trajectory. Intersubjective contexts arc understood in terms of their local meanings, their gender and ethnic/racial relations, as well as the mobilisation of values, desires and resources through friendship and social networks, as well as professional and family relations.

The personal resources and trajectories that the model highlights as important can usefully be accessed through an analysis of 'everyday scene narratives' (Paiva 2005, 2007). Within these narratives, desire, attitudes and knowledge resulting from different discourses (such as the scientific or the religious) are frequently in tension with one another. An analysis at social and programmatic levels requires attention to be focused on cultural traditions; access to justice, leisure, education, jobs, housing and healthcare; the presence (or absence) of non-discriminatory policies and political liberties; and the overall political climate with respect to gender, sexual

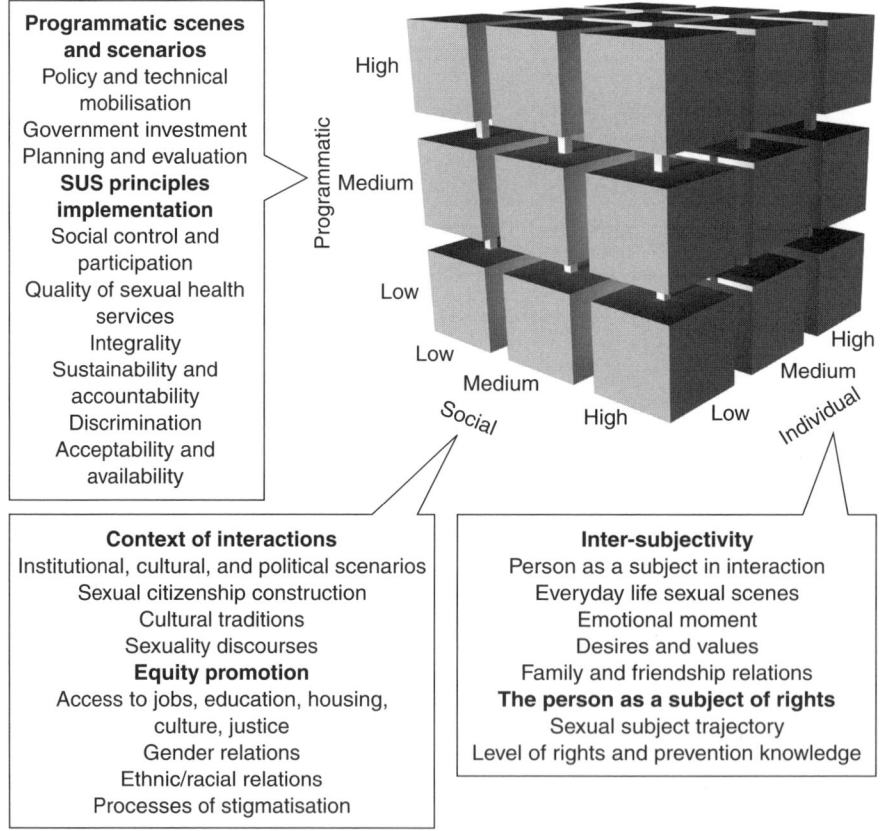

Figure 44.1 HIV-related vulnerability and human rights: individual, social and programmatic levels.

orientation, religion and race. All these factors impact strongly on the attainment of *cidadania* or citizenship.

Within such a framework, evaluation becomes part of the process of changing individual, programmatic and social vulnerability. Researchers are not external to the process and the reflective and analytic skills of those who participate in programmes are one of its main 'outcomes' (Paiva 2005; Benzaken *et al.* 2007).

Young people living with HIV

Promoting young people's sexual health and sexual citizenship poses important challenges in Brazil as elsewhere. Teenage sexual health is rarely engaged on its own terms through a dialogical approach in which young people participate as subjects and rights holders. In the Brazilian Estatuto da Criança e do Adolescente (Statute on Children and Adolescence) (Brazil 1990) as well as in the Convention on the Rights of the Child (UNICEF 1989), sexuality is discussed as an issue of protection – against violence, sexual exploitation and pornography. More usually, sexuality is discussed in the health promotion literature as an issue of protection against pregnancy and sexually transmitted infections.

As part of a larger project to enhance care for people living with HIV in the state of São Paulo (Segurado *et al.* 2003; Paiva *et al.* 2003; Paiva *et al.* 2007), the experiences of young people living with HIV were assessed within the vulnerability framework. The goal was to identify and understand healthcare and psychosocial support needs in terms of young people's own perspectives and the fulfilment of their rights, both individually and collectively as citizens (Ayres *et al.* 2006). In-depth interviews were conducted with 22 HIV-positive young people aged 10 to 20 years of age, and with 13 carers of other HIV-positive young people (many of whom did not know their serostatus) of the same age group. Participants were selected from five HIV and AIDS reference hospitals and clinics.

Lived experiences

Stigma and discrimination were frequently reported by young people and their carers – within the family, in the neighbourhood, at school and in healthcare services (Ayres *et al.* 2006). Diagnosis and disclosure were key events in respondents' accounts, and people's lives could be divided into the moment before and the moment after they were first informed about their HIV serostatus and began to experience stigmatisation.

At the point of diagnosis, young people who had acquired HIV through sexual transmission were most usually regarded as 'irresponsible'. One girl was called *leviana* (irresponsible) by her ante-natal care doctors, and several others reported being depressed and reluctant to commence treatment (Paiva *et al.* 2004). One young man interviewed would not talk about his mode of infection and his healthcare workers suspected sexual abuse. All young people were under 16 years old when diagnosed, and some were already sick, with broader social and programmatic scenarios having affected their vulnerability. The violations of rights had clear impacts on how care was provided, and on young people's psychosocial wellbeing and self-care.

Many HIV-positive children grew up without knowing their HIV serostatus. It was only the imminence of sexual debut that triggered the need to break the news.

Many had grown up in an era when long-term survival was not considered possible, and disclosure had been assumed to expose them to unnecessary suffering. Some carers indicated that surviving from day to day had been an achievement. However, now that young people were of sexual reproductive age, parents and guardians felt they needed to do something.

Underpinning carers' anxieties were issues of sex and sexuality. Many were worried about infection of probable partners, and how young people would cope with stigma and rejection in later life. Moreover, foster caretakers, family members and most health professionals did not feel comfortable talking about sex. Some were not even happy to 'think about it', a somewhat paradoxical response given that discourses of sex in Brazil are generally liberal, the media are open about sexual issues, and HIV prevention in schools stresses condom use. Carers' narratives indicated that they had been trained to treat diseases and infection not to offer comprehensive care. Their accounts revealed anxieties about the content of sexuality education, and how best this could be undertaken:

> He was flirting with a girl, he was dating, so Dr. M.A. [the nurse] told me: 'Now you need to disclose that he is HIV positive. He is dating!'
> (Eva, mother of a boy aged 17 infected by a blood transfusion)

> If you do [not use a condom], you will be prosecuted, you may even be arrested … So, it is not cruel to say this … this is … a reality.
> (Martha, a residential care worker at a foster home)

> [S]he has been asking: 'Can't I have children?' […] And there is always the dating thing … So I talked to her, the question of a relationship with a boyfriend, that she had the risk, when the time for first sexual intercourse arrived … that there is this question of condom use, or she could pass it to her partner.
> (John, adoptive father of a 12-year-old girl infected through parent-to-child transmission)

Lived sexual experience

In the accounts given by interviewed young people, love and dating emerged prominently as key issues. HIV-positive young people wanted to have sexual relationships and wanted to have children:

> It is not a problem for me to have the *illness* […] The problem is I don't know how to live without a woman … this is not sexual, it is psychological […] I am going out, everything is perfect … but then the need arises to talk to her […] Then I panic! … And I love children, babies, all those sort of things! If somebody accepts me, we may adopt … because … I want a normal family.
> (Heitor, 19 years old)

> Dating, for real, was only once. But we mess around sometimes, when we go out … that's normal … I thought it was better not to tell any of the girls I went out with, just to be careful, to take precautions [through condom use].
> (Xandi, 16 years old)

Many young people interviewed had sexual partners and had begun having sex before they were 15 years old. They reported consistent condom use, but not without some occasional difficulty. Some did not have the information they needed. Low levels of HIV prevention awareness among young interviewees, especially concerning parent-to-child transmission, was unexpected:

> I know ... there are medications for not transmitting HIV. And condoms. The medication is something that the women have, I think there are pills, so she won't be pregnant. What else? Do you know how to use them? I don't know anything.
>
> (Beto, 16 years old)

When dating or going out with someone, the majority of young people would choose not to tell their life stories or to disclose their HIV status to boyfriends or girlfriends. 'Trusting to tell' was the coping strategy adopted with partners, friends and peers. Respondents reported waiting until they felt secure they were loved and cared for:

> [If I told him], he might suddenly break up with me, that kind of thing, right?
>
> (Ana, 14 years old)

> Until I find this person ... I would like to keep it secret [...] It was difficult to use condoms in the beginning, getting used to the penis being tight with a condom. [...] I want a child, but do not want to infect my woman. It wouldn't feel right.
>
> (Xandi, 16 years old)

> I use condoms ... dating is great, but he doesn't know about my problem and I don't need to tell him until I feel more confident.
>
> (Vivian, 13 years old)

The desire to have a family and raise children emerged strongly in many interviews, but was accompanied by ambiguity and fear:

> Well, I would like to have a child. But it's ... not even because of the HIV that I don't want to, but because I'm afraid. If you have HIV, you have to do a C-section and so on, and I'm very scared of that. I prefer to adopt a child, you know? [There are] so many children in the world, give them an opportunity to have a family.
>
> (Sara, 15 years old)

People living with HIV: sexual health and rights

This study and others conducted among adults living with HIV in São Paulo in the last decade raises important concerns about the violation of many of the rights highlighted in the WHO's definition noted earlier. Other research reports similar concerns among adults living with HIV – poor levels of knowledge about sexual and vertical transmission and prevention strategies, violations of reproductive rights including lack of support for parenthood, and abusive C-sections without the provision of information on other options (Paiva *et al.* 2003). Study findings reveal that all too often people living with HIV are perceived as potential dangers to others, especially when it comes to sex and sexuality. Crucially, they are not seen as 'reproductive people', but rather as infected people who are to be treated as infectious. Young people living with HIV face further problems since 'adolescents' are rarely viewed as agents of their sexuality, as sexual subjects fighting for their sexual rights. This has consequences not only for quality of life and the fulfilment of citizenship, but also for the prevention of new infections.

A recent study conducted with young women living with HIV in Brazil, Ethiopia and Ukraine described similar experiences to those that we have encountered in São Paulo. Stigmatisation, problems of disclosure, poor access to counselling and support, these are just a few of the difficulties facing young people. Information and counselling was most usually provided too little and too late – when girls were already pregnant, for example, and doctors reported continuing to sterilise HIV-positive women and to deny support for parenthood desires (Engender Health/UNFPA 2006).

Young people living with HIV are people with rights. To provide healthcare that only pays attention to the management of HIV infection and survival is insufficient. Sexuality is both a desire and a challenge. If omission prevails and young people's full care needs are not met, the need for information and access to resources will not go away, and young people will simply enter into sexual relationships without proper information and support. As programmatic vulnerability increases, so too do individual and social vulnerability. Health authorities and carers should be held accountable when rights violations occur, not only persuaded not to 'behave badly', as one carer suggested.

The dreams and aspirations reported here are not about viral events, neither are they those of sick people without a life. They focus not only on HIV transmission and HIV prevention, but on bigger issues than this, namely hopes and aspirations for the future. Young people's sexuality experiences are enacted according to different meanings and scripts, in relation to culture and through different life histories and life obstacles. In the context of effective treatment, HIV is just one factor of many impinging on young people's lives. Nevertheless, it remains true that across most of the world young people are not supposed to act as sexual beings, and are not conceived of as being entitled to sexual rights.

In Brazil, there have been some positive developments of late. These include not only growing recognition of the rights of people living with HIV to comprehensive care and prevention that includes efforts to support their sexual citizenship and the development of an active national network of young people living with HIV. As individual, programmatic and social vulnerability are targeted, the challenge now is to use study findings to further support and strengthen the options available to young people who are living with HIV.

Notes

1 The 2002 Technical Consultation on Sexual Health convened by the WHO Department of Reproductive Health and Research in collaboration with the Department of Child and Adolescent Health and the prevention team of the Department of HIV/AIDS, brought together over 60 international and national experts on sexuality and sexual health-related issues from all regions of the world.
2 See www.usp.br/nepaids for more details on these studies.

References

Ayres, J. R., Paiva, V., França Jr., I., Gravato, N., Lacerda, R., DellaNegra, M. *et al.* (2006) 'Vulnerability, Human Rights and Comprehensive Healthcare Needs of Young People Living With HIV/AIDS', *American Journal of Public Health*, 96: 1001–6.

Benzaken, A. S., Garcia, E. G., Sardinha, J. C. and Paiva, V. (2007) 'Community-based Intervention to control STD/AIDS in the Amazon Region', *Revista de Saúde Pública*, 41 (Suppl. 2): 118–26.

Berkman, A., Garcia, J., Muñoz-Laboy, M., Paiva, V. and Parker, R. (2005) 'A Critical Analysis of the Brazilian Response to HIV/AIDS: Lessons Learned for Controlling and Mitigating the Epidemic in Developing Countries', *American Journal of Public Health*, 95 (7): 1162–72.

Brazil (1990) Statute of the Child and Adolescent, Law No. 8, 069, 13 July 1990. Treats of the Statute of the Child and Adolescent, and Other Measures; available at www.eca.org.br/ecai. htm (accessed 14 November 2008).

Engender Health/UNFPA (2006) 'Sexual and Reproductive Health Needs of Women and Adolescent Girls living with HIV – Research Report for Qualitative Findings from Brazil, Ethiopia and Ukraine, Brazil/Ethiopia/Ukraine'; available at www.unfpa.org/upload/lib_pub_file/619_filename_srh-of-hiv-positive-women.pdf (accessed 7 November 2008).

Frederick, T., Thomas, P., Mascola, L., Hsu, H. W., Rakusan, T., Mapson, C. *et al.* (2000) 'Human Immunodeficiency Virus-infected Adolescents: A descriptive Study of older Children in New York City, Los Angeles County, Massachusetts, and Washington, DC', *Pediatric Infectious Disease Journal*, 19 (6): 551–5.

Gagnon, J. and Parker, R. (1995) 'Conceiving Sexuality', in Gagnon, J. and Parker, R. (eds) *Conceiving Sexuality: Approaches to Sex Research in a Postmodern World*, New York: Routledge.

Gruskin, S. and Tarantola, D. (2005) 'Health and Human Rights', in Gruskin, S., Grodin, M. A. and Marks, S. P. (eds) *Perspectives on Health and Human Rights*, London: Routledge.

Gruskin, S., Ferguson, L. and O'Malley, L. (2007) 'Ensuring Sexual and Reproductive Health for People Living with HIV: An Overview of Key Human Rights, Policy and Health Systems Issues', *Reproductive Health Matters*, 15 (29): 4–26.

Kmita, G., Baranska, M. and Niemiec, T. (2002) 'Psychosocial Intervention in the Process of Empowering Families with Children Living with HIV/AIDS – A Descriptive Study', *AIDS Care*, 14 (2): 279–84.

Lusti-Narasimhan, M., Cottingham, J. and Berer, M. (2007) 'Ensuring the Sexual and Reproductive Health of People Living with HIV: Policies, Programmes and Health Services', *Reproductive Health Matters*, 15 (29): 1–3.

Mann, J. M. and Tarantola, D. J. (1998) 'Responding to HIV/AIDS: A Historical Perspective', *Health and Human Rights*, 2 (4): 5–8.

Paiva, V. (2005) 'Analysing Sexual Experiences through "Scenes": A Framework for the Evaluation of Sexuality Education', *Sex Education*, 5 (4): 345–59.

Paiva, V. (2007) 'Gendered Scripts and the Sexual Scene: Promoting Sexual Subjects among Brazilian Teenagers', in Parker, R. and Aggleton, P. (eds.) *Culture, Society and Sexuality. A Reader*, 2nd edn, New York: Routledge.

Paiva, V., Ayres, J. R. and França Jr., I. (2004) 'Expanding the Flexibility of Normative Patterns in Youth Sexuality and Prevention Programs', *Sex Research & Social Policy*, 1 (1): 83–97.

Paiva, V., Felipe, E. V., Santos, N., Lima, T. and Segurado, A. C. (2003) 'The Right to Love: The Desire for Parenthood among Men living with HIV', *Reproductive Health Matters*, 11 (22): 91–100.

Paiva, V., Santos, N., França Jr., I., Filipe, E., Ayres, J. R. and Segurado, A. C. (2007) 'Desire to have Children, Gender and Reproductive Rights of Men and Women living with HIV: A Challenge to Healthcare in Brazil', *AIDS Patient Care STDs*, 21 (4): 268–77.

Rotheram-Borus, M. J., Lee, M., Leonard, N., Lin, Y. Y., Franzke, L., Turner, E. *et al.* (2003) 'Four-year Behavioral Outcomes of an Intervention for Parents living with HIV and their Adolescent Children', *AIDS*, 17: 1217–25.

Santos, B. S. (2005) 'Subjetividade, Cidadania e Emancipação', in *Pela Mão de Alice: O social e o Político na Pós Modernidade*, 10th edn, São Paulo: Cortez.

Segurado, A. C., Miranda, L. D. and Latorre, M. R. D. O. (2003) 'Brazilian Enhancing Care Initiative Team – Evaluation of Care of Women living with HIV/AIDS in the State of São Paulo', *AIDS Patient Care and STDs*, 17 (2): 85–93.

UN – United Nations (1995) 'Beijing Platform for Action'; available at www.un.org/women-watch/daw/beijing/platform/ (accessed 7 November 2008).

UNAIDS/Guttmacher Institute (2006) 'Meeting the Sexual and Reproductive Health Needs of People living with HIV', *In Brief 2006 Series*, 6; available at www.unaids.org/en/KnowledgeCentre/Resources/PolicyGuidance/Techpolicies/sexual_repro_technical_policies.asp (accessed 7 November 2008).

UNFPA – United Nations Population Fund (1994) *ICPD Programme of Action*, available at www.unfpa.org/icpd/icpd.cfm (date accessed 7 November 2008).

UNICEF – United Nations Children's Fund (1989) Convention on the Rights of the Child; available at www2.ohchr.org/english/law/crc.htm (accessed 7 November 2008).

WHO – World Health Organisation (1975) 'Education and Treatment in Human Sexuality: The Training of Health Professionals', Geneva: WHO. (WHO Technical Report Series No. 572).

WHO – World Health Organisation (1987) World Health Assembly, Resolution WHA 40.26, Global Strategy for the Prevention and Control of AIDS, 5 May 1987, Geneva: WHO.

WHO – World Health Organisation (2006) 'Defining Sexual Health: Report on Technical Consultation on Sexual Health', Geneva: WHO.

45 The 'queer' politics of homo(sexuality) and matters of identity

Tentative notes in the context of HIV/AIDS

Vasu Reddy

I have discovered that sex is political and that, as moffies and letties, we had to be part of a revolution to change everything. It was the beginning of a life of sex and politics.

(Achmat 1994: 341)

I am a lesbian. I am a black woman. I live in the township. Life is not very easy in the township, but I smile through it even though for me, as a black woman and a lesbian, life sometimes doesn't want to make me smile. I come from a Zulu family where the men get first preference for everything, where they get to rule your life if you are a woman.

(Chan-Sam 1994: 191)

But the formation of gay identity in South Africa is complicated even further by the fact that, at the very time we are beginning to see the emergence of a homosexual people, we are also having to live with HIV infection. The impact of HIV on gay men in South Africa has already been catastrophic [...] Homosexuals in the Aids scenario of southern Africa are a minority amongst those who are infected, a minority that can be safely ignored by the majority and those who hold power.

(Pegge 1994: 301)

If, as Felman and Laub (1992: 115) observe, discourses exist in a state of 'constant obligation' to the 'woes of history', then reading history reinforces an understanding of how identities are continually shaped (and indeed reinvented) by context. Identity formation is crucially about tangible experiences that have some connection to strategies of bearing witness. My understanding is that this could be something that is familiar in the form of *accumulated knowledge*. Such knowledge, I believe, is about the life history of the 'self', constructed by a series of events intimately connected to the 'private' and 'public'. The first and last are issues integrally related to the *bios* (life) in which *history* assumes primary significance in the shaping of *personality*.

Similarly, the real, tangible, personal, historical and politicised experiences of Achmat, Sibongile and Pegge in the epigraphs to this chapter, constitute affirmative statements about living, presence, inclusivity and belonging. These are simultaneously utterances about identity, sexuality, culture, disease, oppression and the power that shapes our identities. These assertions also disclose ongoing contestations about homosexuality that many of us who are sexual minorities experience.

'Belonging' in the queer sense, need not necessarily imply acceptance, tolerance, and indeed complete 'freedom' because the danger of homophobic violence is always a persistent threat within the heteronormative institutions that dominate us. The political is therefore always imminent within matters of sexuality and identity. But the political is also always persistent in matters of life and death as well.

'Political' is a derivation of the word *politiki* (meaning 'politics' in Greek) and *res publicae* (in Latin), which refers to the 'affairs of state'. This definition implies that there are matters that may not be matters of the state, but that do *matter* to the state. Homosexuality is one such issue where the state encroaches on the realm of the 'private'. Politics, following Foucault is a form of practical engagement within social relations. Any conception of politics in relation to identity should also direct us to resistance to oppressive power, which is the sense in which 'queer' is understood.

The construction of the queer, like the subject of feminism, following De Lauretis (1986: 9), is 'a political-personal strategy of survival and resistance that is also, at the same time, a critical practice and a mode of knowledge'. The conditions of queer emergence are closely connected to how identity is invested and mediated by discursive aspects, such as, for example, the juridical, political, civic and literary (see also De Lauretis 1987). Identities are in some sense hybrids and discursive formations. Identities are, following Hall (1995: 65), not essences but rather 'processes that constitute and continuously re-form the subject who has to act and speak in the social and cultural world'. In extending this to the queer subject, identities could be conceived as our sense of ourselves as individual and social beings constructed through structural processes, subjected to the play of history, culture and power rather than being innate and pre-given.

In South Africa, the constitution of queer identity is an important effect of the new (post-apartheid) state. Identity is closely connected to normalising the queer self, and is produced in relation to a type of sexual citizenship that involves negotiating the private and public spheres. I subscribe to the view suggested by Hall and Du Gay (1996: 4) that identities are future oriented, a matter of becoming rather than a being. If identities are indeed about becoming, about formation rather than something already formed, the argument opts for the former.

National identity in South Africa in terms of the post-apartheid project is directed towards recognising differences of a shared and divided history, not as something conflictual, but rather as the basis for facilitating the development of a cohesive 'new' sense of commonality based on celebrating differences. Racial, gender and sexual orientation seem to be some of those differences being advanced as the basis for the development of a national identity. Since the birth of democracy in South Africa on 27 April 1994, many legal hurdles facing lesbians and gays in particular have been overcome, most recently with the legal gift of marriage.

Democratic South Africa brought citizenship rights, especially in the renegotiation of citizenship in the context of potentially divisive factors such as race, ethnicity, language, class, location, gender and sexual orientation, among others. Citizenship, therefore, becomes an important marker in a possible relationship between the individual and the State. The relationship includes fundamental notions of who 'belongs' and who is to be excluded. Belonging and exclusion are factors that reduce or facilitate the negotiation of identities in the nation-building effort.

Thinking sex

Within this social and political vision, much like race, sexuality is an important marker of fundamental differences. Feminism's critique of patriarchy, developments in the liberation of gay and lesbian persons and the impact of HIV and AIDS have all contributed to an understanding of sexuality as less of a social and moral 'given' than a continuously debated source of meaning. Sexuality, especially as we have come to understand it in the twentieth century, appears to be punctuated by sexual panics over 'moral rearmament' in a range of issues from abortion, contraception and marital disharmony to frigidity, homosexuality and AIDS (Mclaren 1999).

Homosexuality (as a crucial component of sexuality) has been given renewed cachet through the demise of the apartheid state. The transition from the criminalisation of homosexuality under apartheid governments, to the 'full' citizenship of gays and lesbians under the present government might confirm our beloved Emeritus Archbishop Desmond Tutu's description of South Africa as a 'remarkable country'.[1] However, the leap from an apartheid exclusionist mentality to a post-apartheid inclusionist approach suggests that the temporal shift is a productive moment in which to reconceptualise how homosexuality is renegotiated as an identity to be included in the post-apartheid democracy.

But, at another level, homosexuality, in its relationship to the promise of inclusivity that typifies the post-apartheid state is also a symptom of complex globalisation that has marked the closing decades of the twentieth century (for example, Altman 2000; Appadurai 1996; Harvey 1990). In this regard, Parker and Gagnon (1995) suggest that it is only by seeking to interpret the specificities of local sexual cultures as they are caught up within the cross-currents of global processes of change that we are able to move past a superficial understanding of sexuality and build a more complex understanding of sexual experience in the contemporary world.

Parker and Gagnon emphasise the value of interpreting sexuality by situating it within the broader processes of history and political economy in order to analyse the tension between an emphasis on local meanings and an understanding of global processes (Parker 1999: 2). One meaning that is emerging in many different political and social situations is the location of sexuality as a human rights issue (see Chapters 35 to 40 in this volume).

In another sense, thinking about homosexuality in the context of identity politics and HIV is also another way to respond to the history of silence that has sought to render our existence invisible. In much the same way as women have been 'hidden from history', to borrow the phrase from Rosemary Tong, we must respond to the heterosexual matrix (Butler 1990), the straight mind (Wittig 1992) and the compulsory heterosexuality (Rich 1980) that informs the hegemonic order of heterosexuality. Such a response reinforces the political implications of understanding our sexuality.

For many of us who may still be secretive, a possible reference point is that of the 'closet, a private (or sub-cultural) space one comes out of to inhabit public space and honestly and with one's identity intact' (Creekmur and Doty 1995: 2). For many in South Africa, the reality of the closet persists despite the many legal gains in our favour. The potentially positive visibility of gays and lesbians is also continually offset by cultural taboos, religious doctrine, the HIV crisis and by those who deploy it to reinforce homophobia, often of a violent kind as manifested in the rape by straight of especially black lesbians in order to 'correct' them. Identity construction may be found in cultural experience that is proscribed by a dominant heterosexual culture that has necessitated critical response, in part developed by feminist scholarship.

'Sexual politics' is a necessary factor in understanding the circuits of power informing identity issues because the gendered hierarchy is sexualised by men. The point is that heteropolar regimes of gender have made sex dangerous for women too. Wilton (1997: 126) explains the division in the following terms:

> The discursive package 'gender' constitutes femininity as inherently passive, responsive, responsible, nurturative and innocent of sexual desire/agency and masculinity as inherently active, initiating, irresponsible, unattached and potent with sexual desire/agency.

The violent effects of the sexualisation of the gender, represented by, for example, the socialised attribute of 'virility' for men within patriarchal institutions (such as the family, culture, religion), are often, for example, rape, sexual harassment, sexual abuse of children, prostitution and homophobia. These practices express and actualise the distinctive power of men over women. Because sexuality is the nexus of relationships between genders, much oppression is mediated and constituted within sexuality.

Rethinking sexuality therefore cannot eliminate the possibilities of *agency*. For Rubin, it is when sexuality, as an abstract concept, moves towards tangible expression (sexual acts, sexual behaviours, sexual choices) that social construction becomes a convincing approach to sexuality. Rethinking sexuality in Rubin's (1984: 267) terms entails reconceptualising the battles and contestations fought over sexuality:

> The realm of sexuality also has its own internal politics [...] They are imbued with conflicts of interest and political maneuvering, both deliberate and incidental. In that sense, sex is always political.

The discourses of homosexuality are in fact spaces of agency that demonstrate 'conflicts of interest' as we have seen over the years in opposition by many within the religious sector, by some politicians and opinion makers. Spaces of agency are related to a focus on the subject of sexuality, both as an object of intellectual inquiry, as well as a lens through which we may understand the many and varied interests that inform sexuality; and similarly how these interests, in turn, shape, reflect and demonstrate resistance in relation to factors that inform homosexuality as a contested sexual practice.

In most African states, homosexuality is still criminalised and actively policed. This criminalisation is fuelled by the notion of the supposed un-Africanness of homosex, despite the overwhelming evidence of its existence in earlier times (see Constantine-Simms 2001; Epprecht 2004; Gevisser and Cameron 1994; Murray and Roscoe 1998). The relevant point here is less the issue of its misrecognition and denial than the fact that homosexuality is aligned along a simplistic heteropatriarchal binary that views homosexuality as acts rather than as an identity. This perception locates homosexuality simply as a perverse desire associated with pathology, and signals a return to a biomedical and non-cultural understanding of human sexuality.

HIV and AIDS

When Pegge (1994: 301) claimed in the epigraph that 'homosexuals in the AIDS scenario of Southern Africa are a minority amongst those who are infected, a minority that can be safely ignored by the majority and those who hold power', he was at best being prophetic about the way we have been treated in responses to the epidemic. The gains made by activism in having our sexual orientation recognised as a legal identity, require the same commitment when we ask for the epidemic to be 'regayed'. Regaying implies that we need to return to an understanding of our sexual behaviour within our sexual subcultures to better understand the programmes needed within our communities.

HIV and AIDS continue to challenge the way we think about sexuality and sexual pleasure. On the African continent, sexuality is problematised via its potential for devastation, from overpopulation to AIDS-related mortalities. Repeated associations of sexuality with disease (especially homosexuality) result in isolation, loneliness and the disclosure of status that often have negative consequences for many women (and men) living with HIV. Contemporary international Aids activism operates at the interface between the 'discursive' and 'material' levels. The former focuses on the meanings of HIV in relation to political economic factors generating profits for pharmaceutical companies. The latter directs attention to the experiences and needs of people living with HIV. Recent international HIV conferences (Bangkok, Toronto, Mexico) represented a face of contemporary global AIDS activism that mediates between gay and lesbian identity-based activism and activism that prioritises socioeconomic justice. It is interesting to note that these conferences cost millions in dollar terms, and while the exchange of ideas and knowledge is not to be disparaged, it is important to recognise that HIV-related research has become an industry in itself.

Beyond the statistical projections of infection, and the considerable costs involved in healthcare, the lack of a cure compounds the problem. But the symbolic meanings attached to AIDS also account for its significance: its juxtaposition and explosion of sex and death, of homosexuality and promiscuity, of injecting drug use and racial/ethnic variation still prevail. Another aspect of the virus concerns the crude categorisations of people who are affected by it: as *innocent victims* ((haemophiliacs, women, children) versus *guilty perpetrators* (promiscuous homosexuals, prostitutes, pimps). Even if such a description may not be part of the mainstream vocabulary, the attitudes and stereotypes reinforcing such categories persist.

Returning to identity and knowledge

Therefore, all engagements with homosexuality or same-sex sexuality as it is increasingly described, whether in research, activism, policymaking cannot escape the circuits of power that matter. All societies, Foucault reminded us, have procedures and techniques whereby the production of discourses are controlled, selected, organised and redistributed within a system of power. The proliferation of discourses in Foucault's (1990: 36) model is not to be viewed as a quantitative phenomenon, but rather in terms of the 'forms of imperatives' imposed. What emerged from his understanding were the legal sanctions that focused on the curtailment of 'unreproductive activities' in order to motivate a 'norm of sexual activity'. For Foucault, unreproductive activities were viewed as peripheral and therefore marginal sexualities, of which homosexuality was one such example. Canonical codes defined homosexual activities as unlawful, thereby relegating the homosexual to Foucault's (1990: 42–3) mind as a 'personage, a past, a case history'. Homosexuality according to Foucault (1990: 43) was constituted from the moment it was characterised:

> Homosexuality appeared as one of the forms of sexuality when it was transposed from the practice of sodomy onto a kind of interior androgyny, a hermaphroditism of the soul. The sodomite had been a temporary aberration; the homosexual was now a species.

The mechanisms of power that operate to suppress (and oppress) the homosexual must therefore be viewed within a broader framework in order to explain the practices that give rise to identity. Building on these themes, queers are constituted as subjects within Foucault's model when subjected to control by power operations. In this system of subjection, Foucault also claims self-knowledge, which is linked to identity, is not lost. The struggles between the subjected and the controlling power give rise to identity formation, especially when the struggles concern resistance against domination and the exercise of power.

In *Gender Trouble: Feminism and the Subversion of Identity,* Judith Butler (1999) calls into the question the category of the subject in a genealogical critique (following the model proposed by Foucault) that demonstrates the subject's emergence within discourse. In an important sense, this text offers a genealogy of the discursive construction of identities and bodies. Her reading is further developed in *Bodies That Matter: On the Discursive Limits of 'Sex'* (Butler 1993a) in which she considers how, within a particular culture, certain bodies come to *matter* more than others. Butler reiterates how the excluded body, the abject body in particular (and by extension the homosexual body), is viewed as potentially disruptive to the symbolic order of viable bodies motivated by the heterosexual matrix. Most crucially, it is not 'heterosexual normativity that produces and consolidates gender' but the 'gender *hierarchy* that is said to underwrite heterosexual relations' (Butler 1999: xii, emphasis added). The 'hierarchy' in question is principally informed by how identities and subjectivity are formed within power structures. In other words, subjecthood is not pre-given, but rather something that is in the process of becoming.

To explain this, Butler turns to the notion of performativity to suggest that gender is more than culturally specific meanings that are inscribed on an already sexed body.[2] In her view, the act, or activity of gender is both intentional and performative where the latter entails public, repetitive actions of movement, gesture, posture, dress, labour, production, interaction with objects and the manipulation of space. The 'performative' in the Butlerian project has less to do with performance than it has to do with 'the *effect* of a regulatory regime of gender difference in which genders are divided and hierarchised *under constraint*' (Butler 1993b: 21, emphasis added).

A recurring theme in Butler's (1999: xxii) work is the question of what it is to be human in processes that determine identities:

What continues to concern me most is the following kinds of questions: what will and will not constitute an intelligible life, and how do presumptions about normative gender and sexuality determine in advance what will qualify as the 'human' and the 'livable'.

Both the 'human' and the 'livable' are central to any construction of queer identities. In asking these questions Butler does not, in my view, abandon experience in favour of verbal politics, but is concerned to assess how we mobilise meanings around identities.

Queer is also closely linked to subject formation and identity. Butler's subject is a linguistic structure that is always in the process of formation. In this way, we could interpret that a subject derives identity through an endless process of becoming. Viewing the queer subject this way does not, in my view, restore the experience of the homosexual, but rather demonstrates how the homosexual is produced as a subject in epistemological terms. By this, I mean that ideas about experience and identity accrue in conceiving homosexuality within discourses of power and performativity in marked contrast to the reductiveness in interpreting identities as fixed and immutable essences within heteronormative models.

If Butler's heterosexual matrix is to be understood in terms of the cultural assumptions that shape, construct and configure the homosexual, Sedgwick's 'epistemology of the closet' likewise reinforces the transitivity of sexual identities that imply identities are formed in relation to specific contexts. Sedgwick (1994: 1) proposes that major nodes of thought and knowledge in the twentieth century have been framed, structured and fractured by what she terms the homo/heterosexual binary as a site of much contestation. Her view is applicable insofar as she claims that institutionalised taxonomic discourses (such as the medical, legal, literary and psychological) structure same-sex desire, and these discourses, she claims, are marked by inequality and contest.

For Sedgwick, the closet as a defining structure of gay oppression in the 'privacy' (and thus secrecy) it imposes on homosexuals can be read as opposite to 'coming out' (into the visible and into the public) as a 'private' secret to be disclosed. The closet may be viewed as a space that reveals much about the oppression within heteronormativity. The notion of an epistemology of the closet is a key analytical tool for Sedgwick (1994: 19) which derives, in part, from a 'homosexual panic'. The latter for Sedgwick (1994: 19–20) constitutes an artificial and 'individualising assumption' to pathologise homosexuals in a type of 'socially sanctioned prejudice'.

This type of panic is not a new occurrence. It may be traced to similar 'moral panics' like those that characterised AIDS in the early days of the epidemic, and also diseases such as syphilis in the nineteenth century (cf. Gilman 1988). Central to this panic are the following influences: myth, popular assumption and religion (Watney (1997). Panics give rise to bitter cultural and political battles over sexuality which constructs certain groups and individuals (such as homosexuals) as outlaws by labelling them immoral.

Sedgwick's concept of the 'homosexual panic' is relevant to the current day construction of identities in Southern Africa insofar as her concept motivates the anxieties and crystallises the fears of homophobes. For Sedgwick (1993: 8), 'queer' is an open mesh of possibilities, gaps, overlaps, dissonances and resonances that emerge in discursive formations. It is therefore necessary to hold on to 'identity matters' concerning our sexuality, especially as we engage subcultures within 'same-sex sexuality' that may not necessarily be openly gay or lesbian, or may well simply self-identify as 'heterosexual' but who may simply be (through no fault of their own making) engaged in sex with their same gender.

Postscript: returning to the personal

The question of 'freedom' is a valid concern that reminds us, in the context of Butler's notions of the human and livable, and about the future for queer identities. We have much work to do. To be queer can also imply whether one lives or dies. Sometimes we have choices, sometimes there is none, and sometimes we may have internalised our own homophobia to the extent that we lack the desire to live. While the political comprises networks of relations that obtain between institutions and their representations, identities and the urgency to mobilise against all forms of oppression that threaten us, must be foremost in whatever work we do to advance and improve the lives of sexual minorities. I received such a lesson from my late friend.

Ronald Louw was my friend at university where we worked. He called me 'skattie' (a camp term of endearment in Afrikaans meaning 'darling') because he was intrigued that I studied Afrikaans. Like me, he was gay. He was white, acknowledged his middle-class roots and despised any form of discrimination. We were the closest of friends, comrades in pursuing justice on human rights (especially in the gay and lesbian communities). We worked together on the National Coalition for Gay and Lesbian Equality and established together with Nonhlanhla Mkhize the Durban Lesbian and Gay Community Centre. We also had wonderful conversations about politics, the law and justice and regularly engaged in what a mutual friend described as 'gay men's rituals' in the form of dinner parties at our respective homes.

Ronald died on 26 June 2005 at the age of 47. He had been a much loved and respected member of the university community since 1993 when he joined the law faculty. As an Assistant Dean, Head of the School of Law, and University Proctor, he was an ethical and principled person who fought for equality and social justice. His family, friends, colleagues and students all miss him very much. Six weeks before Ronald died, he fell ill and was hospitalised. Doctors tested to find out what was wrong and discovered he had AIDS. He said that he regretted not having a test sooner. During the last week of his life, Ronald said to me that when he was better, he wanted to run a campaign at the University of KwaZulu Natal encouraging students and staff to get tested. One year later, his wish for a campaign has been fulfilled, even though he is not here to participate as he had wanted to.

Why did Ronald not have an HIV test sooner? Before he fell ill, he told his friends that he would not get a test because he did not need to. Often when people say that they do not need a test, the real reason is that they are afraid. Ronald wanted to spread the message that, even though getting a test can be frightening, it should be an essential part of everyone's healthcare routine. Ronald was filled with terror, not about his sexuality (he celebrated it with gusto). He was filled with dread about confronting HIV and denied himself a test until it was too late.

In all of this there is something to be said about Ronald's life, work and death (and the significance for my ongoing learning and activism). Although born into relative privilege, Ronald gave of his energies and talents to the cause of changing society and the upliftment of others. The combination of vision with the capacity to give it practical effect made him a leader. His contributions and the imprint he leaves on many lives serve as inspiration for the future. Ronald's memory demands that we reaffirm and intensify the struggle for freedom, equality, dignity and social justice.

Likewise, my ongoing work reflects a commitment to issues of diversity, difference, dignity and social justice. In a traditional approach to teaching and research we are indoctrinated to prioritise the rational and the cognitive, aspects to be separated from emotional and the personal. If, as suggested at the beginning, that our experiences are never completely 'objective' but rather inscribed by subjective truths that enable us constantly to bear witness to the experiences that shape us, then the modalities of learning are similarly for me shaped by an opposition to the tyranny of objective fallacies. I cannot separate myself from the activity of learning. I am obligated to account for the personal and the private as *values* in the learning project. It is imperative for me to remember Ronald's life as an important lesson to understand what he stood for, to analyse his fears, his shortcomings in order for us to learn from such experiences.

Our experiences cannot be separated from the 'emotions' that inform our memories. Emotion, in its etymological sense denotes, from Latin, a performative mode: *emovere* (to disturb) and *movere* (move). Such a relationship is necessary for learning: emotions are able to reflect personality and experience in both an ontological and epistemological sense. I continue to use Ronald's life history and experiences in my work and conversations to better understand myself, my interaction with people and the world around me.

Therefore, if one way of reading, interpreting and understanding the conditions of possibility that give rise to queer identity is concerned with investigating relations of the past, another form is concerned with narrating and interrogating a future.

Notes

1 'Ours is a remarkable country. Let us celebrate our diversity, our differences [...] South Africa wants and needs the Afrikaner, the English, the coloured, the Indian, the black [...] Let us move into the glorious future of a new kind of society where people count, not because of biological irrelevancies or other extraneous attributes, but because they are persons of infinite worth created in the image of God. Let that society be a new society – more compassionate, more caring, more gentle, more given to sharing – because we have left the past for a deeply divided society characterised by strife, conflict, untold suffering and injustice and are moving to a future founded on the recognition of human rights, democracy and peaceful coexistence and development opportunities for all South Africans, irrespective of colour, race, class, belief or sex'. (Archbishop Desmond Tutu in *Star*, 1998: 3)
2 Butler develops her ideas on performativity, in part based on the work of Sedgwick (see for example, Parker and Sedgwick 1995).

References

Achmat, Z. (1994) 'My Childhood as an Adult-Molester: A Salt River Moffie', in Gevisser, M. and Cameron, E. (eds) *Defiant Desire: Gay and Lesbian Lives in South Africa*, Johannesburg: Ravan Press.
Altman, D. (2000) *Global Sex*, Chicago: University of Chicago Press.

Appadurai, A. (1996) *Modernity at Large: Cultural Dimensions of Globalization*, Minneapolis and London: University of Minnesota Press.

Butler, Judith (1990) *Gender Trouble: Feminism and the Subversion of Identity*. New York and London: Routledge.

Butler, J. (1993a) *Bodies that Matter: On the Discursive Limits of 'Sex'*, New York and London: Routledge.

Butler, J. (1993b) 'Critically Queer', *GLQ*, 1 (1): 17–32.

Butler, J. (1999) *Gender Trouble: Feminism and the Subversion of Identity*, 2nd edn, New York and London: Routledge.

Chan-Sam, T. (1994) 'Five Women: Profiles of Black Lesbian Life on the Reef', in Gevisser, M. and Cameron, E. (eds) *Defiant Desire: Gay and Lesbian Lives in South Africa*, Johannesburg: Ravan Press.

Constantine-Simms, D. (ed.) (2001) *The Greatest Taboo: Homosexuality in Black Communities*, Los Angeles and New York: Alyson Books.

Copjec, J. (ed.) (1994) *Supposing the Subject*, London: Verso.

Creekmur, C. K. and Doty, A. (eds) (1995) *Out in Culture: Gay, Lesbian, and Queer Essays on Popular Culture*, London: Cassell.

Cullinan, K. (2004) 'The Loneliness of Zwe', *Sunday Times*, 12 September: 21.

De Lauretis, T. (ed.) (1986) *Feminist Studies/Critical Studies*, London: Macmillan.

De Lauretis, T. (1987) *Technologies of Gender: Essays on Theory, Film and Fiction*, London: Macmillan.

Epprecht, M. (2004) *Hungochani: The History of a Dissident Sexuality in Southern Africa*, Montreal: McGill-Queen's University Press.

Felman, S. and Laub, D. (1992) *Testimony: Crises of Witnessing in Literature, Psychoanalysis, and History*, New York: Routledge.

Foucault, M. (1990) *The History of Sexuality: An Introduction* (trans. R. Hurley), Harmondsworth: Penguin.

Gevisser, M. and Cameron, E. (eds) (1994) *Defiant Desire: Gay and Lesbian Lives in South Africa*, Johannesburg: Ravan Press.

Gilman, S. L. (1988) *Disease and Representation: Images of Illness from Madness to AIDS*, Ithaca NY: Cornell University Press.

Hall, S. (1995) 'Fantasy, Identity, Politics', in Carter, E., Donald, J. and Squires, J. (eds) *Cultural Remix: Theories of Politics and the Popular*, London: Lawrence & Wishart.

Hall, S. and Du Gay, P. (eds) (1996) *Questions of Cultural Identity,*. London: Sage.

Harvey, D. (1990) *The Condition of Postmodernity*, Cambridge, MA and Oxford: Blackwell.

McLaren, A. (1999) *Twentieth-Century Sexuality: A History*, Oxford: Blackwell.

Murray, S. O. and Roscoe, W. (eds) (1998) *Boy-Wives and Female Husbands: Studies of African Homosexualities*, New York: St. Martin's Press.

Parker, A. and Sedgwick, E. K. (eds) (1995) *Performativity and Performance*, London and New York: Routledge.

Parker, R. G. (1999) *Beneath the Equator: Cultures of Desire: Male Homosexuality, and Emerging Gay Communities in Brazil*, London and New York: Routledge.

Parker, R. G. and Gagnon, J. H. (eds) (1995) *Conceiving Sexuality: Approaches to Sex Research in a Postmodern World*, New York and London: Routledge.

Pegge, J. (1994) 'Living with Loss in the best Way we know how: AIDS and Gay Men in Cape Town', in Gevisser, M. and Cameron, E. (eds) *Defiant Desire: Gay and Lesbian Lives in South Africa*, Johannesburg: Ravan Press.

Rich, A. (1980) 'Compulsory Heterosexuality and Lesbian Existence', *Signs*, 5 (4): 631–60.

Rubin, G. (1984) 'Thinking Sex: Notes for a Radical Theory in the politics of Sexuality', in Vance, C. S. (ed.) *Pleasure and Danger: Exploring Female Sexuality*, New York: Routledge & Kegan Paul.

Sedgwick, E. K. (1993) *Tendencies*, Durham, NC: Duke University Press.

Sedgwick, E. K. (1994) *Epistemology of the Closet*, Harmondsworth: Penguin.

Star (1998) 'Report of the Truth and Reconciliation Commission', 2 September: 4.

Watney, S. (1997) *Policing Desire: Pornography, AIDS and the Media*, 3rd edn, London: Cassell.

Wilton, T. (1997) *Engendering AIDS: Deconstructing Sex, Text and Epidemic*, London: Sage.

Wittig, M. (1992) *The Straight Mind and Other Essays*, Boston, MA: Beacon Press.

46 Immigration and LGBT rights in the USA

Ironies and constraints in US asylum cases

Héctor Carrillo

Every year, more than one million foreign nationals become permanent residents in the USA. A report from the Department of Homeland Security stated in 2006 that 'nearly two thirds (or 63 per cent) were granted permanent residence based on a family relationship with a US citizen or legal permanent resident of the United States' (Jefferys 2007a: 1). Among them a considerable number were the spouses of US citizens (339,843 people in 2006) and still others were spouses of legal permanent residents (Jefferys 2007a). This means that being or becoming the spouse of a US citizen or legal resident constitutes the single largest path through which foreign nationals immigrate legally to the USA today.

These figures are of enormous significance for US citizens and foreign nationals involved in same-sex binational relationships. Lesbian, gay, bisexual and transgender (LGBT) US citizens and legal immigrants are barred from sponsoring their same-sex partners for immigration purposes (Schulzetenberg 2002; Howe 2007).[1] Cymene Howe (2007: 96) has noted that the 1996 Defense of Marriage Act (DOMA) 'continues to prohibit same-sex binational marriage claims because, for immigration purposes, the DOMA legislation defines marriage as a relationship between a man and a woman'. This same act has perpetuated a form of state discrimination toward a considerable proportion of American citizens (Reed 1996). Ironically, in 1993 the US government began to grant visitor visas to the same-sex partners of non-immigrant foreigners who are legally in the country. The poignant consequence is that long-term non-immigrant foreigners have been conferred a right that is not extended to US citizens or legal immigrants (Schulzetenberg 2002).

Taken together, these policies symbolise the unequal position of sexual minority populations. Most importantly, as a result of these policies the most common path for immigration to the USA among adults has been rendered unavailable to gay and lesbian foreign nationals unless they break the law and engage in sham heterosexual marriages. Furthermore, because it is often much more difficult to obtain other types of immigrant visa that are based on employment or other forms of family-sponsored immigration, the possibilities for LGBT individuals to immigrate to the USA legally are greatly reduced.

LGBT immigrants have had to explore alternative avenues to pursue legal immigration to the USA. Because many of them have been badly mistreated due to their sexual orientation in their countries of origin, beginning in the late 1980s they and their lawyers began to test whether they could attain permanent residency through asylum. These efforts coincided with a federal policy change in 1990 that ended the exclusion of homosexual foreign nationals from the USA (a policy that had been put in place by two separate US Immigration Acts in 1917 and 1952) (Bennett 1999). That same year, the Board of Immigration Appeals granted asylum to a gay Cuban immigrant by the name of Toboso-Alfonso who convincingly claimed that he had been persecuted in Cuba due to his sexual orientation and feared future persecution if he returned (Russ IV 1998; Cantú *et al.* 2005).

Since this first successful case, a growing number of LGBT individuals have obtained immigrant visas through asylum in the USA. As one legal scholar has recently noted: 'Owing to a number of recent developments, US asylum law is one of the most hospitable legal arenas for lesbian, gay, bisexual and transgender ("LGBT") litigants' (Landau 2005: 237). However, being granted asylum is not easy.

In this chapter, I examine the use of asylum as an immigration strategy for LGBT immigrants in the USA. Based on the existing legal literature on the topic, I discuss the practical limitations of this strategy and, at a more conceptual level, the problematic nature of assumptions about homosexuality that typically accompany LGBT asylum cases. Successful arguing of these cases often has involved great oversimplification in ways that disregard the nuance and complexity found in anthropological and sociological studies of same-sex sexualities around the world. My discussion refers to cases in the USA, although this legal strategy has also been used in other rich countries that have large immigrant communities from the developing world. While aspects of the analysis may be generalisable, the specific implementation of LGBT asylum varies from country to country, reflecting the characteristics of local legal systems and policies. Therefore my conclusions should be taken to apply only to the US experience.

The issues that I discuss here are relevant to both sexual minority men and women. It is striking, however, that most successful cases of LGBT asylum have involved gay men and male-to-female transgender individuals (Millbank 2003; Neilson 2005b). One possible explanation for this disparity is that lesbian lifestyles, like those of other women, often are less public than those of men (Chisholm 2001; Millbank 2003; Neilson 2005b).

The challenges of asylum for LGBT immigrants

Making asylum work for LGBT applicants in the USA has been an arduous process for immigration lawyers. Asylum decisions are made at various institutional levels within the US legal system. Petitions are made to the Department of Homeland Security, where an asylum officer approves or denies the petition. Denied applicants who do not have a valid legal status in the USA are placed on removal procedures and referred to an immigration judge in the Department of Justice, who can uphold or overturn the decision by the asylum officer. If the immigration judge upholds the denial, an appeal can be filed with the Board of Immigration Appeals, and if the appeal fails the petitioner's lawyer can then try to bring the case to the US Court of Appeals (Leitner 2004; Randazzo 2005; Jefferys 2007b).

Since the 1990 Toboso-Alfonso case, which was decided by the Board of Immigration Appeals (Henes 1994; Russ IV 1998; Bennett 1999; Landau 2005), other published cases have marked important turning points in the history of LGBT asylum. In 1993, for the first time, an immigration judge granted asylum directly on the basis of sexual orientation. This was the case of Marcelo Tenorio, a gay man from Brazil. The case also constituted the first time that an immigration judge recognised homosexuals as members of a 'particular social group' that is targeted for persecution, which is a requirement of asylum law (Henes 1994; Davis 1999; Anderson 2001; Landau 2005). However, the Tenorio case was not deemed to establish a legal precedent that immigration judges were obliged to recognise. One year later a Mexican man, José García, was granted asylum on the same grounds – the first time that LGBT asylum was granted directly by the Inmigration and Naturalisation Service[2] rather than at a higher level (Randazzo 2005; Cantú *et al.* 2005). Soon afterward, Attorney General Janet Reno ordered immigration boards to adopt *Matter of Toboso-Alfonso* as precedent (Henes 1994; Bennett 1999; Landau 2005; Randazzo 2005).

As part of the Tenorio case, the immigration judge deemed homosexuality to be an immutable characteristic that the applicant cannot reasonably be expected to change (Bennett 1999; Randazzo 2005). Demonstrating persecution due to an immutable characteristic is another requirement to establish grounds for asylum. This early discussion in LGBT asylum cases of whether homosexuality is an immutable characteristic involved some degree of consideration of the still largely unresolved questions about whether sexual orientation is innate or a matter of personal choice (Henes 1994; Queer Law 1999). Questions about immutability were central to LGBT asylum cases during the 1990s. But in 2000, in the case of Hernández-Montiel, the Ninth Circuit Court of Appeals set precedent by ruling that both sexual orientation and sexual identity are immutable characteristics (Martin 2001).

The need to legally establish the immutability of homosexuality required a pragmatic form of oversimplification. It required those supporting LGBT asylum to side with essentialist and biological views of homosexuality as innate. This alignment, which has become common in the pursuit of other forms of LGBT rights in the USA (Epstein 1987), leaves little room for consideration of social constructionist nuance in relation to the aetiology of sexual orientation, which would be perceived as muddying the arguments about immutability.

With the need to prove membership in a particular social group out of the way, individual applicants must still make a convincing case that they were persecuted by the state (or by state inaction) due to their sexual orientation and that they have had a well-founded fear of persecution should they return to their home country. This additional requirement has led immigration courts to ask questions about whether the persecution occurs nationwide, i.e. whether the applicant could return to a different part of the country and not fear persecution. Here, a second kind of oversimplification became necessary. Applicants typically have been forced to engage in a wholesale vilification of their countries of origin, so as to not leave any room for the suggestion that they could go back and not be persecuted (Wei and Satterthwaite 1998; Solomon 2005).

Government lawyers have increasingly utilised reports of the changing conditions with regard to LGBT rights in various countries as proof that the fear of persecution is not well founded. Conceptually, the problem is that the question is simply put in either/or terms, and without leaving much room for nuance about the diversity of same-sex experiences that exist within specific countries. As a result, home countries appear flat and homogeneous, which runs contrary to everything that anthropological and sociological studies of homosexuality have revealed about the variety of LGBT experiences within and among countries.

The limitations of this approach become readily apparent if we consider the treatment of LGBT people in the USA itself. It would not be hard to argue that per-

secution toward LGBT people exists in the USA – in other words, that LGBT persecution exists in the very same country being asked to grant asylum to those escaping
LGBT persecution. Several scholars have offered examples of such persecution,
including the exclusion of gays from the military, the Defense of Marriage Act and
even specific, very dramatic, cases such as one involving a Mexican transgender
woman who, after being denied asylum, was placed on deportation procedures in a
detention centre in Florida, where she was repeatedly raped by her prison guard
(Halatyn 1998; Russ IV 1998; Miluso 2004; Symposium 2000/2001; Martin 2001;
Solomon 2005). Indeed, some of the experiences that LGBT people have could be
construed as evidence of widespread persecution toward LGBT people in this
country, and perhaps could constitute grounds for asylum cases elsewhere if US citizens were to migrate. But, by definition, LGBT asylum cases in the USA must
present that country as enlightened, and the applicants' home countries as backward, which some legal analysts and social scientists have depicted as a revival of a
colonialist mentality (see Rahman in Wei and Satterthwaite 1998; Long 2000/2001;
Cantú *et al.* 2005).

The problem of subjectivity in asylum decisions

An additional problem confronting asylum seekers is that, for the most part, LGBT
asylum cases are adjudicated by asylum officers and immigration judges who have
full discretionary power (Morgan 2006). The possible pitfalls of such discretionary
power – in terms of the adjudicators' biases – are not exclusive to such cases.
However, in this particular case the adjudicators' negative views on homosexuality
(possibly including their own homophobia) may pose a particularly difficult barrier
to overcome. As one legal analyst has put it: '[I]t really depends on the asylum
officer and the immigration judge. You can tell from the moment you sit down.
Sometimes the officers or judges are not accepting of gay claims' (Neilson, quoted
in Pfitsch 2006: 73).

The subjectivity involved in the adjudicators' decisions seems further compounded by their own culturally specific views about what constitutes homosexuality, which may strongly inform their interpretations of specific cases. Lavi Soloway,
of the Lesbian and Gay Immigration Rights Task Force (Soloway 2000/2001),
illustrates this issue well with the example of an immigration judge who could
not understand that in a case involving sex between men only the partner who
identified as gay (who was effeminate and whose sexual preferences included
being penetrated) was persecuted, while his masculine, non-gay-identified male
partners were not. This forced the applicant and his lawyer to lecture the judge on
culturally based interpretations of homosexuality (Soloway 2000/2001). In the end,
this judge understood that the disparity in stigma according to sexual roles did not
minimise the validity of the applicant's claims, but other judges could have concluded the opposite: that the lack of stigmatisation of the masculine partner meant
that (1) the persecution of homosexuals was not wholesale in that country; (2) that
effeminate men could avoid persecution by acting masculine; and (3) that this
applicant's persecution was caused by his acting effeminately and making his difference public.

LGBT applicants and their lawyers often find themselves in the position of needing
to educate immigration judges about cross-cultural models of homosexuality. But, in

an ironic twist, the achievement of this sort of 'cultural sensitivity' on the part of judges also has led to a different form of oversimplification. Once judges see gender-based forms of homosexual interaction as a different cultural model, they may reify it and decide, for instance, that masculine gay men in any given country are not 'gay enough' – that they are *never* stigmatised and thus are by definition ineligible for asylum (Hanna 2005; Morgan 2006).

This divergence in adjudicators' interpretations about the degree of stigmatisation of masculine and feminine gay men has been consequential in recent landmark cases. In 2000 the Ninth Circuit Court established precedent by adding the term 'sexual identity' to the definition of particular social group, which in one case, that of Hernández-Montiel, they described as 'gay men with a female sexual identity' (Leonard 2000: 560; see also Martin 2001; Hanna 2005; Randazzo 2005). This new definition created an opening for transgender individuals to submit asylum petitions (Neilson 2005a). As a result, in 2004, based on that same definition, an applicant named Reyes-Reyes, who identified as transgender, was granted asylum. But the shift seems to have had considerable negative consequences in cases involving masculine gay men. In the 2005 case of Soto Vega, the applicant was denied asylum by the Board of Immigration Appeals because 'he appeared too stereotypically heterosexual' (Hanna 2005: 249).

Immigration lawyers are now assessing the potential for success in gay male asylum cases, based in part on subjective perceptions of the clients' degree of masculinity or femininity. But this contradicts the notion that all homosexuals are part of a particular social group. The case of one man who participated in my recent ethnographic study with Mexican gay and bisexual immigrants illustrates this case.[3] Discussing why he had been unable to pursue asylum as a bisexually identified man, he said:

> They didn't give me any hope … because I identify as bisexual. They said 'it would be hard'… because I don't look effeminate. They said, 'You don't have a good argument to say that you can't go back to your country'. They said, 'You actually scared me, because you look so straight' … So they had thought of me as straight. And I say, 'Well, I am not very feminine, I don't like to show it' … I am quite reserved and I only tell the person [the man] that I want to have sex with.

In this quotation, this man refers to another subjective barrier that gender-conformant gay, bisexual and lesbian asylum seekers now face: individuals often choose to hide their same-sex sexual attraction in their home countries precisely to avoid persecution, although at the price of not being able to live their sexual orientation openly (Hanna 2005). But adjudicators may interpret their ability to pass as evidence that if they returned to their countries of origin they would not face persecution so long as they keep their sexual orientation private (Henes 1994; Hanna 2005; Morgan 2006). Critics of this argument compare it to saying that political dissidents or religious minorities could avoid persecution by hiding their political or religious affiliations, which runs contrary to the spirit of asylum law (Henes 1994).

Overall, the problem with these kinds of subjective or discretionary judgment is that adjudicators may use their own personal beliefs, stereotypes and biases in deciding who is credible, who is gay, who is gay enough and so forth, and these informal criteria appear to severely impact the outcomes of individual cases. Furthermore, because the legal system tends to create black and white scenarios in relation to the nature of sexual orientation that leave little room for any shades of grey, in arguments about what constitutes credible homosexuality and stigma attorneys and adjudicators regularly resort to oversimplifications that inadequately account for the complexities of sexual attraction, gender roles and social stigma.

Conclusion

It is unclear what may happen to asylum as an LGBT immigration strategy in the USA as the conditions surrounding homosexuality in other countries change, and as LGBT people around the world successfully achieve rights that may surpass those available in the USA. In this sense, the central assumption that requires asylum cases to construct the USA as enlightened and the countries where immigrants come from as backward is extremely problematic. Demonstrating generalised persecution of homosexuals is slightly easier in cases involving countries where homosexuality is still illegal, or where the state engages in overt forms of persecution of LGBT people (or clearly fails to protect LGBT people from persecution). By contrast, the situation is becoming more complicated when immigrants come from countries where LGBT people have been successful at achieving some rights or forms of legal and state protection. In those countries, just as in the USA, persecution of LGBT people may still be widespread, and there may be many situations in which particular individuals cannot return to their places of origin without fear of persecution due to their sexual orientation.

Furthermore, countries other than the USA may have better conditions in relation to some LGBT issues but not others. In this sense, the irony is that a US LGBT citizen who experiences persecution within the USA for not being allowed to serve in the army or to get married to a same-sex partner might find relief by moving to a country where those rights exist. But similarly, citizens from those same countries might not want to return to their countries of origin out of fear of police harassment.

The limitations of asylum seem particularly poignant in the case of binational same-sex couples that involve a US citizen or permanent resident. While their heterosexual counterparts can sponsor their spouses for immigration purposes via a comparatively simpler process, pursuing asylum for the foreign partner may be the only available alternative for some of these couples to live together in the USA. Ironically, that very fact might constitute sufficient evidence for them to request asylum elsewhere on the basis of state discrimination and persecution.

Notes

1 In recent years, immigration courts have offered conflicting decisions about what constitutes a same-sex or opposite-sex marriage in cases involving binational couples in which one or both of the partners is a transgender person. At stake are questions about whether the country or US state where the marriage took place recognises the marriage as valid, whether to consider the gender of the transgender partner at birth or at the time of marriage, and how to make decisions consistent with the requirements of federal immigration

policy and with the Defense of Marriage Act (see Haines 2005; Lorenz 2005; Immigration Equality and Transgender Law Center 2006; Wenstrom 2008).

2 The Immigration and Naturalization Service became US Citizenship and Immigration Services in 2003, at which point it moved from the Department of Justice to the newly created Department of Homeland Security.

3 This quotation is from an interview conducted for the Trayectos Study, a large ethnographic research project of sexuality and HIV risk among Mexican gay immigrant men in San Diego, California. For this study, my research team and I interviewed 150 men, including self-identified gay and bisexual Mexican immigrant men, US-born Latino men (who constituted a comparison group) and US-born sexual/romantic male partners of Mexican men. The study also included participant observation in locations where Mexican gay and bisexual immigrants socialise. Trayectos was funded by Award Number R01HD042919 from the National Institute of Child Health and Human Development. The content is solely the responsibility of the author and does not necessarily represent the official views of the National Institute of Child Health and Human Development or the National Institutes of Health.

References

Anderson, K. (2001) 'Expanding and Redefining "Membership within a Particular Social Group": Gender and Sexual Orientation Based Asylum', *New England International and Comparative Law Annual*, 7: 243–7.

Bennett, A. G. (1999) 'The "Cure" that Harms: Sexual Orientation-Based Asylum and the Changing Definition of Persecution', *Golden Gate University Law Review*, 29 (Spring): 279–309.

Cantú Jr., L., Luibhéid, E. and Stern, A. M. (2005) 'Well-Founded Fear: Political Asylum and the Boundaries of Sexual Identity in the U.S.–Mexico Borderlands', in Luibhéid, E. and Cantú Jr., L. (eds) *Queer Migrations: Sexuality, U.S. Citizenship, and Border Crossings*, Minneapolis: University of Minnesota Press.

Chisholm, B. J. (2001) 'Credible Definitions: A Critique of U.S. Asylum Law's Treatment of Gender-Related Claims', *Howard Law Journal*, 44 (Spring): 427–80.

Davis, T. J. (1999) 'Opening the Doors of Immigration: Sexual Orientation and Asylum in the United States', *Human Rights Brief*, 6: 19–20.

Epstein, S. (1987) 'Gay Politics, Ethnic Identity: The Limits of Social Constructionism', *Socialist Review*, 93/94 (July–September): 9–54.

Haines, J. L. (2005) 'Fear of the Queer Marriage: The Nexus of Transsexual Marriages and U.S. Immigration Law', *New York City Law Review*, 9: 209–47.

Halatyn, L. H. (1998) 'Political Asylum and Equal Protection: Hypocrisy of United States Protection of Gay Men and Lesbians', *Suffolk Transnational Law Review*, 22 (Winter): 133–61.

Hanna, F. (2005) 'Punishing Masculinity in Gay Asylum Claims', *Yale Law Journal*, 114 (January): 913–20.

Henes, B. F. (1994) 'The Origin and Consequences of Recognizing Homosexuals as a "Particular Social Group" for Refugee Purposes', *Temple International and Comparative Law Journal*, 8 (Fall): 377–401.

Howe, C. (2007) 'Sexual Borderlands: Lesbian and Gay Migration, Human Rights, and the Metropolitan Community Church', *Sexuality Research & Social Policy*, 4 (2): 88–106.

Immigration Equality and Transgender Law Center (2006) *Immigration Law and Transgender People*, available at: www.transgenderlawcenter.org/pdf/Immigration%20Law%20-%20 English%20fact%20sheet.pdf (accessed 16 November 2008).

Jefferys, K. (2007a) 'U.S. Legal Permanent Residents: 2006', Annual Flow Report: March 2007, Washington, DC: Department of Homeland Security, DHS Office of Immigration Statistics; available at www.dhs.gov/xlibrary/assets/statistics/publications/IS4496_LPRFlow Report_04vaccessible.pdf (accessed 5 November 2007).

Jefferys, K. (2007b) 'Refugees and Asylees: 2006',Annual Flow Report: May 2007, Washington,

DC: Department of Homeland Security, DHS Office of Immigration Statistics; available at www.dhs.gov/xlibrary/assets/statistics/publications/Refugee_AsyleeSec508Compliant. pdf (accessed 5 November 2007).

Landau, J. (2005) '2003 Lavender Law Conference: "Soft Immutability" and "Imputed Gay Identity": Recent Developments in Transgender and Sexual Orientation Asylum Law', *Fordham Urban Law Journal*, 32 (March): 237–63.

Leitner, R. C. (2004) 'A Flawed System Exposed: The Immigration Adjudicatory System and Asylum for Sexual Minorities', *University of Miami Law Review*, 58 (January): 679–99.

Leonard, A. S. (2000) 'Chronicling a Movement: A Symposium to Recognize the Twentieth Anniversary of the Lesbian/Gay Law Notes Edited by Professor Arthur S. Leonard', *New York Law School Journal of Human Rights*, 17: 415–564.

Long, S. (2000/2001) 'Sex Crime, Thought Crime', panel discussion comments in *Symposium Proceedings: Recent Developments in International Law. Review of Law and Social Change*, 26: 169–99.

Lorenz, R. D. (2005) 'Transgender Immigration: Legal Same-Sex Marriages and their Implications for the Defense of Marriage Act', *UCLA Law Review*, 53 (2): 523–59.

Martin, J. H. (2001) 'The Ninth Circuit's Review of Administrative Questions of Laws in the Immigration Context: How the Court in Hernandez-Montiel v. INS Ignored Chevron and Failed to Bring Harmony to "Particular Social Group" Analysis', *George Mason Law Review*, 10 (Fall): 159–82.

Millbank, J. (2003) 'Gender, Sex and Visibility in Refugee Claims on the Basis of Sexual Orientation', *Georgetown Immigration Law Journal*, 18 (Fall): 71–110.

Miluso, B. (2004) 'Family "De-Unification" in the United States: International Law Encourages Immigration Reform for Same-Sex Binational Partners', *George Washington International Law Review*, 36: 915–46.

Morgan, D. A. (2006) 'Not Gay Enough for the Government: Racial and Sexual Stereotypes in Sexual Orientation Asylum Cases', *Law & Sexuality: A Review of Lesbian, Gay, Bisexual, and Transgender Legal Issues*, 15: 135–61.

Neilson, V. (2005a) '2003 Lavender Law Conference: Unchartered Territory: Choosing and Effective Approach in Transgender-Based Asylum Claims', *Fordham Urban Law Journal*, 32 (March): 265–89.

Neilson, V. (2005b) 'Globalization, Security and Human Rights: Immigration in the Twenty-First Century: Homosexual or Female? Applying Gender-Based Asylum Jurisprudence to Lesbian Asylum Claims', *Stanford Law & Policy Review*, 16: 417–44.

Pfitsch, H. V. (2006) 'Homosexuality in Asylum and Constitutional Law: Rhetoric of Acts and Identity', *Law & Sexuality: A Review of Lesbian, Gay, Bisexual, and Transgender Legal Issues*, 15: 59–89.

Queer Law (1999) 'Current Issues in Lesbian, Gay, Bisexual and Transgendered Law', *Fordham Urban Law Journal*, 27: 279–433.

Randazzo, T. J. (2005) 'Social and Legal Barriers: Sexual Orientation and Asylum in the United States', in Luibhéid, E. and Cantú Jr., L. (eds) *Queer Migrations: Sexuality, U.S. Citizenship, and Border Crossings*, Minneapolis: University of Minnesota Press.

Reed, C. M. (1996) 'When Love, Comity, and Justice Conquer Borders: INS Recognition of Same-Sex Marriage', *Columbia Human Rights Law Review*, 97 (28): 97–134.

Russ IV, J. A. (1998) 'The Gap between Asylum Ideals and Domestic Reality: Evaluating Human Rights Conditions for Gay Americans by the United States' Own Progressive Asylum Standards', *U.C. Davis Journal of International Law & Policy*, 4 (Winter): 29–72.

Schulzetenberg, M. (2002) 'Article: U.S. Immigration Benefits for Same Sex Couples: Green Cards for Gay Partners?', *William and Mary Journal of Women and the Law*, 9 (Fall): 99–117.

Solomon, A. (2005) 'Trans/Migrant: Christina Madrazo's All-American Story', in Luibhéid, E. and Cantú Jr., L. (eds) *Queer Migrations: Sexuality, U.S. Citizenship, and Border Crossings*, Minneapolis: University of Minnesota Press.

Soloway, L. (2000/2001) 'Sexual Orientation-Based Asylum Claims and Federal Immigration Law', panel discussion comments in *Symposium Proceedings: Recent Developments in International Law. Review of Law and Social Change*, 26: 169–99.

Wei, T. and Satterthwaite, M. (1998) 'Shifting Grounds for Asylum: Female Genital Surgery and Sexual Orientation', *Columbia Human Rights Law Review*, 29 (Spring): 467–531.

Wenstrom, K. (2008) '"What the Birth Certificate Shows": An Argument to Remove Surgical Requirements from Birth Certificate Amendment Policies', *Law and Sex*, 17: 131–61.

47 'In the life' in diaspora

Autonomy/desire/community

Jafari Sinclaire Allen

For some time now, I have been interested in chronicling and theorising everyday agency among those who find themselves the targets of state oppression and more general forms of approbation on grounds of gender, sexuality and race, and therefore strategically use or recast their interpellated otherness, or deviance. In her essay 'Deviance as Resistance: A New Research Agenda for the Study of Black Politics', Cathy J. Cohen (2004) critiques African American studies' politics of respectability and suggests that the reputed deviance of queers, single mothers and state aid recipients – in the eyes of policymakers, but also scholars and civil society leaders – makes them multiply vulnerable, not only as unruly subject-citizens, but also outside of cultural boundaries.

In a similar vein, M. Jacqui Alexander (2005) has argued that some bodies, such as those of the lesbian and the 'prostitute', cannot be included as citizens in former colonies of the Caribbean precisely because they embody sexual agency and eroticism radically out of step with the aspirations of the nation to advertise itself as independent, developed, disciplined and poised to join in the number of putatively 'civilized' states. Resonant with Cohen, Alexander pushes us to be mindful of 'whether such bodies are offered up ... in an internal struggle for legitimation' (2005: 36). She observes that not only is the Third World subject denied voice in narratives of sexual encounter, but also that state interpellations of the subject's identity are constructed precisely at the interstices of potential struggle. Alexander has shown that like the USA, postcolonial states in the Caribbean and Latin America may also [re]deploy violently heterosexist policies and pronouncements that underscore the patriarchal control of women, sex workers and LGBT (lesbian, gay, bisexual and transgender) and queer individuals. My own recent research in Cuba and experiences at home in the USA (Allen 2007, 2010) impel taking seriously her entreaty to attend to how 'not just *any* body can be a citizen [anymore]' (Alexander 1994: 5).

In thinking of the state's sexualisation (racialisation and gendering) of particular bodies, we should not aim to paint the state with a brush so wide that distinctions between socialist and liberal, or between (post)colonial and imperial, north and south are effaced. There are crucial distinctions that condition and structure the ways in which a state – any state – attempts to regulate particular bodies, and as Roderick Ferguson observes in his queer of colour critique, 'both bourgeois and revolutionary practices were conceived through heteropatriarchy' (2004: 10). These related insights of black feminist and queer of colour critique: first, that heteropatriarchy is left in place in Marxist and otherwise revolutionary societies, and, second, that the state – all states, at least in the Americas – depend on racialised heteropatri-archy to constitute and maintain themselves in the global hierarchy of states, are key to understanding the current situation and to theorising spaces beyond it.

These questions go to the heart of larger questions of subjectivity: who is recog-nised as a person within a nation-state; and with what rights, privileges and expecta-tions? Moreover, In the USA and the Caribbean, non-state actors like families, religious, cultural and even feminist organisations often make strange bedfellows in thcir support for these projects of respectability. Their shared interest is to discip-line individuals, but also their nations' putative racialised unruliness, relative to the north and the west. This presents both a set of political problems across black diaspora, and a theoretical puzzle. Is there any place where (the benefits and recog-nition of) citizenship can accrue to the unruly – the 'prostitute', the homosexual, the transgender person or the black? And what calculus emerges when these raced and sexed categories of, for example non-national, deviant, non-ethnic racial subject or merely 'other' are compounded? Failing inclusion as a properly hygienic citizen or subject, where is the place for the black queer, for example?

Perhaps most pressing, however, is the question whether, if in fact blacks and queers, for example, cannot be full citizens in the neoliberal sense, can they at least be *free*? While anthropologists typically attend to the particularities of place and dif-ference, the concept of diaspora – connection, movement, self- and world making – helps us to think about historically global structures of dominance and resistance, possibilities afforded or not by individual states, and therefore allows us to highlight and imagine spaces of freedom beyond these constraints.

Moving away from the falsely dichotomous rights debate, for which in any case, work by Bell and Binnie (2000) and others have already provided insightful reviews, the challenge here lies in identifying within these contexts prospects for sexual cit-izenship and erotic autonomy. While sexual citizenship refers, generally, to notions of positive rights secured by states within in an international human rights context, Alexander's (1997: 1) notion of 'erotic autonomy' suggests a *belonging to* oneself which is beyond state interpellations, inscriptions and exclusions. Such a notion is connected to Lorde's (1984) idea of deep longing or erotic subjectivity, which is at once self-possessed or personal, and interdependent, connected and committed to enlarging human capacity for social justice. This is especially important to people of African descent – particularly those of minority sexuality – due to the (at least) double bind of putative deviance and the instability of rights, citizenship, participa-tion and inclusion in formal decision making. Black lesbians, bisexuals, transgen-ders and queers must at once challenge discursive and material practices, through organised legal and political work, but also look beyond state and civil society.

Throughout the black diaspora, practices of loving friendship and erotic connec-tion may offer a powerful tool toward healing from the multiple and compounded traumas of race/sex terror. This constitutes, for example, what Kempadoo and Doezema (1998) and others (e.g. Piedra 1992) look for when they talk of Caribbean 'sexual resistance'. It evidences Joseph Beam's (1983: 230) famous assertion that 'black men loving black men is the revolutionary act of the 1980s', and instantiates what I theorise in my book, *¡Venceremos?: Sexuality, Gender and Self-making in Cuba*, as a 'larger freedom' (Allen 2010). Here, I argue that gendered, raced and sexed self-making within the sites I investigate in Cuba is impelled not only by interaction with global discourses and foreigners, but also most pointedly by erotic desire of individuals and group desire. Before there can be discussion about sexual rights, subjects and (erotic) autonomy of African and African descended subjects, or we enjoin this proposal to attend to both sexual citizenship and erotic autonomy toward a larger freedom, articulated through on the ground friendship networks of same-gender loving[1] black people, we must first confront the logics of value that inhere in arguments of sexual deviance or unruliness that makes some potential citizen subjects ineligible or inappropriate, relative to a so called 'universal' subject.

Among people of African descent, poor people and otherwise under-siege populations, sexuality is putatively always in a state of crisis – most often interpellated as deviant, dangerous, unnatural (e.g. Moynihan 1967; Frazier 1966, 1967; Carby 1987) and un-national (e.g. Ortiz 1987; 1995; Lubiano 1997). Given, on one hand, the real experience of sexual repression of Africans and their descendants – legalised kidnapping and torture, forced reproduction, rape, coercion, for example – and, on the other, material, historical and behavioural patterns that have been deemed deviant, such as female-headed households, extended families, age and class egalitarian relationships, early sexual behaviour, for example; I want to suggest that to be black is to be always already seen as 'queer', relative to an understanding of subjectivity based on Western ideals of property, gender and sexual propriety.

Not only are black subjects always already queer relative to normative western ideals of the person, but also, same-gender loving people from the global south who negotiate but do not wholly capitulate to what Cymene Howe (2002: 237) has called the 'universal queer subject', discursively fall, in both time and space (Boellstorff 2007), outside narrowly western and northern middle-class gay constructions of family, lesbian, gay and queer, and of gay rights. One may ask, for example, if homosexual Cubans exist (and, of course, they do) what do we make of the fact that a gay tourist cannot attend a gay bar or tea dance in Havana – rainbow flags waving in the Caribbean breeze? Is the absence of gay political and cultural organisations in Cuba proof positive of repression of homosexuals by the Cuban state? Is this a reflection of machismo or evidence of Third World underdevelopment?

Roger Lancaster points out that we must not look for 'obvious equivalents to the North American experience' (1997: 192) in the experiences of same-gender loving people in other locales. This would betray ethnocentrism that arrogantly positions 'gay' and 'lesbian' identity as the only or most appropriate way to express same-gender loving erotic subjectivities, and by extension, 'proper' – read liberal – political subjectivity. Looking for obvious equivalents or arranging experiences in an evolutionary trajectory starting with 'pre-gay' (Altman 1996) and progressing forward, positions gay rights as the singular trajectory through which political subjectivity of same-gender loving people can be appropriately expressed. However, the yearning expressed by black same-gender loving people in black queer literatures, on stage, in political organising and at the club, is for autonomous – not isolated or separatist – spaces of black queerness, in which we begin to make sense of the complexity and singularity of black experience. This often does not always neatly conform to gay rights paradigms or coming out narratives in which the family of origin is traded in for another set of necessarily antagonistic affiliations.

For example, while as Chauncey (1994) and others point out, gay enclaves were constituted in the Castro in San Francisco and West Village of New York City in postwar USA, signalling a separate gay, largely male community, politics and culture, this has not been the case for people of colour. The politics of these communities are intersectional – concerned with issues of economic advancement, healthcare and racial discriminations, for example, as much or more than struggle for gays in the military or gay marriage. Black queers largely retain not only affective ties to extended families of origin, but also economic ties and residential proximity to black and people of colour neighbourhoods institutions and issues (Battle and Cohen 2003; Dang and Frazer 2005).

As we heed Alexander's (2002: 91) eloquently warning to 'become fluent in each other's histories', we must also attend to the ways this crucial project of mutual literacy is in danger of being rendered a platitude of multiculturalism in which 'diversity' – silently colouring within the lines of the status quo – comes to stand in for social justice, without the historical memory, hard work or honest dialogue that Alexander advocates. Between the mid-1970s and the late 1980s, important ruptures took place, across the globe. This was the beginning of Reaganism and Thatcherism's *longue durée*, the encroachment of neoliberalism and spectacularisation of the global marketplace heralding the postmodern moment. During this moment in the USA, during the onset of the HIV epidemic, black lesbian and gay political organising, literatures and other expressive practices emerged, pushing notions of the erotic beyond hetero sex and reproduction. Examples include the historical connections forged between the black feminist movement and black gay and lesbian organising and critique (Allen 2007; Ferguson 2004; Smith 1998); depictions of black gay and lesbian life that forcefully stressed the importance of families of origin and families of choice; and black queer activism that symbolically and substantively reinforces notions of black belonging (Allen op. cit.). Early and still existing black queer organisations in the USA, such as African Ancestral Lesbians United for Societal Change (AALUSC, founded as Salsa Soul Sisters), Gay Men of African Descent (GMAD), Affinity (Social Services), ADODI and others, emphatically insist on being part of black communities within the USA, and extend in many cases – rhetorically or materially – to other sites in the African diaspora.

Still, rather than encourage work that takes up and pushes this cross-cultural, intergenerational and cross-genre entreaty to, as Foucault asserts 'use one's sexuality henceforth to arrive at a multiplicity of relationships' (1996: 135), recent influential work in queer studies is characterised by its anti-relationality and its stance against futurity. Lee Edelman's (2004) *No Future: Queer Theory and the Death Drive* offers a forceful and eloquent example of this. Although Edelman elegantly recaptures some of the innovative potential of queer theory by tracing cultural shifts of white middle-class gay men toward the so-called mainstream, he proceeds without an analysis of the experiences and intellectual production of people of colour and women, who face co-constitutive racial, sexual and gender hierarchies. Further, following Lacanian theory, in which the real is an effect of language and not to be confused with reality, everyday suffering and death is of little concern in *No Future*. Indeed, *No Future* betrays a brand of scholarly refusal to recognise the complexity of the lifeworlds of those for whom sexual liberation alone will not guarantee freedom, and at the same time, for whom rights discourses hold great symbolic value, but seem to have had limited material purchase since the 1960s. To extend Alexander's theorisation of the state's simultaneous sexualisation, racialisation and gendering of particular bodies, not every child – and almost no black children – resemble The Child in Edelman's polemic.

My own work suggests that black queer writing, support groups and other liminal spaces of survival and potential, like the underground black queer club, are key sites for the exploration of desire, autonomy and community. We take up Cohen's charge to draw *blackprints* of collective resistance by those whose lives 'are indicative of the intersection of marked identities and regulatory processes, relative powerlessness and limited and contradictory agency' (2004: 28). Collective resistance can sometimes be quite direct, such as the physical resistance of black and Latina drag queens, which initiated the Stonewall Riots against oppressive police practices heralding the gay liberation[2] movement, or maroon communities throughout the Americas, in which enslaved and formerly enslaved individuals battled colonial troops. More often, however, challenges are more fugitive. They may occur quickly, silently or incomprehensibly loudly, and in places where no one is looking. Here, Victor Turner's concept of communitas, an often momentary experience of what Durkheim would call 'collective effervescence', or coming together, might be useful. Could the transcendence experienced in moments of communitas on the dance floor move to transgression of hegemonic rule; then *in the life,* can we actually transform ourselves enough to transform our communities and our world? Considering the pace with which technologies of global capital, the state and powerful cultural institution dehumanise by simultaneously atomising and aggregating individuals throughout the globe, these are significant epistemological, spiritual and cultural transgressions, if not yet community resistance.

A number of scholars, activists and artists have contributed moving narratives and convincing arguments that illuminate and articulate this politics of the erotic. For example, black feminist theorists and creative writers such as Alice Walker (1982) and Dionne Brand (2000) have imagined erotic friendship among black women as a way for them to know they were not crazy, as a salve against the daily onslaught of racialised misogyny, gendered racism and heterosexism, and as a way to go about the work of personal and social transformation. This vision of raising consciousness, mending wounds, moving between one place and another, and making new worlds, is the work of friendship. These visions of interdependence and passion are evident across spaces of the black diaspora, in fiction and non-fiction and also on the ground – in clubs and other sacred circles, on stage and between individuals.

Consider that, at least for black diasporic same-gender loving persons, to be homosexual, or more to the point, to be queer, is to build loving friendships and networks of friends outside not only a symbolic discourse in which they are always already invisibilised or muted, but also *once removed* from extended heteropatriarchal bio-families, where the violences of racism often echo and reproduce themselves in homes in which protection from concurrent gendered and sexed trauma cannot be assured. One must 'cross lines', 'break backs' in work, 'conjure theirselves' something new (Bridgforth 2004: 49), since heterosexist structures do not fit, or refuse to accommodate them. This work is often done between friends *in the life* – within marginal spaces like support groups and in the dark of the club – sweat pouring and with pleasure in mind. Those with whom Gloria Wekker (2006) worked used the phrase 'I had gone to seek my life (mi libi)' (132) to talk about mati work and networks of people who engaged in it. Here, we can see that *the life* speaks to facts of blackness throughout diaspora, which condition similar circumstances and set the horizon for a limited number of combinations of action. In my own research in Cuba, respondents and friends easily understood that in the USA, as in Cuba, *el ambiente*, the scene – the life – is at once used to denote spaces of extra-legality and potential danger, as well as trans, gay and lesbian space. In both Cuba and the USA, these non-mutually exclusive spaces often overlap (Allen 2007). This life in between, constrained as it is by racialised, classed and sexualised violence of the state, of global capital and of the anxieties of desperate in-group elites; is also a site of potential freedom, most centrally, because it has to be.

In Michel Foucault's essay 'Friendship as a Way of Life' (1996: 135), he attempts to push the focus of the gay individual to a collective project of sociality. He avers that it would be better to ask oneself:

> [W]hat relations, through homosexuality, can be established, invented, multi-plied, and modulated … the problem is not to discover in oneself the truth of one's sex, but, rather, to use one's sexuality henceforth to arrive at a multiplicity of relationships.

We can also thus think of this mode of life as another facet of Gloria Anzaldúa's (1999) concept of a troubled but productive point of multiple contact and possibil-ities, namely, *nepantla*. What might we learn from black diasporic erotic subjectivi-ties that underscore friendship and communal connection within those interzones? While to be homosexual is pitched as if it is about individuality and 'coming out' of established heteronormative structures and logics, but not necessarily into anything at all, what if we think of queer as precisely not about individualism and moving outside, but as a project of constituting interstitial outsider perspectives, as queers of colour have demonstrated in everyday experience, and in literature?

In Cuba, state apparatus attempts to construct particular types of revolutionary practice through political education or indoctrination. But whereas political educa-tion asks individuals to memorise, rote, from established texts; consciousness raising, or to conscientise, is to interrogate the living texts of individuals' lives. Patricia Hill Collins (1990) uses the nineteenth-century US reformer and mystic Sojourner Truth to illustrate a related point. Pointing out that Truth constantly travelled – migrating across geographic, racial, religious and other borders, Hill Collins writes 'no [T] ruth was possible without a variety of perspectives on any given particularity' (1990: 23). One night, my respondent Delores ran through a litany of negations of the expectations attached to the cultural, political and national identities interpellated for her, as a Cuban woman of African descent:

> I am not the Revolutionary woman who goes to FMC [Cuban Women's Federa-tion] meetings and dresses the children for Pioneros camp … I am not the Afro-Cuban who wears *colares* [Yoruba necklaces representing gods to whom the wearer is consecrated] goes to toques [sacred drumming rituals] or does folk-loric anything … I am not a stunning mulata *fina* or a selfless negrita, nor the only occasional lesbian who performs for men.

This practice of disidentification (Muñoz 1999) is a crucial first step, in order to first demystify, then strategically re-articulate parts of the knowledges that each so-called identity position brings. For Delores, this process of raising consciousness began in weekly discussion groups hosted by a black American political exile living in Cuba, then expanded through her participation in gatherings of lesbian and bisexual women.

I am not saying here that Delores learned to become black, or a woman or an out lesbian in these spaces. In fact Delores does not consistently identify as a black lesbian. However, through evaluating her own experience and those of others around her, she reasoned a cogent and supportable critique of dynamic interlocking structures of state, cultural and global power that find her multiply oppressed, but which at the same time offers her a variety of roadmaps toward liberation (or at least moments of 'liberty'). Through conversations with others, Delores was able to compare what she formerly thought of as her own singular and non-relatable story, to that of others who were similarly situated. Delores' practice of radical becoming begins at disidentification, but is only enabled or operationalised by the constitution of a space of critical enunciation, in which competing narratives are debated and performed publicly. That is, while the process is understood to be deeply personal and 'private' in many ways, it is precisely not individualistic in its politics, motivations and intentions. Individual desire is honoured and at the same time understood to flourish only in the context of a community (building enterprise).

Finally, friendship, Foucault argued, is potentially liberatory because it interrupts that which makes homosexuality 'disturbing' to heteropatriarchal sensibilities (and to racialised heteropatriarchal structures):

> [T]hat individuals are beginning to love one another – there's the problem. The institution is caught in a contradiction; affective intensities traverse it which at one and the same time keep it going and shake it up.
>
> (Foucault 1996: 137)

Such an idea is quite close to my notion of erotic subjectivity, following Audre Lorde. Erotic subjectivity – deeper understandings and compulsions of the body and soul – simultaneously embodying/invoking sex and death, works toward not only transgressing, but transcending and finally transforming hegemonies of global capital, the state and of bourgeois, limited and limiting notions of gender, sexuality or blackness, for example. Here, I am not claiming that this is a sufficient or final step, but rather necessary as a crucial line in the architecture of resistance. To follow Lorde (1983), through friendships and collective discussion, black queers in Cuba, USA and elsewhere 'evaluate those aspects honestly in terms of their relative meaning within their lives' (82). Instantiating her entreaty to 'not to settle for the convenient, the shoddy, the conventionally expected, nor the merely safe' (ibid). Especially at this moment in which there is so little 'safety'.

Note

1 This neologism was coined by the black queer activist Cleo Manago (c. 1995) to mark a distinction between 'gay' and 'lesbian' culture and identification, and black men and women who have sex with members of the same sex. While scholars continue to use gay, lesbian and queer, for example, and the US Centers for Disease Control, for example, uses MSM (men who have sex with men), same-gender loving has important resonance on the ground, in urban communities in the USA.

References

Alexander, M. J. (1994) 'Not Just (Any) Body Can Be a Citizen: The Politics of Law, Sexuality and Postcoloniality in Trinidad and Tobago and the Bahamas', *Feminist Review*, 48, 5–23.

Alexander, M. J. (1997) 'Erotic Autonomy as a Politics of Decolonization: An Anatomy of Feminist and State Practice', in Alexander, J. and Mohanty, C. T. (eds) *Feminist Genealogies, Colonial Legacies, Democratic Futures*, New York: Taylor & Francis.

Alexander, M. J. (2002) 'This Bridge we call Women: Radical Visions for Transformation', in *Remembering This Bridge, Remembering Ourselves: Yearning, Memory, and Desire*, New York: Taylor & Francis.

Alexander, M. J. (2005) *Pedagogies of Crossing: Meditations on Feminism, Sexual Politics, Memory, and the Sacred*, Minneapolis: University of Minnesota Press.

Allen, J. S. (2007) 'Crucil Plimpsest: Re-introducing *Brother to Brother*', in Hemphill, E. (ed.) *Brother to Brother: New Writing by Black Gay Men*, Washington, DC: Redbone Press.

Allen, J. S. (2010) ¡*Venceremos?: Sexuality, Gender and Black Self-making in Cuba*, Durham, NC: Duke University Press.

Altman, D. (1996) 'Rupture or Continuity? The Internationalization of Gay Identities', *Social Text*, 48: 77–94.

Anzaldúa, G. (1999) *La Frontera/Borderlands*, San Francisco: Aunt Lute.

Battle, J. and Cohen, C. (2003) 'Say it Loud, I'm Black and I'm Proud: Black Pride Survey 2000', Los Angeles: National Gay and Lesbian Task Force.

Beam, J. (1983) 'Brother to Brother: Notes from the Heart', in Hemphill, E. (ed.) *Brother to Brother: New Writing by Black Gay Men*, Los Angeles: Alyson Books.

Bell, D. and Binnie, J. (2000) *The Sexual Citizen: Queer Politics and Beyond*. Cambridge: Polity Press.

Boellstorff, T. (2007) 'When Marriage Falls: Queer Coincidences in Straight Time', *GLQ*, 13: 2–3.

Brand, D. (2000) *In Another Place, Not Here*, New York: Grove Press.

Bridgforth, S. (2004) *Love/Conjure/Blues*, Washington, DC: Redbone Press.

Carby, H. V. (1987) *Reconstructing Womanhood*, New York: Oxford University Press.

Chauncey, G. (1994) *Gay New York: Gender, Urban Culture, and the Making of the Gay Male World, 1890–1940*, New York: Basic Books.

Cohen, C. J. (2003) 'Punks, Bull Daggers and Welfare Queens: The real radical Potential of "Queer" Politics', *GLQ*, 3: 437–85.

Cohen, C. J. (2004) 'Deviance as Resistance: A New Research Agenda for the Study of Black Politics', *Du Bois Review*, 1, 27–45.

Collins, P. H. (1990) *Black Feminist Thought; Consciousness, Knowledge, and the Politics of Empowerment*, Boston, MA: Heinemann.

Cossman, B. (2007) *Sexual Citizens: the Legal and Cultural Regulation of Sex and Belonging*, Stanford, CA: Stanford University Press.

Dang, A. and Frazer, S. (2005) *Black Same-Sex Households in the United States: A Report from the 2000 Census*, 2nd edn, Los Angeles: National Gay and Lesbian Task Force.

Edelman, L. (2004) *No Future: Queer Theory and the Death Drive*, Durham, NC: Duke University Press.

Ferguson, R. A. (2004) *Aberrations in Black: Toward a Queer of Color Critique*, Minneapolis: University of Minnesota Press.

Foucault, M. (1996) 'Friendship as a Way of Life', in *The Essential Works of Foucault 1954–1984, Volume 1 – Ethics: Subjectivity and Truth* (trans. R. Hurley), New York: New Press.

Frazier, E. F. (1966) *The Negro Family in the United States*, Chicago: University of Chicago Press.

Frazier, E. F. (1967) *Black Bourgeoisie*, New York: Collier.

Howe, C. (2002) 'Undressing the Universal Queer Subject: Nicaraguan Activism and Transnational Identity', *City and Society*, 14: 237–79.

Kempadoo, K. and Doezema, J. (eds) (1998) *Global Sex Workers: Rights, Resistance, and Redefinition*, New York and London: Routledge.

Lancaster, R. N. (1997) 'Sexual Positions: Caveats and Second Thoughts on "Categories" ', *The Americas*, 54: 1–16.

Lorde, A. (1983) 'Tar Beach', in Smith, B. (ed.) *Home Girls: A Black Feminist Anthology*, New York: Kitchen Table-Women of Color Press.

Lorde, A. (1984) *Sister Outsider: Essays and Speeches*, New York: Trumansburg.

Lubiano, W. (1997) 'Black Nationalism and Black Common Sense: Policing ourselves and Others', in Lubiano, W. (ed.) *The House that Race Built*, New York: Pantheon Books.

Manago, C. (1995) Public Address at Black Nations/Queer Nations Conference, City University of New York.

Moynihan, D. (1967) *The Negro Family: The Case for National Action*, Washington, DC: Government Printing Office.

Muñoz, J. E. (1999) *Disidentifications: Queers of Color and the Performance of Politics*, Minneapolis: University of Minnesota Press.

Ortiz, F. (1987) *Los Negros Brujos*, Havana: Editorial de Ciencias Sociales.

Ortiz, F. (1995) *Los Negros Esclavos*, Havana: Cubanas Ediciones.

Piedra, J. (1992) 'Loving Columbus', in Jara, R. and Spadaccini, N. (eds) *Amerindian Images and the Legacy of Columbus*, Minnesota: University of Minnesota Press.

Smith, B. (1998) *The Truth that Never Hurts: Writings on Race, Gender, and Freedom*, New Brunswick, NJ: Rutgers University Press.

Spillers, H. J. (2003) *Black, White, and in Color: Essays on American Literature and Culture*, Chicago: University of Chicago Press.

Turner, V. W. (1969) *The Ritual Process: Structure and Anti-Structure*, London: Aldine.

Walker, A. (1982) *The Color Purple*, New York: Pocket Books.

Wekker, G. (2006) *The Politics of Passion: Women's Sexual Culture in the Afro-Surinamese Diaspora*, New York: Columbia University Press.

48 Black lesbian gender and sexual culture

Celebration and resistance

Bianca D. M. Wilson

> It is clear … that rather than a lesbian community per se, there exists now a whole lesbian society comprised of different lesbian communities.
>
> (Rothblum and Sablove 2005: xvi)

The notion that there are several forms of lesbian community in the USA, distinguished by the racial, ethnic, socioeconomic class and regional diversity that characterises the country, has been reflected in multiple studies of communities of same-gender loving women[1] (Lapovsky-Kennedy and Davis 1993; Morris 2005; Rabin and Slater 2005). While there are few studies that have attempted to examine the cultural systems of these lesbian communities, empirical research (see, e.g. Lapovsky-Kennedy and Davis 1993) and published personal narratives (see, e.g. Hampton 1981; Nestle 1984) on the ways lesbian community life has been organised reveal lesbian gender expression as a persistent and core feature of lesbian sexual culture.

Sexual discourse theory holds that one way to understand a group's sexual culture is to examine the ways people speak about sex and sexuality, as well as the messages they report hearing from various institutions (e.g. family, school, religion) (Schifter and Madrigal 2001). Within this framework, a researcher approaches the study of sexual culture as a dynamic construct by purposively examining both dominant and less dominant discourses regarding sex, and through the expectation that cultures do not remain the same across time.

There is relatively little empirical research on lesbian gender expression. The few researchers who study lesbian gender have focused most on butch and femme identity development processes (see, e.g. Hiestand and Levitt 2005). Of the studies on lesbian gender, fewer still included significantly black lesbians, despite documentation of the prominence of lesbian gender roles in historical or narrative accounts of black lesbian communities (see, e.g. Garber 1989; Davis 1998; Lorde 1983; Peddle 2005; Smith 1992; Walker 2001).

This absence of research on sexual lives and gender among black lesbians possibly reflects what Hammond (2002) describes as the absence of black queer women's experiences from dominant sexual discourses and the silencing of black female subjectivity. An exception is an in-depth qualitative study of a community of black lesbians in New York City (Moore 2006) that identified three categorisations of gender among black lesbians, including femme, transgressive and gender blender. Moore's study was an important step in the direction of documenting an often ignored segment of US culture, black lesbians, with the purpose of understanding how black lesbians view their relationships from their own perspectives. The current study is aimed at adding to this body of research by specifically examining dimensions of black lesbian sexual cultures.

The study

The current study on lesbian gender roles within African-American lesbian communities is part of a larger study, the Black Lesbians' Ideas about Sex and Sexuality (BLISS) study. I designed BLISS to document the defining features of African-American lesbian sexual culture in Chicago, including the beliefs, values and perspectives about sex and sexuality. The work discussed in this chapter aimed to address the following research questions:

1   What function, if any, does lesbian gender play in black lesbian sexual life?
2   How is lesbian gender constructed and understood?
3   What are the ranges of perspectives regarding lesbian gender in black lesbian communities?

The study aims to expand the use of sexual discourse theory to a multiple minority group. In doing so, I seek to demonstrate the complex relationships black lesbians have to sexual messages that are generated within primarily black lesbian spaces, as well as those from the multiple oppressed communities in which they may participate (e.g. women, African-American, lesbian) or through the dominant mainstream (i.e. patriarchal, European-American and heterosexual) US society.

Methods

Setting

No predominantly black lesbian gay bisexual transgender (LGBT) neighbourhood in Chicago exists. However, several black LGBT organisations and groups exist, suggesting a continued resistance against intersecting oppressions and an effort to create empowering, affirmative and culturally specific spaces and institutions for LGBT people of colour. Yet, most of the organisational resources for black gay people in Chicago are through health institutions, which tend to focus primarily on HIV/AIDS services for gay and bisexual men, leaving a dearth of places for black gay people, especially women, that are not focused on issues of disease. Affinity Community Services, one of the only organisations that solely focused on black lesbians and bisexual women and an organisation that has created its own physical space, was a site for my volunteer work as a youth programme chair and board of directors member.

Participants and procedures

I employed a rapid ethnographic assessment methodology (Kluwin *et al.* 2004), including three data collection methods: focus groups, individual interviews and participant observation. Each method offered a unique lens through which to examine African-American lesbian sexual culture. The study involved focus groups (n=9, 26 participants) with African-American lesbians; individual interviews (n=5) with community leaders;[2] and, participant observations (n=10 across four months) at a weekly open-mic night for African-American lesbians. Focus group participants were recruited through snowball sampling techniques and I organised the groups to include women with similar ages and education levels. Across all nine groups, participants ranged in age from 19 to 65 years (M=36.11, SD=11.16) and most had attended some college (n=15; high school graduate, n=2; college graduate, n=8).

I conducted the focus groups using a protocol that was composed of five domains: a) attitudes toward black lesbian community; b) defining sexuality; c) defining sex; d) butch and femme; and e) the influence of various communities (African-American, lesbian and women) on their views about sex. The open mics were important because they provided an opportunity to see how sex and sexuality were talked about outside of the research-directed setting. The individual interviews with community leaders served as an opportunity to validate and expand on the findings from the focus groups and observations.

Because the primary goal of the study was to document sexual discourses more broadly and the prominence of the lesbian gender theme in this study was emergent, I had not anticipated the need to purposively sample participants that represented various lesbian gender categories. As such, the sample is composed primarily of lesbians who reported that they did not currently have a strong or salient lesbian gender identity and the findings should be contextualised by the sample composition.

Analyses

I followed a coding process endorsed by many qualitative researchers (Vaughn *et al.* 1996; Wolcott 1994). NVivo Software was used to organise the data. Most of the analytic process for focus groups and observations was completed prior to conducting the community leader interviews which were used primarily as a way to help further negotiate my interpretation of the coding structure and identify themes that may have been missed in the focus groups and observations. The final step involved integrating all the data and identifying connections between results and theory.

Results and discussion

Using this analytic process, it was possible to identify several aspects of beliefs and practices regarding lesbian gender roles within African-American lesbian sexual culture in Chicago. First, I will describe how specific lesbian gender labels were constructed to create a masculine-feminine gender role dichotomy that functioned to organise sexual life. Then, I will discuss current debates among black lesbians in this community about the prominence of the roles and labels, including evidence of resistance to the polarised dichotomy of these roles. Finally, I present my interpretations of how lesbian gender was given meaning in sexual situations to produce a radical interpretation of gender sex roles. Quotes from focus group participants and community leaders and observation notes are included as evidence of key themes and relevant literature is included to illustrate connections to contemporary theory and research on lesbian gender expression. Pseudonyms are used for focus group participants and community leader interviewees.

One of the main questions of the focus group protocol was: 'Are roles or labels like butch or femme or aggressive or passive important in sex and sexuality? How so or why not?' This question was eventually rephrased to include the term 'stud' as another term for butch since this was the term most often used by participants to describe masculine gender identities, reflecting ethnic differences in masculine identity terminology in the city. Every focus group chose to devote significant time and energy to answering this question. Participants consistently highlighted lesbian gender roles as a key organising construct of African-American lesbian sexual life. Four participants claimed these labels for themselves. Several other participants supported women's adoption of these roles. The ways in which participants spoke about stud and femme categories indicated that these ways of constructing lesbian gender were part of an overarching sexual cultural norm of which all participants were aware. Within every focus group, participants conveyed a sense that the expectation to adopt a label and to operate within the category was a strong message throughout the black lesbian community. Hence, expectations to be a femme or stud appeared to be a sexual cultural script for this black lesbian community. Participants indicated that this cultural script was communicated in several contexts, including romantic relationships and community settings.

The deep roots of the social pressure to date within these roles were also evident within my observations at the open mics. Most women that appeared to be coupled off, as evidenced by them kissing or cuddling with each other, were a clear stud and femme couple. I did not observe any couple that was composed of two women that were traditionally feminine and observed only one couple in which both were dressed and acted in traditionally masculine ways. An inherent aspect of any sexual discourse is the potential disconnect between expected norms and individual trans-gressions against those norms (Parker 1991; Schifter and Madrigal 2001). Recognis-ing the discrepancy between their coupling and the cultural sexual scripts' expectations within black lesbian communities in this city, I asked that couple whether they had experienced negative reactions to their being a couple in which both women appeared masculine identified. They explained that they had received harsh reactions and lack of understanding from other African-American lesbians. However, they felt that they were no longer into labels and loved each other. They had been together for over eight years, and people knew them as an established couple and eventually left them alone.

Constructing the dichotomous stud-femme label system

Specific to sexual practice, participants within groups and individual community leader interviews, as well as my participant observations, provided a rich description of how the stud-femme label translated to the sexual lives of black lesbians in the community.

Masculine expression

Lesbians who expressed a highly traditional masculinised gender were labelled 'hard studs' and hard studs had relatively strict guidelines for sexual practice. For example, participants talked about the 'hard studs that will come out and say, "I don't want my woman to touch me. I want to be the total pleaser"' (Leslie, focus group discussion). Contrasting femmes and 'hard' studs, another participant claims:

> [B]ecause studs mostly in traditional situations, they're usually the one who ini-tiates, they're usually the one, who, if you have oral sex, they usually the one who would initiate having oral sex on that particular person, when they want, on a femme. I know a lot of studs. They don't like to be touched to a certain point, you know, you can touch them in certain places, but you know, you can't really touch them like on, on their, you know, vagina or so things that may make them feel feminine.
>
> (Jay, focus group discussion)

These participants' descriptions of the hard stud with which they were familiar is similar to the stone butch described in the fictional autobiography of Feinberg's (1993) *Stone Butch Blues*. As such, it is possible that the language of 'hard stud' is an ethnic-specific term that denotes a lesbian gender category identified in other ethnic communities. While a few participants who identified themselves as either aggressive, tomboy or dominant volunteered that they usually or rarely allowed part-ners to penetrate them, it is important to note that focus group participants were not asked to describe their own sexual lives. Hence, data from this study cannot confirm or disconfirm the extent to which these 'hard' or 'stone' sexual scripts reso-nated with the sexual practice of the women in the study.

Illustrating how hard stud sexual scripts were understood by many black lesbians in the community, two primary reasons were provided by participants regarding why hard studs would demand that they not be touched during sex. One explanation was that hard studs were not comfortable with the parts of their bodies that defined them as female, mainly their breasts and vaginas. As such, a successful performance of the 'male' role during sex required that the hard stud's female body parts not be touched. Another reason concerned the meaning of being touched and seduced. That is, participants talked about the importance of maintaining the appearance of dominance in the sexual act for hard studs, and how being touched sexually or being the 'bottom' took away that sense of dominance and control. The vulnerabil-ity of being sexually aroused and pleasured threatened the image of the dominant sexual partner. The contrast between these two explanations is significant. The first explanation, *rejecting femaleness*, is similar to the comments made by some transgen-der people regarding discomfort with their biological body parts that dictate main-stream society's current gendering system. However, the second explanation, *maintaining dominance*, is not about denying one's femaleness as expressed through the body but instead about accepting a view that being sexually pleasured and aroused by another makes a person vulnerable. Being vulnerable does not fit the hegemonic masculine image, and hence does not fit with the image of a true stud.

This study was designed to examine sexual discourses – essentially, how black les-bians discussed sex and what cultural level sexual scripts were recognised in the community. While examining conflicts between cultural level norms and individual behaviour was not the aim of the current study, some participants noted that there is some evidence of transgression. Participants in two focus groups discussed studs they knew who had recently had vaginal sex with men and had children, behaviours that did not fit into the masculine lesbian gender identity role. It is quite likely that many African-American studs and ultra-femmes alike engaged in sexual behaviours that transgressed expected community norms (beyond the mainstream norms they already transgress through sexual orientation and gender presentation), as was found in a study of the level of congruence between butch global presentation and actual self-presentation in sexual settings within a predominantly white sample (Rosenzweig and Lebow 1992).

Feminine expression

Within the masculine/feminine dichotomy that was discussed by participants, there were also the 'pillow princesses' and 'ultra-femmes' at the other end of the lesbian gender spectrum. Similar to the hard stud category, these extreme femme labels have clear sexual behaviour roles. Ultra-femme was a label given to women who expressed themselves in high-fashion feminine ways, usually including heels, makeup and contouring or revealing clothing. Relevant to the current study, pillow princess was a special label for the ultra-femme that alluded to the sexual context. In particular, this label described a lesbian who prefers to be the receiver of sexual pleasure and acts, such as having oral sex performed on her. She is not expected or likely to perform any sexual acts on her partner. In a sexual encounter, the expectation is that ultra-femmes are the ones who will be vaginally penetrated with sex toys or fingers. While not all participants spoke to the relationship between sexual penetration and femme identities, one group agreed that a requirement to being labelled femme was that an individual liked penetration. It is notable that outside of acknowledging that this role may be a little selfish, no pathology related to body image or gender identity was ascribed to the role of pillow princess. In general, it was the role of hard stud that engendered the most resistance, as will be described in the next section.

Debate within the community about lesbian gender

As Burch (1998) has noted, some activists and theorists argue that the adoption of femme and stud roles and labels is an attempt to replicate the gendered sexual norms in which lesbians were raised in the mainstream heterosexual society. Several community leaders and focus group participants thought similarly. For example, in one focus group, Wanda talked about the differences between white and black lesbians that she saw:

> They are, and not just whites, but [also] other non-African-American lesbians see it as we are just two women that love each other. Whereas blacks say we are two women that love each other, however we do have roles. You know, and we are trying to in a sense maybe ascribe to a heterosexual way of life, or way of operating, in our relationship.

Kendra, a community leader who works in lesbian and gay health arenas, also reported that she felt that femme and butch labels appear to mimic traditional gender roles. However, she cautioned against the assumption that mimicking traditional gender roles automatically made lesbian gender label expression 'artificial'.

In contrast to those who disliked lesbian gender labels, some participants embraced them wholeheartedly in their own romantic and erotic lives. For example,

Gail, who proudly discussed her identification as femme and as a member of the 'butch-femme community', also conveyed to the group that their was a renaissance in the butch-femme movement that included reconfiguring butch and femme to mean more than a replication of heterosexual gender roles. She felt that contemporary butch-femme communities were more egalitarian than they had been when she was younger, where femmes were no longer placed in a subservient or domestic role.

Despite the large role that lesbian gender played in organising black lesbian sexual life, every focus group discussion revealed individuals' (within the group or people known by group participants) conscious and purposeful rejection of femme and stud labels/roles. There were several strategies used to reject the femme and stud categories within African-American lesbian communities: refusing to label oneself, feeling bothered by labels, feeling hopeful that the cultural scripts will change and avoiding hanging out with people who like labels. In one focus group discussion, Sheri said in response to a comment from another group participant:

> I agree with that ... [I] don't identify in any of those butch/femme things. It is a mystery to me ... I don't disapprove of it, it just isn't who I am ... the role thing, it makes me a little nervous, but I realise that it's out there. That other folks are, that's who they are. And I understand the politics around those roles. But I don't choose it for myself.

As illustrated by this quote and many others in the study, some participants refused the labels for themselves and also expressed being bothered or irritated with the community trend to adopt labels. However, they also conveyed acceptance or tolerance for those that chose the labels, and for some, the choice to refuse labels for oneself was not incongruent with having an attraction to women who possess the characteristics those labels define.

In addition, several poets at the open mics spoke about struggling against expectations to label oneself in terms of lesbian gender. For example, one poet who enrolled into the study so that I could quote her poem speaks of wanting to drop these labels as she professes her attraction to a straight girl:

> [T]he first time I laid eyes on you
> my heart and soul despised of you
> wondering why I couldn't dine with you
> spend a little time with you
> share a piece of mine with you
> but that was on a Sunday
> one day I took time to clear my mind of each and every thought of you
> the fucked up labels that I brought to you ...
> like STUD and FEMME,
> DYKE and SHEM.
> Just being me was a crime you see
> cause I'm a FEMME living
> STUD LOVING
> thought you was my woman till you said you was my husband?????
> Damn! our lifestyle is complex

that's what leaves the straight ones vexed
thinking we all play roles and can't be role models.

(V-love)

Another poet who was interviewed as a community leader, Warrior, also expressed frustration and anger at being pressured into the label of stud or femme. As soon as I asked her to respond to my preliminary findings suggesting that lesbian gender roles were consistently discussed as a unique feature of African-American lesbian sexual culture, she commented that she wanted to resist the evidence that the phenomenon of butch and femme belongs to 'us' (i.e. black lesbians).

It was in the theme of lesbian gender that forms of resistance, an expected characteristic of sexual discourses (Schifter and Madrigal 2001), were most evident throughout the larger study. As noted earlier, resistance strategies ranged from individual choices to not identify with femme or stud roles, to open rejection of other lesbians who chose those identities. Most of the resistance discussed centred on critiquing the strictness of role expectations, not on lesbian gender expression per se. However, in cases where the frustration was directed specifically at those who identified with gender labels, the discontent was with masculine women, not the femmes. This theme has been observed in other work documenting the experiences of black studs and aggressives (Moore 2006). This is notable because it indicates that resistance against femme-stud lesbian gender expression is not an unqualified rejection of all black lesbians who express themselves in gendered ways. Unlike the conscious movement toward androgynous images which have characterised many middle-class white lesbian communities (Taylor and Rupp 1993), the black lesbians in this study who disagreed with lesbian gender roles were not arguing for the lack of all gendered expression. Instead, the resistance was centred on the rejection of masculine women, studs, who dare to transgress the Eurocentric mainstream cultural expectations for female feminine expression, as well as a possible mainstream black women's cultural expectations of women to operate somewhere between the realm of gender-blending and feminine expression.

Between the extremes

Despite a consistent description of femme and stud at the 'extremes' of lesbian gender expression, participants also discussed several labels that fell between the ultra- femme-hard stud ends of the continuum, such as 'soft stud' and 'aggressive femme'. Labels like these represented lesbians that blended both masculine and feminine ways in their public expression and/or sexual behaviours, but with a purposeful leaning toward either a more masculine or feminine identity. The common use of these terms appears contrary to the reports that there were dominant expectations of highly masculine or highly feminine modes of expression. Yet, the sets of sexual discourses that comprise a group's sexual culture are inherently contradictory and often disjointed from one another (Schifter and Madrigal 2001). There was a collective acknowledgment that dominant sexual discourses in black lesbian communities emphasised an expectation for choosing identities representing opposite sides of a single feminine-masculine continuum. Yet, this expectation did not prevent the expression of informal, less dominant sexual scripts that created room for blending characteristics along both masculine and feminine continua, similar to the 'gender blender' category found in Moore's (2006) study.

One of the community leader interviewees, Kendra, who was in her forties, asserted that the creation of new labels is one form of resistance to the strict dichotomy of stud and femme that arose out of the 'old school' African-American lesbian sexual culture. While the data in this study did not support this participant's suggestion that strict dichotomies were an artefact of only older African-American lesbian culture, the development and adoption of more labels, and thus a broader spectrum of role opportunities, could at minimum represent a quasi-organised movement towards changing an enduring dominant gendered sexual discourse among black lesbians.

A radical side to lesbian gender sex roles

Although many focus group participants, community leaders and poets at the open mics argued that studs and femme roles were replications of heterosexual male and female sexual relationships, the sexual scripts for 'hard studs' and 'pillow princesses' appear to turn the traditional conceptualisation of fe/male sex roles on its head. US heterosexual men may be expected to be the sexual aggressors (as studs were described to be by participants), but they are typically not socialised to view sexual pleasure of *their female partner* as the primary outcome (Maines 1999). Similarly, whereas pillow princesses and other femmes appear to fall in line with heterosexual conceptualisations of sexual roles for women where the woman's role is the passive and non-assertive partner, they represent radical departures in other respects. In particular, participants indicated that ultra-femmes and pillow princesses fully expected that the sexual act ended with their sexual climax. This appears to be a reconceptualisation of the connection between femininity and sexual prowess, deeming the feminine partner as the primary physical beneficiary. In essence, the feminine partner is best viewed as *receptive*, rather than passive (Burch 1998).

Conclusions

African-American lesbians in this study conveyed a set of sexual beliefs, attitudes and behaviours that influenced what types of sex they had, whom they dated and their behaviour within romantic relationships. This study highlighted that femme and stud roles were a dominant norm operating within this African-American lesbian community, yet there were also clearly informal and less dominant sexual discourses that included an integration of masculine and feminine forms of representation. Participants expressed various reactions to dominant scripts regarding lesbian gender roles, including celebration of the erotic power of lesbian gender as well as various forms of resistance.

While the intent of this study was more explicitly focused on sex than Moore's (2006) study of black lesbians, many of the findings related to dating and community expectations around partner choices were similarly reported in the two studies. The similarities of these two studies' findings from different cities, as well as several of the personal narratives discussed earlier, suggest that there may be a persistent sexual cultural script shared among black lesbians. These scripts may be rooted in an interpretation of African-American traditions. The ways in which these similarities are a function of the interaction between race, gender, sexuality and urban living is not known and warrants further investigation. Additional research focusing on significant intracultural or intragroup differences will contribute greatly to theory that accurately represents the diversity of experiences and perspectives among this group which has traditionally been silenced around sex and sexuality.

Notes

1 I use the term 'same-gender loving' women to refer to women who partner and have sex with women. This is a term that has emerged within US African-American gay and lesbian communities to represent the range of labels that may describe non-heterosexual peoples and to counter Eurocentric gay and lesbian terminology.
2 Community leaders were selected for their experience in working within black lesbian communities or because of their work as sexual health educators in ethnically diverse lesbian communities. Due to confidentiality, the individual demographics are not provided, however, they collectively comprise a group of community organisers, artists, religious leaders, public health directors and sex workshops facilitators.

References

Burch, B. (1998) 'Lesbian Sexuality/Female Sexuality: Searching for Sexual Subjectivity', *Psychoanalytic Review*, 85: 349–72.

Davis, A. (1998) *Blues Legacies and Black Feminism: Gertrude 'Ma' Rainey, Bessie Smith, and Billie Holiday*, New York: Pantheon Books.

Feinberg, L. (1993) *Stone Butch Blues*, Los Angeles: Alyson Books.

Garber, E. (1989) 'A Spectacle in Color: The Lesbian and Gay Subculture of Jazz Age Harlem', in Duberman, M. B., Vicinus, M. and Chauncey Jr., G. (eds) *Hidden from History*, New York: NAL Books.

Hammond, E. M. (2002) 'Black (W)holes and the Geometry of Black Female Sexuality', in Mui, C. and Murphy, J. (eds) *Gender Struggles: Practical Approaches to Contemporary Feminism*, Lanham, MD: Rowman & Littlefield.

Hampton, M. (1981) 'Mabel Hampton', in Nestle, J. (ed.) *The Persistent Desire: A Femme-Butch Reader*, Boston, MA: Alyson Books.

Hiestand, K. R. and Levitt, H. M. (2005) 'Butch Identity Development: The Formation of an Authentic Gender', *Feminism & Psychology*, 15: 61–85.

Lapovsky-Kennedy, E. and Davis, M. (1993) *Boots of Leather, Slippers of Gold: The History of a Lesbian Community*, New York: Routledge.

Lorde, A. (1983) 'Tar Beach', in Smith, B. (ed.) *Home Girls: A Black Feminist Anthology*, New York: Kitchen Table-Women of Color Press.

Kluwin, T., Morris, C. and Clifford, J. (2004) 'A Rapid Ethnography of Itinerant Teachers of the Deaf', *American Annals of the Deaf*, 149 (1): 62–72.

Maines, R. (1999) *The Technology of Orgasms: 'Hysteria', the Vibrator, and Women's Sexual Satisfaction*, Baltimore, MD: Johns Hopkins University Press.

Moore, M. R. (2006) 'Lipstick or Timberlands? Meanings of Gender Presentation in Black Lesbian Communities', *Signs: Journal of Women in Culture & Society*, 32: 113–39.

Morris, B. (2005) 'Negotiating Lesbian Worlds: The Festival Communities', in Rothblum, E. and Sablove, P. (eds) *Lesbian Communities: Festivals, RVs, and the Internet*, Binghamton, NY: Harrington Park Press.

Nestle, J. (1984) 'The Fem Question', in Vance, C. (ed.) *Pleasure and Danger: Exploring Female Sexuality*, London: Pandora Press.

Parker, R. (1991) *Bodies, Pleasures, and Passions*, Boston, MA: Beacon Press.

Peddle, D. (2005) *The Aggressives* [motion picture], available from Seventh Art Releasing, Los Angeles, CA.

Rabin, J. and Slater, B. (2005) 'Lesbian Communities across the United States: Pockets of Resistance and Resilience', in Rothblum, E. and Sablove, P. (eds) *Lesbian Communities: Festivals, RVs, and the Internet*, Binghamton, NY: Harrington Park Press.

Rosenzweig, J. M. and Lebow, W. C. (1992) 'Femme on the Streets, Butch in the Sheets? Lesbian Sex-roles, Dyadic Adjustment, and Sexual Satisfaction', *Journal of Homosexuality*, 23: 1–20.

Rothblum, E. and Sablove, P. (eds) (2005) *Lesbian Communities: Festivals, RVs, and the Internet*, Binghamton, NY: Harrington Park Press.

Schifter, J. and Madrigal, J. (2001) *The Sexual Construction of Latino Youth*, New York: Haworth Hispanic/Latino Press.

Smith, B. (1992) 'The Dance of Masks', in Nestle, J. (ed.) *The Persistent Desire: A Femme-Butch Reader*, Boston, MA: Alyson Books.

Taylor, V. and Rupp, L. (1993) 'Women's Culture and Lesbian Feminist Activism: A Reconsideration of Cultural Feminism', *Signs*, 19: 32–61.

Vaughn, S., Schumm, J. S. and Sinagub, J. (1996) *Focus Group Interviews in Education and Psychology*, Thousand Oaks, CA: Sage.

Walker, L. (2001) *Looking like What you Are: Sexual Style, Race, and Lesbian Identity*, New York: New York University Press.

Wolcott, H. (1994) *Transforming Qualitative Data Description, Analysis and Interpretation*, Thousand Oaks CA: Sage.

Index